Bile Acids in Gastroenterology
Basic and Clinical Advances

FALK SYMPOSIUM 80

Bile Acids in Gastroenterology
Basic and Clinical Advances

EDITED BY

A.F. Hofmann
Division of Gastroenterology
Department of Medicine (0813)
University of California
San Diego, La jolla
CA 92093-0813
USA

G. Paumgartner
Medizinische Klinik II
Klinikum Grosshadern der
Universität München
Marchioninistr. 15
D-81377 München
Germany

A. Stiehl
Midizinische Universitätsklinik
Bergheimer Str. 58
D-69115 Heidelberg
Germany

Proceedings of the 80th Falk Symposium (XIII International Bile Acid Meeting), held in San Diego, California, USA, September 30–October 2, 1994

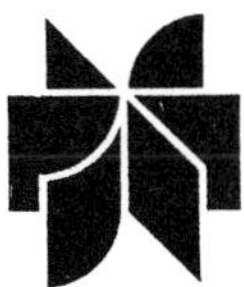

KLUWER ACADEMIC PUBLISHERS
DORDRECHT / BOSTON / LONDON

Distributors

---

for the United States and Canada: Kluwer Academic Publishers, PO Box 358,
Accord Station, Hingham, MA 02018-0358, USA
for all other countries: Kluwer Academic Publishers Group, Distribution
Center, PO Box 322, 3300 AH Dordrecht, The Netherlands

A catalogue record for this book is available from the British Library

ISBN 0-7923-8880-1

Contents

SECTION III: BILE ACID BIOSYNTHESIS

SECTION IV: BILE ACID TRANSPORT: HEPATIC

CONTENTS

SECTION V: BILE AND TRANSPORT: BILIARY AND INTESTINAL

SECTION VI: PHYSIOLOGICAL ACTIONS OF BILE ACIDS

SECTION VII: CYTOTOXICITY AND IMMUNOLOGY OF BILE ACIDS

SECTION VIII: BILE ACIDS AND BILIARY STONE DISEASE

SECTION IX: BILE ACIDS IN THERAPY

List of Principal Authors

A. Amelsberg
Division of Gastroenterology
Department of Medicine (T-013)
University of California San Diego
La Jolla
CA 92093-0813
USA

W. F. Balistreri
Division of Pediatric Gastroenterology and
  Nutrition
Children's Hospital Center
Elland & Bethesda Avenues
Cincinatti
OH 45229-2899
USA

A. Benedetti
Department of Gastroenterology
CP538
University of Ancona
I-60100 Ancona
Italy

U. Beuers
Medizinische Klinik II
Klinikum Grosshadern der Universität
  München
Marchioninistr. 15
D-81377 München
Germany

J. L. Boyer
Department of Medicine and Liver Center
Yale University School of Medicine
333 Cedar Street
New Haven
CT 06510
USA

J. Y. L. Chiang
Department of Biochemistry and
  Molecular Pathology
Northeastern Ohio University College of
  Medicine, PO Box 95
Rootstown
OH 44272
USA

D. E. Cohen
Department of Medicine
Brigham and Women's Hospital
75 Francis Street
Boston
MA 02115
USA

J. M. Crawford
Department of Pathology
Brigham and Women's Hospital
75 Francis Street
Boston
MA 02115
USA

P. A. Dawson
Department of Internal Medicine
Division of Gastroenterology
Bowman Gray School of Medicine
Medical Center Boulevard
Winston-Salem
NC 27157
USA

J. M. Donovan
Brockton/West Roxbury VA Medical
  Center
Division of Gastroenterology
1400 VFW Parkway
West Roxbury
MA 02132
USA

LIST OF PRINCIPAL AUTHORS

R. H. Dowling
United Medical and Dental Schools of
  Guy's and St. Thomas' Hospitals
Gastroenterology Unit, 18th Floor
Guy's Tower
Guy's Hospital, London SE1 9RT
UK

K. A. Einarsson
Department of Medicine
Unit of Gastroemterology and Hepatology
  K63
Huddinge University Hospital
S-141 86 Huddinge
Sweden

E. Evans
Departments of Pathology and Physics
University of British Colombia
Vancouver
BC V6T 1W5
Canada

R. Fried
Department of Gastroenterology
University Hospital
Petersgraben 4
CH-4031 Basel
Switzerland

G. J. Gores
Center for Basic Research in Digestive
  Diseases
Mayo Clinic and Mayo Foundation
Rochester
MN 55905
USA

L. R. Hagey
Department of Medicine, 0813
University of California, San Diego
La Jolla
CA 92093-0813
USA

D. M. Heuman
Division of Gastroenterology
Medical College of Virginia
MCV Station Box 711
Richmond
VA 23298-0711
USA

R. P. Hjelm
Los Alamos National Laboratory
Los Alamos
NM 87545-1663
USA

A. F. Hofmann
Division of Gastroenterlogy
Department of Medicine (0813)
University of California, San Diego
La Jolla
CA 92093-0813
USA

T. Iida
College of Engineering
Nihon University
Koriyama
Fukushima-ken 963
Japan

D. Keppler
Deutsches Krebforschungszentrum
Abteilung für Tumorbiochemie
Im Neuenheimer Feld 280
D-69120 Heidelberg
Germany

W. Kramer
SBU Metabolism
Hoechst Aktiengesellschaft
D-65926 Frankfurt
Germany

G. Kurz
Institut für Organische Chemie und
  Biochemie der Universität
Albertstr. 21
D-79104 Freiburg
Germany

P. J. Meier
Abteilung für Klinische Pharmakologie
Medizinische Klinik
Universitätsspital
Rämistr. 100
CH-8091 Zürich
Switzerland

C. B. O'Brien
8th Floor, Gates Building
Hospital of the University of Pennsylvania
3400 Spruce Street
Philadelphia
PA 19104-4283
USA

R. P. J. Oude Elferink
Department of Gastrointestinal and Liver
  Diseases
Academic Medical Centre
Meibergdreef 9
NL-1105 AZ Amsterdam
The Netherlands

LIST OF PRINCIPAL AUTHORS

G. Paumgartner
Medizinische Klinik II
Klinikum Grosshadern der Universität
  München
Marchioninistr. 15
D-81377 München
Germany

M. Podda
Istituto Scienze Biomedicine
Ospedale S. Paolo
Via di Rudini 8
I-20142 Milano
Italy

R. E. Poupon
Service d'Hépato-Gastro-Entérologie
Hôpital Saint-Antoine
184 Rue de Faubourg Saint Antoine
F-75571 Paris Cedex 12
France

A. Roda
Dipartimento di Scienze Farmaceutiche
Universita di Bologna
Via Belmeloro 6
I-40126 Bologna
Italy

A. J. Sanyal
Gastroenterology and Hepatology
Medical College of Virginia
MCV Station 980711
Richmond
VA 23298-0711
USA

K. D. R. Setchell
Clinical Mass Spectrometry Center
Children's Hospital Medical Center
3333 Burnet Avenue
Cincinnati
OH 45229
USA

M. L. Shiffman
Hepatology Section
Medical College of Virginia
Box 980711
Richmond
VA 23298-0711
USA

J. Sjövall
Department of Medical Biochemistry and
  Biophysics
Karolinska Institutet
S-71 77 Stockholm 60
Sweden

A. Stiehl
Medizinische Universitätsklinik
Bergheimer Str 58
D-69115 Heidelberg
Germany

A. Stolz
LAC-USC 11–221
University of South California
2025 Zonal Avenue
Los Angeles
CA 90033
USA

R. T. Stravitz
Medical College of Virginia
Box 980678, MCV Station
Richmond
VA 23298
USA

S. Tazuma
1st Department of Internal Medicine
Hiroshima University School of Medicine
1-2-3 Kasumi-cho, Minami-ku
Hiroshima 734
Japan

U. Töx
Abteilung Innere Medizin IV
Medizinische Klinik der Universität
Bergheimer Str. 58
D-69115 Heidelberg
Germany

P. Tso
Department of Physiology
Louisiana State University Medical Center
1501 Kings Highway
Shreveport
LA 71130-3932
USA

P. C. Van de Meeberg
Department of Gastroenterology
University Hospital Utrecht
PO Box 85500
NL-3508 GA Utrecht
The Netherlands

R van der Meer
Department of Nutrition
Netherlands Institute for Dairy Research
PO Box 20
NL-6710 BA Ede
The Netherlands

H. J. Verkade
Department of Pediatrics
University of Groningen
Academic Hospital, PO Box 30.001
NL-9700 RB Groningen
The Netherlands

Z. R. Vlahcevic
Division of Gastroenterology
Medical College of Virginia
MCV Station Box 711
Richmond
VA 23298-0711
USA

Foreword

This volume contains the contributions of the speakers at the 13th International Bile Acid Meeting which was held at the Del Coronado Hotel, San Diego, California from 29 September to 2 October, 1994. The symposium was a satellite meeting to the 10th World Congress of Gastroenterology which followed immediately afterwards in Los Angeles. As with previous International Bile Acid Meetings, the meeting was sponsored by the Falk Foundation e.V., Freiburg, Germany.

The Del Coronado Hotel has already celebrated its centennial; therefore it is a historic hostelry by San Diego standards. The hotel has always attracted celebrities, and it was there that a young king of England met Wallis Warfield, and decided to abdicate in order to obtain her hand in marriage. On the beautiful beach in front of the hotel, Marilyn Monroe and Jack Lemmon filmed 'Some Like It Hot!'. San Diego has now become more than a city of beautiful ocean beaches and a magnificent bay; it is the home of several world-famous scientific institutions such as the University of California at San Diego, the Scripps Clinic Research Institute, and the Salk Institute, as well as many biotechnology companies. The San Diego Zoo is known for its Center for Research on Endangered Species, as well as its imaginative housing of an extraordinary collection of diverse animals, and it was in San Diego that the first symposium on the peaceful use of atomic energy was convened. This led to the design of the first atomic reactor here in San Diego.

Bile acid research has involved an ever-widening spectrum of disciplines during the past few decades. In selecting speakers for this meeting, Drs Paumgartner, Stiehl and I attempted to include most of those areas where substantial progress has been made since the last meeting two years ago. The meeting began with chemical aspects of bile acids, including recent discoveries of new bile acids in vertebrates, as well as successful syntheses of uncommon natural bile acids and their isomers and epimers. Bile acid interactions with membranes were discussed, and a new model of the mixed bile acid–digestive product, micelle, was disclosed, based on small-angle neutron scattering. Much progress was reported regarding the molecular biology of cholesterol 7α-hydroxylase, the rate-limiting enzyme in bile acid biosynthesis. The programme then turned to bile acid transport by the hepatocyte and the ileal enterocyte; cloning of key transporters has been a major scientific advance. In an extraordinary *tour de force*, Kramer and his colleagues described a successful research programme aimed at developing non-absorbable inhibitors of the ileal transporter, to be used in the treatment of familial hypercholesterolaemia. Toxicological aspects of bile acids were considered. The binding of luminal bile acids by freshly formed calcium phosphate was reviewed, and a new function of bile acids – to enhance calcium and iron absorption – was presented. New concepts of the mechanism of biliary lipid secretion have been elucidated by creating genetically engineered mice. The remarkable ability of ursodeoxycholic acid conjugates to abolish cholesterol absorption from the perfused intestine was described.

The latter part of the meeting was concerned with the use of bile acids in therapy. Diseases that were discussed including biliary stone disease, cholestatic liver disease, inborn errors of bile acid metabolism, graft-versus-host disease, and hepatitis C, where ursodeoxycholic acid is being used as an adjunct to interferon therapy.

At the moment bile acid research is alive and well, even though it is growing relatively slowly. As yet bile acids have achieved only a modest commercial success. The widespread acceptance of laparoscopic cholecystectomy as a definitive treatment of cholesterol gallbladder stones has diminished early enthusiasm for medical dissolution therapy. In cholestatic liver disease the effect of ursodeoxycholic acid on liver histology is relatively modest, although there is little doubt that the compound is extraordinarily safe. Certainly, the most spectacular success of bile acids in therapy has been for bile acid replacement in the exceedingly rare inborn errors of bile acid biosynthesis. Bile acid transport inhibitors were described for the first time at this meeting, introducing the concept of bile acid 'antagonists'. This area may have considerable commercial potential.

The high point of the Bile Acid Symposium was the presentation of the Windaus Prize, sponsored by the Falk Foundation. This year's recipient – Z. Reno Vlahcevic – received the prize for a lifetime achievement in bile acid research. In particular, the work of Vlahcevic and his colleagues has elucidated mechanisms of control of the rate-limiting enzymes for bile acid biosynthesis.

The 500 participants in this symposium felt that it was very exciting from a scientific standpoint. All of us were grateful that we could gather and exchange ideas in such pleasant surroundings. The superb organization of the meeting resulted from the combined efforts of a local firm, Professional Conference Management (Cass Jones, Christine Kowalski, Pam Wilger and Jennifer Smith) and the Congress organization of the Falk Foundation (Silvia Maresch, Birgitte Oess, and Katja Trommer). Those of us working in the field of bile acid research are unanimous in believing that we are most fortunate to have the continued sponsorship of these meetings by the Falk Foundation. The Falk Foundation was the idea of the late Hans Popper, but its continuing success stems from the talent and imagination of its director, Dr Herbert Falk, who celebrated his 70th birthday earlier this year. The 13th International Bile Acid Meeting was the first Falk symposium to be held in the United States, and we hope that we have continued the tradition of superb science, flawless organization, and delightful social programmes that have been the dominant features of so many Falk Symposia.

ALAN F. HOFMANN, MD
La Jolla, California, 1994

Section I
Chemical aspects

1
New, natural bile acids: implications for bile acid evolution

L. R. HAGEY, C. D. SCHTEINGART and A. F. HOFMANN

INTRODUCTION

Vertebrate bile salts display considerable variation between species, making these end-products of cholesterol metabolism unique among low molecular endobiotics in their biodiversity. The specific biochemical pathways selected by vertebrates not only to dispose of cholesterol but also to convert it into a molecule capable of functioning as a biliary stimulant and digestive aid, can be viewed as evolutionary experiments resulting in different bile acid structures that are able to function perfectly well in the appropriate animal. In an attempt to make biological sense out of the structural differences found in the vertebrate bile salts of different species, a programme was developed with the following aims: (a) to examine bile salts in species not previously studied, to expand our knowledge of the full range of bile salt diversity; (b) to generate hypotheses to account for the diversity of bile salts; and (c) to test whether biliary bile acid composition is a biochemical trait that provides useful information about evolutionary relationships. This latter aim was pursued with great tenacity and skill by the late G. A. D. Haslewood[1].

ANALYTICAL PROCEDURES

Bile samples were obtained from deceased animals, many from the San Diego Zoo, and collected during routine autopsy. Samples obtained from facilities outside the borders of the United States were imported using a veterinary import permit. Gallbladder contents were sampled by puncture and aspiration; hepatic bile was collected from the common bile duct. Bile samples were diluted in several volumes of reagent-grade isopropanol immediately after collection, to prevent bacterial degradation and to precipitate biliary proteins.

TLC (thin-layer chromatography) was used to separate and isolate individual classes of bile salts (unconjugated, glycine amidates, sulphates, glucuronides and taurine amidates). Individual bile salts were visualized using functional group specific sprays[3]. Conjugated bile acids were analysed by HPLC (high-pressure liquid chromatography). Unconjugated and deconjugated bile salts were analysed using GC-MS (gas chromatography – mass spectrometry) as methyl esters, methyl ester acetates, or as methyl ester trimethylsilyl derivatives. Additional mass spectral information was obtained using negative-mode LSIMS (liquid secondary ion mass spectrometry) and by proton and carbon NMR (nuclear magnetic resonance).

RESULTS AND DISCUSSION

Most bile alcohols and acids contain $3\alpha,7\alpha$-dihydroxy substituents on the steroid nucleus and are found with one of three types of side-chains. The first is a branched iso-octane side-chain with a terminal alcoholic group (in C_{27} bile alcohols); the second is the same branched iso-octane side-chain with a terminal carboxylic acid group (in C_{27} bile acids); and the third is an isopentane side-chain, also with a terminal carboxylic acid group (in C_{24} bile acids). Previously, it had been believed that the occurrence of C_{27} bile alcohols was restricted to primitive fish and amphibians, and that only modern animals formed C_{24} and C_{27} bile acids. However, an examination of bile from several ancient mammals (elephants, manatees, and the rock hyrax) found that all lacked bile acids and instead contained C_{27} bile alcohol sulphates[4]. As shown in Fig. 1 for the African Forest Elephant, the major bile alcohol was $3\alpha,7\alpha,25,27$-tetrahydroxy-5β-cholestane (peak B). The acetonide (peak C) of the C_{27} bile alcohol was also formed, a technique used to confirm the presence of hydroxyl groups at positions 25 and 27. In addition to this tetrahydroxy bile alcohol, the manatee[5] and rock hyrax also contained $3\alpha,6\alpha,7\alpha,25,27$- and $3\alpha,6\beta,7\alpha,25,27$-pentahydroxy bile alcohol sulphates. These mammals are all evolutionarily related, and the common presence of such unique bile alcohols fully supports the hypothesis that cholanoid structure can provide information on species relationships.

When we began our work, at least six types of additional (third group) nuclear hydroxylations were known to occur: 1α (rare, marsupials); 2β (rare, fish); 6α (rare, in pigs, rodents, and ancient mammals); 6β (rare, in rodents and ancient mammals); 12α (common in many animals, including primates, bovids, and carnivores); and 16α (common in snakes).

Since then we have discovered one new type of hydroxylation, 1β-hydroxylation, and one new family of bile acids (see below). Pyrek and his colleagues have discovered 15α-hydroxylation in Australian marsupials (personal communication). Bile salts with four nuclear substituents were never predominant in our experience. For certain C_{24} and C_{27} bile acids, one additional hydroxy substituent was found to occur on the side-chain and up to two additional hydroxy substituents occur on the side-chain of C_{27} bile alcohols. Most natural bile acids were conjugated with either glycine, taurine, or taurine derivatives. Bile alcohols were invariably conjugated with sulphate.

An examination of birds from different families has led to the finding that 16α-hydroxychenodeoxycholic acid was a common and characteristic bile acid for this large vertebrate group[6]. The dominance of 16α-hydroxychenodeoxycholic acid in the biliary bile acids of six representative birds (from three different

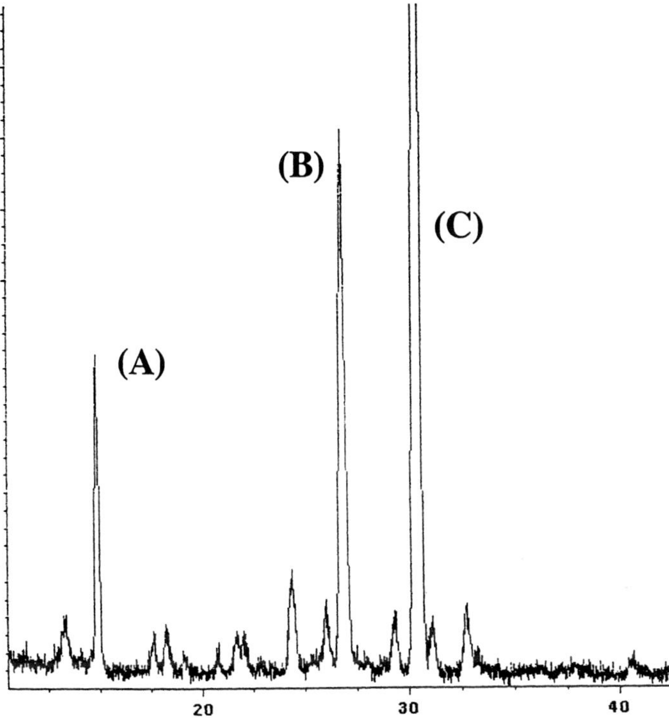

Fig. 1 Capillary GLC profile of the trimethylsilyl methyl esters of bile alcohols from the African Forest Elephant. Peak identification: (**A**) Cholesterol; (**B**) $3\alpha,7\alpha,25,27$-tetrahydroxy-5β-cholestane; and (**C**) $3\alpha,7\alpha,25,27$-tetrahydroxy-5β cholestane acetonide

families) is shown in Table 1.

16α-Hydroxychenodeoxycholic acid was observed in the avian families Balaenicipitae (Shoebill Stork), Carthartidae (condors), Falconidae (falcons), Alcedinidae (kingfishers), Turdidae (thrushes), Laridae (terns), and Spheniscidae (penguins)[2]. Hydroxylation at nuclear position 16α- is not a new discovery, having been previously observed in snakes (forming pythocholic acid, $3\alpha,12\alpha,16\alpha$-trihydroxy-$5\beta$-cholan-24-oic acid)[1]. However, a bile acid with the combination of hydroxylation groups at nuclear positions 3α-, 7α-, and 16α- has not been previously reported. This pattern of hydroxylation occurs in both C_{24} and C_{27} bile acids, and such bile acids may be considered a new bile acid class.

The predominant bile acid for a representative sample of fruit pigeons and doves is the simplest C_{24} primary bile acid, chenodeoxycholic acid[7]. A previously unrecognized hydroxylation site 1β-, in the bile acid nucleus was identified. The natural occurrence of the bile acid 1β-hydroxychenodeoxycholic acid ($1\beta,3\alpha,7\alpha$-trihydroxy-5β-cholan-24-oic acid) found in these birds had not been described in any other species except neonatal humans. The biliary bile acid composition of six fruit pigeons and doves that contained meaningful levels of the bile acid 1β-hydroxychenodeoxycholic acid is summarized in Table 2.

Table 1 16α-Hydroxychenodeoxycholic acid in the biliary bile acids of selected birds

	Bile acid composition (%)		
Avian Family	*3α,7α*	*3α,7α,16α*	*3α,7α,12α*
Ardeidae (Herons)			
Cattle Egret	5	95	0
Great Blue Heron	6	94	0
Pelecanidae (Pelicans)			
Eastern Brown Pelican	20	80	0
Pink Back Pelican	61	33	6
Tytonidae (Owls)			
Thailand Bay Owl	17	80	3
Barn Owl	33	61	6

Table 2 Biliary bile acid composition of selected fruit pigeons and doves

	Bile acid composition (%)		
Common name	*3α,7α*	*1β,3α,7α*	*Glycine*
Spotted Imperial Pigeon	50	50	58
Celebes Imperial Pigeon	61	39	51
Merrill's Fruit Dove	77	23	53
Marche's Fruit Dove	89	11	46
Wompoo Fruit Dove	91	9	29
Black-chinned Fruit Dove	92	8	57

Many fruit pigeons and doves lack a caecum, and it is significant that the common secondary bile acids lithocholic acid and deoxycholic acid were not detected. Also shown in Table 2 is the observation that fruit pigeons conjugate bile acids with glycine. Among vertebrates, glycine conjugation is rare, and all birds (except this small family) conjugate their bile acids with taurine.

SUMMARY

The presence of unique bile alcohols and the absence of bile acids is shared in common by three groups of evolutionarily related ancient mammals (elephants, manatees, and the rock hyrax).

A new bile acid, 3α,7α,16α-trihydroxy-5β-cholan-24-oic acid, is prevalent in vertebrate bile. In parallel with the common names of other bile acids, listed in Table 3, we have called it 'avicholic acid' to signify that it is a class* that has to date been identified only in birds (class Aves).

---

*The term 'class' is used because the 7β epimers, the 7-deoxy, and the 3,7, or 12-oxo derivative may be considered to belong to the same class.

Table 3 C24 bile acid classes

'Default' hydroxyl groups	Third hydroxyl group	Trivial name of class
$3\alpha,7\alpha$	none	'chenodeoxycholic'
$3\alpha,7\alpha$	12α-	'cholic'
$3\alpha,7\alpha$	6α-	'hyocholic'
$3\alpha,7\alpha$	6β-	'muricholic'
$3\alpha,7\alpha$	16α-	'avicholic'
$3\alpha,7\alpha$	1β-	(no name proposed)

A new site of hydroxylation (1β-) has been identified in the biliary bile acids of pigeons and fruit doves. Although nearly all birds conjugate their bile acids with taurine, certain pigeons and fruit doves also conjugate their bile acids with glycine.

References

1. Haslewood GAD. The biological importance of bile salts. Amsterdam: North-Holland; 1978.
2. Hagey LR. Bile acid biodiversity in vertebrates: chemistry and evolutionary implication. PhD thesis. University of California, San Diego. San Diego, CA, 1992.
3. Dawson RMC, Elliott DC, Elliott WH, Jones KM. Data for biomedical research. New York: Oxford University Press; 1969.
4. Hagey LR, Schteingart CD, Ton-Nu H-T, Rossi SS, Hofmann AF. Unique bile alcohols (3,6,7,25,27-pentahydroxy cholestanes) and absence of bile acids are a common feature of three ancient mammals. Hepatology. 1993;18:177A.
5. Kuroki S, Schteingart CD, Hagey LR et al. Bile salts of the West Indian Manatee *Trichechus manatus latirostris*: novel bile alcohol sulfates and absence of bile salts. J Lipid Res. 1988;29: 509–52.
6. Hagey LR, Schteingart CD, Ton-Nu H-T, Hofmann AF. 16α-Hydroxychenodeoxycholic acid, a new major bile acid in birds. Hepatology. 1993;18:305A.
7. Hagey LR, Schteingart CD, Ton-Nu H-T, Hofmann AF. Biliary bile acids of fruit pigeons and doves (Columbiformes): presence of 1β-hydroxychenodeoxycholic acid and conjugation with glycine as well as taurine. J Lipid Res. 1994;35:2041–8.

2
Synthesis of uncommon bile acids

T. IIDA, T. NAMBARA and F. C. CHANG

INTRODUCTION

In recent years considerable attention has been directed to the site of origin, pathways of biosynthesis and metabolism, physiological significance, and excretory routes of 'uncommon', 'tentatively identified' and/or 'unidentified' bile acids in humans in connection with hepatobiliary diseases[1-5]. In addition to five common bile acids of 5β-cholanoic acid series [lithocholic (LCA), chenodeoxycholic (CDCA), ursodeoxycholic (UDCA), deoxycholic (DCA), and cholic (CA) acids; **1–5**] (Chart 1), patients with hepatobiliary diseases, and newborn infants and fetuses, excrete a variety of uncommon bile acids in biological materials such as bile, serum, urine, faeces, meconium and amniotic fluid. Possible implication of bile acids in the development of colon cancer has also stimulated interest in the identity of uncommon metabolites of the conventional bile acids[6-8].

The uncommon bile acids differ from the common bile acids in the number, position and stereochemical configuration of the hydroxyl groups at positions C-1, C-2, C-3, C-6, C-7 and/or C-12 in the 5β-steroid nucleus (normal, A/B-*cis*) and at C-20, C-22 and C-23 in the side-chain; they also include the analogous acids of the 5α-series ('allo', A/B-*trans*), bile acids with various functional groups (e.g. oxo group and double bond) at different positions, and 'short-chain' C_{20}–C_{23} and 'long-chain' C_{27}–C_{29} bile acids.

The existence of new and unusual bile acids in human biological materials has usually been characterized or elucidated only by gas chromatographic–mass spectrometric (GC-MS) analysis. Therefore, a number of 'unidentified' and/or 'tentatively identified' bile acids, as well as uncommon ones, have been reported in the literature. Unequivocal proof of their identification and existence, however, had to await chemical synthesis and demonstration of identity of the isolated compounds with synthetic ones. The availability of these uncommon bile acids as authentic specimens also provides a unique opportunity to study the physical, chemical, biological and physicochemical properties of such organic molecules. This chapter covers new, convenient and improved methods for the syntheses of some classes of biologically important bile acids in humans, particularly for the epimers of conventional bile acids and their 5α-analogues,

Common bile acids and their epimers

	R1	R2	R3	
1.	α-OH	H	H	(LCA)
2.	α-OH	α-OH	H	(CDCA)
3.	α-OH	β-OH	H	(UDCA)
4.	α-OH	H	α-OH	(DCA)
5.	α-OH	α-OH	α-OH	(CA)
6.	β-OH	H	H	(*iso* LCA)
7.	β-OH	α-OH	H	(*iso* CDCA)
8.	β-OH	β-OH	H	(*iso* UDCA)
9.	β-OH	H	α-OH	(*iso* DCA)
10.	α-OH	H	β-OH	
11.	β-OH	H	β-OH	
12.	β-OH	α-OH	α-OH	(*iso* CA)
13.	α-OH	β-OH	α-OH	(ursocholic acid)
14.	β-OH	β-OH	α-OH	(*iso* ursocholic acid)
15.	α-OH	α-OH	β-OH	
16.	α-OH	β-OH	β-OH	

Δ^5**-Unsaturated bile acids**

	R1	R2
17.	H	H
18.	α-OH	H
19.	β-OH	H
20.	H	α-OH
21.	α-OH	α-OH

Allo **bile acids**

	R1	R2	R3	
22.	α-OH	H	H	(*allo* LCA)
23.	β-OH	H	H	(*allo iso* LCA)
24.	α-OH	α-OH	H	(*allo* CDCA)
25.	β-OH	α-OH	H	(*allo iso* CDCA)
26.	α-OH	β-OH	H	(*allo* UDCA)
27.	β-OH	β-OH	H	(*allo iso* UDCA)
28.	α-OH	H	α-OH	(*allo* DCA)
29.	β-OH	H	α-OH	(*allo iso* DCA)
30.	α-OH	H	β-OH	
31.	β-OH	H	β-OH	
32.	α-OH	α-OH	α-OH	(*allo* CA)
33.	α-OH	β-OH	α-OH	
34.	β-OH	β-OH	α-OH	

Chart 1 Bile acids identified in human biological materials

and 1β-, 2β-, 4β- and 6-hydroxylated bile acids. The structures of these bile acids identified in human biological materials are shown in Chart 1.

GENERAL PROCEDURES FOR THE SYNTHESIS OF UNCOMMON BILE ACIDS

Selective protection of hydroxyl groups

As previously discussed by Belle[9], the synthesis of uncommon bile acids, starting from the readily available conventional bile acids, may be first based on protecting some of the hydroxyl groups by substitution. The selective protection is achieved by utilizing the differences in the reactivity against acylation,

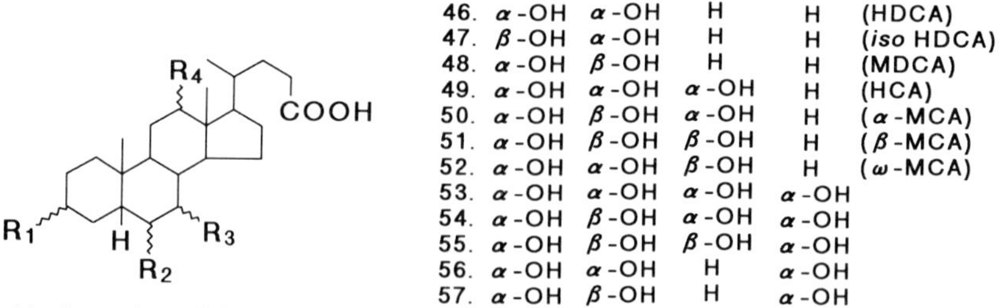

1β-Hydroxylated bile acids

	R1	R2	R3	R4
35.	H	H		
36.	α-OH	H		
37.	β-OH	H		
38.	H	α-OH		
39.	α-OH	α-OH		

2β-Hydroxylated bile acids

	R1	R2	R3	R4
40.	H	H	H	
41.	α-OH	α-OH	H	
42.	H	α-OH	α-OH	

4β-Hydroxylated bile acids

	R1	R2	R3	R4
43.	H	H		
44.	α-OH	H		
45.	α-OH	α-OH		

6-Hydroxylated bile acids

	R1	R2	R3	R4	
46.	α-OH	α-OH	H	H	(HDCA)
47.	β-OH	α-OH	H	H	(iso HDCA)
48.	α-OH	β-OH	H	H	(MDCA)
49.	α-OH	α-OH	α-OH	H	(HCA)
50.	α-OH	β-OH	α-OH	H	(α-MCA)
51.	α-OH	β-OH	β-OH	H	(β-MCA)
52.	α-OH	α-OH	β-OH	H	(ω-MCA)
53.	α-OH	α-OH	α-OH	α-OH	
54.	α-OH	β-OH	α-OH	α-OH	
55.	α-OH	β-OH	β-OH	α-OH	
56.	α-OH	α-OH	H	α-OH	
57.	α-OH	β-OH	H	α-OH	

Chart 1 *Continued*

etherification and oxidation of the certain hydroxyl groups present in the 5α- or 5β-steroid nucleus, depending upon their axial or equatorial nature and steric hindrance. For this purpose formylation, acetylation, trifluoroacetylation, propionylation, carbethoxylation, tosylation and mesylation, and tetrahydropyranyl and *tert*-butyldimethylsilyl etherifications are frequently used for bile acid synthesis. For example, the formylation of CDCA proceeds without selectivity to give the corresponding performate, which in turn is partially hydrolysed with saturated methanolic ammonia to afford the 7-monoformate[10], whereas carbethoxylation gives only the 3-monocathylate[9] (Scheme 1). On the

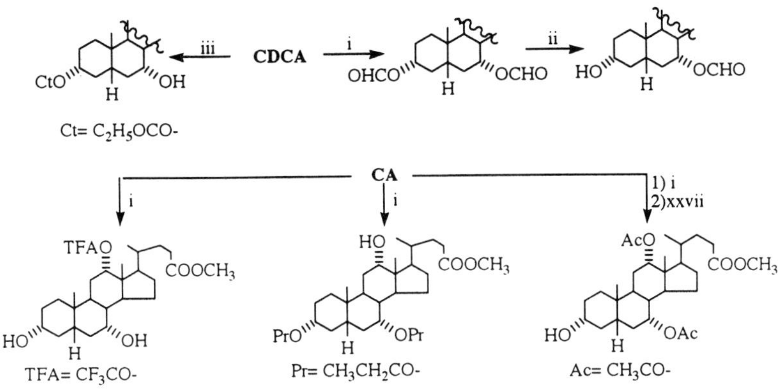

Ct= C$_2$H$_5$OCO-

Scheme 1 Selective acylation of hydroxyl groups

TFA= CF$_3$CO-

Pr= CH$_3$CH$_2$CO-

Ac= CH$_3$CO-

TBDMS= *tert*-butyldimethylsilyl

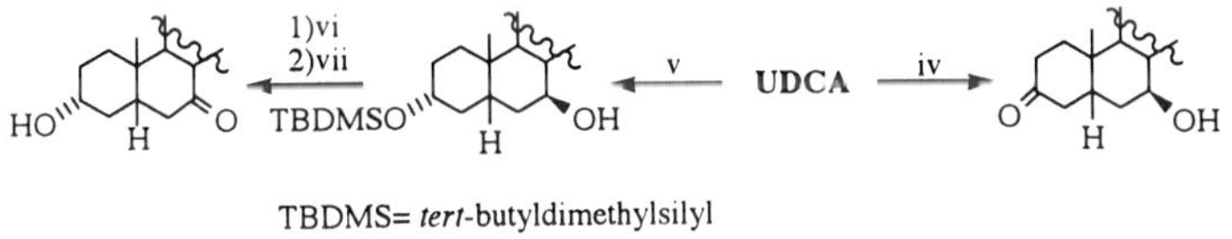

Scheme 2 Selective oxidation of hydroxyl groups

other hand, acylation of CA affords the different types of protected CA derivatives, depending upon the choice of acylating agents[11]. The desired hydroxyl-protected bile acids thus obtained may be used for subsequent reactions.

Regioselective oxidation of hydroxyl groups

Silver carbonate on Celite (Ag$_2$CO$_3$/Celite), a reagent which is used to oxidize selectively hydroxyl groups only at certain positions in a number of polyhydroxylated compounds, was found to react with bile acids to give the corresponding 3-oxo derivatives in good yields[12]. For example, Ag$_2$CO$_3$/Celite oxidation of UDCA having two equatorially oriented hydroxyls at both the C-3 and C-7 positions affords only the corresponding 3-monoketone, whereas the 7-monoketone is prepared via the 3-*tert*-butyldimethylsilyl ether derivative of UDCA[13] (Scheme 2). Analogously, oxidation at C-3 of bile acids having a vicinal 3,4-glycol structure with pyridinium chlorochromate (C$_5$H$_5$NH·ClCrO$_3$) affords exclusively the 3-oxo derivatives[14]. A highly regioselective conversion of 3-hydroxy steroids in the 5α- and 5β-series to the corresponding 1,4-dien-3-ones as key intermediates in steroid synthesis is attained by treatment with iodoxybenzene/benzeneselenic anhydride in boiling toluene[15].

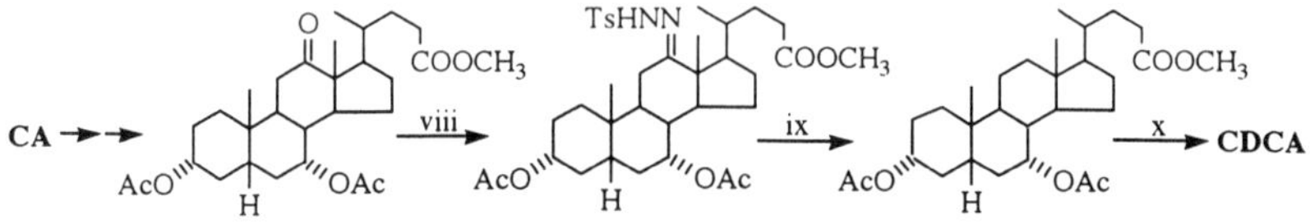

Ac= CH₃CO-; Ts= *p*-CH₃C₆H₄SO₂-

Scheme 3   Reduction of oxo to methylene groups

Reduction of oxo to methylene groups

The reduction of ketones to the corresponding methylene analogues, a key transformation in organic synthesis, has been attained by use of the Huang-Minlon modification of Wolff–Kishner reduction[9]. However, the reaction still has several drawbacks, especially when performed with ketones having other functional groups unstable in the rather extreme conditions of temperature and alkalinity. A highly convenient method for the elimination of oxo groups from bile acids has been developed by us[16]. The reactions involved are the high-yield formation of the tosylhydrazone derivatives of oxo-bile acids and subsequent reductive cleavage with sodium borohydride (NaBH₄) in acetic acid[17]. The two-step procedure represents a mild and simple method for the selective deoxygenation of oxo-bile acids having alkoxycarbonyl groups and possibly also acyloxy groups without concomitant hydrolysis of these latter groups. We have successfully applied this procedure to the preparation of CDCA from CA, which proceeds through easily prepared, well-defined intermediates and afforded a pure product in good yield (30% from CA) without requiring a column chromatographic purification step, in contrast to previous procedures[18] (Scheme 3).

Stereoselective reduction of oxo to hydroxyl groups

The reduction of oxo- to the hydroxyl-compounds has been studied extensively by many investigators[9,19]. Depending on the reducing agents and on the reaction conditions, either α- or β-alcohols, or an epimeric mixture may be obtained.

Scheme 4 shows new stereoselective agents for use in the reduction of 3-, 7- and 12-oxocholanoates. *tert*-Butylamine-borane complex (t-C₄H₉NH₂•BH₃)[20] and potassium *tri-sec*-butylborohydride (*K*-Selectride)[21,22] were found to be effective reducing agents for 3-ketones. With t-C₄H₉NH₂•BH₃, 3-ketones in the 5β-series are converted into the corresponding 3α-alcohols[14,23,24], whereas with *K*-Selectride they are reduced to the axial 3β-epimers[24]; the reverse is true for the 5α-series[22]. Both the reduction reactions proceed much more cleanly and stereoselectively than with the previous reagents, NaBH₄ and catalytic hydrogenation[9].

Previous synthesis of 7α- and 7β-alcohols from 7-ketones was attained by NaBH₄ and metallic sodium in propanol reductions, respectively[9]. A less basic reductant, zinc borohydride [Zn(BH₄)₂][19], and a new dissolving metal agent, potassium in *tert*-amyl alcohol[25], are attractive reducing agents on 7-ketones. By carrying out the reduction using Zn(BH₄)₂, the axial 7α-hydroxy products are

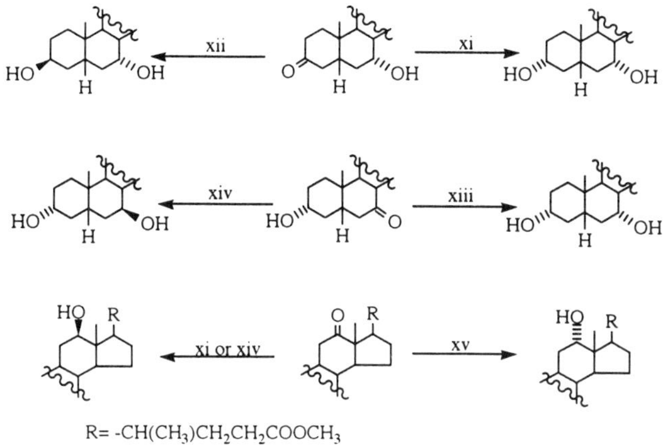

R= -CH(CH$_3$)CH$_2$CH$_2$COOCH$_3$

Scheme 4 Stereoselective reduction of oxo to hydroxyl groups

obtained without concurrent hydrolysis of the C-24 ester group[26,27]. On the other hand, potassium/t-amyl alcohol stereoselectively reduces 7-ketones to the equatorial 7β-epimers[26,27].

According to previous research the most feasible route to 12β-hydroxy acids was by Raney nickel catalytic hydrogenation of the appropriate 12-ketones[9,28], but the method was less stereoselective and produced numerous by-products, probably due to the steric hindrance of the side-chain. The high equatorial selectivity found in the reduction of 3-oxo to 3α-ol by t-C$_4$H$_9$NH$_2$·BH$_3$ and 7-oxo to 7β-ol by potassium/t-amyl ketones mentioned above was selectively applied to 12-ketones. Thus, t-C$_4$H$_9$NH$_2$·BH$_3$[29-31] and potassium/t-amyl alcohol[32] proved to be excellent reducing agents for 12β-hydroxy synthesis; both the reduction reactions are simple, rapid and straightforward. It was also found that the NaBH$_4$/PdCl$_2$ agent[33], instead of traditional NaBH$_4$ alone, stereoselectively reduces 12-ketones to the corresponding axial 12α-hydroxy isomers[34,35].

Inversion reaction of hydroxyl groups

As discussed above, conventional syntheses of epimeric alcohols involve reduction of the appropriate ketones, produced by selective oxidation, to the corresponding epimeric mixtures which are usually separated by chromatography. The syntheses herein discussed do not proceed through intermediary ketones. At present three epimerization reagents for hydroxyl groups are successfully applied to bile acid synthesis, namely N,N-dimethylformamide (DMF)[36], potassium superoxide (KO$_2$)/18-crown-6 ether[37,38], and diethyl azodicarboxylate (DEADCAT)/triphenylphosphine/formic acid[39,40].

As shown in Scheme 5, an equatorial 3α-hydroxy bile acid ester, via the tosylate, undergoes DMF inversion reaction to give the corresponding axial 3β-formate, which in turn is hydrolysed to the desired 3β-epimer[28,41]. Analogously, the 3α-tosylate, when subjected to KO$_2$/crown ether treatment in dimethyl-sulphoxide (DMSO), suffers inversion at C-3, accompanied by simultaneous

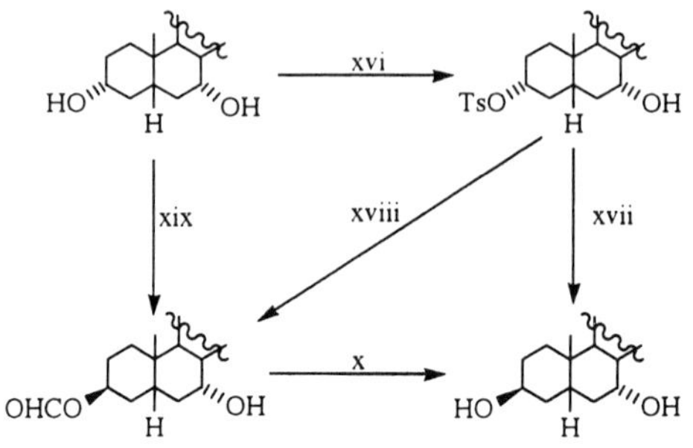

Scheme 5 Inversion reactions of 3α- *to* 3β-hydroxyl groups

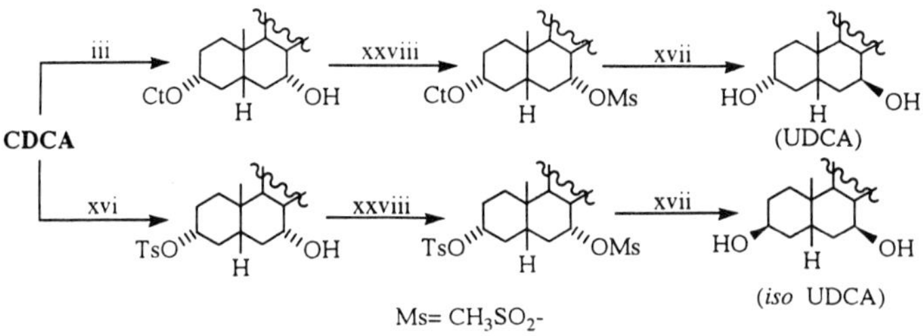

CDCA

Ms= CH_3SO_2-

Scheme 6 Synthetic route from CDCA to UDCA and *iso*-UDCA

hydrolysis of the acyloxy and ester groups to give the 3β-epimer in one step[30,41]. Direct reaction of the 3α-hydroxyl compound by treatment with DEAD-CAT/triphenylphosphine/formic acid gives the inverted 3β-formate which, on hydrolysis, is converted to the 3β-epimer[26,32,42,43].

On the other hand, inversion of a 7α-hydroxyl group succeeds only by KO_2/crown ether reaction with the appropriate 7α-mesyloxy derivative[30,41]. By applying this procedure a facile and clean conversion of CDCA to UDCA which does not involve the reduction of an intermediary 7-ketone has been developed[44] (Scheme 6). Analogously, reaction of methyl 3α-tosyloxy-7α-mesyloxy-5β-cholanoate with KO_2/crown ether results in the simultaneous inversion at both the 3- and 7-positions and hydrolysis of the acyloxy groups at C-3 and C-7 and the ester group at C-24, forming *iso*-UDCA (3β,7β-dihydroxy acid; **8**) in one step[41]. Therefore, these inversion reactions are highly efficient methods of obtaining the desired epimers of bile acids.

SYNTHESIS OF BIOLOGICALLY IMPORTANT UNCOMMON BILE ACIDS

The synthesis of these bile acids is usually attained by starting from the abundantly available common bile acids. By the choice of some of the above-mentioned reactions and reagents it may be possible to synthesize almost all of the naturally occurring bile acids. This is useful either to identify 'unidentified' and 'tentatively identified' acids or to gain full details on their preparation, and subsequent isolation from the biological materials.

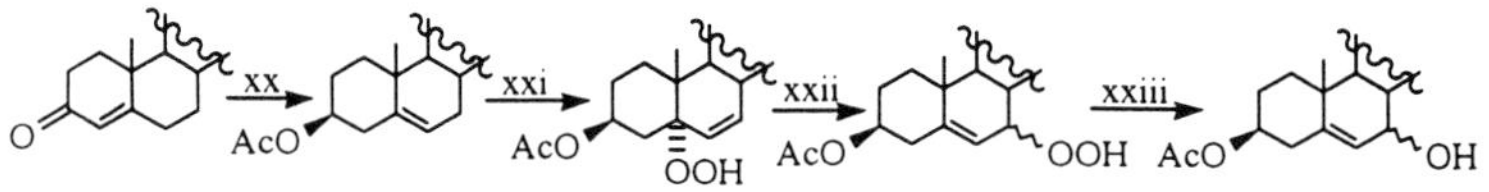

Scheme 7 Synthetic route to Δ^5-unsaturated bile acids

Synthesis of the epimers of common bile acids

Eneroth *et al.* have identified a number of epimeric mono-, di- and trisubstituted 5β-cholanoic acids as minor metabolites in human faeces by GC-MS analysis[45-47]. The presence of other epimeric bile acids in urine[48], serum[49] and bile[50,51] has also been reported. Most of these identified bile acids include the epimers (**6–16**) of the common bile acids and their oxo-derivatives.

We have prepared a series of the stereoisomeric 3,7- and 3,12-dihydroxy- (**7–11**) and 3,7,12-trihydroxy-5β-cholanoic acids (**12–16**) using essentially the general procedures discussed above[30,41,52]. The 3,7-dihydroxy stereoisomers have also been synthesized by an alternative route[49].

Synthesis of Δ^5-unsaturated bile acids

3β-Hydroxy-5-cholenoic acid (**17**) was first isolated as an unusual bile acid from the urine of infants with biliary atresia by Makino and Sjövall[53]. This unsaturated bile acid has subsequently been found as a major component in the urine of patients suffering cholestasis[54], and in human meconium[55]. Excretion of significant amounts of analogous 3β,7α-dihydroxy-5-cholenoic acid (**18**) in human bile[56,57], 3β,7β-dihydroxy-5-cholenoic acid (**19**) in urine[48], 3β, 12α– dihydroxy-5-cholenoic acids (**20**) in serum[58], and 3β,7α,12α-trihydroxy-5- cholenoic acid (**21**) in bile, urine and faeces[57,59] has also been reported. These Δ^5- unsaturated bile acids as authentic samples, especially **18** and **19**, are synthesized from appropriate 3-oxo-Δ^4 intermediates through the Δ^6-5α-hydroperoxides and Δ^5-7-hydroperoxides[60] (Scheme 7).

Synthesis of *allo* bile acids

Allo bile acids, historically of key importance in the elucidation of the structural and stereochemical relationships between the 5α- and 5β-series, are products isolated from some vertebrates[61] and from human biological fluids[1-4], and are also attractive starting materials for the synthesis of various 5α-bile alcohols present in lower vertebrates[62]. However, *allo* bile acids, although known for many years and with several reported methods for preparation[61], are not easily available products.

Allo LCA was first characterized as the major saturated monohydroxylated 5α-cholanoic acid in the urine of an infant with biliary atresia[53]. Subsequently, *allo* CDCA (**24**), *allo* DCA (**28**) and *allo* CA (**32**) and their epimers (**23, 25, 27, 29–31, 33, 34**) have also been detected as constituents of patients with hepatobiliary diseases or colon cancer[6,47,63,64].

Basically, two allomerization (5β to 5α) procedures are used for *allo* bile acid syntheses[61]. The first involves treatment of 3-hydroxy 5β-compounds with Raney

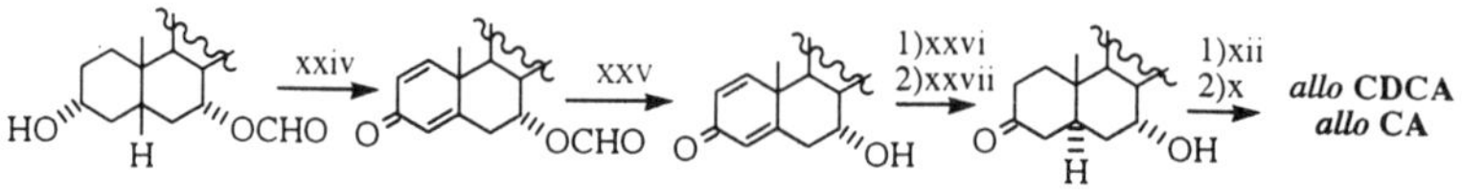

Scheme 8   Synthetic route to *allo* CDCA and *allo*CA

nickel in boiling p-cymene; the second synthesis consists of the reduction of 3-oxo-Δ^4 compounds by lithium/liquid NH_3. By using the latter procedure we have reported new synthetic routes to the stereoisomeric 3,7- and 3,12-dihydroxy- and 3,7,12-trihydroxy-5α-cholanoic acids[35,65,66]. The method, however, still had drawbacks, particularly for the preparation of *allo* CDCA (**24**) and *allo* CA (**32**) having a sterically hindered 7α-hydroxyl group. Hence, a high-yield and regioselective method for the synthesis of these compounds has also been developed[67]. As shown in Scheme 8, the key steps in the synthesis are: (1) simultaneous oxidation–dehydrogenation reaction of protected 3α-hydroxy 5β-bile acids with iodoxybenzene catalysed by benzeneselenic anhydride; (2) reductive allomerization at C-5 of the 1,4-dien-3-oxo-hydroxy acids with lithium/liquid NH_3; and (3) subsequent reduction of the resulting 3-oxo 5α-compounds with K-Selectride (total yields *ca.* 30%). A similar procedure has also been reported by Zhu *et al.*[68].

1β-Hydroxylated bile acids

1β-Hydroxylated metabolites of CDCA, DCA and CA [1β,3α,7α- and 1β,3α,12α-trihydroxy- and 1β,3α,7α,12α-tetrahydroxy-5β-cholanoic acids (**36, 38, 39**), respectively] have been detected for the first time by GC-MS analysis of the urine of patients with liver diseases by Sjövall and his co-workers[47,69]. The tetrahydroxy acid (**39**) was also characterized as a major component in the meconium[70] and urine of healthy human newborns[71]. The stereochemical configurations of the hydroxyl groups were elucidated by metabolic[72,73] and microbial[74] studies. The complete structure of these compounds was finally established by ^{1}H and ^{13}C nuclear magnetic resonance (NMR) analysis of **39** isolated from human urine[75] and by direct comparison with synthetic samples[76]. Subsequently, these 1β-hydroxylated bile acids were isolated in significant amounts in the urine, meconium, umbilical cord blood and amniotic fluid from neonates or infants[77–80], and in the urine, serum, faeces and liver tissue from patients with liver diseases[81–85]. The occurrence of 1β-hydroxylated metabolites of LCA (**35**)[73] and UDCA (**37**)[82,85,86] in humans has also been disclosed. These polar bile acids have been considered particularly advantageous for excretion of bile acids in the fetal and neonatal periods. In particular, a marked increase in the amount of 1β-hydroxylated CA (**39**) excreted in the urine during infancy and pregnancy suggests an important pathway of bile acid synthesis during development.

A novel trihydroxylated C_{24} bile acid was isolated from the gallbladder bile of the Australian opossum, *Trichosurus vulpecula* (Lesson)[87]. This acid, named as vulpecholic acid, was identified as the C-1 epimer of **38**, 1α,3α,7α-trihydroxy-5β-cholanoic acid.

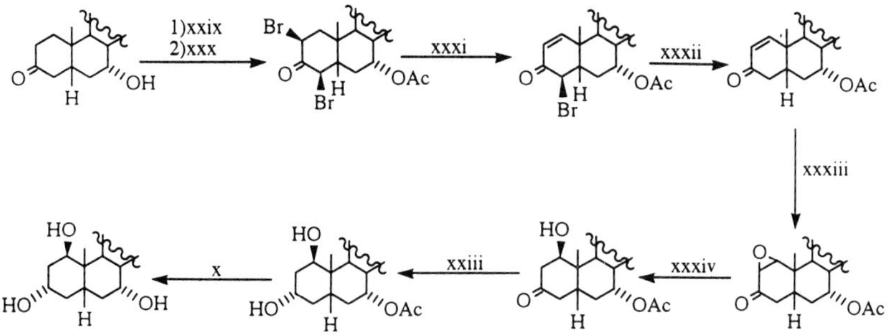

Scheme 9 Synthetic route to 1β-hydroxylated bile acids

1β-Hydroxylated bile acids (**35, 36, 38, 39**) as authentic specimens have been synthesized by Tohma *et al.*[76]. As shown in Scheme 9, the Δ^1-unsaturated ketones were prepared from 3-oxo bile acid esters via dehydrobromination of the 2,4-dibromides with lithium carbonate/lithium bromide, and oxidized with alkaline hydrogen peroxide to give the 1β,2β-epoxyketones. Reductive cleavage of the epoxyketones with chromous acetate and subsequent reduction with NaBH$_4$ afforded the 1β,3α-dihydroxy compounds, which were hydrolysed to the 1β-hydroxylated bile acids. A synthetic procedure for 1α-hydroxylated bile acids has also been reported[88].

2β-Hydroxylated bile acids

Several 2-hydroxylated bile acids with a vicinal 2,3-glycol structure have been identified in human biological samples by GC-MS. The 2β-hydroxylated metabolite of CA, 2β,3α,7α,12α-tetrahydroxy-5β-cholanoic acid (**42**), has been characterized as a minor component of the gastric contents of neonates with intestinal obstruction[89] and in the amniotic fluids of pregnant women[90]. Analogous 2β,3α,6α,7α-tetrahydroxy-5β-cholanoic acid (**41**) has also been tentatively identified as a common constituent in urine from healthy newborns[71,91]. Gustafsson *et al.* have investigated the biotransformation of [24-^{14}C]LCA by the microsomes from human fetal liver and clarified the formation of a 2-hydroxylated LCA (**40**)[73].

2β-Hydroxylated LCA, CDCA, DCA and CA with a diequatorial *trans*-2,3-glycol structure have been prepared from the respective parent compounds[23] (Scheme 10). The principal reactions involved were: (1) bromination of 3-oxo formylated bile acids in DMF; (2) simultaneous rearrangement and substitution of the resulting 4β-bromo-3-oxo derivatives to the 2β-acetoxy-3-oxo compounds with potassium acetate[92]; and (3) reduction to the 2β-acetoxy-3α-hydroxy compounds with t-C$_4$H$_9$NH$_2$·BH$_3$.

4β-Hydroxylated bile acids

Recently, Setchell *et al.* have reported the isolation from human fetal gallbladder bile of a novel bile acid, which accounted for 5–15% of the total biliary bile

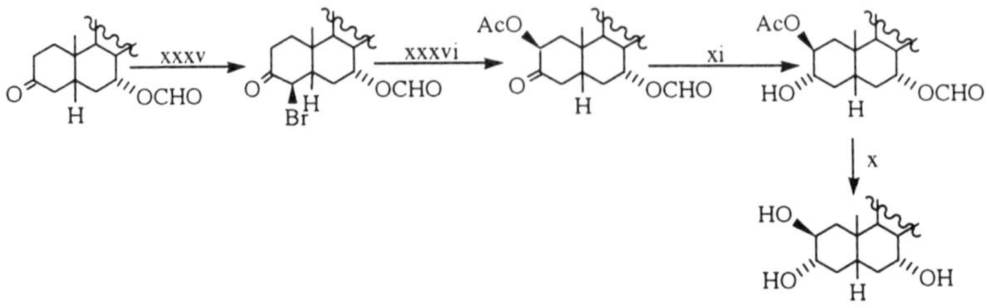

Scheme 10 Synthetic route to 2β-hydroxylated bile acids

acids in early gestation[93]. This novel bile acid was unambiguously characterized by partial chemical synthesis as 3α,4β,7α-trihydroxy-5β-cholanoic acid (**44**), having a diequatorial *trans*-3,4-glycol structure[94,95]. Analogous 4β-hydroxylated LCA (**43**) and CA (**45**) have also been detected in the meconium and faeces of healthy newborn infants. The presence of these bile acids in the amniotic fluids from healthy pregnant women[90] and in human urine[96] has also been reported. In more recent work, Strandvik *et al.* have detected other atypical 4-hydroxylated bile acids as minor components from the urine of neonates, and their structures were tentatively identified by GC-MS analysis as the C-3 epimers of **44** and **45**, 3β,4β,7-trihydroxy- and 3β,4β,7α,12α-tetrahydroxy-5β-cholanoic acids[91]. The above findings indicate the existence of a biotransformation pathway of 4β-hydroxylation.

The 4β-hydroxylated derivatives of LCA, CDCA, DCA and CA and their 3β-epimers as authentic samples have been synthesized by us from their respective parent compounds[10] (Scheme 11). The principal reactions employed were: (1) β-face *cis*-dihydroxylation of Δ^3 intermediates with osmium tetroxide catalysed by *N*-methylmorpholine *N*-oxide; (2) selective oxidation at C-3 of the 3β,4β-diols with $C_5H_5NH \cdot ClCrO_3$; and (3) stereoselective reduction of the 3-monoketones with t-$C_4H_9NH_2 \cdot BH_3$. Recently, the stereoselective acetoxylation at the 4 β-position of 3-oxo compounds with lead tetra-acetate in the presence of boron trifluoride in acetic acid has also provided a short route to the desired acids[97].

6α- and 6β-Hydroxylated bile acids

Various 6-hydroxylated bile acids, especially at the 6α-position, have recently been isolated in significant amounts from biological materials excreted by patients with hepatobiliary diseases and by newborn infants and in fetus, along with 1β-hydroxylated bile acids mentioned above[1–4]. The concurrent occurrence of the 6- and 1β-hydroxylated bile acids is of keen current interest in biological and metabolic studies.

Hyocholic acid (HCA, 3α,6α,7α-trihydroxy-5β-cholanoic acid; **49**), one of the earliest 6α-hydroxylated bile acids known, was isolated first by Haslewood from pig bile[98]. This triol, having a vicinal *cis*-6,7-glycol structure, also presents as a major urinary metabolite of CDCA in patients with cholestatic liver diseases[47,51,69,72,78,81–83] and in newborn infants and fetus[70,90,91,93]. The C-6 and/or C-7 epimers of HCA, 3α,6β,7α-, 3α,6β,7β- and 3α,6α,7β-trihydroxy-5β-

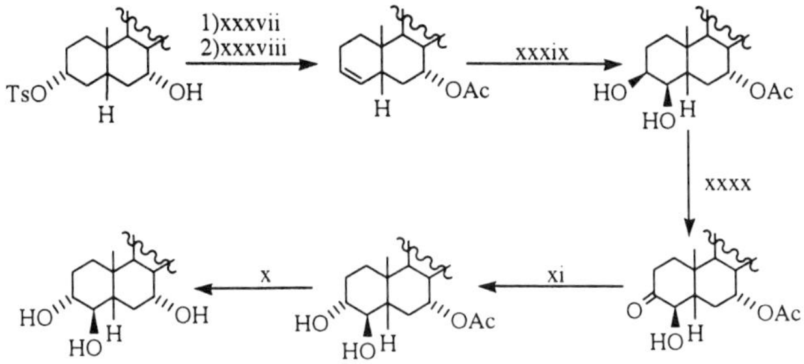

Scheme 11 Synthetic route to 4β-hydroxylated bile acids

cholanoic acids [α-, β- and ω-muricholic acids (MCA) (**50–52**), respectively], have also been excreted in several human species; α-MCA[6], β-MCA[51,99] and ω-MCA[82,86,100].

Hydroxylation at the 6α-position of CA produces 3α,6α,7α,12α-tetrahydroxy-5β-cholanoic acid (**53**), which is a major urinary metabolite in patients with cholestasis[63,72,75,81,83,101]. The presence of epimeric 3α,6β,7α,12α-tetrahydroxy-5β-cholanoic acid (**54**)[72,75] and 3α,6β,7β,12α-tetrahydroxy-5β-cholanoic acid (**55**)[101] in human urine has also been demonstrated.

Other 6-hydroxylated bile acids derived from LCA and DCA and their epimeric analogues have been detected as components of urine from humans and other species, and the following compounds were identified: hyodeoxycholic acid (HDCA, 3α,6α-dihydroxy-5β-cholanoic acid; **46**)[47,73,102–104], *iso*-HDCA (3β,6α-dihydroxy-5β-cholanoic acid; **47**)[6], murideoxycholic acid (MDCA, 3α,6β-dihydroxy-5β-cholanoic acid; **48**)[47,69,103], 3α,6α,12α-trihydroxy-5β-cholanoic acid (**56**)[63,72,104], and 3α,6β,12α-trihydroxy-5β-cholanoic acid (**57**)[47,63,69,103].

Some of the above compounds were unambiguously characterized and identified by direct GC-MS comparison with authentic reference compounds. Others, partially characterized as 3,6-diols, 3,6,7- and 3,6,12-triols or 3,6,7,12-tetrols by GC-MS, still remain uncertain as to stereochemical configuration of their hydroxyl groups and A/B ring junction of the steroid nucleus, and await further characterization.

HCA and its three MCA stereoisomers (**49–52**) were synthesized by Hsia and his co-workers some years ago[105]. We have recently devised an improved procedure for the preparation of **49–52** and their 3β-epimers as potential metabolites[26]. Scheme 12 shows the synthetic route to **49 – 52**. The 6α-bromo-7-ketone as a key intermediate was substituted for a hydroxyl group with potassium hydroxide in methanol to give the α-ketol (6α-OH-7-oxo), and subsequent reduction with Zn(BH$_4$)$_2$ and alkaline hydrolysis afforded HDCA. The bromoketone was converted into the bromohydrin (6α-Br-7α-OH) with Zn(BH$_4$)$_2$, and then treated with zinc powder in acetic acid to give the Δ^6-cholenoate. *cis*-Dihydroxylation of the Δ^6-cholenoate with osmium tetroxide/*N*-methylmorpholine *N*-oxide gave the 6β,7β-dihydroxylated compound, which was hydrolysed to give β-MCA. Epoxidation of the Δ^6-cholenoate with *m*-chloroperbenzoic acid gave the α-epoxide, which was converted into α-MCA with the *trans*-fission of the epoxide by boron trifluoride etherate (or acetic acid)

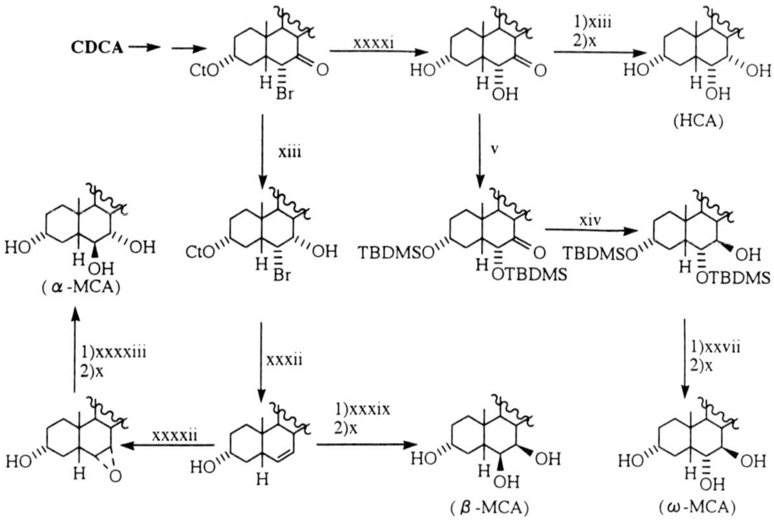

Scheme 12 Synthetic route to stereoisomeric HCA and MCA

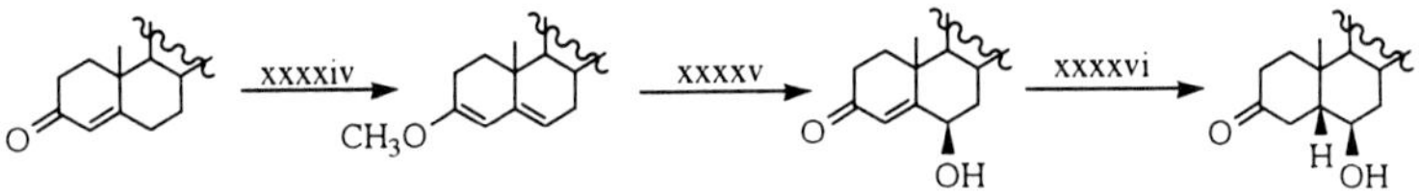

Scheme 13 Hydroxylation at C-6 position

and subsequent alkaline hydrolysis. Finally, treatment of the α-ketol with *tert*-butyldimethylsilyl chloride and successive reduction with potassium/*t*-amyl alcohol afforded ω-MCA after desilylation and alkaline hydrolysis. In a similar manner, the four stereoisomeric $3\alpha,6,7,12\alpha$-tetrahydroxy acids (**53–55** and $3\alpha,6\alpha,7\beta,12\alpha$-tetrol) have been synthesized and characterized by Kurosawa *et al.*[106], Yoshii *et al.*[101], and Iida *et al.*[27].

HDCA (**46**) is historically of particular interest in the interconversion between the two A/B-ring stereochemical types. However, its three possible 5β-stereoisomers (**47, 48** and $3\beta,6\beta$-diol) and their 5α-analogues, although known for many years, are not easily available products in pure forms. We have reported an improved method for the preparation of these 3,6-dihydroxy stereoisomers in both the 5β- and 5α-series[107,108].

Partial syntheses of $3\alpha,6\alpha,12\alpha$-trihydroxy-5β-cholanoic acid (**56**)[109,110] and its 6β-epimer (**57**)[111] have been reported previously. We have recently reported a new method for the preparation of the four possible stereoisomeric $3,6,12\alpha$-trihydroxy-5β-cholanoic acids including the 3β-epimers of **56** and **57**[24]. The key reactions involved a highly stereoselective hydroxylation at the 6β-position of 3-methoxy-3,5-dienes with *m*-chloroperbenzoic acid in aqueous dioxane and catalytic hydrogenation of the resulting 3-oxo-6β-hydroxy-4-enes to the 3-oxo-6β-hydroxy 5β-compounds with palladium on calcium carbonate catalyst in ethanol (Scheme 13).

Some of the unnatural or previously unreported 6-hydroxylated bile acids have also been prepared as potential metabolites. These include $3\alpha,6\beta,7\alpha,12\beta$- and $3\alpha,6\beta,7\beta,12\beta$-tetrahydroxy-5$\beta$-cholanoic acids[112] and stereoisomeric $3\alpha,6,7\beta$-trihydroxy- and $3\alpha,6,7\beta,12\alpha$-tetrahydroxy-5$\alpha$-cholanoic acids[113].

CONCLUSION

This chapter summarizes new and improved methods for the syntheses of uncommon bile acids, the availability of which may serve as reference samples for identifying compounds present in human biological materials and for elucidating pathways of biosynthesis and metabolism and physiological significance. With advances in modern synthetic methods it is possible to prepare bile acid derivatives containing many different functional groups. The synthesis of uncommon bile acids by the chemical transformation of the functional groups in common bile acids has entered a new dimension in the understanding of the chemistry of steroid molecules.

Reagents

i, HCOOH, $(CH_3CO)_2O$, $(CH_3CH_2CO)_2O$ or $(CF_3CO)_2O/CH_3COCl$; **ii**, NH_3, MeOH; **iii**, $ClCOOC_2H_5$, dioxane, pyridine; **iv**, Ag_2CO_3/Celite, toluene; **v**, *tert*-butyldimethylsilyl chloride, imiazole, DMF, pyridine; **vi**, K_2CrO_4, CH_3COOH; **vii**, HCl, acetone; **viii**, *p*-toluenesulphonyl hydrazide, CH_3COOH; **ix**, $NaBH_4$, CH_3COOH; **x**, KOH, MeOH, reflux; **xi**, *tert*-$C_4H_9NH_2$·BH_3, CH_2Cl_2; **xii**, *K*-Selectride, THF, $-40°C$; **xiii**, $Zn(BH_4)_2$, Et_2O; **xiv**, K, *tert*-amyl alcohol, reflux; **xv**, $NaBH_4$, $PdCl_2$, MeOH; **xvi**, *p*-$CH_3C_6H_4SO_2Cl$, pyridine; **xvii**, KO_2, 18-crown-6 ether, DMSO; **xviii**, DMF, 80°C; **xix**, DEADCAT, triphenylphosphine, HCOOH, reflux; **xx**, *tert*-BuOK, CH_3COOH, *tert*-BuOH, $NaBH_4$; **xxi**, photo irradiation in the presence of oxygen and haematoporphyrin, pyridine; **xxii**, $CHCl_3$, reflux; **xxiii**, $NaBH_4$, MeOH; **xxiv**, $C_6H_5IO_2$, $(C_6H_5SeO)_2O$, toluene, reflux; **xxv**, LiOH, MeOH,H_2O; **xxvi**, Li, liquid NH_3, NH_4Cl; **xxvii**, *p*-$CH_3C_6H_4SO_3H$ (or conc. HCl), MeOH; **xxviii**, CH_3SO_2Cl, pyridine; **xxix**, $(CH_3CO)_2O$, *N,N*-dimethylaminopyridine, Et_3N, CH_2Cl_2; **xxx**, Br_2, CH_3COOH; **xxxi**, Li_2CO_3, LiBr, DMF; **xxxii**, Zn, CH_3COOH; **xxxiii**, H_2O_2, NaOH, dioxane, H_2O; **xxxiv**, $Cr(OCOCH_3)_2$, EtOH; **xxxv**, Br_2, *p*-$CH_3C_6H_4SO_3H$, DMF; **xxxvi**, CH_3COOK, CH_3COOH, reflux; **xxxvii**, 2,6-lutidine, reflux; **xxxviii**, $(CH_3CO)_2O$, pyridine; **xxxix**, OsO_4, *N*-methylmorpholine *N*-oxide, *tert*-BuOH, THF, H_2O; **xxxx**, C_5H_5NH·$ClCrO_3$, CH_3COONa, CH_2Cl_2; **xxxxi**, KOH, MeOH; **xxxxii**, *m*-ClC_6H_4COOOH, 4,4′-thiobis-(6-*tert*-butyl-3-methylphenol), 1,2-dichloro-ethane, reflux; **xxxxiii**, BF_3·Et_2O, DMF; **xxxxiv**, *p*-$CH_3C_6H_4SO_3H$, 2,2-dimethoxy-propane, DMF, MeOH, reflux; **xxxxv**, *m*-ClC_6H_4COOOH, dioxane, H_2O; **xxxxvi**, H_2, Pd/$CaCO_3$, EtOH.

References

1. Elliot WH. Metabolism of bile acids in liver and extrahepatic tissues. In: Danielsson H, Sjövall J, editors. Sterols and bile acids. Amsterdam: Elsevier; 1985:303–29.

2. Murphy GM. Serum bile acids. In: Setchell KDR, Kritchevsky D, Nair PP, editors. The bile acids. Chemistry, physiology, and metabolism, Vol. 4: Methods and applications. New York: Plenum Press; 1988:379–403.

3. Back P. Urinary bile acids. In: Setchell KDR, Kritchevsky D, Nair PP, editors. The bile acids. Chemistry, physiology, and metabolism, Vol. 4: Methods and applications. New York: Plenum Press; 1988:405–40.

4. Setchell KDR, Street JM, Sjövall J. Fecal bile acids. In: Setchell KDR, Kritchevsky D, Nair PP, editors. The bile acids. Chemistry, physiology, and metabolism, Vol. 4: Methods and applications. New York: Plenum Press; 1988:441–570.

5. Lester R, Pyrek JS, Little JM, Adcock EW. Diversity of bile acids in the fetus and newborn infant. J Pediatr Gastroenterol Nutr. 1983;2:355–64.

6. Setchell KDR, Gilbert JM, Lawson AM. Fat and cancer. Br Med J. 1983;286:1750.

7. Hikasa Y, Tanida N, Ohno T, Shimoyama T. Faecal bile acid profiles in patients with large bowel cancer in Japan. Gut. 1984;25:833–38.

8. Imray CHE, Radley S, Davis A et al. Faecal unconjugated bile acids in patients with colorectal cancer or polyps. Gut. 1992;33:1239–45.

9. Belle HV. Cholesterol, bile acids and atherosclerosis. Amsterdam: North-Holland; 1965:10–55.

10. Tserng K-Y, Klein PD. Formylated bile acids: improved synthesis, properties, and partial deformylation. Steroids. 1977;29:635–48.

11. Bonar-Law RP, Davis AP, Sanders JKM. New procedures for selectively protected cholic acid derivatives. Regioselective protectin of the 12α-OH group, and t-butyl esterification of the carboxyl group. J Chem Soc (Perkin Trans 1). 1990:2245–50.

12. Tserng K-Y. A convenient synthesis of 3-keto bile acids by selective oxidation of bile acids with silver carbonate-Celite. J Lipid Res. 1978;19:501–4.

13. Goto J, Kato H, Hasegawa F, Nambara T. Synthesis of monosulfates of unconjugated and conjugated bile acids. Chem Pharm Bull. 1979;27:1402–11.

14. Iida T, Momose T, Chang FC, Goto J, Nambara T. Potential bile acid metabolites. 15. Synthesis of 4β-hydroxylated bile acids; unique bile acids in human fetal bile. Chem Pharm Bull. 1989;37:3323–9.

15. Iida T, Shinohara T, Goto J, Nambara T, Chang FC. A facile one-step synthesis of $\Delta^{1,4}$-3-keto bile acid esters by iodoxybenzene and benzeneselenic anhydride. J Lipid Res. 1988;29:1097–101.

16. Iida T, Tamura T, Matsumoto T, Chang FC. Improved conditions for preparation and reductive cleavage of steroidal ketone tosylhydrazones. Synthesis. 1984:957–9.

17. Hutchins RO, Natale NR. Sodium borohydride in acetic acid. A convenient system for the reductive deoxygenation of carbonyl tosylhydrazones. J Org Chem. 1978;43:2299–301.

18. Iida T, Chang FC. Potential bile acid metabolites. 3. A new route to chenodeoxycholic acid. J Org Chem. 1981;46:2786–8.

19. Walker ERH. The functional group selectivity of complex hydride reducing agents. Chem Soc Rev. 1976;5:23–50.

20. Andrews GC. Chemoselectivity in the reduction of aldehydes and ketones with amine boranes. Tetrahedron Lett. 1980;21:697–700.

21. Contreras R, Mendoza L. The reduction of 5α-cholestan-3-one and 5β-cholestan-3-one by some boranes and hydroborates. Steroids. 1979;34:121–4.

22. Tal DM, Frisch GD, Elliott WH. Bile acids LXIX. Selective K-Selectride reduction of 3,7-diketo steroids. Tetrahedron. 1984;40:851–4.

23. Iida T, Komatsubara I, Chang FC, Goto J, Nambara T. Potential bile acid metabolites. 17. Synthesis of 2β-hydroxylated bile acids. Steroids. 1991;56:114–22.

24. Iida T, Tamaru T, Chang FC, Goto J, Nambara T. Potential bile acid metabolites. XVIII. Synthesis of stereoisomeric $3,6,12\alpha$-trihydroxy-5β-cholanoic acids. J Lipid Res. 1991;32:649–58.

25. Giordano C, Perdoncin G, Castaldi G. Reduction of ketones by alkali metals in tertiary alcohols: unexpected cation effect on the stereochemistry. Angew Chem Int Ed Engl. 1985;24:499–501.

26. Iida T, Momose T, Tamura T et al. Potential bile acid metabolites. 14. Hyocholic and muricholic acid stereoisomers. J Lipid Res. 1989;30:1267–79.

27. Iida T, Komatsubara I, Yoda S, Goto J, Nambara T, Chang FC. Potential bile acid metabolites. 16. Synthesis of stereoisomeric $3\alpha,6,7,12\alpha$-tetrahydroxy-5β-cholanoic acids. Steroids. 1990;55:530–9.

28. Chang FC. Potential bile acid metabolites. 2. 3,7,12-Trisubstituted 5β-cholanic acids. J Org Chem. 1979;44:4567–72.

29. Chang FC. Potential bile acid metabolites. 5. 12β-Hydroxy acids by stereoselective reduction. Synth Commun. 1981;11:875–9.
30. Iida T, Chang FC. Potential bile acid metabolites. 7. 3,7,12-trihydroxy-5β-cholanic acids and related compounds. J Org Chem. 1982;47:2972–8.
31. Iida T, Chang FC. Potential bile acid metabolites. 8. 7,12-Dihydroxy- and 7β-hydroxy-5β-cholanic acids. J Org Chem. 1983;48:1194–7.
32. Batta AK, Aggarwal SK, Salen G, Shefer S. Selective reduction of oxo bile acids: synthesis of 3β-, 7β-, and 12β-hydroxy bile acids. J Lipid Res. 1991;32:977–83.
33. Satoh T, Mitsuo N, Nishiki M, Nanba K, Suzuki S. A new powerful and selective reducing agent, sodium borohydride-palladium chloride system. Chem Lett. 1981:1029–30.
34. Iida T, Momose T, Chang FC, Nambara T. Potential bile acid metabolites. 11. Synthesis of stereoisomeric 7,12-dihydroxy-5α-cholanic acids. Chem Pharm Bull. 1986;34:1934–8.
35. Iida T, Shinohara T, Momose T et al. Potential bile acid metabolites. 12. Syntheses of stereoisomeric 3,7,12-trihydroxy-5α-cholanic acids and related compounds. Synthesis. 1986:998–1004.
36. Chang FC, Blickenstaff RT. Acyl amides as epimerization reagents. J Am Chem Soc. 1958;80:2906.
37. Corey EJ, Nicolaou KC, Shibasaki M, Machida Y, Shiner CS. Superoxide ion as a synthetically useful oxygen nucleophile. Tetrahedron Lett. 1975:3183–6.
38. Starks CM, Liotta C. Phase transfer catalysis. Principles and Techniques. New York: Academic Press; 1978:157–69.
39. Bose AK, Lal B, Hoffman WA III, Manhas MS. Steroids. IX. Facile inversion of unhindered sterol configuration. Tetrahedron Lett. 1973:1619–22.
40. Mitsunobu O. The use of diethyl azodicarboxylate and triphenylphosphine in synthesis and transformation of natural products. Synthesis. 1981:1–28.
41. Iida T, Chang FC. Potential bile acid metabolites. 6. Stereoisomeric 3,7-dihydroxy-5β-cholanic acids. J Org Chem. 1982;47:2966–72.
42. Dayal B, Greeley DN, Williams TH, Tint GS, Salen G. Stereospecific synthesis of 3β-hydroxylated bile alcohols. J Lipid Res. 1984;25:646–50.
43. Dayal B, Salen G. Stereospecific synthesis and two-dimensional ^{1}H-NMR investigation of isoursocholic acid. J Lipid Res. 1991;32:1381–7.
44. Iida T, Chang FC. Potential bile acid metabolites. IV. Inversion of 7α-hydroxyl; ursodeoxycholic acid. Lipids. 1981;16:863–5.
45. Eneroth P, Gordon B, Ryhage R, Sjövall J. Identification of mono- and dihydroxy bile acids in human feces by gas–liquid chromatography and mass spectrometry. J Lipid Res. 1966;7:511–23.
46. Eneroth P, Gordon B, Sjövall J. Characterization of trisubstituted cholanoic acids in human feces. J Lipid Res. 1966;7:524–30.
47. Alme B, Bremmelgaard A, Sjövall J, Thomassen P. Analysis of metabolic profiles of bile acids in urine using a lipophilic anion exchanger and computerized gas–liquid chromatography–mass spectrometry. J Lipid Res. 1977;18:339–62.
48. Marschall H-U, Matern H, Wietholtz H, Egestad B, Matern S, Sjövall J. Bile acid N-acetylglucosaminidation. In vivo and in vitro evidence for a selective conjugation reaction of 7β-hydroxylated bile acids in humans. J Clin Invest. 1992;89:1981–7.
49. Maeda M, Ohama H, Takeda H, Yabe M, Nambu M, Namihisa T. Identification of 3β,7β-dihydroxy-5β-cholan-24-oic acid in serum from patients treated with ursodeoxycholic acid. J Lipid Res. 1984;25:14–26.
50. Howard PJ, Gleeson D, Murphy GM, Dowling RH. Ursocholic acid: bile acid and bile lipid dose response and clinical studies in patients with gall stones. Gut. 1989;30:97–103.
51. Nakagawa M, Colombo C, Setchell KDR. Comprehensive study of the biliary bile acid composition of patients with cystic fibrosis and associated liver disease before and after UDCA administration. Hepatology. 1990;12:322–34.
52. Chang FC, Wood NF, Holton WG. 3β,12β-Hydroxycholanic acid. J Org Chem. 1965;30:1718–23.
53. Makino I, Sjövall J. Excretion of 3β-hydroxy-5-cholenoic and 3α-hydroxy-5α-cholanoic acids in urine of infants with biliary atresia. FEBS Lett. 1971;15:161–4.
54. Back P. Identification and quantitative determination of urinary bile acids excreted in cholestasis. Clin Chim Acta. 1973;44:199–207.

55. Back P, Ross K. Identification of 3β-hydroxy-5-cholenoic acid in human meconium. Hoppe-Seyler's Z Physiol Chem. 1973;354:83–9.

56. Hirano K, Harano T, Yamasaki K, Yoshioka D. Isolation of $3\beta,7\alpha$-dihydroxychol-5-en-24-oic and $3\beta,7\alpha$-dihydroxychol-4-en-24-oic acids from human bile. Proc Japan Acad. 1976;52: 453–6.

57. Clayton PT, Leonard JV, Lawson AM et al. Familial giant cell hepatitis associated with synthesis of $3\beta,7\alpha$-dihydroxy- and $3\beta,7\alpha,12\alpha$-trihydroxy-5-cholenoic acids. J Clin Invest. 1987;79: 1031–8.

58. Tohma M, Takeshita H, Mahara R, Kurosawa T, Makino I. Determination of $3\beta,12\alpha$-dihydroxy-5-cholen-24-oic acid and related bile acids in human serum by gas chromatography–mass spectrometry. J Chromatogr. 1987;421:9–19.

59. Ichimiya H, Egestad B, Nazer H, Baginski ES, Clayton PT, Sjövall J. Bile acids and bile alcohols in a child with hepatic 3β-hydroxy-Δ^5-C_{27}-steroid dehydrogenase deficiency: effects of chenodeoxycholic acid treatment. J Lipid Res. 1991;32:829–41.

60. Tohma M, Mahara R, Takeshita H, Kurosawa T. A convenient synthesis of $3\beta,12\alpha$-, $3\beta,7\alpha$-, and $3\beta,7\beta$-dihydroxy-5-cholen-24-oic acids: unusual bile acids in human biological fluids. Steroids. 1986;48:331–8.

61. Elliott WH. Allo bile acids. In: Nair PP, Kritchevsky, D, editors. The bile acids. Chemistry, physiology, and metabolism, Vol. 1: Chemistry. New York: Plenum Press; 1971:47–89.

62. Hoshita T. Bile alcohols and primitive bile acids. In: Danielsson H, Sjövall J, editors. Sterols and bile acids. Amsterdam: Elseiver; 1985:279–99.

63. Thomassen PA. Urinary bile acids in late pregnancy and in recurrent cholestasis of pregnancy. Eur J Clin Invest. 1979;9:425–32.

64. Amuro Y, Hayashi E, Endo T, Higashino K, Kishimoto S. Unusual trihydroxylated bile acids in urine of patients with liver cirrhosis. Clin Chim Acta. 1983;127:61–7.

65. Iida T, Tamura T, Matsumoto T, Chang FC. Potential bile acid metabolites. 9. 3,12-Dihydroxy- and 12β-hydroxy-5α-cholanic acids. J Lipid Res. 1985;26:874–81.

66. Iida T, Momose T, Nambara T, Chang FC. Potential bile acid metabolites. 10. Syntheses of stereoisomeric 3,7-dihydroxy-5α-cholanic acids. Chem Pharm Bull. 1986;34:1929–33.

67. Iida T, Nishida S, Chang FC, Niwa T, Goto J, Nambara T. Potential bile acid metabolites. 21. A new synthesis of allochenodeoxycholic and allocholic acids. Chem Pharm Bull. 1993;41:763–5.

68. Zhu X, Amouzou E, McLean S. Allomerization of cholic acid and conversion to petromyzonol. Can J Chem. 1987;65:2447–9.

69. Bremmelgaard A, Sjövall J. Bile acid profiles in urine of patients with liver diseases. Eur J Clin Invest. 1979;9:341–8.

70. Back P, Walter K. Developmental pattern of bile acid metabolism as revealed by bile acid analysis of meconium. Gastroenterology. 1980;78:671–6.

71. Strandvik B, Wikström S-Å. Tetrahydroxylated bile acids in healthy human newborns. Eur J Clin Invest. 1982;12:301–5.

72. Bremmelgaard A, Sjövall J. Hydroxylation of cholic, chenodeoxycholic, and deoxycholic acids in patients with intrahepatic cholestasis. J Lipid Res. 1980;21:1072–81.

73. Gustafsson J, Anderson S, Sjövall J. Bile acid metabolism during development: metabolism of lithocholic acid in human fetal liver. Pediatr Res. 1987;21:99–103.

74. Carlström K, Kirk DN, Sjövall J. Microbial synthesis of 1β- and 15β-hydroxylated bile acids. J Lipid Res. 1981;22:1225–34.

75. Back P, Fritz H, Populoh C. The isolation of tetrahydroxy bile acids as methyl esters from human urine and their characterization by ^{1}H- and ^{13}C-nuclear magnetic resonance spectroscopy. Hoppe-Seyler's Z Physiol Chem. 1984;365:479–84.

76. Tohma M, Mahara R, Takeshita H, Kurosawa T, Ikegawa S. Synthesis of the 1β-hydroxylated bile acids, unusual bile acids in human biological fluids. Chem Pharm Bull. 1986;34:2890–9.

77. Mahara R, Takeshita H, Kurosawa T, Ikegawa S, Tohma M. Determination of 1β-hydroxylated bile acids and related compounds in human biological fluids by gas chromatography–mass spectrometry. Anal Sci. 1987;3:449–52.

78. Shoda J, Mahara R, Osuga T et al. Similarity of unusual bile acids in human umbilical cord blood and amniotic fluid from newborns and in sera and urine from adult patients with cholestatic liver diseases. J Lipid Res. 1988;29:847–58.

79. Obinata K, Nittono H, Yabuta K, Mahara R, Tohma M. 1β-Hydroxylated bile acids in the urine of healthy neonates. J Pediatr Gastroenterol Nutr. 1992;15:1–5.

80. Wahlén E, Strandvik B. Effects of different formula feeds on the developmental pattern of urinary bile acid excretion in infants. J Pediatr Gastroenterol Nutr. 1994;18:9–19.
81. Shoda J, Osuga T, Mahara R et al. Altered metabolism of bile acids in cholestasis: determination of 1β- and 6α-hydroxylated metabolites. J Chromatogr. 1989;488:315–28.
82. Batta AK, Arora R, Salen G, Tint S, Eskreis D, Katz S. Characterization of serum and urinary bile acids in patients with primary biliary cirrhosis by gas–liquid chromatography–mass spectrometry: effect of ursodeoxycholic acid treatment. J Lipid Res. 1989;30:1953–62.
83. Shoda J, Tanaka N, Osuga T, Matsuura K, Miyazaki H. Altered bile acid metabolism in liver disease: concurrent occurrence of C-1 and C-6 hydroxylated bile acid metabolites and their preferential excretion into urine. J Lipid Res. 1990;31:249–59.
84. Miyara T, Shindo N, Tohma M, Murayama K. Capillary gas chromatography/negative ion chemical ionization mass spectrometry for the quantification of bile acids including 1β-hydroxylated and unsaturated bile acids in serum and urine. Biomed Chromatogr. 1990;4: 56–60.
85. Jönsson G, Hedenborg G, Wisén O, Norman A. Presence of bile acid metabolites in serum, urine, and faeces in cirrhosis. Scand J Clin Lab Invest. 1992;52:555–64.
86. Koopman BJ, Wolthers BG, van der Molen JC, Nagel GT, Kruizinga W. Abnormal urinary bile acids in a patient suffering from cerebrotendinous xanthomatosis during oral administration of ursodeoxycholic acid. Biochim Biophys Acta. 1987;917:238–46.
87. Lee SP, Lester R, Pyrek JS. Vulpecholic acid ($1\alpha,3\alpha,7\alpha$-trihydroxy-5β-cholan-24-oic acid): a novel bile acid of a marsupial, *Trichosurus vulpecula* (Lesson). J Lipid Res. 1987;28:19–31.
88. Herz JE, Ocampo R. Synthesis of 1-hydroxylated bile acids: methyl $1\alpha,3\alpha$-dihydroxy-5β-cholan-24-oate. Steroids. 1982;40:661–4.
89. Clayton PT, Muller DPR, Lawson AM. The bile acid composition of gastric contents from neonates with high intestinal obstruction. Biochem J. 1982,206:489–98.
90. Nakagawa M, Setchell KDR. Bile acid metabolism in early life: studies of amniotic fluid. J Lipid Res. 1990;31:1089–98.
91. Strandvik B, Wahlén E, Wikström S-Å. The urinary bile acid excretion in healthy premature and full-term infants during the neonatal period. Scand J Clin Lab Invest. 1994;54:1–10.
92. Haslewood GAD, Tökés L. Comparative studies of bile salts. A new type of bile salt from *Arapaima gigas* (Cuvier) (family Osteoglossidae). Biochem J. 1972;126:1161–70.
93. Colombo C, Zuliani G, Ronchi M, Breidenstein J, Setchell KDR. Biliary bile acid composition of the human fetus in early gestation. Pediatr Res. 1987;21:197–200.
94. Setchell KDR, Dumaswala R, Colombo C, Ronchi M. Hepatic bile acid metabolism during early development revealed from the analysis of human fetal gallbladder bile. J Biol Chem. 1988;263:16637–44.
95. Dumaswala R, Setchell KDR, Zimmer-Nechemias L, Iida T, Goto J, Nambara T. Identification of $3\alpha,4\beta,7\alpha$-trihydroxy-5β-cholanoic acid in human bile: reflection of a new pathway in bile acid metabolism in human. J Lipid Res. 1989;30:847–56.
96. Goto J, Hasegawa K, Nambara T, Iida T. Gas chromatographic–mass spectrometric determination of 4- and 6-hydroxylated bile acids in human urine with negative ion chemical ionization detection. J Chromatogr (Biomed. Appl.) 1992;574:1–7.
97. Yoshimura T, Mahara R, Kurosawa T, Ikegawa S, Tohma M. An efficient synthesis of 4β- and 6α-hydroxylated bile acids. Steroids. 1993;58:52–8.
98. Haslewood GAD. Comparative studies of 'bile salts'. 9. The isolation and chemistry of hyocholic acid. Biochem J. 1956;62:637–45.
99. Huang CTL, Leeuwen PS-V, Strickland A, Calvin R, Nichols BL. Novel bile acids in serum, urine and duodenal fluid of a child with intrahepatic cholestasis. Fed Proc. 1979;38:1118.
100. Nakashima T, Sano A, Seto Y et al. Unusual trihydroxy bile acids in the urine of patients treated with chenodeoxycholate, ursodeoxycholate or rifampicin and those with cirrhosis. Hepatology. 1990;11:225–60.
101. Yoshii M, Kihira K, Shoda J, Osuga T, Hoshita T. Identification of 3,6,7,12-tetrahydroxy-5β-cholan-24-oic acids in human biologic fluids. Steroids. 1990;55:512–15.
102. Summerfield JA, Billing BH, Shackleton CHL. Identification of bile acids in the serum and urine in cholestasis. Evidence for 6α-hydroxylation of bile acids in man. Biochem J. 1976;154:507–16.
103. Almé B, Nordén Å, Sjövall J. Glucuronides of unconjugated 6-hydroxylated bile acids in urine of a patient with malabsorption. Clin Chim Acta. 1978;86:251–9.

104. Almé B, Sjövall J. Analysis of bile acid glucuronides in urine. Identification of $3\alpha,6\alpha,12\alpha$-trihydroxy-5β-cholanoic acid. J Steroid Biochem. 1980;13:907–16.
105. Hsia SL. Hyocholic acid and muricholic acids. In: Nair PP, Kritchevsky D, editors. The bile acids. Chemistry, physiology, and metabolism, Vol. 1: Chemistry. New York: Plenum Press; 1971:95–120.
106. Kurosawa T, Mahara R, Nittono H, Tohma M. Synthesis of 6-hydroxylated bile acids and identification of $3\alpha,6\alpha,7\alpha,12\alpha$-tetrahydroxy-$5\beta$-cholan-24-oic acid in human meconium and neonatal urine. Chem Pharm Bull. 1989;37:557–9.
107. Iida T, Momose T, Tamura T et al. Potential bile acid metabolites. 13. Improved routes to $3\beta,6\beta$- and $3\beta,6\alpha$-dihydroxy-5β-cholanoic acids. J Lipid Res. 1988;29:165–71.
108. Iida T, Tamaru T, Chang FC, Niwa T, Goto J, Nambara T. Potential bile acid metabolites. 20. A new synthetic route to stereoisomeric 3,6-dihydroxy- and 6-hydroxy-5α-cholanoic acids. Steroids. 1993;58:362–9.
109. Haslewood GAD. Comparative studies of 'bile salts'. II. $3\alpha{:}6\alpha{:}12\alpha$-trihydroxycholanic acid and related substances. Biochem J. 1958;70:551–8.
110. Takeda K, Igarashi K. Bile acids and steroids. XI. Synthesis of $3\alpha,6\alpha,12\alpha$-trihydroxycholanic acid and its oxidation products. J Biochem. 1959;46:1313–22.
111. Ratliff RL, Matschiner JT, Doisy EA Jr, et al. Bile acids. XV. Partial synthesis of the new metabolite of deoxycholic acid, $3\alpha,6\beta,12\alpha$-trihydroxycholanic acid. J Biol Chem. 1961;236:685–7.
112. Aggarwal SK, Batta AK, Salen G, Shefer S. Synthesis of $3\alpha,6\beta,7\alpha,12\beta$- and $3\alpha,6\beta,7\beta,12\beta$-tetrahydroxy-$5\beta$-cholanoic acids. Steroids. 1992;57:107–11.
113. Iida T, Nishida S, Chang FC, Niwa T, Goto J, Nambara T. Potential bile acid metabolites. 19. The epimeric $3\alpha,6,7\beta$-trihydroxy- and $3\alpha,6,7\beta,12\alpha$-tetrahydroxy-$5\alpha$-cholanoic acids. Steroids. 1993;58:148–52

3
Structure – activity relationship studies of new 6α-methyl and 6α-fluoro-ursodeoxycholic acid derivatives

A. RODA, R. PELLICCIARI, G. CANTELLI FORTI, C. CERRÈ,
C. POLIMENI, B. SADEGHPOUR, M. BARALDINI and E. SAPIGNI

INTRODUCTION

Ursodeoxycholic acid (UDCA) has been proven to be useful for dissolution of cholesterol gallstone[1-4] and treatment of chronic cholestatic diseases[5-8]. Its therapeutic efficacy in both conditions, however, is still limited by incomplete bioavailability[9,10] and bacterial biotransformation; moreover, its exact mechanism of action is still poorly understood.

As part of a broad structure – activity relationship study devoted to designing more active UDCA analogues[11-18], we synthesized the two new 6-substituted analogues described in this chapter, with the aim of studying their behaviour to better understand the pharmacokinetics and metabolism of UDCA, and also to evaluate the potential therapeutic efficacy of the two new analogues.

A 6α-methyl group (6-MUDCA) or 6α-fluorine atom (6-FUDCA) was introduced to the UDCA molecule with the aim of limiting intestinal bacterial 7-dehydroxylation of the molecule, and to explore the role of physicochemical properties such as lipophilicity, detergency, H-bonding capacity and polarity, in the pharmacokinetics, metabolism and activity of these molecules.

However, the prevention of intestinal metabolism is not the only determinant of increased bile acid (BA) accumulation in the enterohepatic circulation; thus there was also a need to study how these substitutions influence other factors determining accumulation, such as the kinetics of intestinal absorption, hepatic uptake, secretion and metabolism.

The main physicochemical properties of the two analogues were evaluated, and their pharmacokinetics and metabolism studied in both bile fistula rat and hamster. The analogues and UDCA were infused both intravenously and intraduodenally, and the secretion rates of these and endogenous BA, cholesterol, phospholipids, as well as choleresis, were determined.

The two analogues and UDCA were chronically administered to hamsters in order to study their accumulation in bile under steady-state conditions, as well as to determine any metabolites that would be formed.

Regarding cholesterol gallstone dissolution, their activity was evaluated *in vitro* by measuring their ability to dissolve synthetic cholesterol gallstones in simulated bile. Their potential use for treatment of cholestatic liver disease was evaluated in bile fistula rat: hepatotoxicity was induced by i.v. taurochenodeoxycholic acid infusion, while the analogues were simultaneously infused i.d.; the ability of the analogues to prevent the hepatotoxic effect by reducing ALP and LDH linking in bile, and maintain normal liver histology, was then assessed.

MATERIAL AND METHODS

Chemicals

Synthesis of the 6-methyl and 6-fluoro UDCA analogues

$3\alpha,7\beta$-Dihydroxy-6α-methyl-5β-cholan-24-oic acid (6-MUDCA) and $3\alpha,7\beta$-dihydroxy-6α-fluoro-5β-cholan-24-oic acid (6-FUDCA) were synthesized and purified as described in detail elsewhere[19,20].

Briefly, 6-MUDCA was prepared from the 7-oxo-derivative in which the 3α-hydroxyl was protected with a tetrahydropyranyl group. Six-methylation was carried out using methyl iodide and an appropriate base solvent system. The 6-methyl derivative was deprotected and the 7-keto group selectively reduced to give the 7β-hydroxy derivative.

The 6-FUDCA analogue was also prepared from 6-methyl-7-ketolithocholate. The 7-keto group was converted to the corresponding silyl enolether followed by fluorination with Selectfluor™. The reduction with sodium borohydride followed by epimerization of the 7α-hydroxy group produced the 6-FUDCA analogue. All the other BA were purchased from Sigma (St Louis, MO, USA). All the studies below reported were carried out using the sodium salts of both UDCA and analogues obtained by titration with $NaHCO_3$ and freeze-drying.

Analytical procedures

Total BA, phospholipids and cholesterol were determined as reported elsewhere[21–23]. The qualitative and quantitative composition of BA in bile or other matrices was determined using various chromatographic procedures as previously described[24]. The BA were evaluated by HPLC using a reverse-phase C-18 column connected on line with two different detectors: an evaporative light-scattering mass detector[24] and with a mass spectrometer with an electrospray interface (Trio 2000-Fisons Instruments, UK). A mass spectrum of each BA was obtained giving the molecular weight of the $[M-H]^-$ BA ion directly. With this system, endogenous BA, synthetic analogues and metabolites can be accurately identified without any prederivation procedure.

Physicochemical properties

The critical micellar concentration (CMC) was determined by surface tension measurements[25]. The lipophilicity was evaluated by a conventional N-octanol/buffer partition coefficient procedure, as previously described, and by retention on C-18 HPLC[26]. Other properties, such as water-solubility and pK_a were evaluated as previously reported[27].

In vitro studies

Stability towards bacterial 7-dehydroxylation was evaluated in human stools under anaerobic conditions as previously described[19]. Briefly, the studied BA were incubated with stool homogenates under nitrogen at 37°C; at 0, 4, 8, 16, 20, 24 and 72 h the reaction was stopped with 30% NaOH and the BA were subsequently isolated with C-18 solid-phase extraction and analysed by HPLC[24]. The rate of biotransformation of 6-MUDCA and 6-FUDCA was calculated and compared with UDCA and other naturally occurring BA.

Acute in vivo studies

The hepatic metabolism and biliary secretion was evaluated in both bile fistula rat and hamster[11]. The studied BA were infused both i.v. and i.d. at a dose of $10\,\mu\text{mol}\,\text{min}^{-1}\,\text{kg}^{-1}$ over 1 h; hepatic bile was collected for 3 h at 30-min intervals. The bile flow rate was measured and the concentration of BA, phospholipids and cholesterol determined enzymatically. The qualitative and quantitative biliary BA composition was evaluated by HPLC with a light-scattering mass detector and by HPLC-MS with electrospray interface. The secretion rate of the lipids and individual BA was then calculated and expressed in $\mu\text{mol}\,\text{min}^{-1}\,\text{kg}^{-1}$. From the kinetic profiles, mean $\pm$ SD secretion rate and relative time (S_{max} and T_{max}), as well as mean residual secretion rate (RS) were evaluated.

Chronic study

The studied BA were administered for 3 weeks to Golden Syrian hamster ($100-120\,\text{g}$; $n = 6$ for each group) at a daily dose of 50 mg/kg by gavage. Control animals received only the vehicle (water).

At the end of the treatment, gallbladder bile was collected for the determination of total BA, phospholipids and cholesterol; BA composition was evaluated by HPLC.

Table 1 Physicochemical properties of the studied analogues and those of natural occurring bile acids ($pK_a = 5$ for all bile acids)

BA	WS (μmol/l)	CMC (mmol/l)	CMpH	C-18 rK'	logP$_{A-}$	Albumin binding (%)
6MUDCA	28	17	7.8	1.32	2.30	80
6-FUDCA	72	22	7.3	0.69	1.45	90
UDCA	8	26	8.4	1.00	2.21	91
CA	273	10	6.7	1.40	1.10	70
CDCA	27	6	7.6	3.88	2.25	92
DCA	28	7.5	7.3	4.02	2.65	95

WS = water solubility; CMC = critical micellar concentration; CMpH = critical micellar pH; rK' = hydrophilicity; logP$_{A-}$ = octanol/water partition coefficient of the BA ionized form

Pharmacological activity

6-MUDCA

The ability of this analogue to dissolve cholesterol gallstones[19] was evaluated in simulated bile composed of 100 mmol/l total BA (taurocholic acid, TCA) and 10 mmol/l lecithin (control study). Fifty per cent of the TCA was replaced by 6-MUDCA and by UDCA. A synthetic cholesterol gallstone (cholesterol monohydrate/calcium carbonate 90/10 w/w, 10 mm diameter) was added and incubated at 37°C. Every day for 3 weeks a small aliquot was taken, filtered and analysed for cholesterol concentration. The rate of cholesterol dissolution and cholesterol holding capacity was then calculated.

6-FUDCA

Pharmacological activity was evaluated in bile fistula rat: its ability to prevent the hepatotoxicity induced by i.v. administration of taurochenodeoxycholic acid when co-infused i.d. was assessed and compared with that of UDCA[28]. TCDCA was infused i.v. at a dose of 8μmol min^{-1}kg^{-1} and the analogues simultaneously infused i.d. at a dose of 8μmol min^{-1}kg^{-1}. Bile was collected at 15-min intervals for 3 h and analysed for LDH and ALP activities. Total and individual BA were analysed by HPLC-MS: bile flow (μl min^{-1}kg^{-1}) was also calculated.

RESULTS AND DISCUSSION

The main physicochemical properties in aqueous solution of the two new BA are listed and compared with those of other naturally occurring BA in Table 1. 6-MUDCA is much more lipophilic than UDCA as a result of having one more carbon atom in the 6-position, and also because of the lipophilic properties of the methyl group as a whole. In contrast, 6-FUDCA is slightly more hydrophilic than UDCA, due to the presence of the 6-fluorine atom; this substituent has a strong electron-withdrawing effect that introduces more polarity than a methyl group but less, for example, than would a hydroxyl group.

The critical micellar concentrations (CMC) of both compounds are slightly lower than that of UDCA, but these values are still in the range indicative of poor detergency (in the same order of magnitude as UDCA, but much higher than that of CDCA; Table 1).

The effect of the methyl group on micellar formation must be studied further: the methyl group facilitates hydrophobic interaction, but the steric effect and other factors could be also important.

The effect of the fluorine atom is more complex: while this substituent resembles a hydroxy group in polarity and Van der Waals volume, it is more lipophilic[29–30].

We believe that the main effect of the fluorine atom is due to its strong electronic effect, and from the fact that it acts only as an H acceptor, in contrast to −OH which has both acceptor and donor capacity. Since H bonds are responsible for micellar growth, the particular bonding capacity of the fluorine atom could explain its CMC value. Another relevant consideration is the CMpH of the two analogues: 6-MUDCA, and particularly 6-FUDCA, have lower CMpH values than UDCA (i.e. they require a lower pH to dissolve).

As can be seen from Fig. 1, both analogues are very stable towards 7-dehydroxylation. The 6-methyl analogue is essentially unmetabolized by intestinal bacteria, confirming steric hindrance by the 6-methyl group of the OH group in 7-position. 6-FUDCA is slightly metabolized, but only after 24 h of incubation. The C−F bond is very stable: indeed, the fact that it is poorly metabolized suggests that the fluorine atom induces an electronic and, to a lesser extent, steric hindrance to 7-dehydroxylation enzyme activity. The effect of the fluorine atom is slightly greater than that of an OH group; indeed, hyocholic acid is metabolized more slowly than cholic acid. However, attentive comparison must be done with ω-muricholic acid $(3\alpha,6\alpha,7\beta)$.

When acutely administered i.v. or i.d. to rats and hamsters, both 6-MUDCA and 6-FUDCA were transported well by the intestine, taken up by the liver and secreted in bile. The maximum secretion rate, time peak and cumulative recoveries in bile are reported in Table 2.

The behaviour of both analogues regarding hepatic amidation and transport processes is slightly different in the two animal species. When the S_{max} values after i.v. and i.d. administration in the two animal species were compared, we found that both analogues presented similar values, which are also close to those of UDCA, suggesting that they are transported well by the intestine and the liver, at least as well as the parent molecule. No major effects on bile flow, biliary cholesterol or phospholipid secretion rates were observed when compared with UDCA.

Good intestinal absorption, as evaluated by the biliary secretion rate after i.d. infusion of UDCA, was facilitated by administration as a sodium salt (rather than the acid form[32–34]).

The two analogues were efficiently secreted in both species, exclusively as glycine and taurine amidates; at the dose administered, no other hepatic metabolites were identified by HPLC−mass spectrometry. When infused i.v. in the rat, 6-FUDCA is essentially secreted only as taurine amidates (with a very efficient transport maximum), whereas 6-MUDCA, like UDCA, is also secreted amidated with glycine.

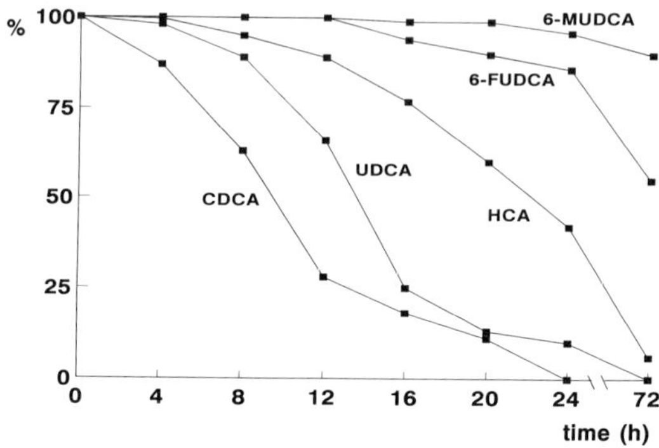

Fig. 1 Metabolism of the studied bile acids when incubated in human stool under anaerobic conditions. Results are expressed as quantity of original molecule recovered as a percentage of the total bile acids present after incubation

When 6-MUDCA, 6-FUDCA and UDCA were chronically administered to hamsters, their accumulation in gallbladder bile was respectively 25%, 60% and 15% of total BA (Fig. 2).

After administration of UDCA, a large amount of this compound could be epimerized to form chenodeoxycholic acid, probably accounting for its low accumulation in bile. On the contrary, 6-FUDCA and, to a lesser extent, 6-MUDCA, are more efficiently accumulated in bile, without metabolite formation, as demonstrated by HPLC analysis of bile.

These results suggest that the prevention of 7-dehydroxylation or, in more general terms, 7-metabolism, is an efficient way to increase the accumulation of a BA. However, other factors are responsible for analogue conservation, since 6-MUDCA is better accumulated than UDCA, but not as well as 6-FUDCA. Since both analogues were amidated with glycine and taurine during steady-state chronic feeding, it is the pharmacokinetics of these latter compounds that most importantly influence its effects. Their intestinal transport, in particular, is quite different from that of the administered unconjugated form of the drugs, i.e. it is active rather than passive. Specific interactions due to the effect of the introduced substituents with the ileal transport system are important, and must be studied in more detail.

When present in simulated bile as 50% of total BA (50% TCA), 6-MUDCA is able to increase both the rate and efficiency of cholesterol monohydrate dissolution. This effect is higher than that of UDCA, as shown in Table 3.

When co-infused i.d. with TCDCA, 6-FUDCA efficiently prevents the linking in bile of ALP and LDH and maintains sustained bile flow. The effect is similar to, or better than, that given by UDCA, particularly on choleresis and TCDCA transport, evidenced by the TCDCA secretion rate. 6-MUDCA is poorly efficient in preventing this hepatotoxic effect.

Table 2 Biliary bile acid secretion parameters in bile fistula rat and hamster after i.v. or i.d. administration of the studied bile acids at a dose of $10\,\mu\mathrm{mol\,min^{-1}\,kg^{-1}}$. Values are the mean $\pm$ SD of six animals

BA	Rat								Hamster							
	S_{max} (μmol min^{-1} kg^{-1})		T_{max} (min)		R_s (μmol min^{-1} kg^{-1})		Recovery (%)		S_{max} (μmol min^{-1} kg^{-1})		T_{max} (min)		R_s (μmol min^{-1} kg^{-1})		Recovery (%)	
	i.d.	i.v.	i.d.	i.v.	i.d.	i.v.	i.d.	i.v.	i.d.	i.v.	i.d.	i.v.	i.d.	i.v.	i.d.	i.v.
6-MUDCA	1.40±0.29	1.96±0.55	90–180	90	0.91±0.08	0.61±0.12	49±9	51±8	1.47±0.20	1.79±0.77	90–150	120	1.19±0.10	1.02±0.15	52±8	57±7
6-FUDCA	5.76±1.38	3.77±1.72	60	60	0.94±0.28	0.57±0.12	100±7	60±9	1.34±0.05	1.01±0.02	60–180	60–210	0.76±0.21	0.60±0.18	47±8	32±4
UDCA	2.68±1.30	3.80±1.30	60	60	0.80±0.17	0.44±0.11	68±7	65±9	2.25±0.71	1.98±0.55	60	120	0.69±0.05	0.48±0.13	41±6	42±7
Saline	1.25±0.49	0.98±0.18	60	60	0.50±0.21	−0.55±0.23	–	–	0.47±0.16	0.35±0.08	60	60	0.18±0.03	0.18±0.03	–	–

S_{max} = maximum secretion rate; T_{max} = time at S_{max}; R_s = residual secretion rate

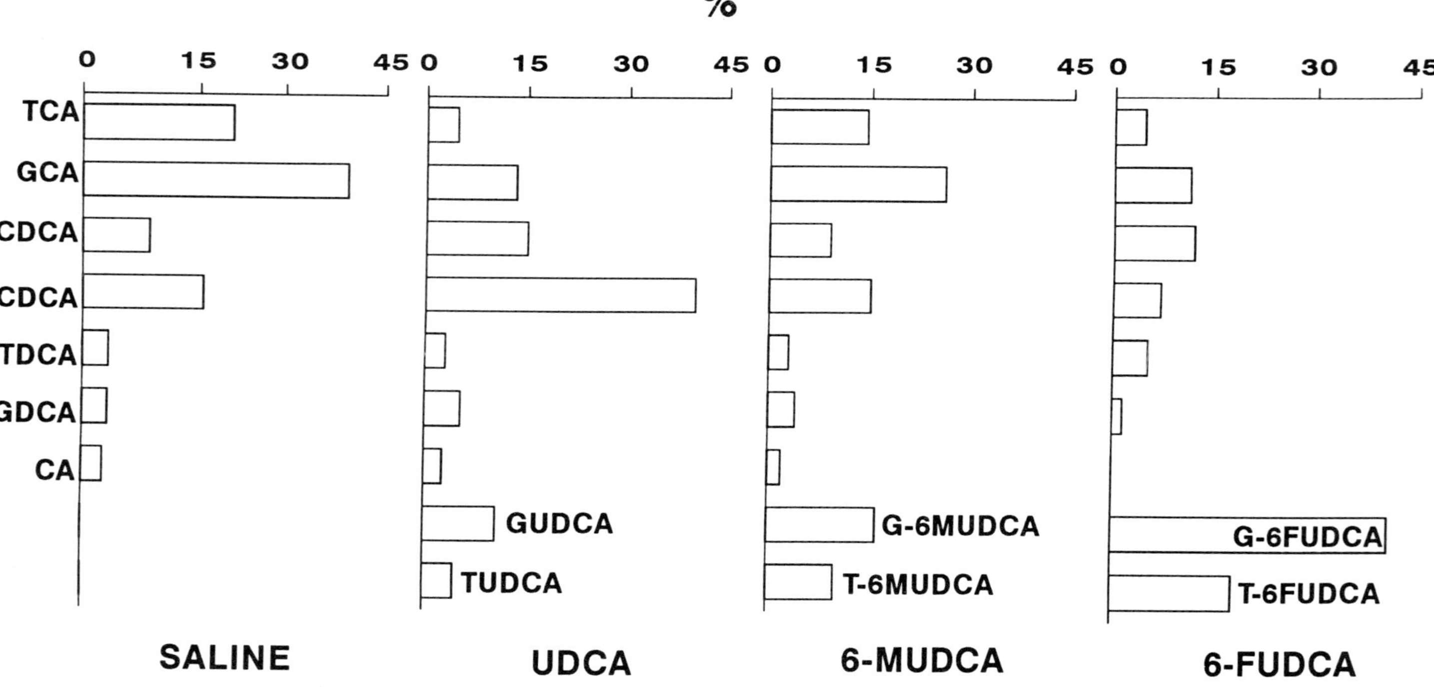

Fig. 2 Bile acid composition of hamster gallbladder bile after 3 weeks of chronic feeding at a dose of 50 mg/kg per day of 6-MUDCA, 6-FUDCA, and UDCA. Each point is a mean value of six animals

Table 3 *In vitro* cholesterol monohydrate dissolution kinetic in simulated bile solution (100 mmol/l of taurocholic acid, 10 mmol/l purified egg lecithin) 50% enriched with the 6-methyl analogue and the parent compound. Each value is the mean ± SD of five experiments

BA	*Dissolution rate (mmol/l per day)*	*Cholesterol-holding capacity (mmol/l)*
6-MUDCA	1.10 ± 0.20	4.0 ± 0.6
UDCA	0.42 ± 0.05	3.2 ± 0.2
Control	0.16 ± 0.03	2.0 ± 0.3

CONCLUSIONS

The results obtained on the two 6-substituted analogues suggest that the introduction of either a methyl group or a fluorine atom is an efficient way to prevent 7-dehydroxylation, by steric or electronic hindrance, respectively. The two substituents, each with unique properties, modify the physicochemical properties of the original UDCA molecule in different ways. 6-MUDCA is more lipophilic than UDCA, though it has similar mild detergency. This fact is compatible with its faster and more efficient passive intestinal absorption on isolated rabbit ileum (data not reported). The 6-MUDCA analogue dissolves cholesterol gallstone *in vitro* and more efficiently than UDCA, but it is not able to prevent the hepatotoxic effects induced by TCDCA in rat, as could have been predicted by its physical properties.

6-FUDCA, like 6-MUDCA, enters the enterohepatic circulation and is amidated by the liver to form glycine and taurine conjugates. Despite the presence of a 6-fluorine atom, its passive intestinal absorption is similar to that of UDCA, suggesting that this substituent, owing to its being only an H-bond acceptor, does not limit this process as an −OH group would (CA vs. CDCA, for example). The most important finding was the efficient accumulation of 6-FUDCA with chronic feeding in the hamster, much higher than 6-MUDCA or UDCA. This result could depend on several factors, three of the more probable being good active intestinal transport of its glycine and taurine amidated forms, good metabolic stability, and very high and efficient hepatic transport maxima.

The lower CMpH values of 6-FUDCA with respect to 6-MUDCA and UDCA also contribute to better conservation of the molecules by facilitating solubilization, or preventing precipitation, in the intestinal tract.

6-FUDCA is very efficient in preventing the hepatotoxic effects induced by TCDCA; it could act by enhancing the TCDCA transport maximum, thus reducing the concentration and the time in which liver cells are exposed to TCDCA. The three-fold increase in TCDCA transport maximum is also paralleled by increased choleresis with respect to control and UDCA groups.

In conclusion, 6-MUDCA shows considerable potential for use in cholesterol gallstone dissolution, and 6-FUDCA for treating cholestatic liver disease; obviously, more detailed study in different animal models and in humans is required.

References

1. Makino J, Shinizaki K, Nakagawa K, Yoshino K. Dissolution of cholesterol gallstones by long-term administration of ursodeoxycholic acid. Jpn J Gastroenterol. 1975;72:690–702.
2. Roda E, Bazzoli F, Morselli AM *et al*. Ursodeoxycholic acid versus chenodeoxycholic acid as cholesterol gallstone dissolving agents: a comparative randomized study. Hepatology. 1982;2:804–10.
3. Bacharach WH, Hofmann AF. Ursodeoxycholic acid in the treatment of cholesterol cholelithiasis. Dig Dis Sci. 1982;27:737–61,833–56.
4. Fromm H, Roat JW, Gonzalez V, Sarva RP, Farivar S. Comparative efficacy and bile effects of ursodeoxycholic and chenodeoxycholic acids in dissolving gallstones. A double blind controlled study. Gastroenterology. 1983;85:1257–64.
5. Leuschner U, Fisher H, Kurtz W *et al*. Ursodeoxycholic acid in primary biliary cirrhosis: results of a controlled double-blind trial. Gastroenterology. 1989;96:1268–74.
6. Poupon R, Chretien Y, Poupon RE, Ballet F, Calmus Y, Darnis F. Is ursodeoxycholic acid an effective treatment for primary biliary cirrhosis? Lancet. 1987;1:834–46.
7. Stiehl A, Raedsch R, Mommerell B. The effect of ursodeoxycholic acid in primary biliary cirrhosis. Gastroenterology. 1988;94:595.
8. Hofmann AF, Popper H. Ursodeoxycholic acid for primary biliary cirrhosis. Lancet. 1987;2:398–9.
9. Parquet M, Metman EH, Raizman A, Rambaud JC, Berthaux N, Infante N. Bioavailability, gastrointestinal transit, solubilization and faecal excretion of ursodeoxycholic acid in man. Eur J Clin Invest. 1985;15:171–8.
10. Stiehl A, Raedsch R, Rudolph G. Acute effects of ursodeoxycholic and chenodeoxycholic acid on small intestinal absorption of bile acids. Gastroenterology. 1990;98:424–8.
11. Roda A, Grigolo B, Roda E *et al*. Quantitative relationship between bile acid structure and biliary lipid secretion in rat. J Pharm Sci. 1988;77:596–605.
12. Roda A, Grigolo B, Pellicciari R, Natalini B. Structure–activity relationship studies on natural and synthetic bile acid analogs. Dig Dis Sci. 1989;34:1–12.
13. Roda A, Grigolo B, Minutello A, Pellicciari R, Natalini B. Physicochemical and biological properties of natural and synthetic C-22 and C-23 hydroxylated bile acids. J Lipid Res. 1990;31:289–98.
14. Roda A, Aldini R, Grigolo B *et al*. 23-methyl-3α,7β-dihydroxy-5β-cholan-24-oic acid: dose response study of biliary secretion in rat. Hepatology. 1988;8:1571–6.
15. Pellicciari R, Cecchetti S, Natalini B, Roda A, Grigolo B, Fini A. Bile acids with cyclopropane containing side chain. I. Preparation and properties of 3α,7β-dihydroxy-22,23-methylene-5β-cholan-24-oic acid. J Med Chem. 1984;27:746–9.
16. Pellicciari R, Cecchetti S, Natalini B, Roda A, Grigolo B, Fini A. Bile acids with cyclopropane containing side chain. II. Synthesis and properties of 3α,7β-dihydroxy-22,23-methylene-5β-cholan-24-oic acid-N-2-sulfoethyl amide. J Med Chem. 1985;28:239–42.
17. Roda A, Grigolo B, Aldini R *et al*. Bile acids with a cyclopropyl-containing side chain. IV. Physicochemical and biological properties of the four diastereoisomers of 3α,7β-dihydroxy-22,23-methylene-5β-cholan-24-oic acid. J Lipid Res. 1987;28:1384–97.
18. Pellicciari R, Natalini B, Cecchetti S *et al*. Bile acids with a cyclopropyl-containing side chain. III. Separation, identification and properties of all the four stereoisomers of 3α,7β-dihydroxy-22,23-methylene-5β-cholan-24-oic acid (CUDCA). J Med Chem. 1988;31:730–6.
19. Roda A, Pellicciari R, Cerrè C *et al*. New 6-substituted bile acids: physicochemical and biological properties of 6α-methyl ursodeoxycholic acid and 6α-methyl-7-epicholic acid. J Lipid Res. 1994;35(In press).
20. Roda A, Pellicciari R, Polimeni C *et al*. Metabolism, pharmacokinetics and activity of a new 6-fluoro analog of ursodeoxycholic acid in rat and hamster. Gastroenterology. 1995 (In press).
21. Fausa O. Quantitative determination of serum bile acids using a purified 3α-hydroxysteroid dehydrogenase. Scand J Gastroenterol. 1975;10:747–51.
22. Roda A, Festi D, Sama C *et al*. Enzymatic determination of cholesterol in bile. Clin Chim Acta. 1975;64:337–41.
23. Roda A, Geminiani S, Rossi R, Festi D, Roda E, Barbara L. Enzymatic determination of phospholipids in bile. Lab J Res Med. 1981;2:119–22.
24. Roda A, Cerrè C, Simoni P, Polimeni C, Vaccari C, Pistillo A. Determination of free and

amidated bile acids by high-performance liquid chromatography with evaporative light scattering mass detection. J Lipid Res. 1992;33:1393–402.

25. Roda A, Hofmann AF, Mysels KJ. The influence of bile salt structure on self association in aqueous solutions. J Biol Chem. 1983;258:6362–70.

26. Roda A, Minutello A, Angellotti MA, Fini A. Bile acids structure–activity relationship: evaluation of bile acid lipophilicity using 1-octanol/water partition coefficient and reverse phase HPLC. J Lipid Res. 1990;31:1433–43.

27. Roda A, Fini A. Effect of nuclear hydroxy substituents on aqueous solubility and acidic strength of bile acids. Hepatology. 1984;4:72–6.

28. Heuman DM, Mills AS, McCall JB, Hylemon PB, Pandak WM, Vlahcevic ZR. Conjugates of ursodeoxycholate protect against cholestitis and hepatocellular necrosis caused by more hydrophobic bile salts: *in vivo* studies in the rat. Gastroenterology. 1991;100:203–11.

29. Hansch C, Leo A. Substituent constants for correlation analysis in chemistry and biology. New York: Wiley, 1979.

30. Yang GZ, Lien EJ, Guo ZR. Physical factors contributing to hydrophobic constant π. Quant Struct Act Relat. 1986;5:12–19.

31. Van de Waterbeemed H, Testa B. The parametrization of lipophilicity and other structural properties in drug design. Advances in drug research. New York: Academic Press; 1987;16:85–225.

32. Dietschy JM, Salomon HS, Siperstein MD. Bile acid metabolism. I. Studies on the mechanisms of intestinal transport. J Clin Invest. 1966;45:832–46.

33. Aldini R, Roda A, Lenzi P, Ussia G, Vaccari C. Bile acid active and passive ileal transport in the rabbit: effect of luminal stirring. Eur J Clin Invest. 1992;22:744–50.

34. Roda A, Roda E, Marchi E *et al*. Improved intestinal absorption of an enteric-coated sodium ursodeoxicholate formulation. Pharm Res. 1994;11:642–7.

Section II
Physicochemical aspects

4

Structure of mixed micelles present in bile and intestinal contents based on studies of model systems

R. P. HJELM, P. THIYAGARAJAN, C. SCHTEINGART,
A. F. HOFMANN, H. ALKAN-ONYUKSEL and HUONT-THU TON-NU

INTRODUCTION

The form and structure of the particles found in mixed aqueous colloids of bile salts with phosphatidylcholine (PC) has been of considerable interest as models of the morphology of particles present in native bile. The interest stems from the insight provided by studies of these mixtures into the structure–function relationships of the transport and processing of lipophilic materials from the liver, and in the intestine; in the action of pancreatic lipase; and in the role that particle shape may play in the adsorption of hydrolysed dietary lipids through the endothelial layer of the intestinal mucosa. The interest in these systems also extends to problems in medicine and pharmacology, such as in the development of drug therapies for certain types of gallstones, and issues of bioavailability of some oral formulations which may be affected by drug interactions with bile.

Our present understanding of these systems has its roots in the classical studies of Donald Small[1,2] and his collaborators on the cholate–egg yolk phosphatidyl-choline (EYPC)–water system. Their work showed a complex phase map containing various liquid crystalline phases and an isotropic phase (as defined by observations using polarized light microscopy) where there is sufficient bile salt present to break up PC lamellar phases (Fig. 1). The microstructure of the isotropic phase became the subject of considerable study, which showed this consisted of at least three regions[3–5]: a region containing a mixture of simple bile salt micelles and mixed bile salt–PC micelles; a region containing only mixed micelles; and a region containing mixed vesicles (Fig. 1). Light-scattering studies showed that as solutions initially containing mixed micelles are diluted there is a substantial growth of the mixed micelles. The mixed micelle size appeared to diverge at the concentration where the mixed micelle to vesicle transition occurred[3], the so-called divergence line (Fig. 1). As the system is further diluted the vesicles decrease in size[6]. Although detailed models were

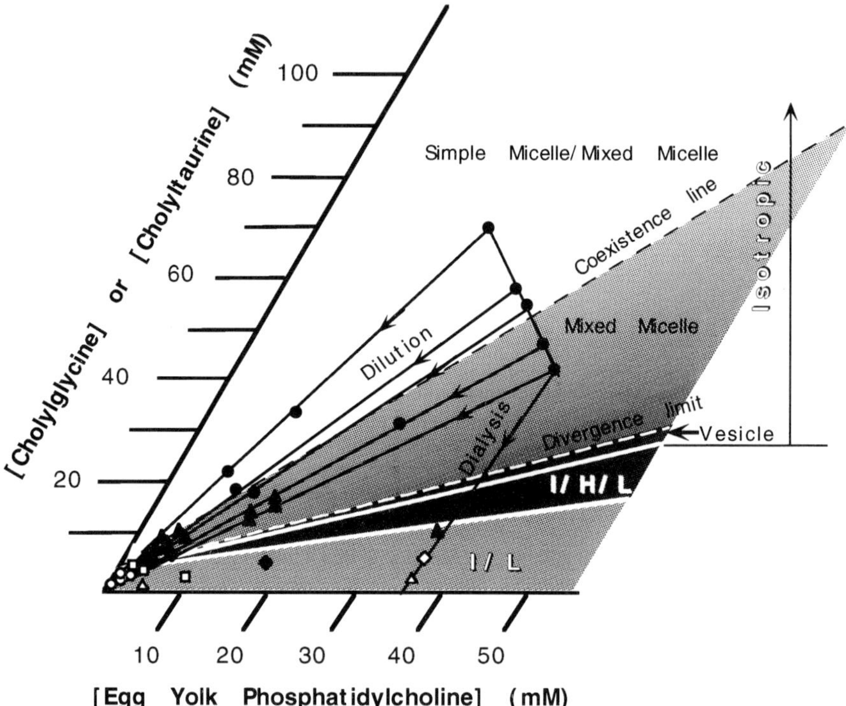

[Egg Yolk Phosphatidylcholine] (mM)

Fig. 1 The cholyltaurine–EYPC–water phase map at high water content. Figure redrawn from Cabral and Small[35] showing the structure of the phase map at high water content. White, solid lines separate the isotropic from the isotropic–hexagonal–lamellar (I/H/L) triphase (dark grey) from the isotropic–lamellar (I/L) biphase (light grey). Dashed lines in the isotropic phase separate the simple micelle–mixed micelle region (coexistence line), from the mixed micelle region (light grey), and the mixed micelle region from the vesicle region (divergence limit). Points are compositions measured in the cholylglycine phase map by SANS. Lines indicate where dilution or dialysis was used to prepare samples from stocks. Symbols indicate particle forms and are the same as for Fig. 5

proposed for the structure of the mixed micelles[2,3,7], there were no definitive data to indicate the correct model.

What was missing were definitive measurements using probes of the most relevant length scales for micelle structure from about 1 nm to a few tens of nm. This could be afforded by small angle X-ray (SAXS) or neutron-scattering (SANS) techniques. SAXS was attempted, but the low contrast of the lipid relative to water, and the relatively low X-ray intensities available, limited measurements to solutions with high total lipid concentrations[8]. SANS, on the other hand, can take advantage of the large contrast that is available when lipids are present in solutions containing D_2O. As a consequence, even very dilute bile salt–PC solutions could be measured at relatively modest neutron sources.

The first SANS experiments clarified our concepts of particle form in the mixed micelle region of the isotropic phases. The measurements showed that at certain compositions mixed micelles are present that are locally rigid rods, about 2.7 nm in radius[9]. The particle growth observed by the light-scattering studies[3] is due to rod elongation, the radius of the rod being unchanged as the sample is diluted to the concentration-induced vesicle transition point[9].

In this chapter we review the picture of particle form and structure obtained from SANS measurements of dilute cholylglycine (CG)–EYPC solutions and cholyltaurine (CT)–dipalmitoylphosphatidylcholine (DPPC) solutions[9–12]. We also show the results of new work on dilute CG–monoolein (MO) aqueous mixtures. The latter results suggest that the particle forms observed in the CG–EYPC solutions are conserved, regardless of the extensive differences between the MO and EYPC structures.

MATERIALS AND METHODS

Preparation of bile salt–phosphatidylcholine mixtures

All bile salt–PC mixtures were prepared by coprecipitation followed by the addition of D_2O buffer to make a 50 g/l stock, as described elsewhere[9]. Samples are prepared for measurement by dilution or dialysis (Fig. 1) of this stock. Samples of CG and MO are made by similar methods, taken up in D_2O buffer and diluted.

Small-angle neutron scattering

SANS is the measurement of scattering intensity $I(Q)$ at a momentum, Q, transferred to the neutron as a result of a scattering event in the sample. Q is related to the incident neutron wavelength, λ, and to the scattering angle, 2θ, as

$$Q = \frac{4\pi}{\lambda} \sin \theta$$

The scattering intensity is normalized to sample thickness and total lipid concentration, so it is expressed as differential cross-section per unit mass ($m^2 g^{-1}$). The instruments, methods of measurement and data reduction are described in earlier publications[13–15].

Analysis of the scattering data and determination of particle shape

There are certain features of the scattering profile that are indicators of particle form. To understand particle form we use Q-domains where the scattering can be approximated by what are known as the Guinier expressions, after A. Guinier, who pointed out the validity of the first of these approximations[16]. When the Q-domain is sufficiently small relative to the radius of gyration, R_g, which is a measure of the particle size, the scattering is approximated by

$$I(Q) = \Delta M_0 \exp\left(\frac{Q^2 R_g^2}{3}\right) \tag{1}$$

Here the factor ΔM_0 is the contrast-weighted total scattering mass of the particle and is directly related to the particle composition by equation (4), below. If the particle is rod-like, then there is a domain at larger Q where another Guinier approximation holds[17,18]:

$$I(Q) = \pi \Delta m_0 Q^{-1} \exp \left(\frac{Q^2 R_c^2}{2} \right) \qquad (2)$$

where R_c is the radius of gyration of the rod cross-section and Δm_0 is the contrast-weighted scattering mass per unit length along the rod. Finally, if the particle is either a flat sheet[19] or is a sheet closed into a vesicle[20], then there is a Q-domain where the final Guinier approximation applies

$$I(Q) = 2\pi \Delta \mu_0 Q^{-2} \exp (Q^2 R_d^2) \qquad (3)$$

Here R_d is the radius of gyration of scattering density along a line perpendicular to the sheet central plane. The prefactor, $\Delta \mu_0$, is the contrast-weighted scattering mass per unit area in the sheet.

Measurements over different Q-domains probe spatial density fluctuations in the sample over different length scales. The length scales probed go as Q^{-1}; thus a particle that appears as a point at low Q, making equation (1) applicable, can appear locally as a rod (equation (2)) or a sheet (equation (3)) over larger Q where the intraparticle structure is apparent.

By fitting the appropriate Q-domains to one of the Guinier forms of equations (1–3) we can show that the scattering is consistent with a particular particle form. The resulting determination of the corresponding radius of gyration gives a measure of the particle size.

The determination of the contrast-weighted scattering mass per unit length in rod-like mixed micelles gives information on the particle composition[12], as

$$\Delta m_0 = n_L N \; \frac{\{\Delta \rho_B V_B \gamma^{-1} + \Delta \rho_L V_L\}^2}{\{[\Gamma^{-1} W_B + W_L]\}} \qquad (4)$$

The V are molecular volumes; the $\Delta \rho$ are contrasts; and the W are formula weights. The subscript B shows the quantity corresponds to the bile salt; L, the swelling lipid (PC or MO). N is Avogadro's constant, Γ is the molar ratio of bile salt to PC or MO in the solution, and γ is the ratio in the particles. Hence the number of swelling lipid molecules per unit length, n_L, can be determined if γ is known. These are taken from the measurements of Spink $et\ al.$[21] and Duane[22] for the PC systems and from the data of Hofmann[23] for MO solutions. The corresponding values for total surfactant densities are determined from $n_0 = n_L(1 + \gamma^{-1})$.

RESULTS

Particle morphology in dilute cholylglycine–egg yolk phosphatidylcholine solutions: the structural phase map

With these analytical tools we can examine the scattering obtained from solution at different cholylglycine and EYPC concentrations. These are produced by dilution or by a combination of dialysis and dilution experiments (Fig. 1). All of the samples that we consider in detail here have compositions that are in the mixed micelle part of the isotropic region of CT–EYPC–water system[3] (Fig. 1)

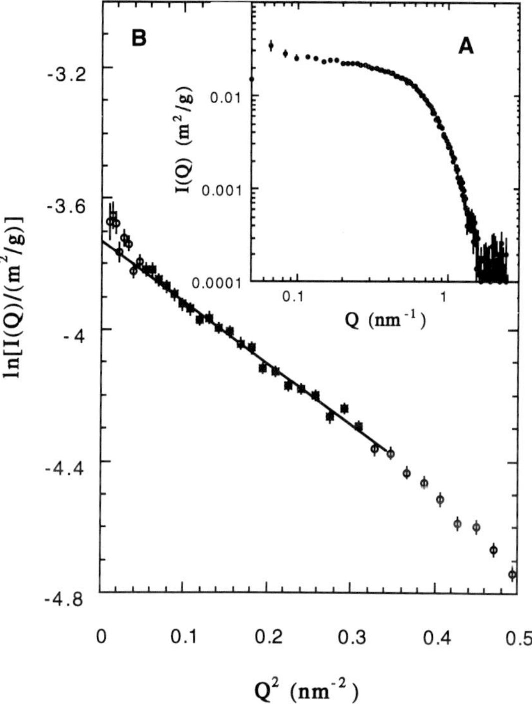

Fig. 2 Scattering from globular micelles present at high total lipid concentrations and Guinier analysis of the data. A: Scattering from a solution of CG–PC at 16.7 g/l total lipid and Γ=0.5. B: Guinier analysis of data shown in A: O, data; (____), fit of equation (1) over $0 < Q^2 < 0.3$ nm^{-1}

Table 1 Structural parameters from scattering analysis of globular mixed micelles

Mixture	C_{lipid} (g/l)	ΔM_0 (10^{-4} m^2/g)[a]	R_g (nm)[a]
EYPC-cholylglycine[b]	16.7	240 (10)	2.41 (0.03)
Monoolein–cholylglycine	10.0	188 (1)	2.29 (0.04)

[a]Numbers in parentheses are root mean square uncertainty in the regression
[b]See text for abbreviations

or in the isotropic–hexagonal or isotropic–hexagonal–lamellar phases of the cholate–EYPC–water mixtures[1,2] (Fig. 1).

At the highest concentrations the scattering is characteristic of globular particles (Fig. 2). The scattering approaches that expected from equation (1) at low Q, with a characteristic R_g of 2.4 nm (Table 1). A spheroid with this radius of gyration would have a radius of about 3.0 nm. The form of the scattering is not quite as expected, as the condition of completely independent particles in solution uncorrelated in position and orientation is not met. Thus there are interparticle interactions present that lower the scattering slightly below that expected according to equation (1). For small interactions these effects have been analysed[24,25], but we do not do so here, as we find interaction effects to be highly variable in the CG–EYPC solutions at these concentrations. Thus the parameters

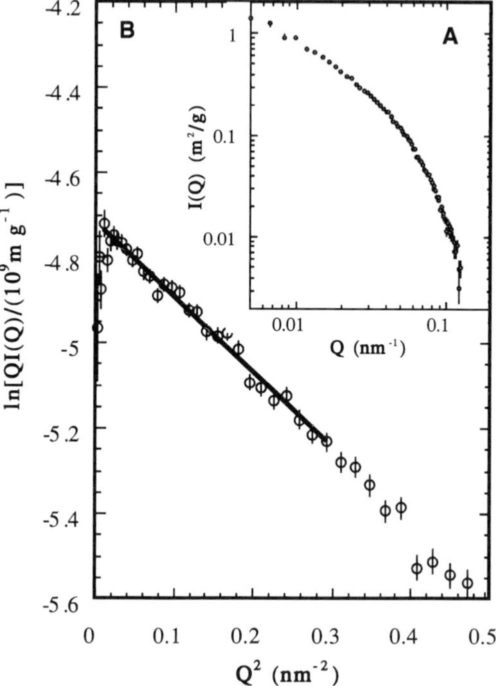

Fig. 3 Scattering from rod-like micelles. **A**: SANS from an EYPC–CG solution at 10 g/l total lipid and $\Gamma = 0.5$, containing rod-like micelles. **B**: Guinier analysis modified for a rod-like form (equation (2)) of the data in A: O, data; (____), fit of equation (1) over $0.02 < Q^2 < 0.3 \, \mathrm{nm}^{-2}$

from the analysis of Fig. 2 given in Table 1 should be considered as approximate.

As the concentration is reduced, the form of the scattering changes taking on the form of a long, locally rigid rod. This is seen by the form of the scattering that approaches the form given by equation (2) in Fig. 3. The R_c determined from several such analyses on a variety of mixtures[9–12] are given in Table 2. The rod radii derived from these values is 2.5–2.7 nm regardless of the PC–bile salt mixture used[9–12]. This observation has been confirmed by SANS measurement of EYPC–deoxycholyltaurine solutions[25]. Dynamic light-scatter-ing (DLS) and static light-scattering (SLS) measurements, which probe longer length scales than observed here, show that the micelles are semiflexible rods[24]. This interpretation of the global structure is consistent with the SANS result, which probes more local structure.

When the concentration is reduced further, the scattering changes form considerably (Fig. 4). The intensity at low Q becomes substantially larger, and the peaks are seen at larger Q. This is the scattering signature of a vesicle. On further dilution the form of the scattering indicates smaller and smaller vesicles.

At concentrations intermediate between those where rod-like scattering and vesicle scattering are observed the samples show scattering that indicates the presence of both types of particles. This is illustrated in Fig. 4, which suggests a biphase of rods and vesicles. The existence of a mixed micelle–vesicle biphase

Table 2 Phosphatidylcholine and total lipid density in rod-like micelles found in mixtures of phosphatidylcholines and bile salts

Mixture	Γ	[lipid] (g/l)	γ^{1}	R_c (nm)[a]	n_L^a (nm)$^{-1}$	n_0^a (nm)$^{-1}$
DPPC–cholyltaurine[b]	0.6	4.00	0.35	1.71 (0.07)	9	11
	0.6	3.33	0.33	1.73 (0.06)	10	15
	0.6	2.86	0.31	1.89 (0.04)	12	15
EYPC–cholylglycine[b]	0.5	5.0	0.45	1.91 (0.02)	10	14.5
	0.56	5.0	0.40	1.92 (0.02)	10	14
	0.8	10	0.30	1.90 (0.02)	10	13
	0.8	8.3	0.34	1.84 (0.02)	10	13
	0.8	7.1	0.28	1.92 (0.02)	10	13
	0.9	10	0.29	1.90 (0.02)	9	12
EYPC–chenodeoxycholylglycine	0.8	1.7	0.22	1.90 (0.03)	11	13
Monoolein–cholylglycine	1.2	4.0	1.32	1.59 (0.02)	10	17

[a]Numbers in parentheses are root mean square uncertainty in the regression
[b]See text for abbreviations

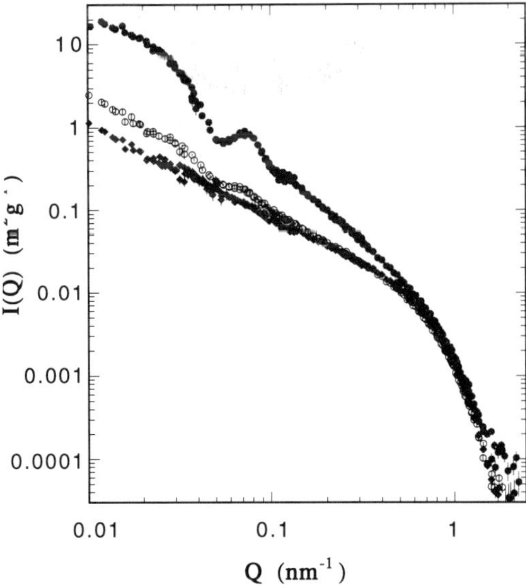

Fig. 4 Scattering from a dilution series through the mixed micelle–vesicle biphase region. EYPC–CG solution, Γ=0.8; ◆, 6.25 g/l; O, 5.6 g/l; ●, 5.0 g/l

was first pointed out in cryotransmission electron microscopy studies of sonicated phosphatidylcholine liposomes back-titrated with either octanyl glycoside or cholate[26,27].

The phase map, which is the result of analyses using the same methods as shown in Figs 2–4 and in Fig. 10 (below, is shown in Fig. 5. One striking feature of the map is that the particle forms are largely dependent on the amount of bile salt present, and much less so on the concentration of EYPC. This result suggests that the relatively large solubility of the CG is the determining factor in the

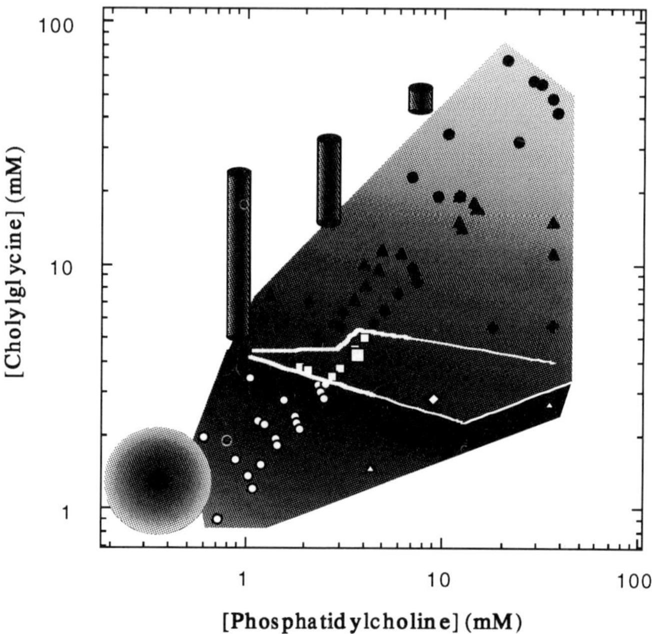

Fig. 5 Structural phase map for cholylglycine–EYPC–water mixtures. The forms of micelles and vesicles observed at different aqueous compositions of cholylglycine and egg yolk phosphatidylcholine. ●, Globular mixed micelles; ▲, elongated mixed micelles; ◆, long rod-like micelles; □, rod-like mixed micelles and mixed vesicle coexisting; ○, mixed vesicles; ◇, coexisting rod-like and sheet-like forms; △, sheet-like forms. Micelle or vesicle size is indicated by light (small) to dark (large) shading. Thick lines show boundaries between mixed micelle and biphase and biphase and mixed vesicle regions determined from the data. Thin lines are extension of these lines into areas that are not so well determined experimentally. The particle shapes are shown schematically

observed differences in particle form. EYPC–CG solutions at the same compositions as the upper part of the isotropic–lamellar–hexagonal (I/H/L in Fig. 1) triphase of the EYPC–cholate–water mixture at high EYPC concentrations are turbid. They show scattering characteristic of elongated and rod-like molecules. When the CG concentration is lowered to the isotropic–lamellar phase (I/L in Fig. 1), the scattering becomes characteristic of mixed rods and sheet-like objects (Figs 1 and 5). At the lowest CG concentrations sheet-like scattering only is observed. In the dilute corners (Figs 1 and 5) the solutions become opalescent at the concentration-induced vesicle transition. The scattering is characteristic of vesicles. Further dilution of the solutions causes them to clear and form smaller vesicles.

Particle structure

The structure of mixed micelles

The form of the micelles was easily derived from the scattering curves. The arrangement of the micelle components is not directly obtained from the above studies, but can be obtained from measurements where the head group of the PC is specifically deuterated. Because EYPC cannot readily be deuterated we used DPPC, which can be deuterated at the 9-hydrogens of the PC methyls. This allows us to consider how the rod-like PC is arranged in the rod-like micelle. There are only two general models for this system.

The first model, which we shall call the stacked disc model, proposed by Shankland[7], consists of mixed micelle discs stacked one on the other, like a stack of coins, to form the rod-like micelle. Each micelle disc has a structure first proposed by Small[2], and consists of a discoid bilayer of PC surrounded by a ribbon of bile salt. In this model the rods grow with dilution by association of small pre-formed micelles. It is not clear, however, what is the driving force of association, if we assume that the repartitioning of bile salt is mainly responsible for micelle growth.

The second model was first proposed for the structure of rod-like micelles in the hexagonal phase[28,29], and was subsequently shown to be consistent with concentration-dependent rod growth observed by exclusion chromatography experiments[30]. Here the PC is arranged radially along the rod with the head group outward along the surface of the rod. The bile salt is arranged parallel to the rod surface between the PC head groups and acts as a wedge, providing the required radial curvature between the PC. According to this picture for the rod-like micelles in solution[30] the ends of the micelle are capped with bile salts to stabilize the structure in the aqueous environment. The presence of the end caps provides a driving force to lengthen the rods when the system is diluted, repartitioning the bile salt into the aqueous bulk phase[30]. We term this the radial-shell model.

The deuterium labelling and SANS provide a ready means of distinguishing between these two models. Since the sample is measured in D_2O the deuterated DPPC head will have lower contrast against the D_2O than the protonated counterpart. Consequently, the apparent radius of the rod would appear smaller in the deuterium-labelled sample if the radial-shell model applies, and would appear unchanged if the stacked disc model applies.

The apparent radii of the protonated and deuterated samples are measured using the Guinier analysis for rod-like forms of equation (2), using the relationship between R_c and the apparent rod radius given by $R = \sqrt{2}R_c$. The measurements give smaller values for R_c for the deuterated sample, consistent with the radial-shell model (Fig. 6).

We can take this analysis one step further by considering the relationship between Δm_0 and R_c for each model, and comparing this with the observed values. In this we calculate the apparent radii of the rods given the measured R_c. The value of Δm_0 is calculated for each model using equation (4) given the radius and the aggregation number densities, n_L and n_0. Figure 7 shows the results of the calculations for the two models, and compares these with the measured R_c and Δm_0. The computed values for the radial-shell model provide a better fit of the data. The importance of deuteration in discriminating between the two models is seen when we consider the effects on the value of V_B on the calculation. In comparing the data from the deuterated samples with the expectations from the two models, the radial-shell model always fits the data far better than the stacked disc model: the radial-shell model calculation gives values that correspond well to the observed values when the smallest bile salt volumes[31] (0.52 nm^3) are

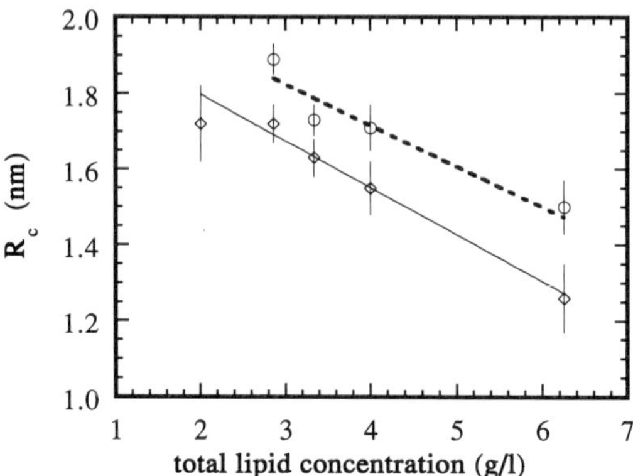

Fig. 6 Concentration-dependence of the cross-sectional radius of gyration. $\bigcirc$, DPPC-CT mixture; $\diamondsuit$, DPPC-d_9-CT mixture. Linear fits to the data (_ _ _ _), for DPPC mixtures; and (____), for DPPC $-d_9$ mixtures

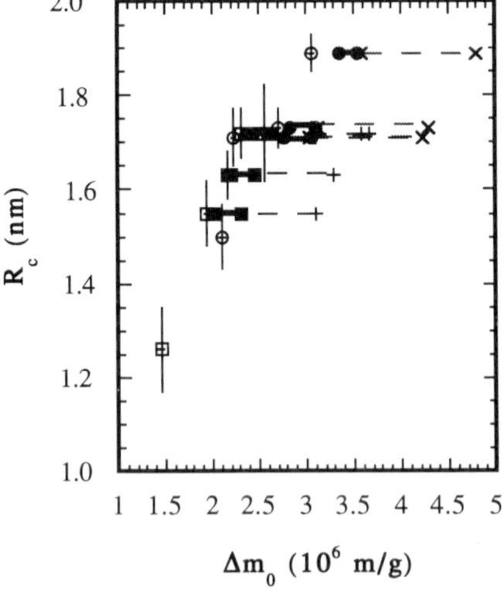

Fig. 7 Cross-sectional radius of gyration verses the contrast-weighted scattering mass per unit length. Measured values of R_c for the mixtures containing protonated and deuterated DPPC are plotted versus computed (see text) and measured values of Δm_0. Data, $\square$, deuterated–DPPC–CT solutions, $\bigcirc$, protonated-DPPC–CT solutions. Values calculated from models: Range of values for the shell model, $\blacksquare$—$\blacksquare$, for solutions with deuterated DPPC, and $\bullet$—$\bullet$, for solutions with protonated-DPPC. Stacked disc model, $\times$—$\times$, for solutions with deuterated-DPPC, and $+$—$+$, for solutions with protonated-DPPC. Values on the left of each range were obtained when V_{BS} is assumed[30] to be 0.52 nm³, values on the right of each range[31] are when V_{BS}=0.77 nm³ is assumed

assumed. In the case of samples with protonated PC the radial-shell model fits the observations far better than the stacked disc model if large[32] (0.77 nm³) or intermediate (0.6 nm³) values (derived from the data of Small[32]) for V_B are assumed. However, the two models fit the data for the protonated samples equally well if the smallest V_B value is assumed.

The question arises as to the generality of this model. This was tested by again using equation (4) for a rod-like form to derive n_L. These values are shown for the DPPC–choltaurine mixtures and different EYPC–CG and EYPC–chenodeoxycholylglycine solutions in Table 2. The values have been revised slightly upward from those published earlier[12], as somewhat smaller values of the molecular volume of the bile salt in the range $0.52-0.6\,nm^3$ are used in this calculation. These values are more consistent with measurements on cholate and chenodeoxycholate[31] and on cholyltaurine[32] than those used previously[12]. We find that for all cases considered n_L is about 10 phosphatidylcholine molecules per nm. This value is higher than that determined from light-scattering studies[24] of 7.7.

We have devised a model, shown in Fig. 8, which explains one way in which the locally rigid rods are assembled, and which accounts for the SANS[12] observations and for the measurements of the molar ratio of PC and bile salts in the mixed micelles[21,22]. In this model the PC is arranged with its axis perpendicular to the rod axis. The hydrophilic tails are partitioned into a core region of the rod. The PC hydrophilic head groups constitute the outer shell of the structure. The bile salt molecules are at the interface between the core and the shell region, with the long molecular axis parallel to the micelle rod axis. The head group and the hydrophilic side of the bile salt face upward into the shell region.

The structure of vesicles

We consider the structure of the vesicles found in the solvent corner of the phase map (Fig. 5). The issue we consider is whether the vesicle wall is likely to be a lipid bilayer. We use three analyses of the SANS data to answer this question.

The first method involves the use of the Guinier law for sheets (equation (3)) to derive the thickness and lipid packing per unit area in the vesicle. Such an analysis is shown in Fig. 9, from which it is determined that the value of R_d is about $1.1\,nm$, corresponding to a vesicle shell thickness, t, of about $3.8\,nm$. Normally a value of $5\,nm$ is anticipated for a phosphatidylcholine bilayer, but the relatively low contrast of the phosphatidylcholine head group relative to D_2O is likely to reduce that apparent thickness.

We can also fit the entire scattering curve to a vesicle scattering law, given by

$$I(Q) = \Delta M_0 \, \frac{9}{Q^2(R^3 - r^3)^2} \, [R^2 j_1(QR) - r^2 j_1(Qr)]^2 \tag{5}$$

The vesicle radius, R, and the vesicle inner radius, $r = R - t$, along with the factor ΔM_0, are the fitted parameters. The j_1 are first-order spherical Bessel functions. We fit equation (5) to the data taking into account the resolution of the instrument[9,14], from which we see that the vesicle wall thickness is about $4.0\,nm$ (Table 3)[9]. It is evident from Fig. 10 that equation (5) does not completely account for the observed scattering, the residual being due to polydispersity in vesicle size.

Finally, we can ask how the apparent radius given by the analysis in Fig. 10, and summarized in Table 3, correlates with the scattering extrapolated to $Q = 0$. From equation (4) we readily see that ΔM_0 is proportional to the aggregation

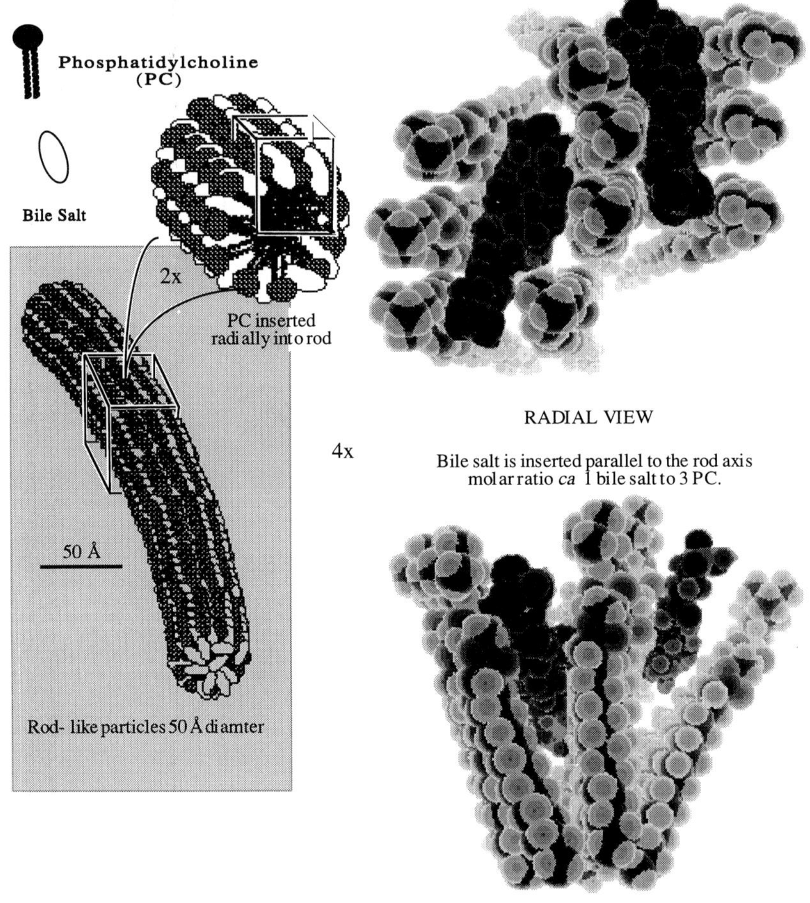

Fig. 8 Space-filling model illustrating one way that phosphatidylcholine and bile salts can be arranged in rod-like mixed micelles. Schematic of a semi-rigid rod-like mixed micelle inside greyed area. Box indicates a segment of a radial-shell mixed micelle rod expanded 2-fold. Possible molecular arrangement of a few PC (light-shaded) and bile salt (cholyltaurine; dark-shaded) molecules. The fatty acid chains shown in extended conformations are oriented perpendicularly to the rod axis. The head groups face outward in the solvent. The choline methyls are outermost. These are the groups that were deuterated. The arrangement of the bile salt with its axis parallel to the rod axis is inferred by measured values of γ[21,22] that suggest that approximately three DPPCs are associated with each bile salt. The bile salt acts as a wedge in only one direction. In this model the side of the bile salt with the three hydroxyl groups faces outward toward the solvent

number; hence the particle volume. Thus, in the limit of a thin shell, $\Delta M_0 \propto R^2$. From Fig. 11 we see that this expected relation holds[9].

From these three lines of evidence we conclude that the PC is arranged as a single bilayer structure in the vesicle. The conclusion that bilayer vesicles are present at the lowest total lipid concentrations is consistent with the evidence

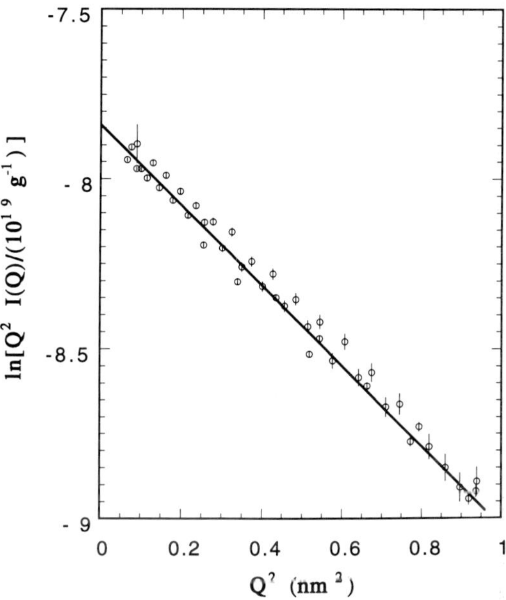

Fig. 9 Guinier analysis modified for sheet-like forms of a sample containing vesicles. Guinier analysis modified for a sheet-like form (equation (3)) of the data in Å: O, data; (____), fit of equation (1) over $0.1 < Q^2 < 1\,\mathrm{nm}^{-2}$

Table 3 Fitted parameters for vesicles

Lipid (g/l)	ΔM_0 (m²/g)	Radius (nm)	Shell thickness (nm)
2.5	320	27.7	4.0
2.0	180	20.2	4.4
1.67	140	17.8	4.4
1.43	110	16.2	4.4
1.0	94	14.4	4.6

available from DLS[3,6] and NMR[33] data. The data given here present the strongest evidence of the existence of vesicles under these conditions.

MONOOLEIN – CHOLYLGLYCINE MIXTURES

An approach towards understanding the determinants of self-assembly in the bile salt-swelling lipids is to consider the particle structure mixed colloids of bile salt and MO. MO differs from the long-chain PCs in being a neutral lipid with a single oleate chain. The physiological importance of these mixtures stems from the observation that MO is formed in the small intestine from the action of pancreatic lipase on triglyceride; thus these studies are also aimed towards an understanding of the physiological importance of colloid particle form and structure in bile. We consider samples at compositions in the isotropic domain of

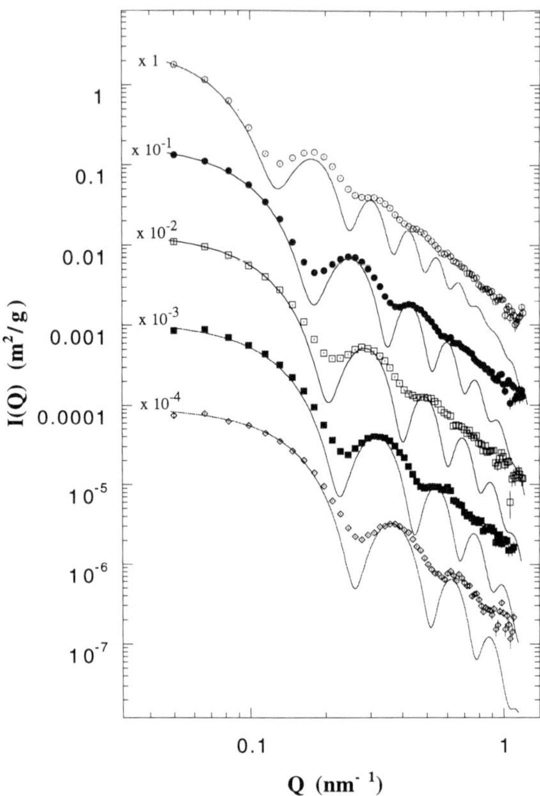

Fig. 10 Vesicle form factors fitted to scattering data. EYPC–CG solutions at ○, 2.5 g/l; ●, 2.0; □, 1.76 g/l; ■, 1.43 g/l; ◇, 1.0 g/l. _____, data fitted to vesicle form factors using the parameter given in Table 3

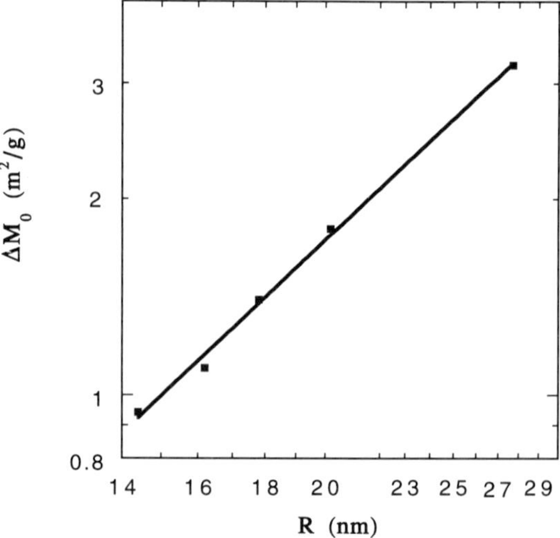

Fig. 11 Scaling of vesicle $I(0)$ with vesicle radius: Vesicle fit parameters taken from Table 3. ■, data; _____, fit to power law $I(0) = R^{1.9}$

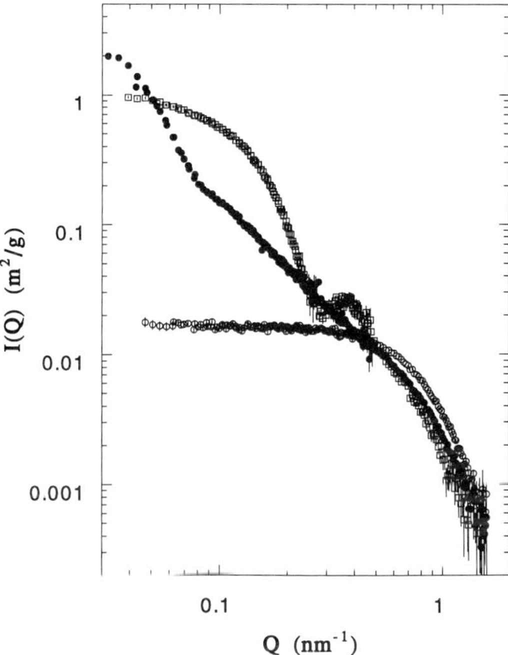

Fig. 12 Examples of scattering from CG–MO mixtures at different lipid concentrations. Cholylglycine and monoolein at $\Gamma = 1.2$. $\bigcirc$, 10 g/l; $\bullet$, 4.0 g/l; $\square$, 2.0 g/l

the phase map, in which previous NMR and DLS[34] studies of the CT–MO–water system have revealed globular micelles and vesicles.

Figure 12 shows some examples of scattering observed in CG–MO mixtures at $\Gamma = 1.2$. This ratio is chosen, as it gives the same stoichiometry of fatty acid moieties to bile salt molecules as found in the DPPC mixtures used in the deuteration studies cited above[12]. There are striking similarities between the SANS observed in the CG–MO solutions and the CG–EYPC counterparts.

At the highest concentrations the shape and magnitude of the scattering from the two types of mixtures are similar, suggesting the same size and shape of the micelles. This impression is strengthened by comparison of the R_g and ΔM_0 values from the Guinier analysis of equation (1), given in Table 1.

At lower concentrations the mixtures pass into what appears to be a coexistence regime of rod-like forms and vesicles. This is inferred from the existence of two distinct domains in the scattering. At low Q the scattering is suggestive of a vesicle. At higher Q the scattering is more like that expected for a rod. The R_c measured for the rod is slightly less than that measured for the EYPC systems, being 1.6 nm (Table 2). This corresponds to a radius of about 2.3 nm, smaller than 2.5–2.7 nm[9–12] from the R_c of the PC mixtures (Table 2). This observation is understandable in terms of the radial organization of PC or MO discussed above, as MO has a shorter overall extended length than PC. We derive a packing density of monoolein of about 10 nm^{-1} using equation (4) and

Table 4 Vesicle wall parameters from Guinier analysis modified for sheet-like forms

Mixture	Δm_0 $(10^{14}\,g^{-1})$[a]	R_d (nm)[a]	Apparent shell thickness (nm)
EYPC–cholylglycine[b]	5.92 (0.02)	1.1 (0.1)	3.8
EYPC–cholylglycine[b]	7.96 (0.01)	1.1 (0.1)	3.8
Monoolein–cholylglycine	6.6 (0.1)	0.9 (0.1)	3

[a]Numbers in parentheses are root mean square uncertainty in the regression
[b]See text for abbreviations

the value for γ of 1.38 from the solubility studies of Hofmann[23]. This is the same as observed in the PC systems (Table 2).

The characteristic scattering signature of vesicle is evident when the sample is diluted to 2.5 g/l. The Guinier analysis modified for sheet-like forms suggests that the thickness is 3 nm, slightly smaller than that observed for the corresponding phosphatidylcholine mixtures (Table 4). The $\Delta\mu_0$ derived from this analysis is consistent with those obtained in PC vesicles[9–11] (Table 4), suggesting again that the packing of lipids very similar when either the PC or MO is present.

We draw two conclusions on the self-assembly of swelling lipid–CG particles from these results. The first is that neither the two-tailed nature nor the zwitterionic character of the PC is a determinant of the form or structure of the particles in these systems. The second is that the packing densities of lipid in the rod-like forms observed in these systems appear to be the same. Finally, that the forms and structures of MO–CG mixed particles are the same as those of the PC–CG particles suggests that the particle form and structure may be important in the physiological function of bile.

Acknowledgements

This work was conducted under the auspices of the United States Department of Energy. The work benefited from the use of the Low-Q Diffractometer at the Los Alamos Neutron Scattering Center of the Los Alamos National Laboratory, which is supported by the Office of Basic Energy Sciences of the United States Department of Energy under contract W-7405-ENG-36 to the University of California. The work also benefited from the use of the Small-angle Neutron Diffractometer at the Intense Pulsed Neutron Source at Argonne National Laboratory. The facilities at IPNS are funded by the US Department of Energy, BES-Materials Science, under Contract W-31-109-Eng-38. Work at UCSD was supported in part by NIH Grant DK 21506 (to A.F.H.). Measurements on monoolein–cholylglycine was done on NG7SANS at the National Institutes of Standards and Technology. We thank Dr C. Glinka (NIST) for expert help in carrying out these measurements.

References

1. Small DM, Bourgès MC, Dervichian DG. The biophysics of lipidic associations: 1. The ternary systems lecithin-bile salt-water. Biochim Biophys Acta. 1966;125:563–80.

2. Small DM. Physicochemical studies of cholesterol gallstone formation. Gastroenterology. 1967; 52:607–10.

3. Mazer NA, Benedek GB, Carey MC. Quasielastic light scattering studies of aqueous biliary lipid systems. Mixed micelle formation in bile salt–lecithin solutions. Biochemistry. 1980;19: 601–15.

4. Mazer NA, Schurtenberger P, Carey MC, Preisig R, Weigand K, Kanzig W. Quasi-elastic light scattering studies of native hepatic bile from the dog: comparison with aggregative behavior of model biliary lipid systems. Biochemistry. 1984;23:1994–2005.

5. Mazer NA, Carey MC. Quasi-elastic light scattering studies of aqueous biliary lipid systems. Cholesterol solubilization and precipitation in model bile systems. Biochemistry. 1983;22: 426–42.

6. Schurtenberger P, Mazer NA, Kanzig W. Micelle to vesicle transition in aqueous solutions of bile salt and lecithin. J Phys Chem. 1985;89:1042–9.

7. Shankland W. The equilibrium and structure of lecithin–cholate mixed micelles. Chem Phys Lipids. 1970;4:109–30.

8. Müller K. Structural dimorphism of bile salt/lecithin mixed micelles. A possible regulatory mechanism for cholesterol solubility in bile? X-ray structure analysis. Biochemistry. 1980; 20:404–14.

9. Hjelm RP, Thiyagarajan P, Alkan H. A small-angle scattering study of the effects of dilution on particle morphology in mixtures of glycocholate and lecithin. J Appl Cryst. 1988;21:858–63.

10. Hjelm RP, Thiyagarajan P, Alkan H. Particle morphology in mixed glycholate–lecithin colloids. Mol Cryst Liq Cryst. 1990;180A:155–64.

11. Hjelm RP, Thiyagarajan P, Sivia D, Lindner P, Alkan H, Schwahn D. Small-angle neutron scattering from aqueous mixed colloids of lecithin and bile salt. Prog Coll Polymer Sci. 1990; 81:225–31.

12. Hjelm RP, Thiyagarajan P, Alkan H. The organization of phosphatidylcholine and bile salt in rod-like mixed micelles. J Phys Chem. 1992;96:8653–61.

13. Glinka CJ, Rowe JM, LaRock JG. The small-angle neutron scattering spectrometer at the national bureau of standards. J Apply Cryst. 1986;19:427–9.

14. Hjelm RP. Resolution of time-of-flight low-Q diffractometers: instrumental, data acquisition and reduction factors. J Appl Cryst. 1988;21:618–28.

15. Seeger PA, Hjelm RP. Small-angle neutron scattering at pulsed spallation sources. J Appl Cryst. 1991;24:467–78.

16. Guinier A. La diffraction des rayons X aus très petits angles: application a l'étude de phénomènones ultramicroscopiques. Ann Phys. 1939;12:161–237.

17. Luzzati V. Interpretation des measures absolutes de diffusion centrale des rayons x en collimation ponctuelle ou lineaire: solutions de particles globulaires et de bâtonnets. Acta Cryst. 1961;13:939–45.

18. Hjelm RP. The small-angle approximation of X-ray and neutron scatter from rigid rods of non-uniform cross section and finite length. J Appl Cryst. 1985;18:452–60.

19. Porod G. General theory. In: Glatter O, Kratky O, editors. Small-angle scattering of x-rays. New York: Academic Press; 1982:17–52.

20. Knoll W, Haas J, Sturhmann HB, Fuldner H-H, Vogel H, Sackmann E. Small-angle neutron scattering of aqueous dispersions of lipids and lipid mixtures. A contrast variation study. J Appl Cryst. 1981;14:191–202.

21. Spink CH, Müller K, Sturtevant JM. Precision scanning calorimetry of bile salt–phosphatidylcholine micelles. Biochemistry. 1982;21:6598–605.

22. Duane WC. Taurocholate and taurochenodeoxycholate–lecithin micelles: the equilibrium of bile salt between aqueous phase and micelles. Biochem Biophys Res Commun. 1977;74:223–9.

23. Hofmann AF. The function of bile salts in fat absorption. Biochem J. 1963;89:57–68.

24. Egelhaaf SU, Schurtenberger P. Shape transformation in the lecithin–bile salt system: from cylinders to vesicles. J Phys Chem. 1994;98:8560–73.

25. Long MA, Kaler EW, Lee SP, Wignall GD. Characterization of lecithin taurodeoxycholate mixed micelles using small-angle neutron scattering and static and dynamic light scattering. J Phys Chem. 1994;98:4402–10.

26. Vinson PK, Talmon Y, Walter A. Vesicle–micelle transition of phosphatidylcholine and octanyl glycoside elucidated by cryo-transmission electron microscopy. Biophys J. 1989;56:669–81.

27. Walter A, Vinson PK, Talmon Y. Intermediate structures in the cholate–phosphatidylcholine

vesicle–micelle transition. Biophys J. 1991;60:1315–25.
28. Ulmius J, Lindblom G, Wennerstrom H *et al.* Molecular organization in the liquid crystalline phases of lecithin–sodium cholate–water systems studied by nuclear magnetic resonance. Biochemistry. 1982;21:1553–60.
29. Lindblom G, Erikson P-O, Arvidson G. Molecular organization in phases of lecithin–cholate–water as studied by nuclear magnetic resonance. Hepatology. 1984;4:129–33S.
30. Nichols JW, Ozarowski J. Sizing of lecithin–bile salt mixed micelles by size-exclusion high-performance liquid chromatography. Biochemistry. 1990;29:4600–6.
31. Vadnere M, Natarajam, Lindenbaum S. Apparent molar volumes of bile salts in H_2O and D_2O solution. J Phys Chem. 1980;84:1900–3.
32. Small DM. The physical chemistry of the colonic acids. In: Nair PP, Kritchevsky D, editors. The bile acids: chemistry, physics and metabolism. New York: Plenum: 1971:247–354.
33. Stark RE, Gosselin GJ, Donovan JM, Carey MC, Roberts MF. Influence of dilution on the physical state of model bile systems: NMR and quasi-elastic light scattering investigations. Biochemistry. 1985;24:5599–605.
34. Svärd M, Schurtenberger P, Fontell K, Jönsson B, Lindman B. Micelles, vesicles, and liquid crystals in the monoolein-sodium taurocholate-water system. Phase behavior, NMR, self diffusion, and quasi-elastic light scattering studies. J Phys Chem. 1988;92:2261–70.
35. Cabral DJ, Small DM. Physical chemistry of bile. In: Schultz SG, Forte JG, Rauner BB, editors. Handbook of physiology, the gastrointestinal system III, section 6. New York: Waverly Press; 1989:621–62.

5
Lipid bilayer expansion and mechanical disruption in solutions of water-soluble bile acid

E. EVANS, W. RAWICZ and A. F. HOFMANN

INTRODUCTION

Bile acids are shunted from the liver to the intestine to solubilize products of fat digestion. Even though large quantities of bile acid move past cell membranes in the biliary tract and intestine, the linings remain intact in normal conditions with some evidence of perturbation by excess concentrations and less hydrophilic bile acids[1-3]. As recognized for many years, bile acids at high concentrations break up model membranes of pure lipids and solubilize the contents into mixed micelles[4-6]. However, little is known about physical mechanisms of disruption, and especially sublytic degradation of single membrane capsules. Hence, we have used micromechanical methods to directly measure bilayer area expansion – elasticity – and rupture strength on single vesicles following transfer to solutions of a good 'solubilizer', i.e. the trihydroxy bile acid cholylglycine (CG). For the synthetic lecithin stearoyl-oleoyl phosphatidylcholine (SOPC) examined here, reduction in bilayer strength was apparent at concentrations well below levels necessary for complete disruption.

At the most simple level, thermodynamic theory for partitioning of bile acid into the bilayer is predicated on entropy of mixing and the activity contributed by mechanical tension. At the next level, energetic barriers to uptake are included that can arise from electrical charge on the acid group and restriction of bile acid movement across the bilayer. In our experiments we found that increase in vesicle area correlated well with predictions for ideal thermodynamic mixing of CG into *both* layers of the SOPC lipid bilayer. There was no strong barrier to uptake at high solution concentrations. Carried out under controlled tension, the measurements of area change also yielded several important molecular scale properties: the area per molecular complex in the bilayer; the ratio of aggregate size in the bilayer to that in aqueous solution; the small degree of ionization at the surface and an estimate of molecular charge.

METHODS

Vesicles were formed by careful hydration of neutral (SOPC) and neutral + charged (palmitoyl-oleoyl phosphatidylserine, POPS) lipids that had been dried from chloroform:methanol solution onto Teflon (see ref. 7 for details). A non-electrolyte solution of 0.2 mol/l sucrose was used to swell the lipid into very large vesicles with single bilayer membranes. Following stratification by centrifugation a small aliquot of vesicles was resuspended at very dilute concentration in 0.2 mol/l glucose, which provided an index of refraction contrast to enhance visibility by interference microscopy. The final vesicle suspension was loaded into one side of a dual-chamber assembly mounted on the microscope stage. The adjacent chamber contained the aqueous bile acid–buffer solution made with 10 mmol/l HEPES (pH 7), 0.1–12 mmol/l Na^+ glycocholate, and sufficient glucose to give exactly the same osmolarity as the vesicle suspension. The vesicle experiments were performed in solutions of cholylglycine synthesized from chromatographically pure cholic acid following published methods[12]. The material was purified by adsorption chromatography using a silica gel column; the column was eluted with mixtures of methanol–chloroform with stepwise increases in the ratio of methanol to chloroform. Fractions were examined by thin-layer chromatography[13] and only fractions that contained the desired compound were pooled. Purity of the final material was evaluated with HPLC; based on absorbance at 200 nm wavelength[14], the impurity content was less than 2%.

In each test, a cell-size (~20 μm diameter) vesicle was chosen from the suspension by micropipet and transferred to the bile acid solution while held under constant suction pressure. Critical for the test method, vesicle volume was held fixed by osmotic activity of the solution, since the pressure scale for displacing water is several orders of magnitude above pipet suction pressures (i.e. 4 atm >> 0.001 atm). Thus, to minimize evaporation and maintain constant osmotic activity in the unsealed chambers, the assembly was kept at temperatures just above the dewpoint (~16°C), which is about 10°C above the gel–liquid crystalline transition for SOPC.

In a micromechanical test, pipet suction pressure P set the level of tension τ_m in the vesicle membrane as specified by ref. 7,

$$\tau_m = P \cdot R_p / 2(1 - R_p/R_o)$$

where R_p, R_o are the pipet radius and radius of the spherical vesicle segment outside the pipet, respectively. Since the vesicle was pressurized into a spherical shape, changes in length ΔL_p of the projection aspirated into the pipet provided sensitive measurements of area changes, i.e.

$$\Delta A = 2\pi R_p (1 - R_p/R_o)\Delta L_p$$

Therefore, when a vesicle was transferred into an iso-osmotic solution, incorporation of new material into the bilayer was expected to produce an increase in projection length if the lipid content remained fixed. Incorporation of molecules into a bilayer from bile acid solution is demonstrated by the video images shown in Fig. 1. To ensure that the lipid composition was unchanged, and uptake reversible, the vesicle was transferred back to the original solution where

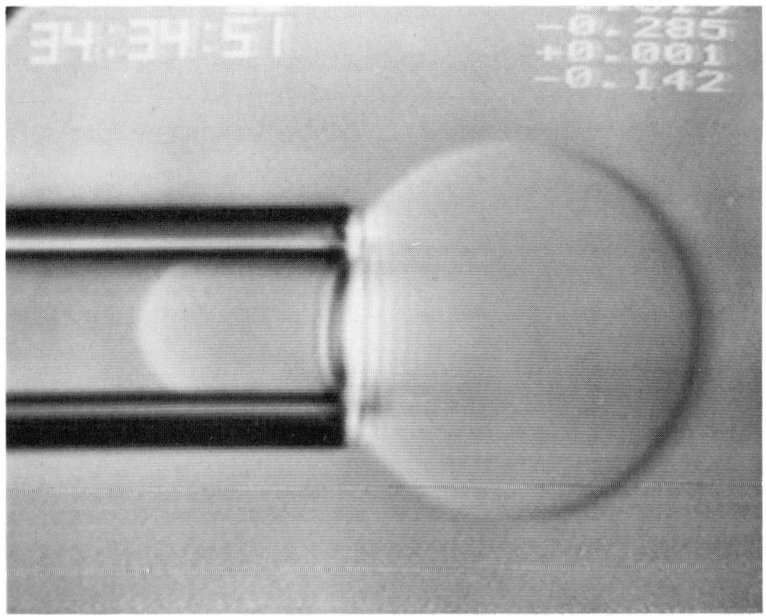

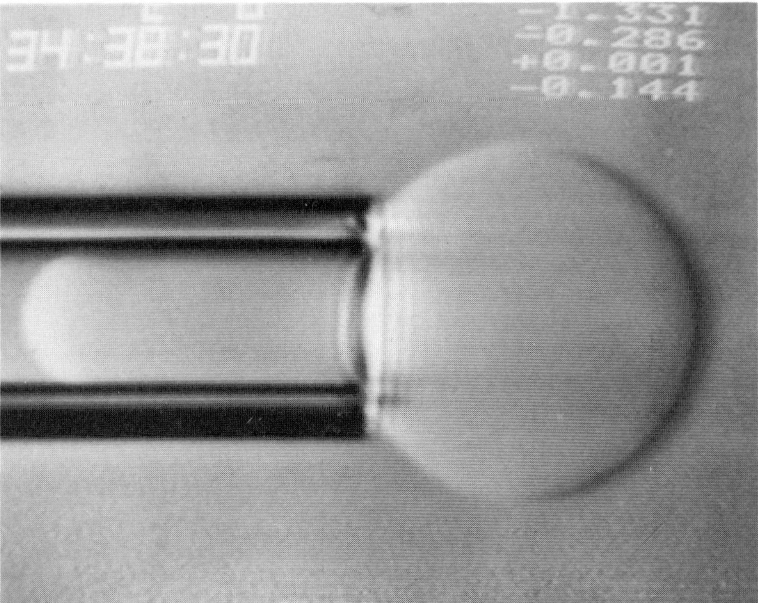

Fig. 1 Videomicrographs of a cell-size ($\sim 20\,\mu$m) SOPC bilayer vesicle suspended in buffer before (above) and after (below) transfer into buffer plus CG in the millimolar range. The increase in projection length inside the pipet is a direct measure of the area expansion by CG insertion into the bilayer, since vesicle volume was fixed by matching osmotic activities of the two solutions

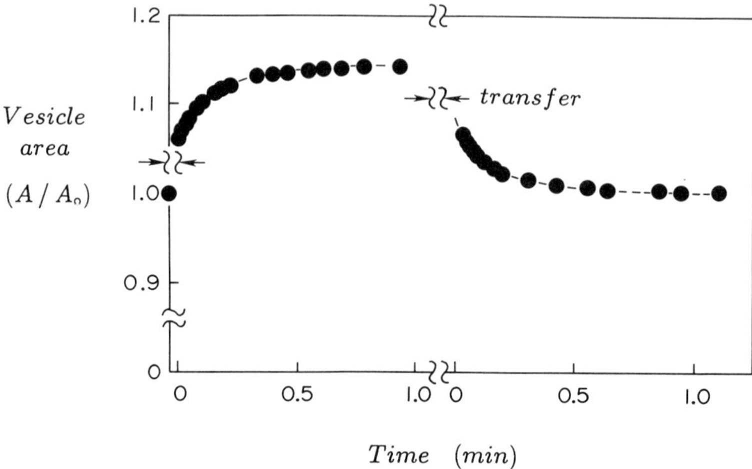

Time   (min)

Fig. 2   Time-course of area expansion when a vesicle was transferred into a 2 mmol/l CG solution followed by area reduction when transferred back to the CG-free buffer solution which demonstrates reversible dynamics of partitioning into SOPC bilayers. (Note: the time breaks at the beginning of each phase represent transfer between chambers on the microscope stage)

the added material could be released. Approach to equilibrium and reversible uptake of bile acid is shown in Fig. 2; the increase in area versus time was found from analysis of projection length. At equilibrium, changes in area of the bilayer with increase in tension represented elastic compressibility of the bilayer. The modulus of elastic compressibility K_A is defined by $\Delta\tau_m/\Delta(A/A_o)$, which reflects both reversible uptake of molecules from solution and elastic stretch of lipid area. Finally, the strength of the bilayer was quantitated by the level of tension necessary to rupture the vesicle at the end of an elasticity test.

RESULTS AND DISCUSSION

Expansion of neutral bilayers by bile acid insertion

Using the procedure shown in Fig. 1 and analysis illustrated in Fig. 2, we examined the uptake of bile acid by SOPC bilayers in a range of concentration from 0.1 to 12 mmol/l CG. Vesicles were so fragile in 8 mmol/l solutions that it was not possible to reach equilibrium; and vesicles disappeared immediately when transferred to solutions of 12 mmol/l CG. However, as shown in Fig. 2, the approach to equilibrium at concentrations below 8 mmol/l was rapid and reversible. In Fig. 3, equilibrium area fractions $\alpha = \Delta A/A$ (where $A = A_o + \Delta A$) are plotted on a logarithmic scale versus vesicle tension for concentrations up to 5 mmol/l. These results are consistent with ideal mixing of CG in the bilayer as characterized by the following relation for thermodynamic equilibrium:

$$1/n_s \cdot \ln(x_s/n_s) + \mu_s^o/kT = \mu_m^o/kT + 1/n_m \cdot \ln(x_m/n_m) - \tau_m \cdot a_s/2kT$$

biased by the activity coefficient for tension applied to the bilayer. [x_s, x_m are the

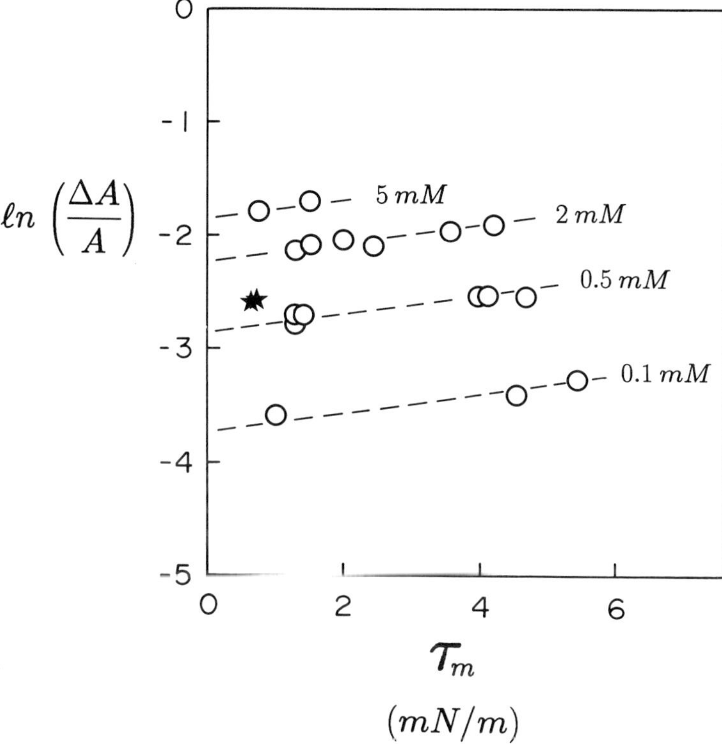

Fig. 3 Logarithm of the fractional increase in area $\alpha = \Delta A/A$ (area change ÷ final area) measured at equilibrium for neutral vesicles transferred at constant tension τ_m into CG solutions. The fraction of CG in the bilayer is observed to increase as the *square root* of the CG concentration. The slope of the linear dependence on tension (dashed lines) yields a molecular area of $\sim 60\,\text{Å}^2$ for CG in the bilayer. The points flagged by stars ($\star$) are data for binding to negatively charged vesicles (7 SOPC: 3 POPS) at 2 mmol/l concentration, which demonstrates the exclusion of weakly ionized CG from the bilayer

mole fractions of bile acid in water and each lipid layer of the bilayer; $\mu_s^{\,\circ}$, $\mu_m^{\,\circ}$ are reference chemical potentials; a_s is the area occupied by a CG complex in a lipid layer; and kT is thermal energy. The factor n_s/n_m represents the ratio of monomer aggregate number in aqueous solution to the number in a bilayer aggregate (only valid if the aggregates have fixed sizes in both phases or if mole fractions and reference potentials are identified as functions of size).] Since $x_m \sim$ the area fraction α in the bilayer and $x_s \sim$ the concentration c_s, in aqueous solution, we see that the data in Fig. 3 obey a single cooperative binding relation,

$$\alpha/\sqrt{c_s} = \text{constant} \cdot \exp\left(\tau_m \cdot a_s/2kT\right)$$

The correlation yields an area per CG complex of about $60\,\text{Å}^2$ in each leaflet of the bilayer. n_m/n_s implies that CG aggregates were predominantly fixed sizes in both phases *and* split in half when partitioning into the bilayer (e.g. probably from dimers in solution to monomers in the bilayer at low ionic strength, as shown by the well-accepted results published in ref. 8).

Ionization of bile acid groups at the neutral bilayer interface

Most intriguingly, there was no strong barrier to uptake that would arise from electrostatic charging of the interface or elastic stretch due to blocked transfer to the inner lipid layer of the bilayer. Both energy potentials increase in proportion to CG uptake and reduce the binding by a factor exp $(-b \cdot \alpha)$. The dimensionless energy coefficient b is given by,

$$b = [e \cdot \partial \psi / \partial \alpha + K_1 \cdot a_s/2]/kT$$

where e is the electric charge on the bound complex, ψ is the electrostatic surface potential, and K_1 is the elastic dilation modulus for the lipid bilayer. If ionized species of bile acid partition into the interface, the surface potential is expected to build up in accordance with Guoy–Chapman theory[9], where the electrostatic barrier $(e \cdot \psi/kT)$ depends on charge density σ_e and ionic strength c_i mol/l) through the following transcendental equation:

$$\sinh (e \cdot \psi/2kT) \approx 136 \ \sigma_e/\sqrt{c_i}$$

Here, the charge density $\sigma_e = e^* \alpha/a_s$ is defined as $\#/Å^2$ and e^* is the average fractional charge of groups added to the surface. (At low potentials the sinh function approaches its argument and the potential becomes proportional to charge density, which is the Debye Huckle approximation.) The elastic potential is predicted by analysis of the differential change in area between inner/outer leaflets that must accompany large expansion of a *smooth* bilayer when material is inserted into only one side. The parameters in both potentials are known except for the fractional charge e^* of groups inserted into the membrane. As such, the two energy scales inside the brackets are readily calculated to be of order 45 $(e^*)^2 kT$ for weak charging in 0.01 mmol/l electrolyte and $16\,kT$ for SOPC bilayer elasticity $(K_1 \approx 210\,mN/m$, ref. 10). Clearly, binding in the millimolar range would be suppressed significantly if acid groups were fully ionized at the surface, or were restricted to insert only in the outer lipid layer of the bilayer.

The absence of strong potentials at high levels of binding was surprising, since about 99.9% of CG is ionized in solution at pH 7 (for $pK_a \sim 4$). Thus, we designed an experiment to determine the proportion of ionized CG groups inserted into the bilayer surface. Using vesicles prepared with 30% negatively charged lipid (7 SOPC: 3 POPS, $\sigma_e \approx 1/200 Å^2$), the surface potential was essentially clamped at $e \cdot \psi/kT \approx 5.2$ in 0.01 mol/l electrolyte. Because of the large potential, the binding energy of ionized groups was anticipated to shift linearly with charge and, thereby, reduce the binding of charged species by a factor of exp $(-5.2 e^*)$. As shown by the data flagged in Fig. 3, binding to charged vesicles in solutions of 2 mmol/l CG was lowered substantially by a factor of exp (-0.4). Assuming that CG groups can be categorized as either ionized or neutral (protonated), we conclude that the reduction in area expansion represented nearly complete exclusion of the ionized species from the charged bilayer. Hence, the ratio of ionized to protonated species appears to be reversed dramatically from 1000 : 1 in solution to 1 : 2 in neutral bilayers. Similar to uptake of acylated glycines and fatty acids by bilayers[9], the affinity for binding protonated CG to the bilayer seems to be much greater than for ionized CG. In most measurements of binding to lipid vesicles the amount of lipid is comparable to the amount of bile acid in

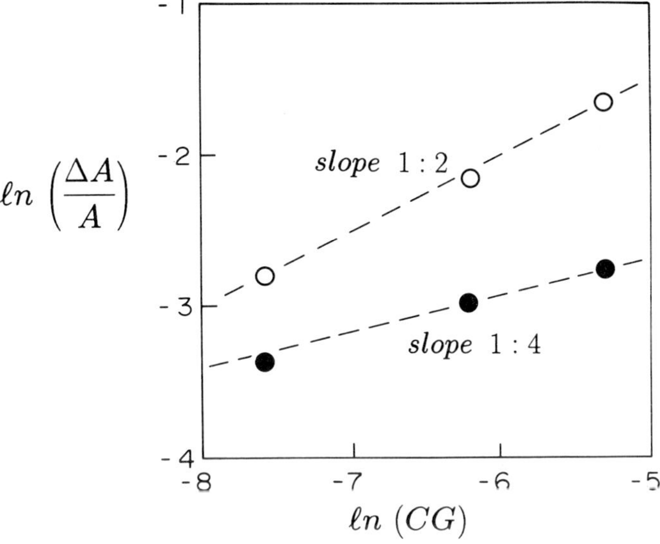

Fig. 4 Logarithm of the fractional increase in area of SOPC bilayer vesicles held at a constant tension of 1mN/M as a function of the logarithm of CG concentration (mmol/l). Data are plotted from experiments with two different CG fractions solubilized in the same 10 mmol/l Na^+, 10 mmol/l HEPES (pH7), 0.1 mol/l glucose buffer. The open circles represent the material synthesized according to the procedures outlined in the Methods section and used throughout this study (cf. Figs 3, 5, 6). Tested for comparison, the closed circles represent the material obtained from a commercial source. The linear behaviour in both cases demonstrates ideal mixing in the bilayer and the difference in slopes exposes the difference in aggregate sizes in solution

the total mixture. Thus, when pH is well above the pK_a of the acid group, the bound fraction of ionized species will approach the fraction in solution[9] and the surface potential will build up to suppress uptake, which gives the impression of saturation binding. By comparison, in single-vesicle experiments, the amount of lipid brought to the test chamber represents total concentrations of only 10^{-12}–10^{-11} mmol/l, which allows each species to establish independent equilibrium with the bilayer. Most likely, preferential uptake of protonated species by the vesicle bilayer accounts for the rapid kinetics of CG monomer transfer between lipid leaflets of the membrane[15]. Also, preferential affinity for protonated species may provide a clue to the difference in uptake by SOPC bilayers found between the two sets of CG solutions (cf. Fig. 4). Small amounts of surface active impurities could affect the aggregation state of a low concentration of protonated CG monomers present at pH levels well above the pK_a of the acid.

Mechanical softening and rupture of bilayers by bile acid

After equilibrium was reached in the CG solution, pressurization of the vesicle produced increases in surface area proportional to bilayer tension that were fully reversible when the pressure was reduced. Slopes of the tension–area data yielded elastic moduli K_A for area compressibility. Starting from the stiff elastic response of an SOPC bilayer in Fig. 5, the measurements show the pronounced

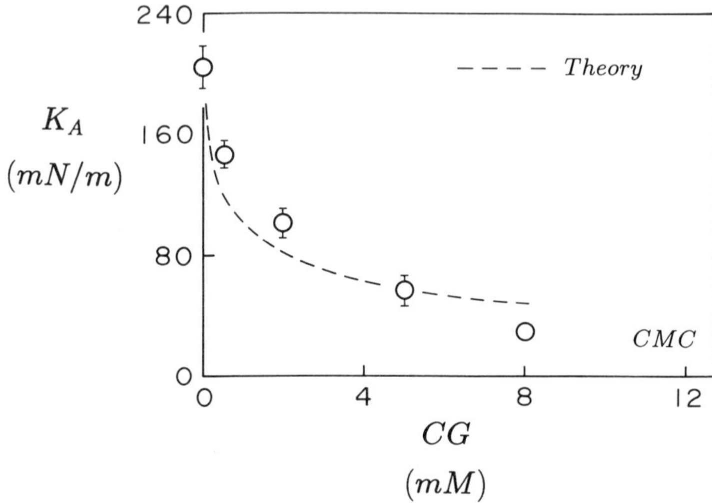

Fig. 5 Elastic moduli K_A for area compressibility of SOPC bilayers in CG solutions determined from measurements of area increase ΔA in response to increase in tension τ_m, i.e. $K_A = A_o(\Delta \tau_m / \Delta A)$. Note that the bilayer is already *softened* significantly at low CG concentrations. The dashed curve is the prediction of *softening* derived from the simple ideal mixing theory described in the text

softening of bilayers even at low CG concentrations. The origin of this striking effect is exposed by the simple thermodynamic model: i.e. bilayer compliance in the bile acid solution involves serial coupling of reversible CG uptake and elastic stretch of the insoluble lipid material. In other words the bilayer acts like a *sponge* that pulls CG out of solution when under tension, and expels CG when the tension is relaxed. Assuming that lipid elasticity is unaffected by the presence of bile acid in the bilayer (i.e. consistent with the *ideal* mixing hypothesis), analysis of the area expansion yields a superposition of compliances in proportion to mole fraction of each surface component,

$$1/K_A \approx (1-\alpha)/K_1 + \alpha/K_s$$

The compliance $1/K_s$ for reversible uptake of bile acid molecules is derived from the relation for equilibrium by differentiating at constant chemical potential (i.e. constant concentration in aqueous solution):

$$1/K_s = 1/(1-x_m) \cdot [\partial(\ln x_m)/\partial \tau_m]_\mu = a_s/2kT(1-x_m)$$

A factor $(1-x_m)$ arises because the derivative is taken with respect to molecular number. The elastic coefficient K_s exposes the ideal gas-like exchange of bile acid with the bilayer. Using the molecular area $a_s \sim 60 \text{ Å}^2$ found from equilibrium binding at constant tension, predictions of elastic moduli for SOPC bilayers in CG solutions are plotted along with the measurements in Fig. 5. (The agreement is good except that the prediction falls slightly below the measured values at low CG concentrations where it should be best. The deviation appears to originate from not providing sufficient time between tension steps to allow diffusive equilibrium with the bilayer when tested at concentrations below millimolar.) As

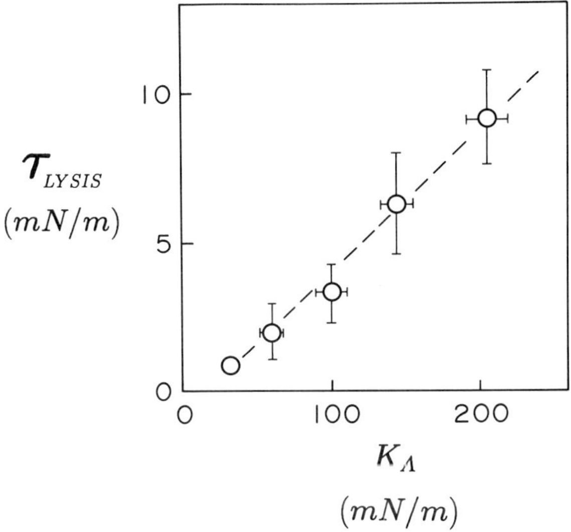

Fig. 6 Correlation of the strength of SOPC bilayers in CG solutions (measured by the level of tension at vesicle lysis) versus elastic modulus of area compressibility. The progressive reduction in strength with *softening* is a universal characteristic found for lipid bilayers of all compositions tested[11], and demonstrates a non-specific mechanism of bilayer degradation in bile acid solutions well below conditions required for dissolution

pipet suction increased, tension reached a level where vesicles lysed, which defined bilayer rupture strength. Measurements of rupture strength versus concentration of CG in solution exhibited the same precipitous decline as seen in Fig. 5 for elastic moduli. Direct correlation of bilayer strength to *softening* is shown in Fig. 6. This material feature appears to be a universal property of bilayers[12], which implies that mechanical tension couples to molecular scale fluctuations in bilayer rupture. Independent of physical origin, the clear message is that *softening* of bilayers through reversible uptake of bile acid significantly diminishes strength even at low concentrations. This could represent an important non-specific mechanism for degradation of cell membranes when exposed to bile acid anions. It is likely that nature has evolved the lipid composition of membrane bilayers to resist this action, which emphasizes a need to examine lipid mixtures with cholesterol and sphingolipids known to increase bilayer cohesion[11].

Acknowledgement

This work was supported in part by grants MT7477 from the Medical Research Council of Canada to E.E. and DK 21506 from the U.S. National Institute of Health plus the Falk Foundation, eV., Germany, to A.H.

References

1. Yousef IM, Barnwell S, Gratton F, Tuchweber B, Weber A, Roy CC. Liver cell membrane solubilization may control maximum secretory rate of cholic acid in the rat. Am J Physiol. 1987;252:84–91.
2. Barnwell SG, Lowe PJ, Coleman R. Effect of taurochenodeoxycholate or tauroursodeoxycholate upon biliary output of phospholipids and plasma-membrane enzymes, and the extent of cell damage, in isolated perfused rat livers. Biochem J. 1983;216:107–11. Barnwell SG, Tuchweber B, Yousef IM. Biliary lipid secretion in the rat during infusion of increasing doses of unconjugated bile acids. Biochim Biophys Acta. 1987;922:221–33.
3. Hofmann AF, Mysels KJ. Bile salts as biological surfactants. Colloids Surf. 1988;30:145–73.
4. Schurtenberger P, Mazer N, Kanzig W. Micelle to vesicle transition in aqueous solutions of bile salt and lecithin. J Phys Chem. 1985;89:1042–9.
5. Schubert R, Schmidt K-H. Structural changes in vesicle membranes and mixed micelles of various lipid compositions after binding of different bile salts. Biochemistry. 1988;27:8787–94. Schubert RK, Beyer K, Wolburg H, Schmidt K-H. Structural changes in membranes of large unilamellar vesicles after binding of sodium cholate. Biochemistry. 1986;25:5263–9.
6. Heuman DM. Tauroursodeoxycholate protects cholesterol-rich model membranes against disruption by more hydrophobic bile salts. In: Paumgartner G, Stiehl A, Gerok W, editors. Bile acids as therapeutic agents. Falk Symposium 58. 1991:237–42.
7. Needham D, Evans E. Structure and mechanical properties of giant lipid (DMPC) vesicle bilayers from 20°C below to 10°C above the liquid crystal–crystalline phase transition at 24°C. Biophys J. 1988;27:8261–9.
8. Small DM. Size and structure of bile salt micelles. In: Goddard ED, editor. Molecular association in biological and related systems. Advances in Chemistry. 1968;84:31–52.
9. Peitzsch RM, McLaughlin S. Binding of acylated peptides and fatty acids to phospholipid vesicles: pertinence to myristoylated proteins. Biochemistry. 1993;32:10436–43.
10. Evans E, Needham D. Physical properties of surfactant bilayer membranes: thermal transitions, elasticity, rigidity, cohesion, and colloidal interactions. J Phys Chem. 1987;91:4219–28.
11. Bloom M, Evans E, Mouritsen OG. Physical properties of the fluid lipid-bilayer component of cell membranes: a perspective. Q Rev Biophys. 1991;24:293–397.
12. Tserng K-Y, Hachey DL, Klein PD. An improved procedure for the synthesis of glycine and taurine conjugates of bile acids. J Lipid Res. 1977; 18:404–7.
13. Hofmann AF. Thin-layer adsorption chromatography of free and conjugated bile acids on silicic acid. J Lipid Res. 1962;2:127–8.
14. Rossi SS, Converse JL, Hofmann AF. High pressure liquid chromatographic analysis of conjugated bile acids in human bile: simultaneous resolution of sulfated and unsulfated lithocholyl amidates and the common bile acids. J Lipid Res. 1987; 28:589–95.
15. Cabral DJ, Small DM, Lilly HS, Hamilton JA. Transbilayer movement of bile acids in model membranes. Biochemistry. 1987;26:1801–4.

6
Calcium affinity for biliary lipid aggregates in model bile: lecithin in mixed micelles and vesicles significantly augments calcium binding by bile salts

J. M. DONOVAN, M. R. LEONARD and M. C. CAREY

INTRODUCTION

Calcium is believed to play a number of important roles in the development of cholesterol gallstones, and is critical for the development of pigment gallstones[1]. In the case of the latter, calcium precipitates with the organic anion unconjugated bilirubin, as well as the inorganic anions phosphate and carbonate, to form the major components of both black and brown pigment gallstones[2,3]. Furthermore, ionic interactions between calcium and polyanionic proteins, including biliary mucin, appear to be involved in the initial stages and growth of both pigment and cholesterol gallstones[4,5]. Calcium is believed to bind principally to bile salts (BS)[6], which are present in bile as monomers, simple BS $\pm$ cholesterol micelles, and BS/lecithin/cholesterol mixed micelles and vesicles[7]. Calcium also accelerates the process of cholesterol crystal formation *in vitro*[8], although the relevance to *in vivo* nucleation and the formation of cholesterol gallstones is uncertain[9,10]. However, the relative distribution of calcium binding to BS in these biliary lipid aggregates was largely unexplored.

We therefore undertook studies to determine how the magnitude of calcium binding can be related to the distribution of particles present in pathophysiologically important regions of the ternary phase diagram of the major biliary lipids (Fig. 1). As the relative BS to egg yolk lecithin (EYL) ratio decreases, and the phase diagram is traversed along a line between 100% BS and 100% EYL, the predominant lipid aggregate changes from simple micelles to mixed micelles to vesicles. As cholesterol is added, the relative composition increases in the vertical direction (Fig. 1), vesicles and/or cholesterol crystals are present in addition to mixed micelles. Experiments were designed to measure calcium bind-

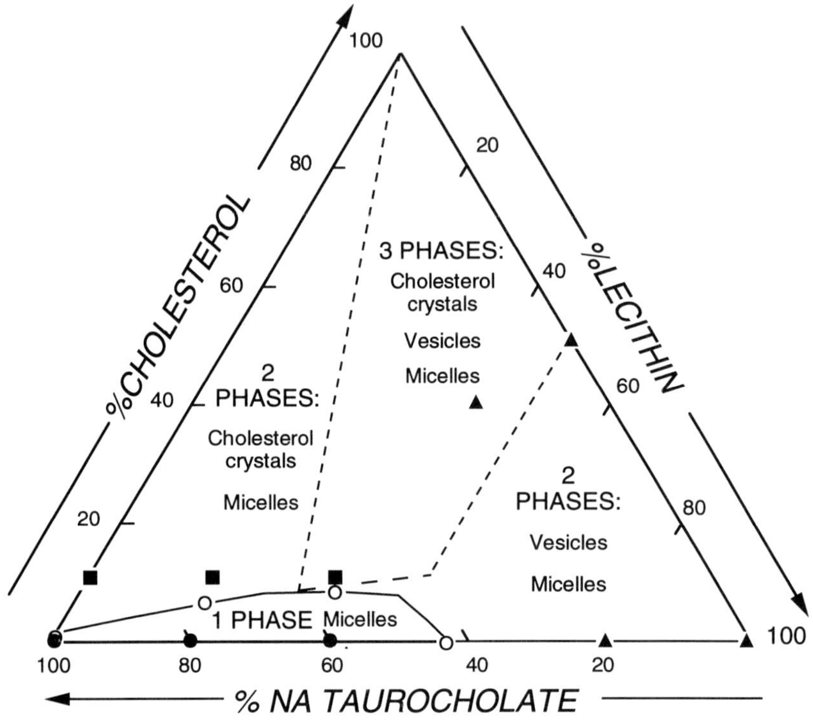

Fig. 1 Phase diagram of taurocholate, EYL and cholesterol at 10% total lipid concentration in the presence of 8 mmol/l $CaCl_2$ plus 126 mmol/l NaCl at 37°C. Phase boundaries ○ were determined by light scattering and polarized light microscopy, and approximated closely those in the absence of calcium (not shown)[11]. With cholesterol contents in excess of the micellar phase, several multiphase zones containing two or three phases exist; principally an aqueous phase with cholesterol monohydrate crystals and/or vesicles and mixed micelles. Systems studied in this work contained either micelles (●), two or three phases with predominantly micelles and cholesterol monohydrate crystals ± vesicles (■) or predominantly vesicles (▲). Reprinted from ref. 12

ing to BS in model systems containing different proportions of simple micelles, mixed micelles, and vesicles, with the goal of determining relative calcium binding to each of these lipid aggregates.

MEASUREMENT OF CALCIUM BINDING

Calcium is present in biological fluids as the divalent ion, which may be free in aqueous solution or complexed to anions. The calcium electrode measures the free calcium concentration, sometimes referred to as 'ionized' calcium, although both free and soluble complexed calcium retain a net charge. This extraordinarily useful tool was developed 25 years ago by James Ross[13], and utilized by Edward Moore and colleagues in landmark studies of biological fluids[14]. The basic principle of the original electrode remains to the present: a reference electrode and an ion-selective electrode are immersed in a calcium-containing solution, and the voltage potential between the two is measured. The Nernst equation predicts that the voltage difference will depend linearly on the logarithm of the free calcium concentration[13,14]. Early electrodes used an organo-phosphate exchanger in an organic matrix, but these electrodes were susceptible to damage by BS and other anionic detergents that could complex with calcium and partition into the organic phase[15]. More recently, neutral molecules that complex calcium, such as ETH1001, have been incorporated into a polyvinyl carbonate matrix[16]. The solid nature of the latter matrix does not allow permeation by BS, and this has thereby minimized the possibility of interference.

The free calcium concentration was measured in model biles composed with 8 mmol/l $CaCl_2$ and 126 mmol/l NaCl, for a total electrolyte ionic strength of 150 mmol/l, at constant temperature (37°C), as detailed in ref. 12. An Orion ion-sensitive electrode based on the principles described by Anker and colleagues[16] (Orion Instruments, Cambridge, MA) was calibrated with a series of $CaCl_2$ standards (0.1–20 mmol/l Ca^{+2}), and exhibited behaviour as predicted by the Nernst equation. In addition to determinations with the calcium electrode at a total calcium concentration of 8 mmol/l, selected measurements were also made using the spectral shift of murexide (5,5′-nitrilodibarbituric acid monoammonium salt) to monitor free calcium content[17].

CALCIUM BINDING TO MONOMERS, SIMPLE AND MIXED MICELLES

To determine the relative magnitude of calcium binding to monomeric as compared to simple micellar BS, we compared calcium binding for the trihydroxy-BS taurocholate and tauroursocholate, and the triketo-BS taurodehydrocholate in systems composed of BS alone. In the case of all three BS, calcium binding was virtually identical, and increased with increasing total BS concentration (data not shown). Despite enormous differences in the relative concentrations of monomers and simple micelles in these systems, calcium binding rose smoothly. Calculated affinity constants (assuming a 1:1 BS:Ca stoichiometry) demonstrated that calcium affinity increased modestly with each increment in BS concentration, and reached a plateau at ≈ 40 mmol/l BS.

Figure 2 shows calcium binding to model micellar biles containing taurocholate with increasing relative amounts of EYL. For each relative BS content, calcium binding increased with total absolute BS concentration. Hence, calcium binding increased with addition of EYL for any fixed BS concentration. Similar trends were observed using the spectral shift of murexide to measure unbound calcium (data not shown; see Appendix in ref. 12). As relative BS concentration was decreased from 100% to 60%, the predominant aggregate changed from simple micelles to mixed micelles (cf. Fig. 7). Measurements of the intermixed micellar/intervesicular BS concentration for this system demonstrated that >90% of the BS are in mixed micelles, rather than as monomers or simple micelles. Hence, mixed micelles are the predominant form in which calcium is bound in physiologically relevant model biles.

Calcium binding in micellar systems containing cholate and its glycine conjugate with varying EYL compositions was compared with taurocholate-

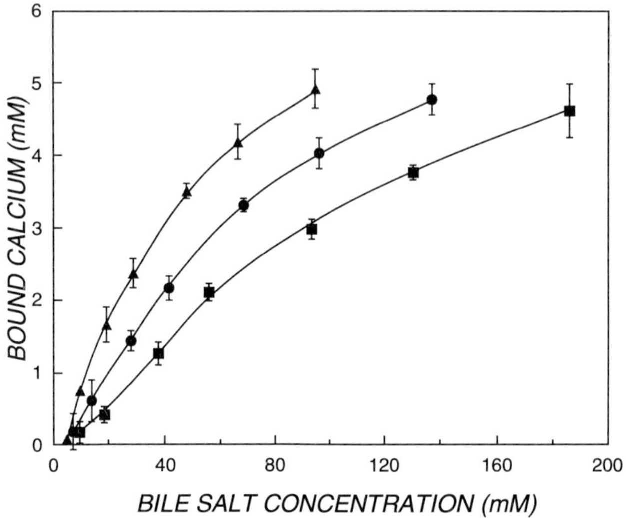

Fig. 2 Dependence of bound calcium on total BS concentration for taurocholate/EYL systems, at BS/(BS+EYL) molar ratios: 1.0 (■), 0.8 (●) and 0.6 (▲). Addition of EYL significantly enhances calcium binding by BS at all taurocholate concentrations. Conditions were 8 mmol/l $CaCl_2$, 126 mmol/l NaCl, and 37°C. Error bars denote standard deviations. Reprinted from ref. 12

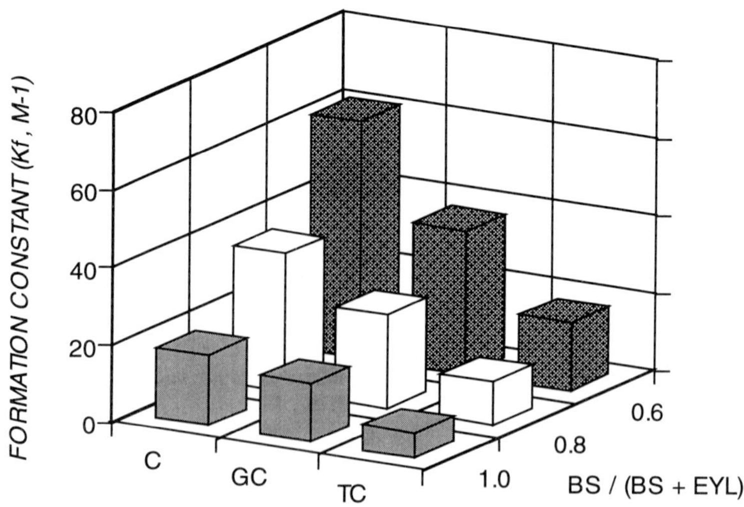

Fig. 3 Formation constants (K_f, in units of l/mol) for calcium binding to 65 mmol/l cholate (C), glycocholate (GC) and taurocholate (TC) as functions of variations in BS/(BS=EYL) ratios (right horizontal axis). In the presence of EYL, all BS displayed enhanced calcium binding. For constant BS/(BS+EYL) ratios, K_f values increased in the order TC<GC<C.

containing systems. All three BS were studied at pH values at which BS were fully ionized. In Fig. 3 the vertical axis displays equilibrium formation constants (l/mol) for calcium binding; the larger values denote increased calcium affinity.

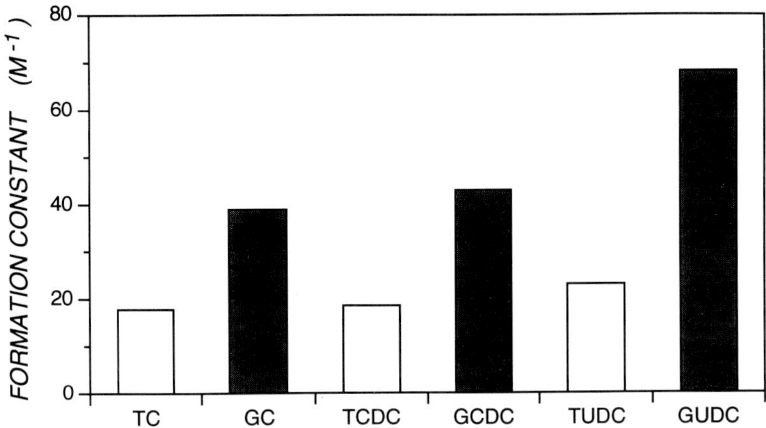

Fig. 4 Formation constants (K_f, l/mol) for calcium binding to 65 mmol/l glycine and taurine conjugates of dihydroxy BS, chenodeoxycholate (GCDC and TCDC) and ursodeoxycholate (GUDC and TUDC), as well as cholate for comparison, at a BS/(BS+EYL) ratio of 0.6. Glycine conjugates uniformly displayed higher affinities for calcium than did taurine conjugates. Conditions were 8 mmol/l $CaCl_2$, 126 mmol/l NaCl, and 37°C

Calcium binding increases as relative BS content falls, and relative EYL content rises at fixed total BS for all three homologues, with the decreasing rank order being cholate > glycocholate > taurocholate. As observed for the taurine conjugate, BS in mixed micelles bind calcium more strongly than BS in simple micelles.

Figure 4 compares formation constants for calcium binding to glycine and taurine conjugates of the dihydroxy-BS chenodeoxycholate and ursodeoxycholate with those of cholate at a BS/(BS+EYL) ratio of 0.6. Glycine conjugates uniformly have higher affinities for calcium than taurine conjugates, as noted previously for pure BS systems[18–20]. The dihydroxy BS, which have higher affinities for calcium than the trihydroxy BS, showed a similar but less pronounced increase in calcium binding in the presence of EYL (data not shown). Caution is advisable because values for glycine-conjugated BS are not true equilibrium values. As shown by Jones and colleagues[21], all glycine conjugates, especially the dihydroxy BS, form insoluble calcium salts of remarkable metastability at physiological concentrations.

As shown in Fig. 5, EYL enhanced calcium binding to a physiological mixture of eight BS[22]. In biles of physiological compositions, most BS are associated with lecithin[22]: hence, calcium is predominantly associated with BS in mixed micelles.

CALCIUM BINDING IN SYSTEMS CONTAINING VESICLES AND/OR CHOLESTEROL CRYSTALS

In native bile, cholesterol-saturated or supersaturated micelles coexist with cholesterol/lecithin vesicles and/or cholesterol crystals[23]. Calcium binding was examined in multiphase systems whose compositions fall above the micellar

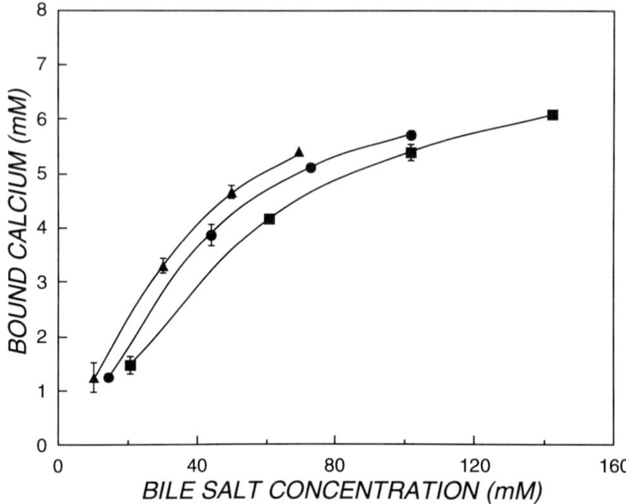

Fig. 5 Calcium binding to model bile systems containing a physiological BS mixture (see text) with BS/(BS + EYL) ratios: 1.0 (■), 0.8 (●) and 0.6 (▲). Conditions were 8 mmol/l $CaCl_2$, 126 mmol/l NaCl, pH ≈8.5, and 37°C. Standard deviations are within symbols or denoted by error bars. Reprinted from ref. 12

zone of the equilibrium phase diagram (see Fig. 1). In these systems, both simple and mixed micelles are supersaturated with cholesterol, but micellar size, as determined by quasielastic light scattering[24], remained unchanged as compared with systems without cholesterol[25]. Calcium affinity was not significantly altered by incorporation of 10 mol% cholesterol into these systems (data not shown). Thus, enhancement of calcium binding by EYL is not influenced by incorporation of cholesterol into mixed micelles, or by cholesterol present as insoluble (crystalline) phases.

Vesicles constitute a quantitatively minor fraction of lipids in supersaturated cholesterol systems at physiological BS content as in the gallbladder[23]. Calcium binding was therefore measured in two-phase, predominantly vesicular, systems of EYL or equimolar EYL/cholesterol with 20 mol% taurocholate. Figure 6A shows bound calcium (normalized per mole BS) on the vertical axis and relative percentage BS on the horizontal axis. As the relative BS/EYL ratio decreased, calcium binding per mole of BS increased and, concomitantly, there was a transition from simple to mixed micelles to vesicles. Figure 6B shows mean hydrodynamic radii of these systems as determined by quasielastic light scattering[24]. Enhanced calcium binding with increased EYL content was not due to calcium binding to EYL alone because, in the absence of BS, neither pure EYL nor EYL/cholesterol vesicles (1 and 3 g/dl) bound appreciable amounts of calcium ions.

PATHOPHYSIOLOGICAL IMPLICATIONS

The relative distribution of BS and bound calcium was calculated from measurements of the intermixed micellar/intervesicular BS concentration[27] and gel

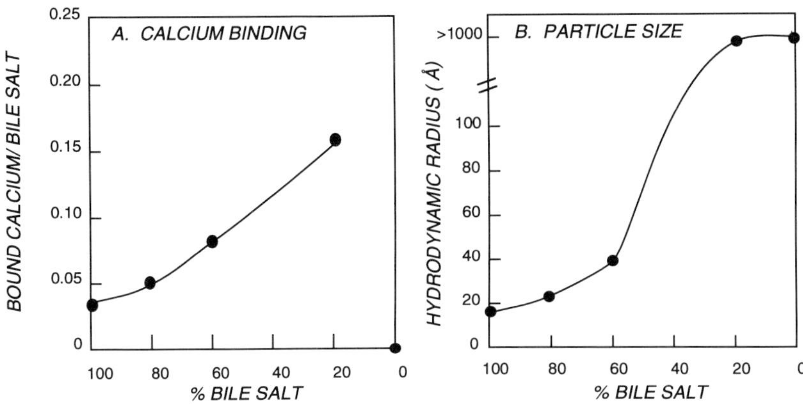

Fig. 6　**A**: Molar ratio of bound calcium per BS molecule for taurocholate/EYL systems. Vesicular systems (% BS/(BS+EYL)<20%) contained EYL vesicles±20 mol% taurocholate. **B**: Mean hydrodynamic radius (previously unpublished, Donovan JM *et al.*), as determined by quasielastic light scattering[24] was not significantly changed as compared with systems in the absence of calcium[26]. Conditions were total lipid concentration of 3 g/dl, 8 mmol/l $CaCl_2$, 126 mmol/l NaCl, and 37°C

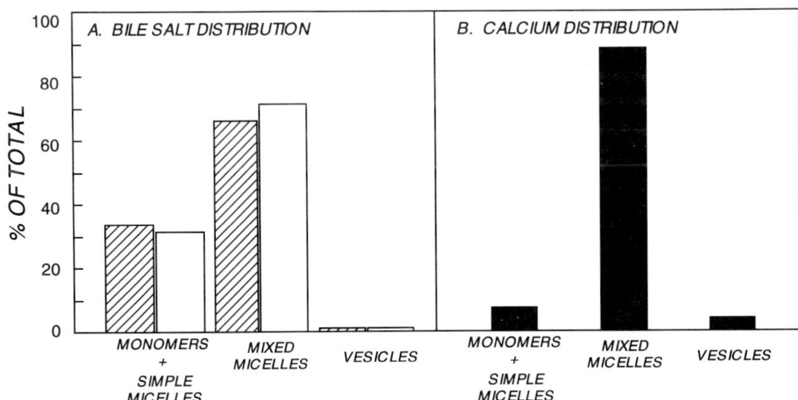

Fig. 7　**A**: Experimentally determined distribution of TC in a model bile of typical physiological composition: 3 g/dl, TC/(TC+EYL)=0.7, 10 mol% cholesterol, at 0 (striped bars) and 8 mmol/l (white bars) $CaCl_2$. **B**: Calculated distribution of bound calcium in the same model bile (solid bars)

filtration chromatography as described in ref. 12 in a model bile composed with 70 mol% taurocholate, 10 mol% cholesterol, at a total lipid concentration of 3 g/dl. Figure 7A shows the distribution of BS among biliary lipid aggregates in the presence and absence of 8 mmol/l calcium. Approximately 70% of the BS are associated with mixed micelles, with the remainder as simple micelles or monomers, and trivial amounts of BS bound to vesicles. Figure 7B depicts the relative amount of calcium bound to monomers and simple micelles, mixed micelles, and vesicles corresponding to the BS distribution in Fig. 7A. In physiological model bile, >90% of the bound calcium is associated with BS in mixed micelles, and not associated with monomers and simple micelles, as was suggested previously[1]. Although, quantitatively, calcium binding to cholesterol/ EYL vesicles is small, the high-affinity binding induced by incorporation of BS may play an important role in aggregation of biliary vesicles by imparting a net negative charge.

In summary, calcium binds unequivocally to BS monomers, but binding affinity is not substantially augmented by simple micelle formation. Lecithin, but not cholesterol, increases calcium binding to all BS contained in biliary lipid aggregates. Thus, both BS and EYL decrease calcium activity in bile, and enhance solublity of calcium-sensitive anions. For physiological biliary lipid compositions most calcium is bound to mixed micelles rather than to monomers or simple micelles. We propose that, even when BS are associated with EYL, the side-chain carboxylic acid or sulphonate group and the steroid ring hydroxyl groups are available to complex with calcium. This requires that BS molecules orient with their steroid ring flat at the aqueous interface, an orientation supported by surface monolayer studies of binary mixtures of dihydroxy-bile acids and a typical biliary lecithin species[28].

These data suggest that BS can induce high-affinity calcium binding to EYL and EYL/cholesterol vesicles that can, under appropriate conditions, crosslink cholesterol-rich vesicles, and hence promote cholesterol crystal and gallstone formation. Calcium binding also decreases calcium activity in bile, and hence can inhibit precipitation of inorganic and organic calcium salts that constitute pigment gallstones. Additionally, high-affinity calcium binding by membrane-bound BS may be responsible for BS-induced enhancement of transmembrane calcium transport[29,30]. Further studies on calcium binding to membrane-associated BS are likely to give insights into mechanisms of cholesterol and pigment gallstone formation as well as BS cytotoxicity.

Acknowledgements

This work was supported in part by research grants DK 36588 and DK 18707, and Center grant DK 34854 from the National Institutes of Health (US Public Health Service), and research funding from the Veterans Administration.

References

1. Moore EW. Biliary calcium and gallstone formation. Hepatology. 1990;12:206–14S.
2. Cahalane MJ, Neubrand MW, Carey MC. Physical–chemical pathogenesis of pigment gallstones. Sem Liver Dis. 1988;8:317–28.
3. Donovan JM, Carey MC. Physical–chemical basis of cholesterol and pigment gallstone formation. Gastroenterol Clin N Am. 1991;20:47–66.
4. Lamont JT, Carey MC. Cholesterol gallstone formation. 2. Pathobiology and pathomechanics. Prog Liver Dis. 1992;10:165–91.
5. Ostrow JD. APF/CBP, an anionic polypeptide in bile and gallstones that may regulate calcium salt and cholesterol precipitation from bile. Hepatology. 1992;16:1493–6.
6. Moore EW, Celic L, Ostrow JD. Interactions between ionized calcium and sodium taurocholate: bile salts are important buffers for prevention of calcium-containing gallstones. Gastroenterology. 1982;83:1079–89.
7. Donovan JM, Carey MC. Inter-mixed micellar/intervesicular (non-lecithin associated) bile salt concentration (IMC) in bile: measurement, effects of physiological variables and pathophysio-

logical implications. In: Paumgartner G, Stiehl A, Gerok W, editors. Bile acids and the hepato-biliary system: from basic science to clinical practice. Dordrecht, The Netherlands: Kluwer; 1993:187–94.

8. Berenson MM, Cardinal JR. Calcium accelerates cholesterol phase transitions in analog bile. Experientia. 1985;41:1328–30.

9. Neithercut WD. Effect of calcium, magnesium and sodium ions on *in vitro* nucleation of human gall bladder bile. Gut. 1989;30:665–70.

10. Gallinger S, Harvey PRC, Petrunka CN, Strasberg SM. Effect of binding of ionised calcium on the *in vitro* nucleation of cholesterol and calcium bilirubinate in human gall bladder bile. Gut. 1986;27:1382–6.

11. Carey MC, Small DM. The physical chemistry of cholesterol solubility in bile: relationship to gallstone formation and dissolution in man. J Clin Invest. 1978;61:998–1026.

12. Donovan JM, Leonard MR, Batta AK, Carey MC. Calcium affinity for biliary lipid aggregates in model biles: complementary importance of bile salts and lecithin. Gastroenterology. 1994; 107:831–46.

13. Ross JW. Calcium-selective electrode with liquid ion exchanger. Science. 1967;156:1378–9.

14. Moore EW. Ionized calcium in normal serum, ultrafiltrates, and whole blood determined by ion-exchange electrodes. J Clin Invest. 1970;49:318–34.

15. Accatino L, Gavilan P. Phospholipids and bile acids as diffusional carriers of Na^+ across nonpolar media. Hepatology. 1988;8:898–903.

16. Anker P, Wieland E, Ammann D, Dohner RE, Asper R, Simon W. Neutral carrier based ion-selective electrode for the determination of total calcium in blood serum. Anal Chem. 1981; 53:1970–4.

17. Scarpa A. Measurements of cation transport with metallochromic indicators. Methods Enzymol. 1979;56:301–8.

18. Gleeson D, Murphy GM, Dowling RH. Calcium binding by bile acids: *in vitro* studies using a calcium ion electrode. J Lipid Res. 1990;31:781–91.

19. Baruch E, Lichtenberg D, Barak P, Nir S. Calcium binding to bile salts. Chem Phys Lipids. 1991;57:17–27.

20. Marteau C, Portugal H, Mathieu S, Pauli AM, Gerolami A. Effect of various bile salts on calcium concentration and calcium carbonate saturation of rat bile. J Hepatol. 1988;7:57–62.

21. Jones CA, Hofmann AF, Mysels KJ, Roda A. The effect of calcium and sodium ion concentration on the properties of dilute aqueous solutions of glycine conjugated bile salts: phase behavior and solubility products of the calcium salts of the common glycine conjugated bile acids. J Coll Interf Sci. 1986;114:452–70.

22. Donovan JM, Jackson AA, Carey MC. Molecular species composition of the inter-mixed micellar/vesicular bile salt concentrations in model bile. Dependence upon hydrophilic–hydrophobic balance. J Lipid Res. 1993;34:1131–40.

23. Donovan JM, Carey MC. Separation and quantitation of cholesterol 'carriers' in bile. Hepatology. 1990;12:94–105S.

24. Cohen DE, Fisch MR, Carey MC. Principles of laser light-scattering spectroscopy: applications to the physicochemical study of model and native biles. Hepatology. 1990;113–21S.

25. Mazer NA, Carey MC. Quasi-elastic light scattering studies of aqueous biliary lipid systems. Cholesterol solubilization and precipitation in model bile solutions. Biochemistry. 1983;22: 426–42.

26. Mazer NA, Benedek GB, Carey MC. Quasielastic light-scattering studies of aqueous biliary lipid systems. Mixed micelle formation in bile salt–lecithin solutions. Biochemistry. 1980;19:601–15.

27. Donovan JM, Jackson AA. Rapid determination by centrifugal ultrafiltration of the inter-mixed micellar/vesicular (non-lecithin associated) bile salt concentrations in model bile: influence of Donnan equilibrium effect. J Lipid Res. 1993;34:1121–9.

28. Fahey DA, Donovan JM, Carey MC. Bile acid–lecithin interactions in mixed monomolecular layers: a powerful tool to investigate bile acid cytoprotection as well as penetrating/perturbing effect on biomembranes. Hepatology. 1993;18:576.

29. Oelberg DG, Wang LB, Sackman JW, Adcock EW, Lester R, Dubinsky WP. Bile salt-induced calcium fluxes in artificial phospholipid vesicles. Biochim Biophys Acta. 1988;937:289–99.

30. Donovan JM, Jackson AA, Zeidel ML. Hydrophobic but not hydrophilic bile salts dramatically increase membrane permeability to calcium in model systems. Gastroenterology. 1994;106: A885.

Section III
Bile acid biosynthesis

7
Presentation of the Adolf Windaus Prize 1994

J. SJÖVALL

It is a great honour for me to present the Adolf Windaus Prize 1994. The prize is awarded for outstanding achievements in the field of bile acid research. It has been donated by the Falk Foundation, and on behalf of all scientists in this field I wish to thank Dr Herbert Falk for his donation and continued support in furthering this field which we find so interesting and important.

Previous presentations have all been made by Professor Gerok, who is unable to be present here in San Diego. Being from Freiburg he usually started with a brief presentation of Adolf Windaus. This is where, in 1901, Windaus started his remarkable research career which led to a Nobel Prize in chemistry in 1928 for 'research into the constitution of the sterols and their connection with the vitamins'. Being in Stockholm I went to the library of the Nobel Committee to read the biography and Nobel lecture of Windaus. Professor Gerok related that on one occasion Windaus refused to be photographed because he found neither time nor pleasure in such activity. I show here an exception to this attitude; it is the official photo from the records of the Nobel ceremonies in 1928.

In those days the Nobel Prize in chemistry was usually given to single individuals. However, the prize for 1927 had been reserved, and was awarded to Heinrich Wieland for 'his investigations of the constitution of the bile acids and related substances'. Wieland and Windaus both came to Stockholm in 1928 to receive their prizes and deliver their lectures.

The lectures are extraordinary reading. How could these men arrive at such results with the methods available? Is this how results of today will be viewed 60 years from now? While the structures of cholesterol and bile acids were wrong at the time Wieland and Windaus received their prizes, alternatives were considered as shown in Wieland's lecture. X-ray results by Bernal, and reinterpretation of some chemical reactions, provided the final keys for the correct structures to be assigned in 1932.

Windaus was quite unknown, except to a narrow circle of chemists, when he received his prize. He had worked on the structure of cholesterol for over 25 years. This must have been a heroic project and not an area in fashion; but Windaus said that a substance that was so widespread in occurrence must be very

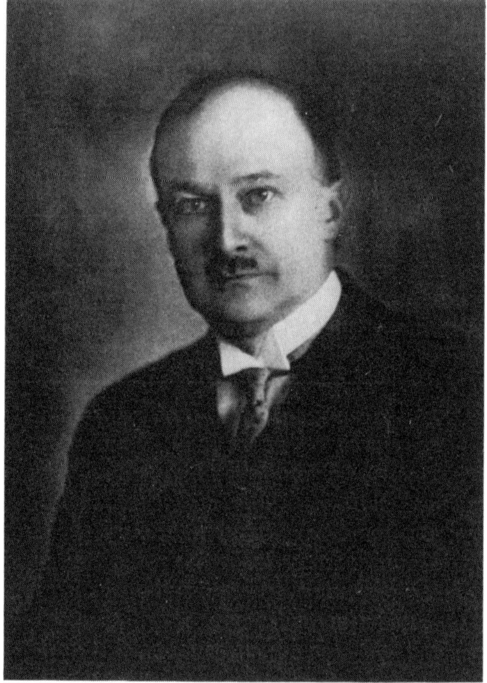

Adolf Windaus

important for the organism. For Windaus, the solving of basic problems came first, and applications were secondary.

However, it is clear both from Wieland's and Windaus' lectures that, without potential applications, research would not be sufficiently supported and funded. Wieland, who discovered the structures of the complexes with deoxycholic acid called choleic acids, said that if it had not been for the potential therapeutic use of this property of deoxycholic acid, 'it would have been impossible to master, with the technical resources of a scientific laboratory, the quantity of initial material required to determine the constitution of the bile acids'. Windaus related what he later called the peculiar and tortuous road to vitamin D that had started in medicine and physiology. When it seemed possible that a sterol was a provitamin D, Windaus was invited by the physiologist Hess, in New York in 1925, to work on the problem, since he was the 'foremost expert in the field of sterols'. Thus, a potential application gave Windaus the opportunity to work on what he thought was important. This led to the discovery of ergosterol as a provitamin D. Then Windaus went on to clarify vitamins D_2 and D_3 and to isolate vitamin D_3 from fish-liver oil. Thus, we can see that fashion and applications influenced basic research in those days, as they do now.

It is a serious responsibility to select a recipient of a prize bearing the name Adolf Windaus. The selection committee, with H. Dowling, W. Gerok, A. Hofmann, G. Paumgartner, D. Small, A. Stiehl and myself, came to the decision to award this year's prize to Z. Reno Vlahcevic, Division of Gastroenterology, Medical College of Virginia.

Dr Vlahcevic was born in Zagreb, Croatia, where he got his MD and early medical training. He then emigrated to the United States, specialized in gastroenterology/hepatology and came to the Medical College of Virginia, where he is now professor and chairman of the division of gastroenterology.

Dr Vlahcevic was not a youth when he entered the field of bile acid research around 1970 under the guidance of Leon Swell. His first studies concerned bile acid kinetics in patients with gallstones. The novel finding that the bile acid pool was diminished in these patients greatly stimulated clinical bile acid research, not least with regard to gallstone dissolution with bile acids. Mechanisms behind this change are still being studied. In the mid-1970s (together with Schwartz and Swell) Dr Vlahcevic published a number of studies concerning cholesterol pools for bile acid synthesis. After measuring the kinetics of labelled cholesterol and mevalonic acid in humans they arrived at a model where most of the bile acids were formed from free cholesterol in lipoproteins, and a small proportion from newly synthesized cholesterol. They also showed that the cholesterol came mainly from high-density lipoproteins. Their work also led to studies of alternative pathways in bile acid biosynthesis, an area which is presently of considerable interest with regard to the control of the degradation of cholesterol of different origin.

In the 1980s Dr Vlahcevic started collaboration with Hylemon and others, to study regulation of bile acid biosynthesis in isolated hepatocytes. This led to the concept of a correlation between bile acid hydrophobicity and feedback inhibition of cholesterol 7α-hydroxylase. Since this time the focus of Dr Vlahcevic's research has been on the regulation of several enzymes in the bile acid biosynthetic pathways. A finding of considerable experimental importance was that the combined addition of dexamethesone and thyroxine greatly increased the activity of cholesterol 7α-hydroxylase and increased the level of its mRNA in isolated rat hepatocytes. This finding made these cells useful for studies of the control of bile acid synthesis, both by feedback mechanisms and by hormones. The hormone combination had a similar effect in the case of 3α-hydroxysteroid dehydrogenase and, in addition, dexamethasone prolonged the half-life time of this enzyme markedly. Dr Vlahcevic and his group are presently very active in the field of regulatory mechanisms. Physiological and biochemical methods are combined with the methods of molecular biology to obtain a comprehensive view of the regulation of bile acid formation and its relationship to the regulation of cholesterol synthesis. Cells and animals are manipulated in different ways with hormones, inhibitors, cholesterol precursors and bile acids. Enzyme activities, half-life times, mRNA levels and transcriptional rates are then measured. Special emphasis has been put on the regulation of cholesterol 7α-hydroxylase. Interesting connections between the synthesis of cholesterol and some of its precursors or metabolites and the transcriptional regulation of cholesterol 7α-hydroxylase have been discovered. This has occurred during the past few years, which have been very productive.

In summary, Dr Vlahcevic has made important contributions to our knowledge about bile acid physiology and biochemistry in the interface between basic and clinical research. He has stimulated an interdisciplinary collaboration that has been very important for the development of the bile acid field. In this process he has helped a number of very talented young scientists to enter the field. The results that have been produced have influenced the directions of bile acid research.

8
Adolf Windaus Prize Lecture: Studies of cholesterol degradative pathways in the rat

Z. R. VLAHCEVIC

I would like to thank the members of the Nominating Committee for selecting me as this year's recipient of the Adolf Windaus Prize. I am certain that there are many other investigators whose contribution to bile acid research was equally deserving of this prize. For this reason I accept the Adolf Windaus Prize with a sense of pride and gratitude, on behalf of all of those who have helped me earn it. I would like to use this opportunity to extend my thanks to Dr Falk who, for over two decades, has provided the best forum for presentation of research in bile acid metabolism. By organizing this and many other meetings, he has done more than any other person or institution in promoting scientific exchange between basic scientists, clinical investigators and clinicians from around the world. I and others have been the beneficiaries of this extraordinary effort, and for this I thank him profoundly.

The acceptance of the Adolf Windaus Prize is enormously gratifying and, for me, it is undoubtedly the crowning moment of my professional career. However, the journey to here has been equally gratifying. It started in 1959 with the decision to emigrate from my native country to the United States in order to start an academic career. This decision was enthusiastically supported by my parents. I now fully appreciate the enormity of this personal sacrifice, and would like to honour their generosity and selflessness by acknowledging it. In the United States I have been assisted by many wonderful individuals, who helped in shaping my career. My thanks go to Dr Henry Stebbins who, upon my arrival as an intern in Salem Hospital, Salem, Massachusetts, was my first mentor. He tutored me in English and taught me the basics of the practice of clinical medicine. Without him I would not have survived the first two trying years in the United States. My lucky streak continued by meeting Ed Moore at the Lemuel Shattuck Hospital in Boston, who dazzled me with his intellect and infected me with enthusiasm for research. He introduced me to clinical investigation and was my first scientific mentor. After completion of my training in gastroenterology/ hepatology I was fortunate to meet Leon Swell, an outstanding scientist who taught me all I know about research. Without him I would not be standing in front of you today.

Fifteen years ago, Phil Hylemon (a recipient of the Adolf Windaus Prize in 1990) and I started a very productive scientific collaboration which is continuing up to this time. He has been a superb friend and collaborator, tireless worker and creative force behind many of our research endeavours. As Chairman of the Division of Gastroenterology at the Medical College of Virginia, I have been in a position to attract to research a number of young and talented investigators such as Chuck Schwartz, Doug Heuman, Mike Pandak and Todd Stravitz, all of whom are working in different aspects of bile research and are now part of our Lipid Research Group in Richmond. Three of them are presenting their data at this meeting. The future of research in cholesterol and bile acid metabolism in our institution will rest on them, and I consider this the greatest accomplishment of my professional career.

My research in bile acid metabolism started in 1967, and for the first 20 years it involved studies in humans. Specifically, I was involved in studies of cholesterol and bile acid metabolism in patients with gallstones and in patients with liver disease. Later I became involved in studies of exchange of cholesterol between plasma and liver with the expressed purpose of determining the sources of cholesterol for bile acid synthesis and biliary cholesterol secretion. I also carried out extensive studies of bile acid biosynthetic pathways in humans. Because of time restriction I will not discuss this earlier work. Instead, I will focus on our recent studies of regulation of cholesterol degradative pathways in the rat.

The synthesis of primary bile acids from cholesterol occurs exclusively in the liver via 'neutral' and 'acidic' bile acid biosynthetic pathways (Fig. 1). The end-products of the neutral pathway are cholic and chenodeoxycholic acids. The conversion of cholesterol to these two primary bile acids involves 14 enzymatic reactions taking place in four different organelles. The initial step in this pathway is conversion of cholesterol to 7α-hydroxycholesterol. This conversion is catalysed by cholesterol 7α-hydroxylase, a microsomal P450 monooxygenase, which is also thought to be rate-determining in the neutral pathway. The first step in the acidic pathway is conversion of cholesterol to 27-hydroxycholesterol. This step is catalysed by sterol 27-hydroxylase, a mitochondrial P450 enzyme. The predominant end-product of this pathway is chenodeoxycholic acid. The contribution of this pathway to total bile acid synthesis is still uncertain. Several recent studies by Princen *et al.*[1], Axelson and Sjövall[2], and our own studies (unpublished data), have indicated that the acidic pathway may contribute as much as 50% of total bile acid synthesis. This chapter will focus on the regulation of cholesterol 7α-hydroxylase and sterol 27-hydroxylase, the two enzymes which initiate the synthesis of bile acids via these two pathways. The studies of regulation of these two pathways are of great importance, since 50% of total cholesterol elimination from the body each day occurs via its conversion to bile acids.

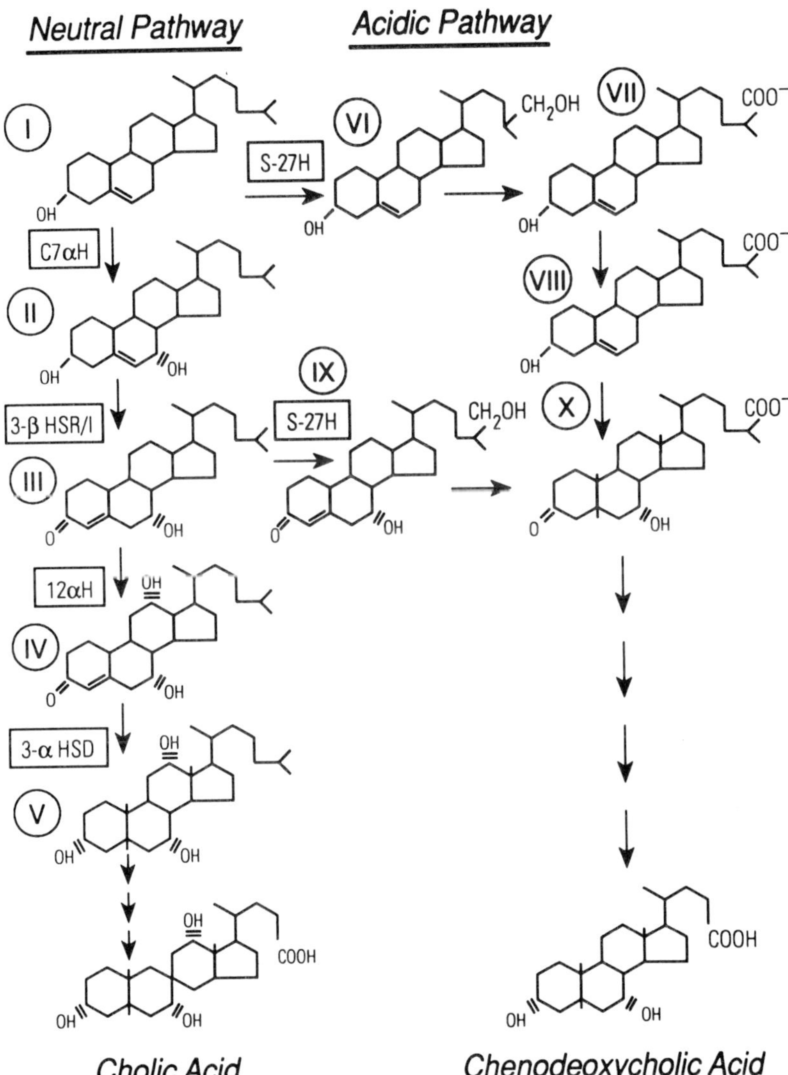

Fig. 1 Neutral and acidic bile acid biosynthetic pathways. Cholesterol 7α-hydroxylase (C7αH) and sterol 27-hydroxylase (S-27) initiate neutral and acidic pathways, respectively. Cholesterol 7α-hydroxylase is also a rate-determining step in the neutral pathway. 3β-Hydroxysteroid oxido-reductase/isomerase (3HSR/I), 12α-hydroxylase (12αH) and 3α-hydroxysteroid dehydrogenase (3αHSD) denoted in this figure are additional enzymes in the neutral pathway, the regulation of which has been studied by our group, but is not reported here. No information is available on the regulation of other enzymes in these two pathways

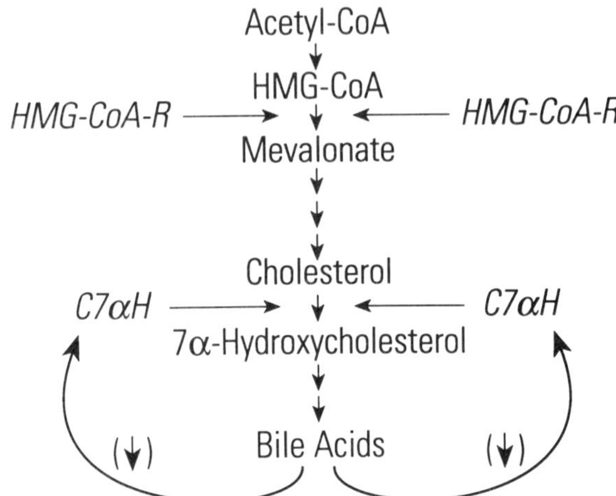

Fig. 2 Regulation of bile acid synthesis: negative feedback control of cholesterol 7α-hydroxylase (C7αH) by bile acids as perceived in 1986. The general consensus was that *all* bile acids down-regulate C7αH. The role of bile acids in the regulation of HMG-CoA reductase was not known

REGULATION OF CHOLESTEROL 7*a*-HYDROXYLASE BY BILE ACIDS

Based on the work of Bergstrom, Danielsson, Mosbach and many others[3], the general consensus in the mid-1980s was that cholesterol 7α-hydroxylase is regulated by *all* bile acids via negative feedback control (Fig. 2). Neither the molecular basis of this regulation nor the effects of other potential regulators on cholesterol 7α-hydroxylase were known at that time. In the mid-1980s Davis *et al.*[4,5] and our group[6] were unable to demonstrate feedback control of bile acid synthesis in primary rat hepatocytes even after addition of supraphysiological concentrations of different bile acids. The lack of feedback regulation of bile acid synthesis in this experimental model was puzzling. Based on data in primary hepatocytes, Davis *et al.*[4,5] postulated that cholesterol substrate availablity may be a more important regulator of cholesterol 7α-hydroxylase than are bile acids. In order to reconcile the discrepancies between the *in vitro* and *in vivo* experiments, we initiated a series of *in vivo* experiments in which we fed seven bile acids of different hydrophobicity to rats with intact enterohepatic circulation, and determined cholesterol 7α-hydroxylase and HMG-CoA reductase-specific activities at the time of sacrifice (Fig. 3). To our surprise, hydrophilic bile acids had no effect on HMG-CoA reductase or cholesterol 7α-hydroxylase-specific activities, while relatively hydrophobic bile acids down-regulated both enzymes in order of progressive hydrophobicity[7]. These data confirmed the existence of negative feedback control of cholesterol 7α-hydroxylase. Thus, for the first time, the specific role of hydrophobic bile acids in the regulation of these two enzymes was recognized (Fig. 4). These studies, however, have not provided any data on the molecular basis of regulation of cholesterol 7α-hydroxylase; nor have they offered any explanation as to why hydrophobic bile acids regulate cholesterol 7α-hydroxylase while hydrophilic bile acids do not.

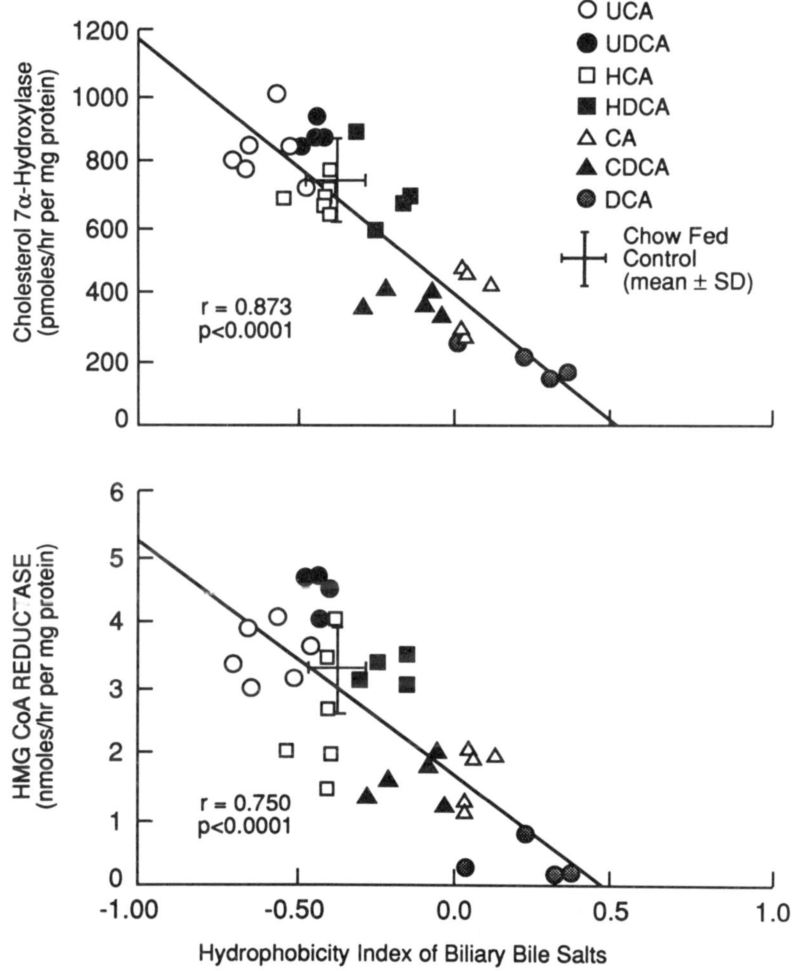

Fig. 3 Down-regulation of cholesterol 7α-hydroxylase and HMG-CoA reductase is exerted *only* by hydrophobic, but not by hydrophilic, bile acids. The down-regulation of both enzymes by hydrophobic bile acids was in order of progressing hydrophobicity

In 1990 three investigators, Okuda, Chiang and Russell, reported almost simultaneously the cloning and sequencing of rat cholesterol 7α-hydroxylase gene coupled with characterization of mRNA and protein[8]. This was a major accomplishment because it provided the opportunity to define the molecular basis of regulation of this important enzyme. In collaboration with Dr Chiang, who provided us with the specific antibody to cholesterol 7α-hydroxylase and cDNA probe, Pandak *et al.* from our laboratory[9] were able to show that cholesterol 7α-hydroxylase-specific activity, enzyme mass, steady-state mRNA levels and transcriptional activity increased 3–5-fold following biliary diversion, and decreased to normal levels following infusion of 36 μmol of taurocholate/100 g

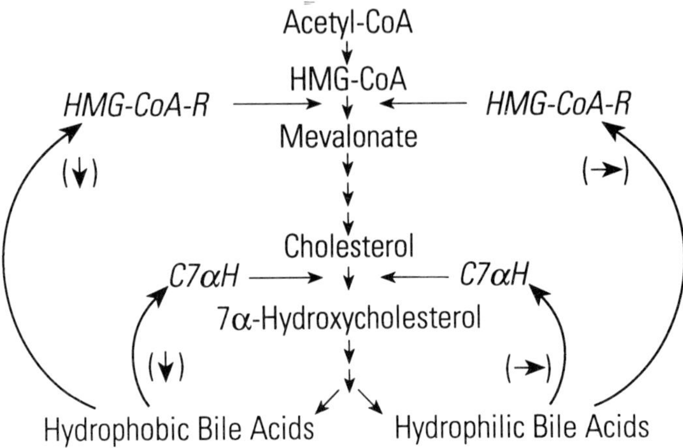

Fig. 4 Regulation of bile acid synthesis (1990): only hydrophobic bile acids down-regulate HMG-CoA reductase and cholesterol 7α-hydroxylase; hydrophilic bile acids have no effect on either enzyme. The molecular basis of regulation of cholesterol 7α-hydroxylase by hydrophobic bile acids was not known

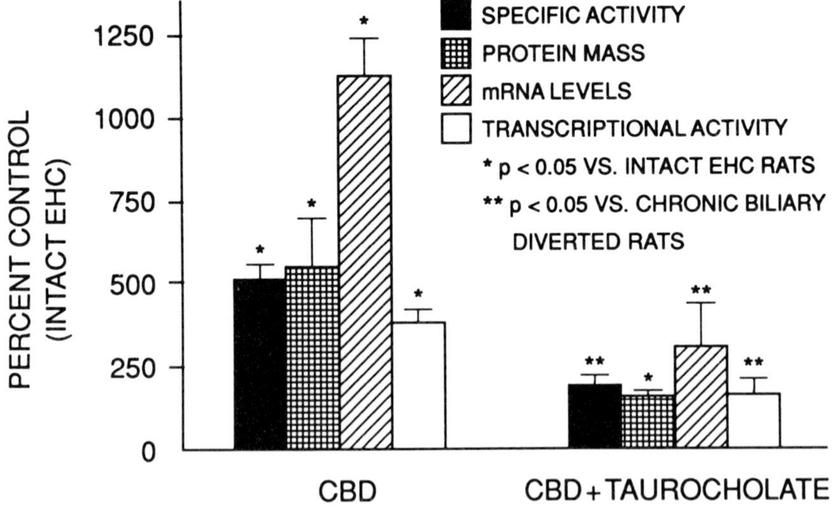

Fig. 5 Effects of chronic biliary diversion and chronic biliary diversion (CBD) plus infusion of taurocholate (CBD+taurocholate; $36\,\mu$mol/10 g rat per hour) on cholesterol 7α-hydroxylase-specific activity, enzyme mass, mRNA levels and transcriptional activity. A marked increase was observed in all four parameters following biliary diversion. Return to almost control level (intact rat) occurred following intraduodenal infusion of taurocholate to rats with chronic biliary diversion. *$p<0.05$ vs. intact EHC rats; **$p<0.05$ vs. chronic biliary diverted rats

rat per hour (Fig. 5). These studies were extended to rats with intact entero-hepatic circulation[10] fed cholestyramine (0.5% in diet) and cholic (1%), cheno-deoxycholic (1%) and deoxycholic (0.5%) acids for 14 days. In the intact rats the specific activity, mRNA levels and transcriptional activity increased 3-fold following cholestyramine feeding. In contrast, cholic, chenodeoxycholic, and

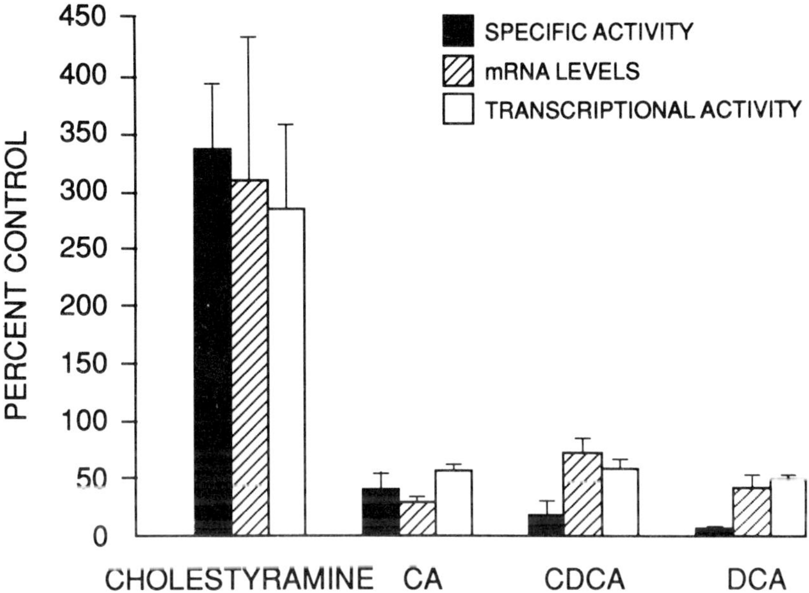

Fig. 6 Effects of cholestyramine (5%) and bile acid feeding (0.5–1.0%) on cholesterol 7α-hydroxylase-specific activity, mRNA and transcription in rats with intact enterohepatic circulation. A marked increase was observed in all three parameters following cholestyramine feeding, and a decrease following feeding of three bile acids (cholic acid = CA; chenodeoxycholic acid = CDCA; and deoxycholic acid = DCA)

deoxycholic acid feeding decreased all three parameters by approximately 50% (Fig. 6). Following these *in vivo* experiments we extended our studies to primary rat hepatocytes, in which we demonstrated that relatively hydrophobic bile acids, taurocholate and taurodeoxycholate, decreased cholesterol 7α-hydroxylase mRNA levels, while a hydrophilic bile acid, tauroursodeoxycholate, had no effect (Fig. 7). Addition of physiological concentrations of taurocholate (50 μmol) to primary rat hepatocytes also caused a 60% decrease in cholesterol 7α-hydroxylase gene transcriptional activity (Fig. 8)[11]. Our data on the regulation of cholesterol 7α-hydroxylase in Hep G2 cells (presented at this meeting in a poster session by Dr Pandak) are in agreement with *in vitro* results obtained in primary rat hepatocytes[12].

Thus, *in vivo* and *in vitro* data (primary rat hepatocytes, Hep G2 cells) have provided evidence that hydrophobic bile acids down-regulate cholesterol 7α-hydroxylase predominantly at the level of gene transcription (Fig. 9). Most studies on the regulation of cholesterol 7α-hydroxylase done by other investigators are consistent with these conclusions. Thus, in 1992, our studies provided additional information on the molecular basis of regulation of cholesterol 7α-hydroxylase by hydrophobic bile acids.

Next, we studied the mechanism of interaction between hydrophobic bile acids and cholesterol 7α-hydroxylase promoter region. Two possible models could explain our previous findings (Fig. 10). In the first ('direct' model), bile acids bind to bile acid receptors, enter the nucleus and bind to a bile acid responsive

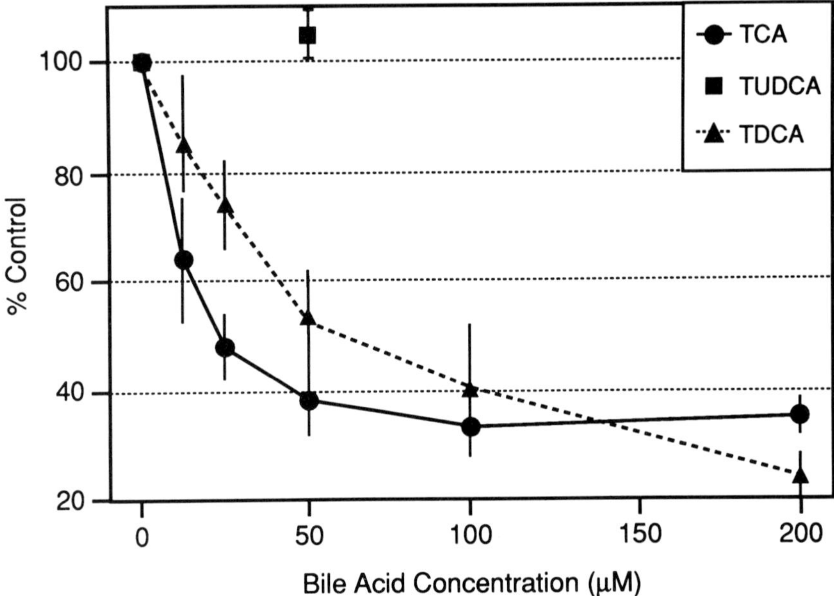

Fig. 7 In primary rat hepatocytes, taurocholate (TCA) and taurodeoxycholate (TDCA) decreased cholesterol 7α-hydroxylase mRNA levels in a concentration-dependent fashion. Tauroursodeoxycholate (TUDCA) had no effect on mRNA levels

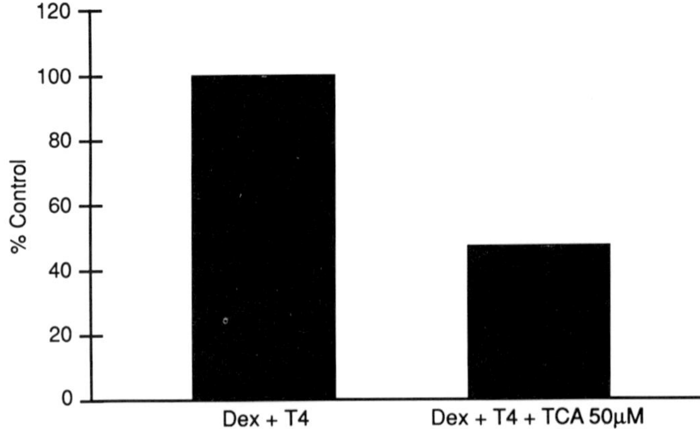

Fig. 8 Addition of taurocholate (TCA; 50 μmol/l) to primary rat hepatocytes decreases cholesterol 7α-hydroxylase transcriptional activity by approximately 60%

element in the 5' flanking region of the cholesterol 7α-hydroxylase gene, which in turn represses cholesterol 7α-hydroxylase gene transcription. In the 'indirect' model bile acids activate a signal transduction cascade, which in turn causes covalent modification of a transacting factor which interacts with cholesterol 7α-hydroxylase promoter and results in the repression of transcription of the cholesterol 7α-hydroxylase gene. Recent data by Dr Stravitz from our group

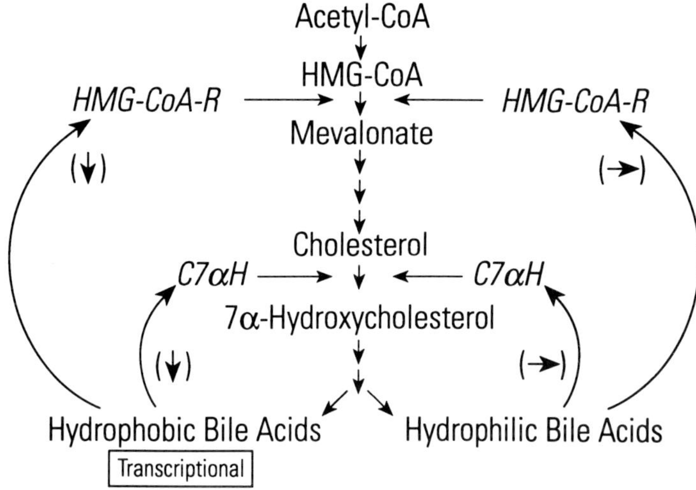

Fig. 9 Regulation of bile acid synthesis (1990): in *in vivo* and *in vitro* experiments, hydrophobic bile acids repress cholesterol 7α-hydroxylase predominantly at the level of gene transcription

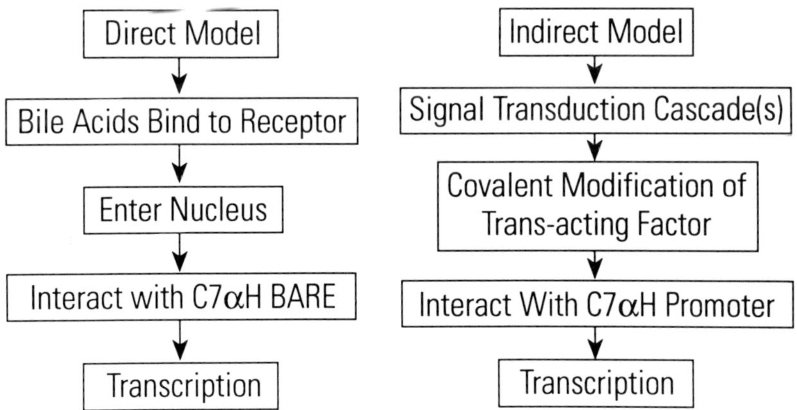

Fig. 10 Two models of possible interaction of hydrophobic bile acids with 5′ flanking region of cholesterol 7α-hydroxylase gene

demonstrate that hydrophobic bile acids down-regulate cholesterol 7αhydroxylase gene transcription *indirectly*, i.e. by activating protein kinase C[13]. These data will be presented by Dr Stravitz at this meeting, and can be reviewed in the proceedings of the meeting.

In order to determine whether down-regulation of cholesterol 7α-hydroxylase requires the presence of bile acids in the enterohepatic circulation, we compared the effects of equimolar infusions of taurocholate (36 μmol/100 g rat liver per hour) *intravenously* and *intraduodenally*. In order to avoid haemolysis, taurocholate was administered intravenously with a large volume of isotonic saline. Two groups of control rats received identical fluxes of taurocholate intra-

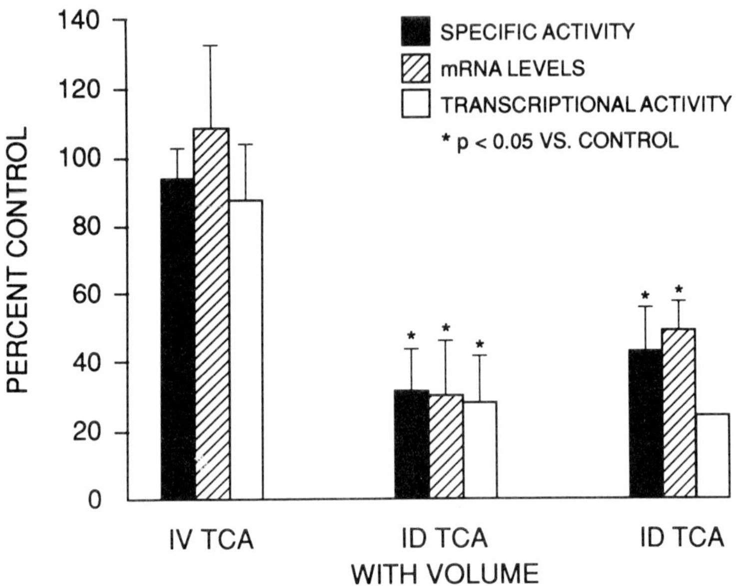

Fig. 11 The effects of intravenous vs. intraduodenal (with and without added volume) infusions of equimolar concentrations of taurocholate (36 μmol/100 g rat per hour) on cholesterol 7α-hydroxylase-specific activity, mRNA levels and gene transcription. There was no evidence of a decrease of cholesterol 7α-hydroxylase-specific activity, mRNA levels or gene transcriptional activity by intravenous administration of taurocholate (IV TCA). As previously observed, marked decreases of all three parameters (50–60%) were observed with intraduodenal infusions of taurocholate (ID TCA with volume and ID TCA)

duodenally with a large volume (identical to the volume received by the rats infused intravenously) and without the added fluid. The bile flow, bile acid secretion and recovery of labelled bile acids was almost identical in all three groups of experimental models. To our surprise the intravenous infusion of taurocholate failed to repress cholesterol 7α-hydroxylase-specific activity, mRNA levels or gene transcriptional activity (Fig. 11). In contrast, equimolar infusions of taurocholate intraduodenally (with or without added volume) repressed all three parameters by 50–60%. We concluded that intestinal circulation of bile acids is necessary to transcriptionally down-regulate cholesterol 7α-hydroxylase. We speculate (Fig. 12) that bile acids in the intestines release a luminal or humoral factor which, in conjunction with hydrophobic bile acids, represses cholesterol 7α-hydroxylase[14]. We are presently investigating the effects of glucagon and enteroglucagon on cholesterol 7α-hydroxylase. The blood levels of these hormones were reported to increase following intestinal perfusion of bile acids. The release of these intestinal hormones by bile acids could explain our finding, particularly since glucagon is a powerful *in vitro* repressor of cholesterol 7α-hydroxylase (see below). Alternatively, bacterial metabolites of cholic acid, such as deoxycholic acid, could down-regulate 7α-hydroxylase as proposed by Stange *et al.*[15]. These possibilities are presently being investigated in our laboratories. However, until these experiments are completed, we postulate that

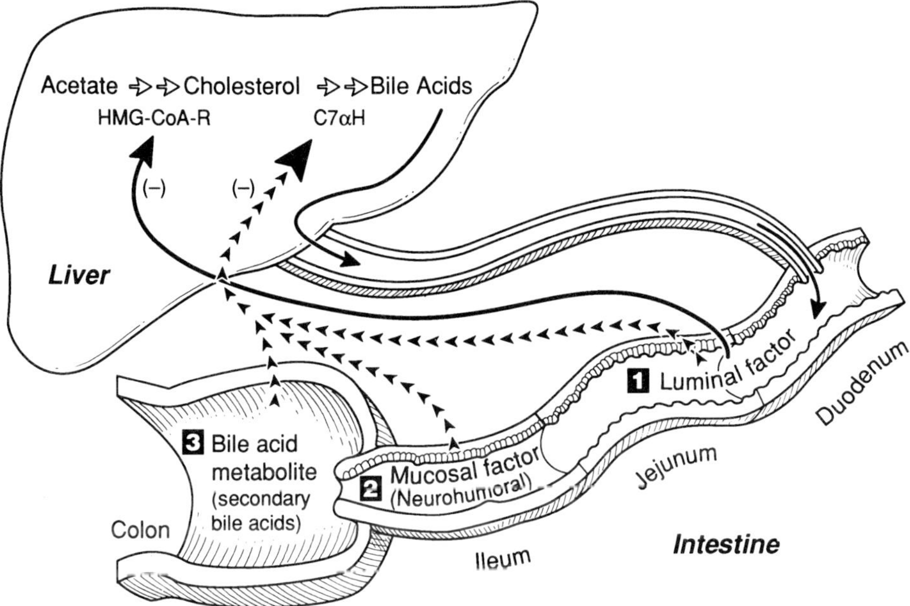

Fig. 12 Possible mechanism by which intraduodenal infusion of taurocholate down-regulates choleterol 7α-hydroxylase

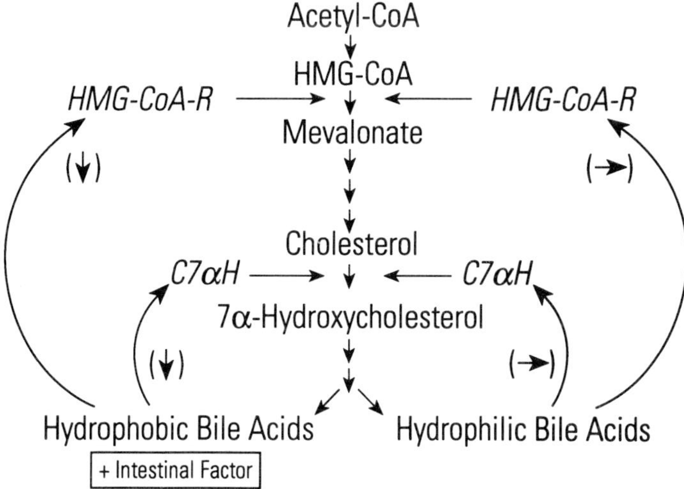

Fig. 13 Regulation of bile acid synthesis (1992): in the *in vivo* situation, enterohepatic circulation of hydrophobic bile acids is prerequisite for down-regulation of cholesterol 7α-hydroxylase. The co-regulation of cholesterol 7α-hydroxylase by hydrophobic bile acids and the putative intestinal factor is postulated

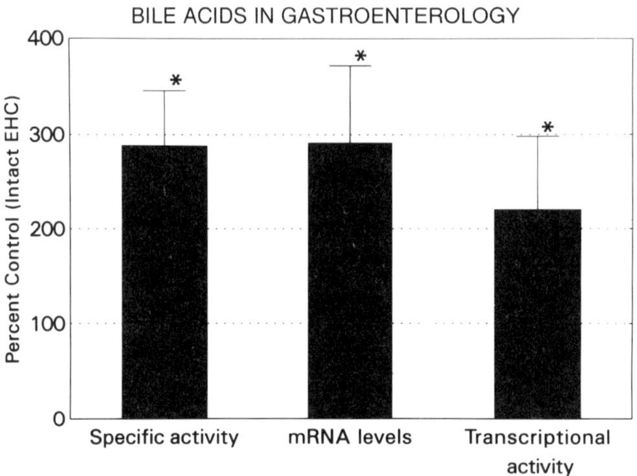

Fig. 14 Specific activity, mRNA levels and transcription of cholesterol 7α-hydroxylase are elevated approximately 3-fold following feeding of a diet high in cholesterol to rats with intact enterohepatic circulation. $*p < 0.05$ vs. respective control

in an *in vivo* situation cholesterol 7α-hydroxylase is regulated by hydrophobic bile acids in tandem with an as yet undefined intestinal factor (Fig. 13).

REGULATION OF CHOLESTEROL 7*a*-HYDROXYLASE BY CHOLESTEROL

At this point there was a need to define the potential role of other effectors on the regulation of cholesterol 7α-hydroxylase. Cholesterol, a precursor of bile acids, most likely plays a role in the regulation of this enzyme. Very few data are available on the role of cholesterol in the regulation of cholesterol 7α-hydroxylase. In 1991 Pandak *et al.*[9] have shown that a high-cholesterol diet increased cholesterol 7α-hydroxylase-specific activity, mRNA levels and transcriptional activity by approximately 3-fold (Fig. 14). However, Björkhem *et al.*[16] provided suggestive evidence that a diet high in cholesterol may result in bile acid malabsorption. Hence, the aforementioned data by Pandak *et al.* could be interpreted as a result of a 'cholestyramine-like' effect of a high-cholesterol diet. In order to circumvent the presumed effect of dietary cholesterol on the intestinal bile acid metabolism, we administered intravenous infusion of mevalonate ($180\,\mu$mol/h) for different time periods (1.5, 3.0, 4.5 and 24h) to rats with intact enterohepatic circulation[17]. At all time periods mevalonate, a precursor of cholesterol which is readily converted to cholesterol, increased cholesterol 7α-hydroxylase-specific activity, mRNA levels and transcription 2–3-fold (Fig. 15). These data suggest that *in vivo* cholesterol may be an important up-regulator of cholesterol 7α-hydroxylase. The role of cholesterol in the regulation of cholesterol 7α-hydroxylase has been studied further in rats with chronic bile fistula with maximal cholesterol and bile acid synthesis. Administration of a single dose of lovastatin, a potent HMG-CoA reductase inhibitor, resulted in a 40% suppression of cholesterol 7α-hydroxylase-specific activity, enzyme mass, mRNA and gene transcriptional activity (Fig. 16)[17]. These data suggest that decrease in cholesterol availability turns off cholesterol 7α-hydroxylase gene transcription. In cultured rat hepato-

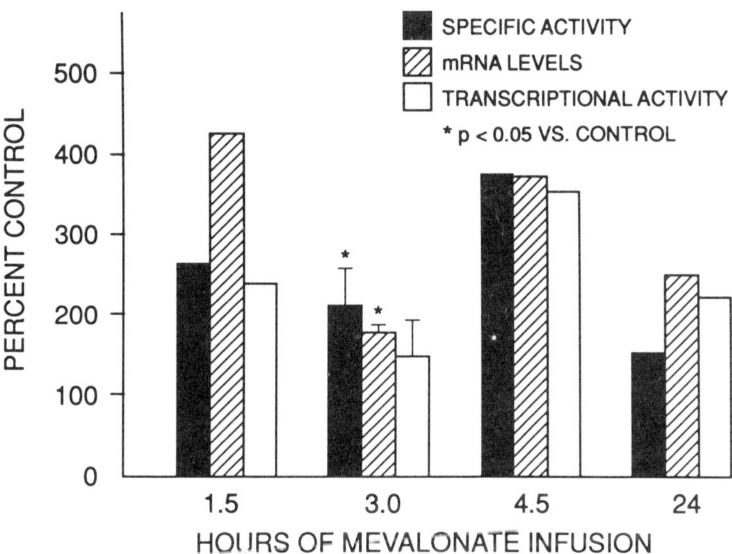

Fig. 15 Specific activities, mRNA levels and transcriptional activities are increased 2–3-fold following intravenous infusion of mevalonate at 1.4, 3.0, 4.5 and 24h in rats with intact enterohepatic circulation. Mevalonate is an intermediate in the cholesterol biosynthetic pathway which is rapidly converted to cholesterol and results in a rapid increase of specific activity, mRNA levels and transcriptional activity. These results are attributed to the excessive formation of newly synthesized cholesterol, and suggest that excess cholesterol turns the cholesterol 7α-hydroxylase gene on. $*p<0.05$ vs. control

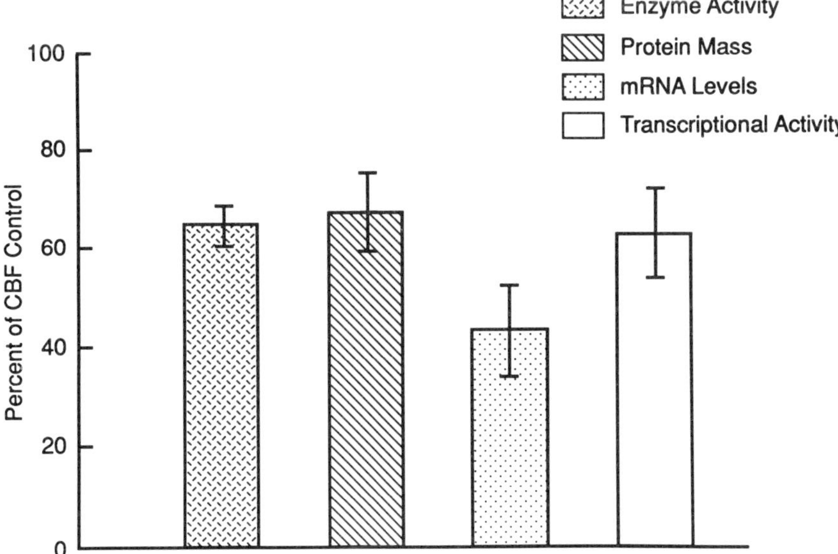

Fig. 16 The effect of a single dose of lovastatin, an inhibitor of HMG-CoA reductase, on cholesterol 7α-hydroxylase specific activity, enzyme mass, mRNA levels and gene transcription in rats with chronic biliary fistula. A 40% decrease in all four parameters was observed at 3h following lovastatin injection. These data suggest that a decrease in the availability of cholesterol turns the cholesterol 7α-hydroxylase gene off

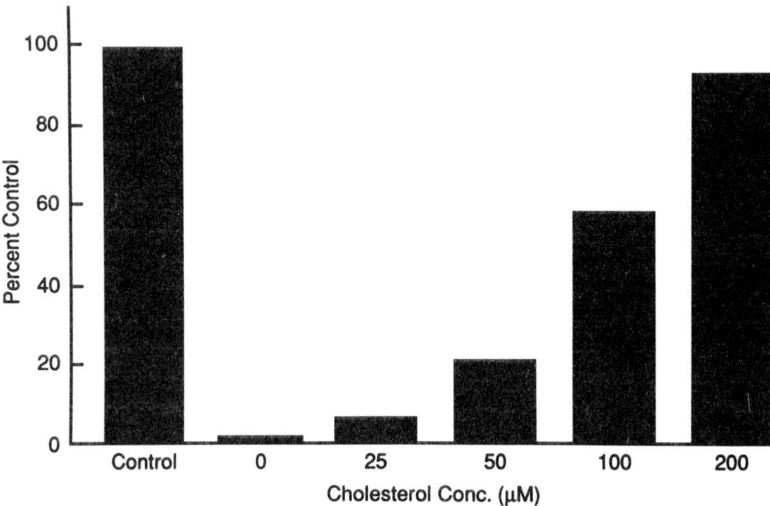

Fig. 17 Addition of squalestatin, a powerful inhibitor of cholesterol synthesis, to primary rat hepatocytes causes almost complete repression of cholesterol 7α-hydroxylase mRNA levels (line 0). These levels returned to normal following addition of increasing concentrations ($25-200\,\mu$mol/l) of cholesterol solubilized in liposomes

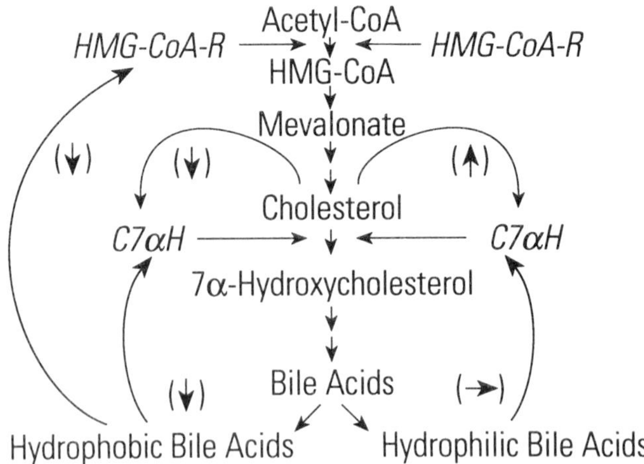

Fig. 18 Regulation of bile acid synthesis (1993): in addition to transcriptional down-regulation of cholesterol 7α-hydroxylase (C7αH) by hydrophobic bile acids, the cholesterol appears to be a potent up-regulator of cholesterol 7α-hydroxylase gene. Excess cholesterol turns the cholesterol 7α-hydroxylase gene on: deficient supply of cholesterol turns the gene off

cytes (fig. 17) squalestatin, a potent inhibitor of cholesterol synthesis, reduced cholesterol 7α-hydroxylase mRNA levels by 90%; the addition of increasing concentrations of cholesterol solubilized in liposomes to primary rat hepatocytes returned cholesterol 7α-hydroxylase mRNA to control levels. These *in vitro* data provided the most convincing evidence so far that, at least in the rat, cholesterol plays an important role in the regulation of cholesterol 7α-hydroxylase[18].

Thus, our *in vivo* and *in vitro* studies have provided strong evidence that, in the rat, cholesterol 7α-hydroxylase is regulated by cholesterol at the level of gene transcription (Fig. 18). When cholesterol is present in excess, cholesterol 7α-hydroxylase gene is turned on, allowing for the conversion of excess cholesterol to bile acids. When cholesterol supply is deficient, cholesterol 7α-hydroxylase is turned off, allowing for preservation of hepatic cholesterol. Thus, it appears that this finely tuned mechanism plays a role in the maintenance of cholesterol homeostasis in the rat. The mechanism by which cholesterol interacts with the 5′ flanking region of cholesterol 7α-hydroxylase is not known. The steroid-responsive element (SRE) CAC (C/G) (C/T) CAC, which has been identified in the promoter region of cholesterol (oxysterols) regulated genes such as HMG-CoA reductase, HMG-CoA synthase and low-density lipoprotein receptors, has not been identified in the cholesterol 7α-hydroxylase gene. However, several modified SRE repeats have been identified in the 5′ upstream region of rat cholesterol 7α-hydroxylase gene. It should be noted that oxysterols repress gene expression in the cholesterol biosynthetic pathway, whereas cholesterol or metabolic products of cholesterol up-regulate cholesterol 7α-hydroxylase in the rat. Thus, different steroid-responsive motifs may be present in the cholesterol 7α-hydroxylase gene. This area of regulation of cholesterol 7α-hydroxylase requires much additional work.

REGULATION OF CHOLESTEROL 7α-HYDROXYLASE BY BILE ACIDS IN THE PRESENCE OF EXCESS CHOLESTEROL

We also studied the interaction between the stimulatory effect of intravenously infused mevalonate ($180\,\mu$mol/h), a known cholesterol precursor and the down-regulatory effects of bile acids on cholesterol 7α-hydroxylase in rats with chronic bile fistula infused with taurocholate intraduodenally ($36\,\mu$mol/$100\,$g rat per hour). In rats with chronic biliary diversion (Fig. 19), intravenous infusion of mevalonate failed to overcome the down-regulatory effects of taurocholate administered intraduodenally[19]. Identical data were obtained in cultured rat hepatocytes in which addition of cholesterol failed to prevent the down-regulation of cholesterol 7α-hydroxylase by added taurocholate (Fig. 20). However, these *in vivo* and *in vitro* data suggest that the repressive effect of taurocholate on cholesterol 7α-hydroxylase is not altered by the availability of excess cholesterol. These conclusions are supported by studies in mice[20]. However, Spady *et al.*[21] showed that diet high in cholesterol can overcome the repressive effects of dietary cholate on cholesterol 7α-hydroxylase. The reason for these discrepancies is not known.

We speculate that cholesterol may be responsible for a basal level of cholesterol 7α-hydroxylase gene expression, while hydrophobic bile acids play a major role in modulating the level of cholesterol 7α-hydroxylase gene expression. The level of cholesterol 7α-hydroxylase gene expression in the liver is ultimately determined by the balance of these two regulatory compounds.

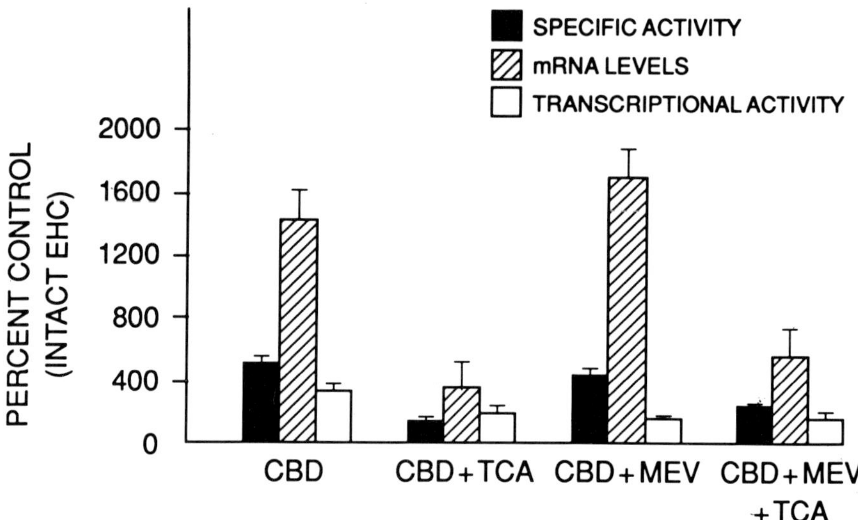

Fig. 19 Interaction of mevalonate (a source of newly synthesized cholesterol) and taurocholate (TCA) on the regulation of cholesterol 7α-hydroxylase-specific activity, mRNA and transcription. As in a previous experiment, TCA decreased all three parameters when infused intraduodenally to rats with chronic biliary diversion (CBD + TCA). Mevalonate (MEV) infusion does not prevent down-regulation of cholesterol 7α-hydroxylase by taurocholate (CBD + MEV + TCA). The mevalonate infusion alone (CBD + MEV) failed to increase significantly cholesterol 7α-hydroxylase-specific activity, mRNA and transcription

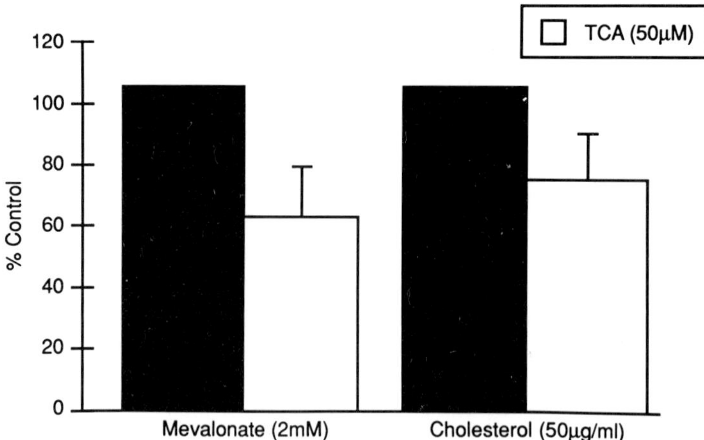

Fig. 20 Addition of mevalonate (2 mmol/l) and cholesterol (50 μg/ml) to taurocholate (TCA 50 μmol/l) added to primary rat hepatocytes failed to restore cholesterol 7α-hydroxylase gene transcriptional activity repressed by TCA

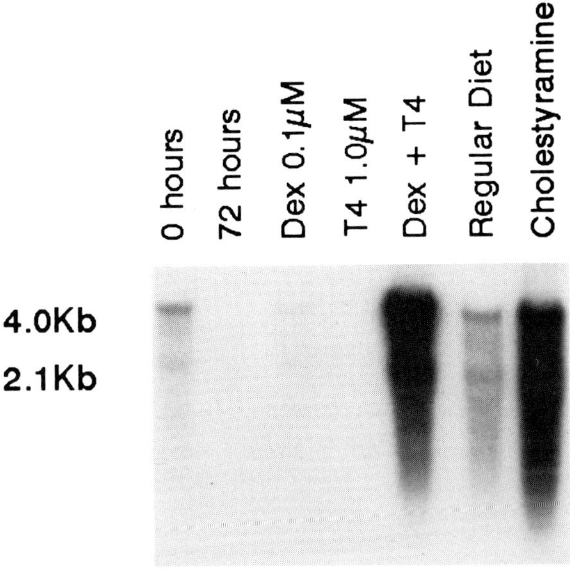

Fig. 21 At 72h after plating, cholesterol 7α-hydroxylase mRNA is not detectable (line 2) when compared to controls (line 1) by Northern blot. Addition of dexamethasone or thyroxine (lines 3 and 4) alone showed no increase in mRNA levels. Addition of combined thyroxine plus dexamethasone increased cholesterol 7α-hydroxylase mRNA levels (line 5) in excess of those found in the whole liver, even in rats fed cholestyramine (lines 6 and 7)

REGULATION OF CHOLESTEROL 7α-HYDROXYLASE BY HORMONES

The role of hormones in the regulation of cholesterol 7α-hydroxylase was suspected because this enzyme undergoes diurnal variation which can be abolished by adrenalectomy. However, no precise studies of regulation of cholesterol 7α-hydroxylase by hormones were in evidence until recently. We were the first to establish that, in the primary rat hepatocytes without addition of appropriate hormones, cholesterol 7α-hydroxylase mRNA was not expressed 72h after plating. These data provided an explanation for the lack of negative feedback control after addition of bile acids in supraphysiological concentrations to primary rat hepatocytes. Addition of physiological concentrations of dexamethasone and thyroxine alone also failed to increase cholesterol 7α-hydroxylase mRNA to detectable levels. However, the addition of both hormones resulted in a marked increase in cholesterol 7α-hydroxylase mRNA which exceeded the levels obtained in whole liver, even in rats pretreated with cholestyramine (Fig. 21)[22]. Addition of dexamethasone plus thyroxine in physiological concentrations also resulted in a 12-fold increase in cholesterol 7α-

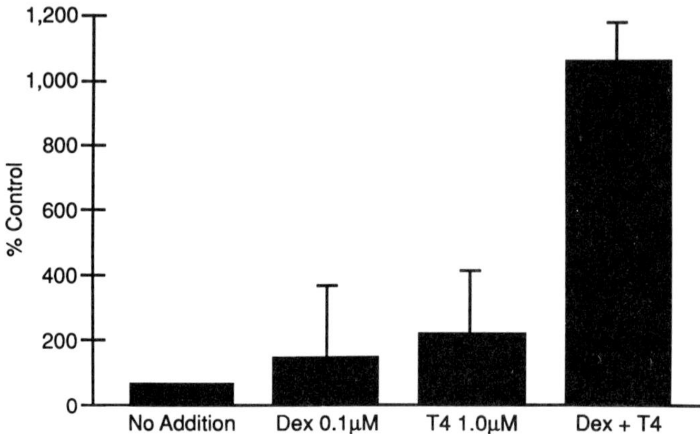

Fig. 22 Addition of dexamethasone plus thyroxine increases cholesterol 7α-hydroxylase transcriptional activity 12-fold. Addition of thyroxine and dexamethasone alone increased transcription 2.5- and 3.5-fold, respectively

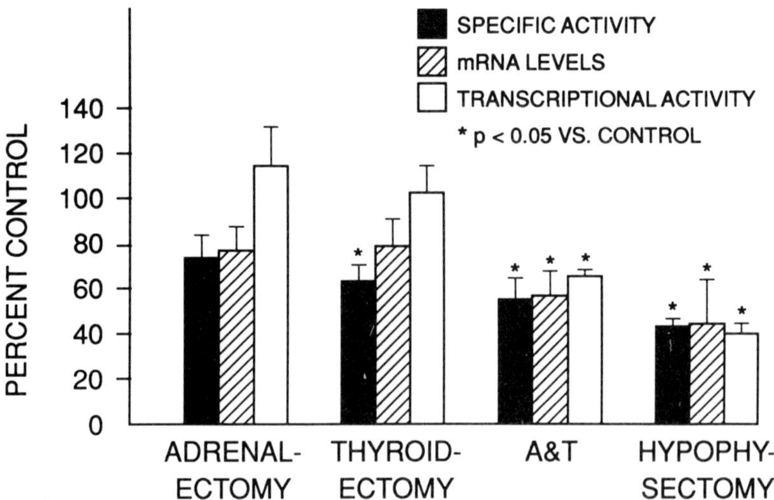

Fig. 23 Specific activities, mRNA levels and gene transcriptional activity are markedly decreased in hypophysectomized and adrenalectomized plus thyroidectomized rats (A&T). No significant change in any of the three parameters was observed in adrenalectomized or thyroidectomized rats. $*p<0.05$ vs. control

hydroxylase gene transcriptional activity (Fig. 22). The underlying mechanism responsible for the synergistic action of these two hormones on cholesterol 7α-hydroxylase transcription is still not clear.

In order to confirm these *in vitro* observations we carried out *in vivo* experiments in which cholesterol 7α-hydroxylase-specific activity, mRNA levels and transcriptional activity were determined in adrenalectomized, thyroidectomized,

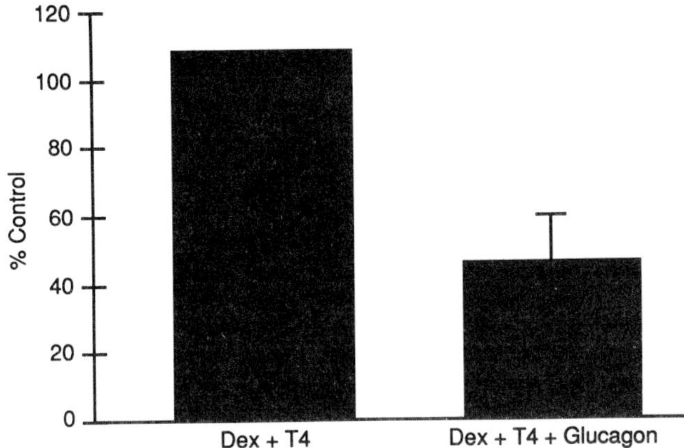

Fig. 24 Addition of glucagon (50 μmol) to primary rat hepatocytes decreased cholesterol 7α-hydroxylase gene transcriptional activity by 60%

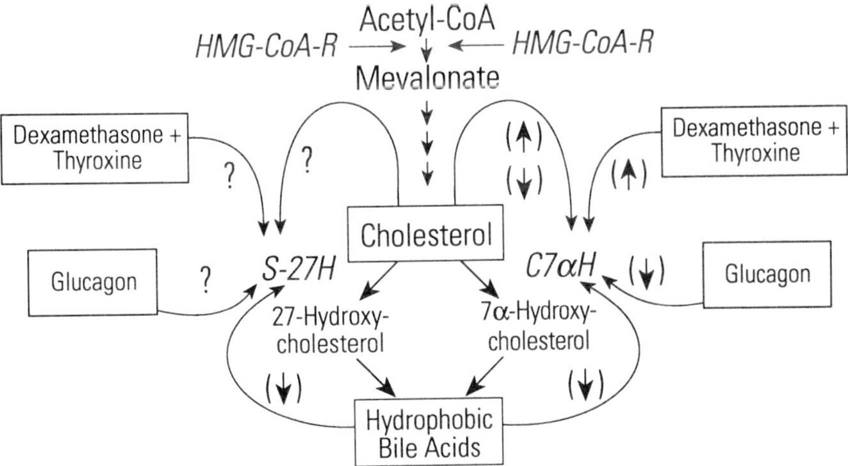

Fig. 25 Regulation of bile acid synthesis (1994): in addition to repressive action of hydrophobic bile acids and stimulatory action of cholesterol on cholesterol 7α-hydroxylase, we have demonstrated that the combination of thyroxine plus glucocorticoids turns on cholesterol 7α-hydroxylase transcription. In contrast, glucagon turns cholesterol 7α-hydroxylase gene off in both *in vitro* and *in vivo* experiments

adrenalectomized plus thyroidectomized, and hypophysectomized rats (Fig. 23). All three parameters were decreased by 50% in rats with combined thyroidectomy plus adrenalectomy, and in the hypophysectomized rats. By contrast, no statistically significant changes in these three parameters were observed in rats with thyroidectomy or adrenalectomy alone[23]. These data clearly demonstrate that *in vivo* cholesterol 7α-hydroxylase is also synergistically regulated by thyroxine and glucocorticoids. In additional experiments in primary rat hepatocytes we have shown that the physiological concentrations of glucagon in near-physiological concentrations decreases cholesterol 7α-hydroxylase gene transcriptional activity (Fig. 24). Similar results were obtained in *in vivo* experiments using constant infusion of glucagon (data not shown).

These *in vivo* and *in vitro* studies provided additional information on the regulation of cholesterol 7α-hydroxylase by different hormones (Fig. 25). The mechanism by which glucocorticoids and thyroxine synergistically interact with cholesterol 7α-hydroxylase promoter region is still not understood. An imperfect direct repeat TGGTCANNNNAGTTCA, which is similar to thyroxine-responsive element (TRA) is highly conserved in the cholesterol 7α-hydroxylase gene. A glucocorticoid half-site response element (GRE) TGTTCT has also been tentatively identified in the promoter region of the cholesterol 7α-hydroxylase gene. However, it remains to be determined whether these postulated sequences mediate regulation by glucocorticoids and thyroxine, thus opening another area for future research.

REGULATION OF STEROL 27-HYDROXYLASE

Sterol 27-hydroxylase catalyses the conversion of cholesterol to 27-hydroxycholesterol, the first committed step in the acidic pathway of bile acid biosynthesis. The same mitochondrial enzyme also initiates side-chain oxidation of bile acid intermediates in the neutral bile acid biosynthetic pathway. The deficiency of this enzyme has been implicated as a major cause of deficient bile acid synthesis in patients with cerebrotendinous xanthomatosis[24]. The enzyme has recently been cloned and characterized[25]. However, very little information is available on its regulation.

I will report our preliminary data on the molecular basis of regulation of sterol 27-hydroxylase by bile acids. In rats with bile fistula, specific activities of sterol 27-hydroxylase and cholesterol 7α-hydroxylase were determined on days 1, 3 and 5 following acute biliary diversion (Fig. 26). A marked increase of sterol 27-hydroxylase-specific activity was observed on days 3 and 5 following biliary diversion. This increase was not as pronounced as that observed with cholesterol 7α-hydroxylase. In rats with intact enterohepatic circulation (Fig. 27), cholestyramine feeding increased sterol 27-hydroxylase-specific activity by about 2-fold while cholic, chenodeoxycholic and deoxycholic acid feeding reduced the specific activities of sterol 27-hydroxylase by 35–40%. Similar data were obtained when we determined sterol 27-hydroxylase steady-state mRNA levels (data not shown). In both instances the repression of sterol 27-hydroxylase was less pronounced than that of cholesterol 7α-hydroxylase. Chenodeoxycholic acid feeding decreased sterol 27-hydroxylase gene transcriptional activity by about 40%, which was less pronounced than that observed with cholesterol 7α–hydroxylase. Lastly, both sterol 27-hydroxylase and cholesterol 7α-hydroxylase undergo diurnal variation; a marked increase in specific activities of both enzymes was observed in mid-dark as compared to mid-light periods (data not shown).

In summary, in the past 8 years we have learned a great deal about the regulation of two enzymes initiating neutral and acidic pathways of bile acid synthesis from cholesterol (Fig. 28). It is apparent from our studies that

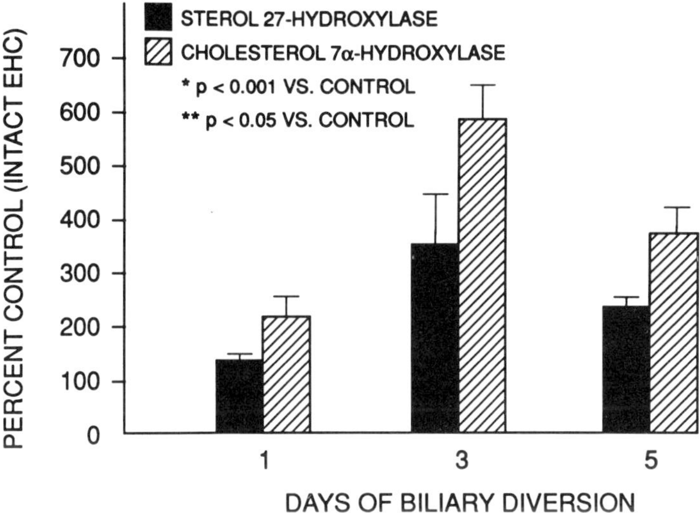

Fig. 26 Following biliary diversion there was an approximately 2-fold increase in sterol 27-hydroxylase specific activity on days 3 and 5. The increase in sterol 27-hydroxylase activity is not as pronounced as that of cholesterol 7α-hydroxylase activity. *$p<0.001$ vs. control; **$p<0.05$ vs. control

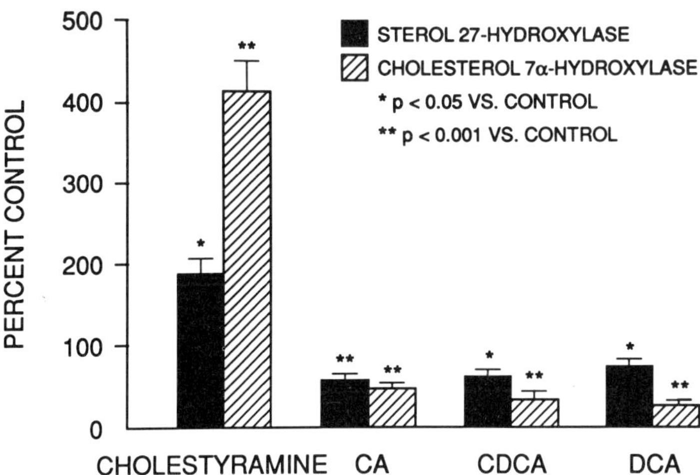

Fig. 27 Cholestyramine feeding increases while feeding of cholic (CA), chenodeoxycholic (CDCA), and deoxycholic acid (DCA) decrease sterol 27-hydroxylase-*specific activity*. The observed changes in specific activities of sterol 27-hydroxylase were less pronounced than those observed with cholesterol 7α-hydroxylase. *$p<0.05$ vs. control; **$p<0.001$ vs.control

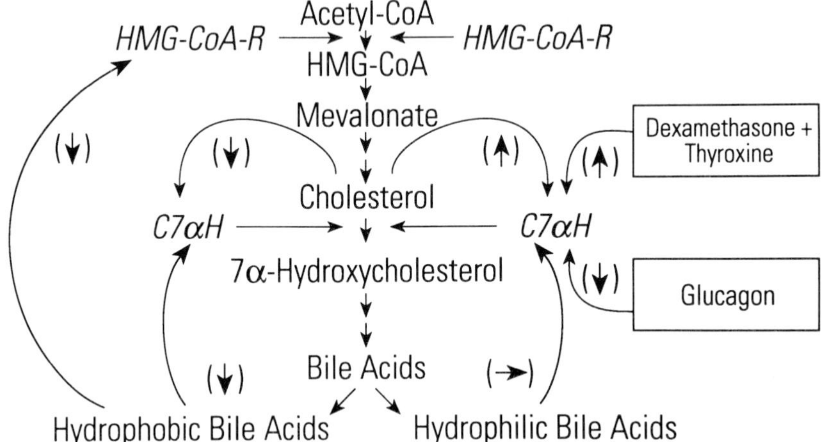

Fig. 28   Regulation of bile acid synthesis (1994): the two initial enzymes in the neutral (cholesterol 7α-hydroxylase) and bile acid biosynthetic pathways (sterol 27-hydroxylase) are both regulated by hydrophobic but not hydrophilic bile acids (negative bile acid biofeedback) at the level of gene transcription. Cholesterol 7α-hydroxylase is also regulated by hormones (glucocorticoids, thyroxine and glucagon) and by cholesterol. The extent of regulation of sterol 27-hydroxylase by different hormones and by cholesterol has not as yet been studied

regulation of cholesterol 7α-hydroxylase involves a number of regulatory factors; all regulators appear to affect cholesterol 7α-hydroxylase at the level of gene transcription. Gene transcription is turned on by cholesterol, thyroxine and glucocorticoids, or by absence or decrease of bile acids in the enterohepatic circulation. Glucagon is a powerful inhibitor of cholesterol 7α–hydroxylase gene transcription both *in vitro* and *in vivo*, but its physiological role has not been fully evaluated. The mechanism by which cholesterol, thyroxine, glucocorticoids and bile acids interact to coordinately regulate cholesterol 7α-hydroxylase gene expression is speculative. It is conceivable that glucocorticoids and thyroxine regulate cholesterol 7α-hydroxylase gene expression via receptor-mediated mechanisms. Hydrophobic bile salts down-regulate cholesterol 7α-hydroxylase by stimulating protein kinase C, which presumably phosphorylates the specific transcription factor turning off the cholesterol 7α-hydroxylase gene transcription. It is conceivable that cholesterol, thyroxine and dexamethasone are responsible for the basal level of cholesterol 7α-hydroxylase gene expression, while hydrophobic bile acid-mediated repression may fine-tune cholesterol 7α-hydroxylase gene transcription.

Sterol 27-hydroxylase, the enzyme responsible for the initiation of the acidic pathway of bile acid synthesis, appears to be down-regulated by hydrophobic bile salts in a negative feedback manner at the level of gene transcription. The negative feedback control of this enzyme is less well pronounced than that of cholesterol 7α-hydroxylase. The role of hormones in the regulation of this enzyme has not as yet been studied, but since its diurnal variation is established, it is probably regulated by glucocorticoids. The role of cholesterol in the regulation of sterol 27-hydroxylase has not as yet been studied. The preliminary data obtained so far provide suggestive evidence that cholesterol 7α-hydroxylase and sterol 27-hydroxylase, the two initial enzymes in the neutral and acidic pathways, respectively, may be regulated in a similar manner.

Acknowledgements

This work was supported by the Veterans Administration and by the National Institutes of Health Program Project (1 P01 DK38030).

References

1. Princen HMG, Meier P, Walthers BG, Vonk R, Kuipers F. Cyclosporine A blocks bile acid synthesis in cultured hepatocytes by specific inhibition of chenodeoxycholic acid synthesis. Biochem J. 1991; 275:501 –5.
2. Axelson M, Sjövall J. Potential bile acid precursors in plasma – possible indicators of biosynthetic pathways to cholic acid and chenodeoxycholic acid in man. J Steroid Biochem. 1990;36:631–40.
3. Vlahcevic ZR, Pandak WM, Heuman DM, Hylemon PB. Function and regulation of hydroxylases involved in the bile acid biosynthesis pathways. In: Davis R, Kern F, editors. Seminars in liver disease, Vol. 12(4). New York. Thieme; 1992:403–19.
4. Davis RA, Hyde PM, Kuan JC, Malone-McNeal M, Archambault-Schexnayder J. Bile acid synthesis by cultured rat hepatocytes: regulation by cholesterol availability. J Biol Chem. 1983; 258:3661–7.
5. Davis RA, Highsmith SE, Malone-McNeal M, Archambault-Schexnayder J, Kuan JC. Bile acid synthesis by cultured hepatocytes: inhibition by mevinolin but not by bile acids. J Biol Chem. 1983;258:4079–82.
6. Kubaska WM, Gurley EC, Hylemon PB, Guzelian P, Gustafsson J, Vlahcevic ZR. Absence of negative feedback control of bile acid biosynthesis in cultured rat hepatocytes. J Biol Chem. 1985;260:13459–63.
7. Heuman DM, Hylemon PB, Vlahcevic ZR. Regulation of bile acid synthesis. III. Correlation between biliary bile salt hydrophobicity index and the activities of enzymes regulating cholesterol and bile acid synthesis in the rat. J Lipid Res. 1989;30:1161–71.
8. Chiang JYL, Vlahcevic ZR. The regulation of cholesterol conversion to bile acids. In: Jefcoate CR, editor. Advances in molecular and cell biology: physiological functions of cytochrome P450 in relation to structure and regulation. 1994;379–91.
9. Pandak WM, Li YC, Chiang JYL et al. Regulation of cholesterol 7α-hydroxylase m-RNA and transcriptional activity by taurocholate and cholesterol in the chronic biliary diverted rat. J Biol Chem. 1991;266:3416–21.
10. Pandak WM, Vlahcevic ZR, Heuman DM, Redford KS, Chiang JYL, Hylemon PB. Effect of different bile salts on the steady-state mRNA levels and transcriptional activity of cholesterol 7α-hydroxylase. Hepatology. 1994;19:941–7.
11. Stravitz RT, Hylemon PB, Heuman DM et al. Transcriptional regulation of cholesterol 7α-hydroxylase m-RNA by conjugated bile acids in primary cultures of rat hepatocytes. J Biol Chem. 1993;268:13987–93.
12. Pandak WM, Stravitz RT, Lucas V, Chiang JYL. Hep G$_2$ cells: a model for studies of human cholesterol 7α-hydroxylase at the molecular level. J Lipid Res. 1994 (Submitted).
13. Stravitz RT, Vlahcevic ZR, Hylemon PB. Repression of cholesterol 7α-hydroxylase transcription by bile acids in cultured rat hepatocytes is mediated through protein kinase C. J Lipid Res. 1995 (in press).
14. Pandak WM, Vlahcevic ZR, Heuman DM, Chiang JYL, Hylemon PB. Down-regulation of cholesterol 7α-hydroxylase and HMG-CoA reductase in the bile fistula rat for intraduodenal but not by intravenous infusion of taurocholate: evidence for an intestinal factor. Gastroenterology. 1994 (In press).
15. Stange EF, Scheibner J, Ditschuneit H. Role of primary and secondary bile acids as feedback inhibitors of bile acid synthesis in the rat in vivo. J Clin Invest. 1989;84:173–80.
16. Björkhem I, Eggertsen G, Andersson U. On the mechanism of stimulation of cholestero 7α-hydroxylase by dietary cholesterol. Biochim Biophys Acta. 1991;1085:329–35.

17. Jones MP, Pandak WM, Hylemon PB, Chiang JYL, Heuman DM, Vlahcevic ZR. Cholesterol 7α-hydroxylase: evidence for transcriptional regulation by cholesterol or metabolic products of cholesterol in the rat. J Lipid Res. 1993;34:885–92.

18. Doerner KC, Gurley EC, Vlahcevic ZR, Hylemon PB. Cholesterol 7α-hydroxylase expression requires cholesterol in primary rat hepatocyte cultures. J Lipid Res. 1994 (Accepted).

19. Pandak WM, Vlahcevic ZR, Chiang JYL, Heuman DM, Hylemon PB. Bile acid synthesis: VI. Regulation of cholesterol 7α-hydroxylase by taurocholate and mevalonate. J Lipid Res. 1992; 33:659–68.

20. Dueland S, Drisko J, Graf L, Machleder D, Lusis AJ, Davis RA. Effect of dietary cholesterol and taurocholate on cholesterol 7α-hydroxylase and hepatic LDL receptors in inbred mice. J Lipid Res. 1993;34:923–31.

21. Spady DK, Cuthbert JA. Regulation of hepatic sterol metabolism in the rat. Parallel regulation of activity and m-RNA for 7α-hydroxylase but not 3-hydroxy-3-methylglutaryl-coenzyme-reductase or low density lipoprotein receptor. J Biol Chem. 1992;267:5584–91.

22. Hylemon PB, Gurley EC, Stravitz RT *et al*. Hormonal regulation of cholesterol 7α-hydroxylase mRNA levels and transcriptional activity in primary rat hepatocyte cultures. J Biol Chem. 1992; 267:16866–71.

23. Vlahcevic ZR, Stravitz RT, Gurley EC, Pandak WM, Hylemon PB. *In vitro* and *in vivo* studies of hormonal regulation of cholesterol 7α-hydroxylase. In: Paumgartner G, Stiehl A, Gerok W, editors. Bile acids and the hepatobiliary system. Lancaster: Kluwer; 1993:33–43.

24. Cali JJ, Hsieh C-L, Francke U, Russell DW. Mutations in the bile acid biosynthetic enzyme sterol 27-hydroxylase underlie cerebrotendinous xanthomatosis. J Biol Chem. 1991;266;7779–83.

25. Andersson S, Davis DL, Dahlbäck H, Jörnvall H, Russell DW. Cloning, structure, and expression of the mitochondrial cytochrome P-450 sterol 26-hydroxylase, a bile acid biosynthetic enzyme. J Biol Chem. 1989;264:8222–9.

9
Molecular mechanism of regulation of cholesterol 7α-hydroxylase gene

J. Y. L. CHIANG, D. STROUP, M. CRESTANI and
DAN-PING WANG

INTRODUCTION

The conversion of cholesterol to bile acids in the liver is a major pathway for disposal of cholesterol from the body[1]. Cholesterol 7α-hydroxylase is the first and rate-limiting enzyme in the bile acid biosynthetic pathway, the activity of which is regulated primarily at the gene transcriptional level by multiple factors, including the bile acid feedback inhibition[2], stimulation by cholesterol[3] and steroid/thyroid hormone[4], and diurnal rhythm[5]. However, the underlying molecular mechanisms of regulations of the *CYP7* gene appear to be very complicated, and not understood at present. To study the regulation of the *CYP7* gene we have recently cloned and sequenced the rat cholesterol 7α-hydroxylase gene[3,6]. Analysis of the proximal promoter of the *CYP7* gene revealed many consensus sequences for liver-enriched transcription factors which are highly conserved in different species[7]. DNase I footprinting assay was applied to map transcription factor binding regions in the promoter[8]. Gel mobility shift assay was then used to study interactions of liver nuclear proteins with footprinted sequences[8].

We have reported that cholesterol 7α-hydroxylase mRNA levels in the human hepatoblastoma cell line, HepG2, could be regulated by known physiological regulators, bile acids[9]. We also established that HepG2 cells were suitable for transient transfection assay of the promoter activity of the *CYP7* promoter/luciferase chimeric gene constructs[9]. This transient transfection assay system was used to map transcription factor binding regions and identified a bile acid response element in the proximal promoter region. Co-transfection assay of *CYP7*/Luc gene constructs with plasmids carrying transcription factor gene was performed to study regulation of the *CYP7* gene by liver-enriched transcription factors.

EXPERIMENTAL PROCEDURES

The rat *CYP7* gene was cloned and sequenced as described previously[6]. DNase I footprinting and electrophoretic mobility shift assay (EMSA) were done as described previously[8]. The 5'-upstream sequence from −3644 to +36 of the rat *CYP7* gene was ligated upstream to a luciferase reporter gene of the plasmid pGL2-Basic, deletion mutants of which were constructed by restriction digestion of unique restriction sites or by polymerase chain reaction. A thyroid hormone response element-like sequence (7αTRE, nt −73 to −55) was linked to a SV40 promoter/luc gene plasmid, pGL2-Promoter, and a clone, p-73/-55LUC-2f, containing a tandem repeat of 7αTRE was selected by sequencing[8].

HepG2 cells were cultured in DMEM:F12 medium supplemented with 10% fetal calf serum as described previously[9]. Cells were plated in six-well cluster plates at a density of $0.7 \times 10^5/cm^2$ (subconfluent cultures) or $1.3 \times 10^5/cm^2$ (confluent cultures) and grown for 24h (subconfluent cultures) or 6 days (confluent cultures) at 37°C in the presence of 5% CO_2 in a humidified incubator. Chimeric gene constructs were transiently transfected into HepG2 cell cultures using the calcium phosphate–DNA co-precipitation method as described[10]. Five micrograms of test plasmid were co-transfected with 0.5 µg of β-galactosidase expression plasmid, pCMVβ, which was used as an internal standard for adjustment of transfection efficiency. Cells were incubated with co-precipitates for 4h, shocked with 15% glycerol and incubated for 42h in serum-free medium or in medium containing bile acids. Luciferase activities of *CYP7*/LUC reporter gene constructs expressed in cell extracts were determined and adjusted for β-galactosidase activity.

To study the effect of liver-enriched transcription factors on the *CYP7* promoter activity, 5 µg of plasmid p-416/+32LUC were co-transfected with 1 µg of expression plasmids carrying transcription factor genes. Transcription factor expression plasmids were the generous gifts of Drs U. Schibler (pSCT/DBP for DBP), W. Chen (pL-H3α for HNF3α; pLEN4S for HNF3β), P. Johnson (pMEXC/EBP for C/EBPα; pMEXCRP2.seq for LAP), and M.-J. Tsai (pTF3A for COUP-TFII).

RESULTS

The structure of *CYP7* gene

The rat cholesterol 7α-hydroxylase gene contains six exons and five introns, which span a minimum of about 10 kb of the genome (Fig. 1). An 8 kb *Sac*I fragment containing a 3644 bp 5'-flanking region and region from exon I to the *Sac*I site of exon IV was sequenced completely[8]. The nucleotide sequences of the 5'-flanking region from −416 to +36 are shown in Fig. 1. Analysis of this proximal promoter revealed many consensus sequence motifs for liver-enriched transcription factors, i.e. hormone response element (HRE, including thyroxine response element, TRE; and glucocorticoid response element, GRE), hepatocyte nuclear factors (HNF, including HNF1, HNF3, HNF4), TGT3, TGT4, albumin D-site binding protein (DBP), CCAAT/enhancer

The Proximal Promoter of Rat CYP7 Gene

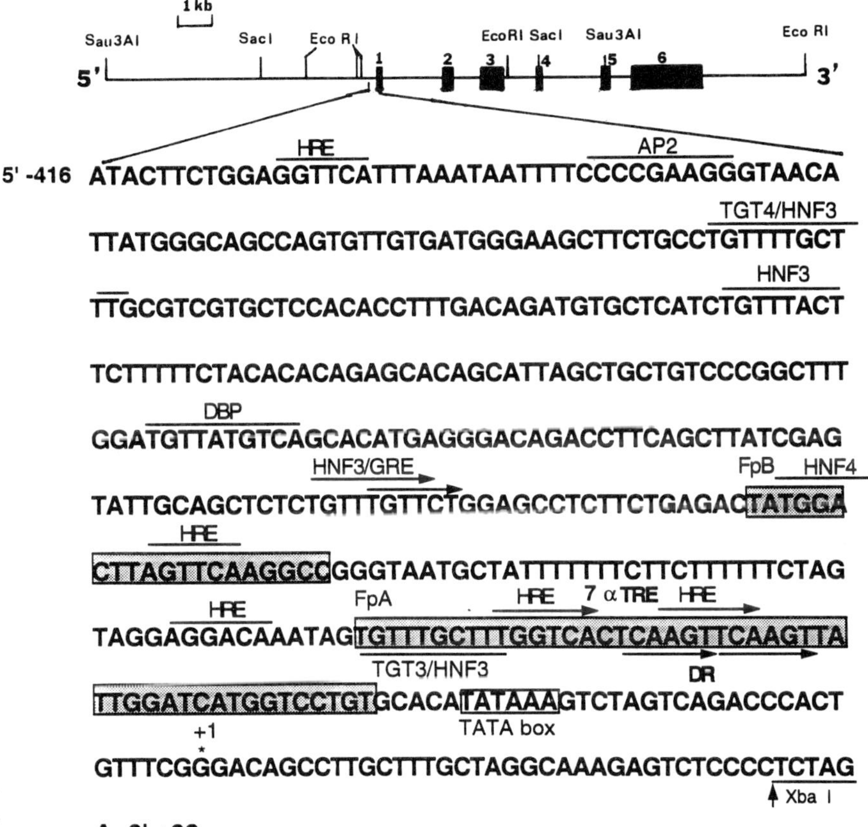

Fig. 1 The rat cholesterol 7α-hydroxylase gene (*CYP7*) structure. Nucleotide sequences in the proximal promoter region, DNase I footprints and putative sequence motifs for liver-enriched transcription factors and nuclear receptors are indicated. HRE, hormone response element, HNF1, HNF4, hepatocyte nuclear factors; 7αTRE, a thyroid hormone response element like HRE direct repeats; DR, a direct repeat sequence; FpA, FpB, DNase I footprints A and B; DBP, albumin D site binding protein; TATA, TATAAA box; TGT3, TGT4, TGTTT(T)GCTTT sequences

binding protein (C/EBP) and AP2. DNase I footprinting assay using rat liver nuclear extracts identified two distinct footprints, FpA (nt −81 to −35) and FpB (nt −148 to −129)[8]. Footprints are sequences protected from DNase I digestion, and thus are potential transcription factor binding regions. FpA contains sequences for TGT3/HNF3, a TRE-like motif 7αTRE, a direct repeat (DR) TCAAGTTCAAGT, and a reversed CCAAT box (ATTGG) which is a potential binding site for C/EBP[8]. TATA box is located at −29. FpB contains a consensus sequence for HNF4 and a HRE. These sequence motifs are highly conserved in the *CYP7* gene of the rat, hamster, human, rabbit and mouse. This conserved proximal promoter must be important in the regulation of the liver-specific expression of the *CYP7* gene.

Transient transfection assay of the *CYP7* promoter activity

To study the regulation of the *CYP7* gene promoter by known physiological regulators such as bile acids, sterols and hormones, the 5′-flanking region from −3644 to +36 of the gene was linked to a luciferase reporter gene (Luc). The chimeric gene construct, p-3644Luc, and its deletion mutants were transiently transfected into the human hepatoblastoma cell line, HepG2. Figure 2 shows the promoter activities of these chimeric gene constructs, which were measured as the adjusted luciferase activity expressed in HepG2 cells. The promoter activity of *CYP7* was quite high in comparison with the standard strong promoter SV40. Transfection efficiency was higher in subconfluent cultures than in confluent culture of HepG2 cells. However, the adjusted promoter activities were higher in confluent than in subconfluent cultures. Deletions of the 5′-upstream sequence increased promoter activity and the −416 fragment was shown to have the highest activity in confluent culture. Repressor sequences apparently were located between −593 and −416 and the region further upstream. Activator sequences were located between 161 fragment was very low, and this region is probably the minimum promoter required for the liver-specific expression of *CYP7* gene transcription.

Identification of a putative bile acid-responsive element

The effects of bile acids on the promoter activities of *CYP7*/Luc chimeric gene constructs were studied to map regions conferring bile acid repression of *CYP7* gene expression. We reported previously that the luciferase activities of these gene constructs were reduced by taurochenodeoxycholic acid (TCDCA) and taurodeoxycholic acid (TDCA), but not by taurocholic acid (TCA) in confluent cultures of HepG2 cell[9]. Shorter promoter constructs showed much less effect by bile acids. We concluded that there were at least two regions which are responsive to bile acid repression. One is located in the −160 region and the others might be located further upstream. In subconfluent cultures, TDCA or TCDCA did not have much effect on the promoter activity. We also reported that the endogenous cholesterol 7α-hydroxylase mRNA levels in confluent cultures of HepG2 cells were reduced by TDCA and TCDCA, but not by TCA or TUDCA[a]. It appeared that hydrophobic bile acids were strong repressors of *CYP7* gene transcription, and bile acid responsiveness may be a developmentally regulated process.

To further identify bile acid responsive element (BARE) in the gene, a 7αTRE fragment was linked upstream to a heterologous promoter SV40/Luc gene, and the effect of bile acids on the promoter activity was studied. As shown in Fig. 3, TDCA significantly repressed 7αTRE/SV40/Luc promoter activity by 80% at $5-10\,\mu\text{mol/l}$. At the same concentration, TDCA did not repress promoter activity of the control plasmid pGL2 promoter which contains a SV40 promoter. However, when the concentration of TDCA was higher than $50\,\mu\text{mol/l}$ it also repressed SV40/Luc promoter activity.

Electrophoretic mobility shift assay revealed a direct repeat sequence in the FpA region which specifically shifted one or two bands in rat or human liver nuclear extracts and these shifted bands were absent when deoxycholate-

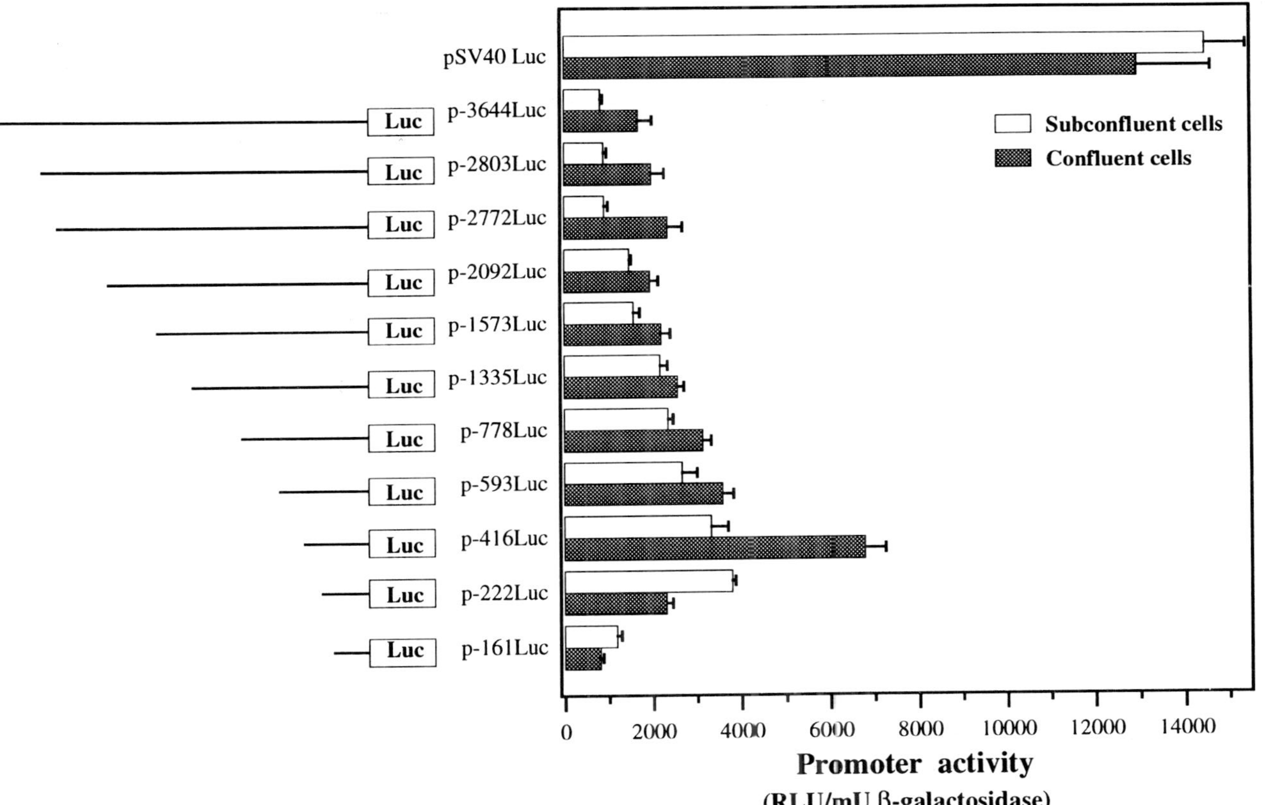

Fig. 2 The promoter activity of rat *CYP7*/luciferase chimeric genes transfected in HepG2 cells. Subconfluent and confluent HepG2 cell cultures were transfected as described under 'Experimental procedures' and incubated for 40 h in serum-free media. At the end of the experiment, cells were harvested and promoter activities were determined as described. Results are expressed as the ratio of luciferase and β-galactosidase activity, and represent the mean ± standard deviation of three determinations. The number of nucleotides from the transcription start site is indicated for each plasmid

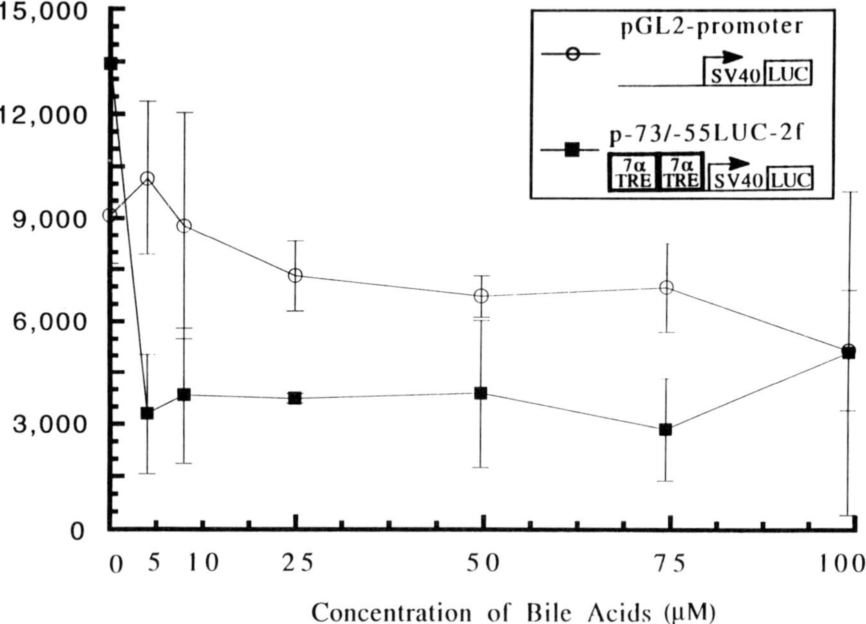

Fig. 3 Effect of taurodeoxycholate on 7αTRE/SV40 promoter activity in HepG2 cells. A plasmid p-73/-55LUC-2f containing a tandem repeat of 7αTRE located upstream of the SV40 promoter/LUC gene was transfected into confluent HepG2 culture. Taurodeoxycholate was added in cultures and incubated for 40 h in serum-free media. Luciferase activities was adjusted for β-galactosidase activity. The ranges of activity are indicated by error bars

treated rat liver nuclear extracts were used in EMSA[8]. Treatment with cholate, cholestyramine or cholesterol did not abolish these gel shifts. The bands shifted by human liver nuclear extracts appeared to be much stronger than those shifted by rat extracts. This direct repeat sequence interacted with a 57 000 protein (p57) in rat and human liver nuclear extracts, which may be a putative bile acid responsive protein (BARP)[8].

Promoter activity of p-416/+32ΔTRE which had the 7αTRE sequence (nt −73 to −55) deleted was much higher than the wild-type plasmid p-416/+32 (Fig. 4). This experiment provides strong evidence that the 7αTRE sequence is a negative regulatory element and the putative binding protein p57 is apparently a strong repressor of *CYP7* gene expression.

Regulation of *CYP7* gene by liver-enriched transcription factors

Our footprinting experiments identified potential regulatory regions which contain many consensus sequence motifs for liver-enriched transcription factors, such as HNF1, HNF3, HNF4, C/EBP, DBP and nuclear receptors such as HNF4, COUP-TF, GR, TRE and retinoic acid receptors, RAR/RXR[8]. We tested the effect of over-expression of these transcription factors on *CYP7* promoter activity. As shown in Fig. 5, co-transfection of plasmids carrying

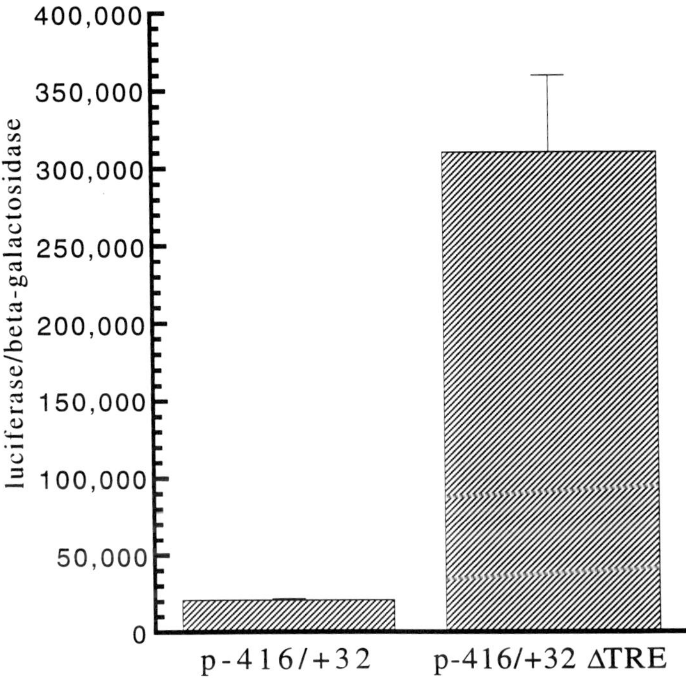

Fig. 4 Effect of deletion of 7αTRE sequence on the *CYP7* promoter activity. p-416/+32 ΔTRE plasmid had nucleotides −73 to −55 deleted from p-416/+32 plasmid. Plasmids were transfected into confluent cultures of HepG2 cells

HNF3 or HNF4 stimulated p-200/+32 by about 2-fold. Liver-specific enhancer binding proteins C/EBPα or C/EBPβ (LAP) stimulated promoter activity by 9- and 5-fold, respectively. DBP, a diurnal regulated transcription factor which was originally identified as albumin D-site binding protein, stimulated p-200/+32 activity by 5-fold. COUP-TFII, a ubiquitous nuclear receptor, strongly stimulated the *CYP7* promoter activity by 8.5-fold.

DISCUSSION

Cholesterol 7α-hydroxylase activity is expressed at a very low level in hepatocytes, and is highly regulated by multiple factors at the gene transcriptional level. The *CYP7* promoter activity is surprisingly high in the transient transfection assay in HepG2 cells. This may be due to the lack of bile acid feedback in the culture system. We demonstrated that enhancer sequences are located in the nt −416 to −162 region. The minimal promoter (from −161 to +32) of the *CYP7* gene is highly conserved in homologous genes, and may be important for liver-specific expression of the *CYP7* gene. The upstream regions of the promoter may also be participating in the regulation of the

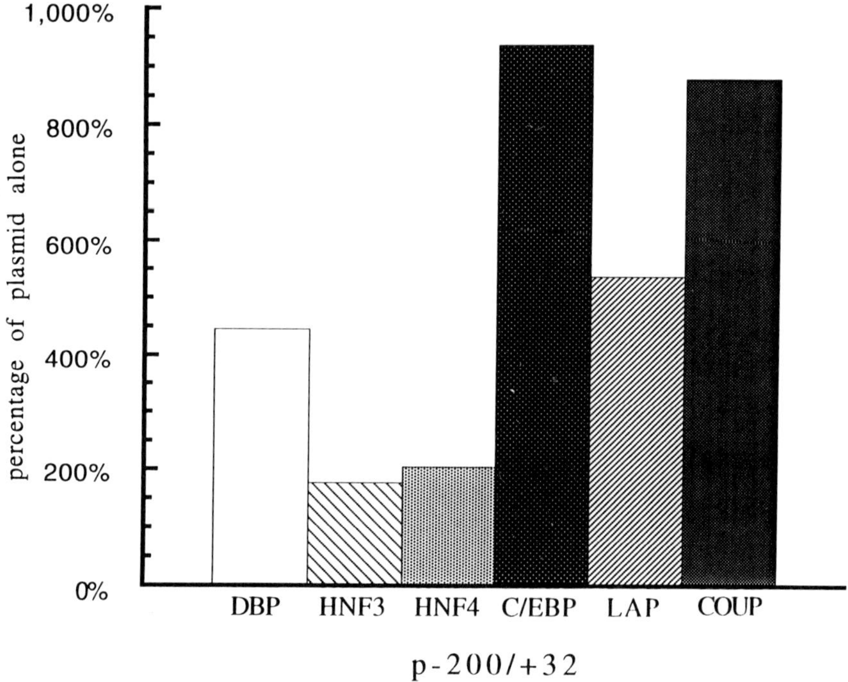

Fig. 5 Effect of co-transfection of liver-enriched transcription factors and COUP-TF on the *CYP7* promoter activity. Five micrograms of p-200/+32 plasmid and 1 µg plasmid carrying transcription factor gene were transfected into confluent cultures of HepG2 cells. Effects of transcription factors on *CYP7* promoter activity were expressed as a percentage of promoter activity without co-transfection with transcription factors

CYP7 gene expression; however, the −416 to +32 region is important in mediating the effects by physiological regulators.

We demonstrated that hydrophobic bile acids are strong inhibitors of *CYP7* gene promoter activity. The 7αTRE sequence could confer bile acid repression of a heterologous promoter and is a strong negative regulatory element. This fragment is a putative bile acid responsive element. The direct repeat sequence in 7αTRE, TCAAGTTCAAGT, is unique and is the binding site of a nuclear protein p57, which is apparently a negative transcription regulator. The upstream sequences which might be involved in conferring the bile acid repression of promoter activity have yet to be identified.

Co-transfection assays demonstrated that HNF3, HNF4, C/EBP, LAP, DBP and COUP-TF are probably involved in the expression of the *CYP7* gene. These liver-enriched transcription factors may bind to consensus sequences which were identified in the *CYP7* promoter. It has been reported that DBP, a diurnal regulated transcription factor, is a strong activator of the *CYP7* gene[5]. DBP was originally identified as an albumin promoter D-site binding protein. It is likely that the diurnal rhythm of cholesterol 7α-hydroxylase activity is regulated by DBP, and the *CYP7* gene is the target gene of DBP. COUP-TF, a well-studied repressor of liver-specific genes, surprisingly stimulated the

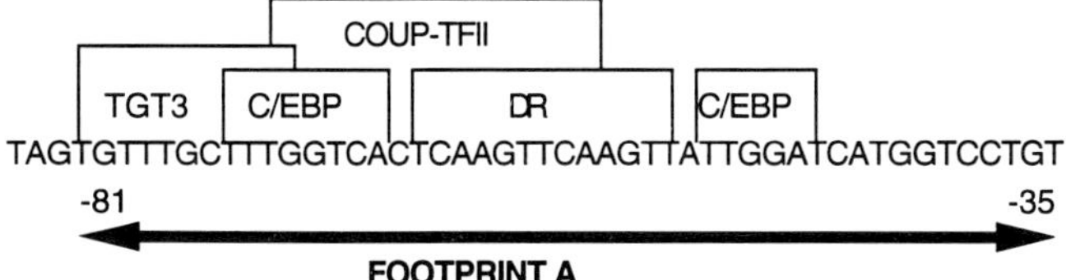

A. Basal Transcriptional Activation

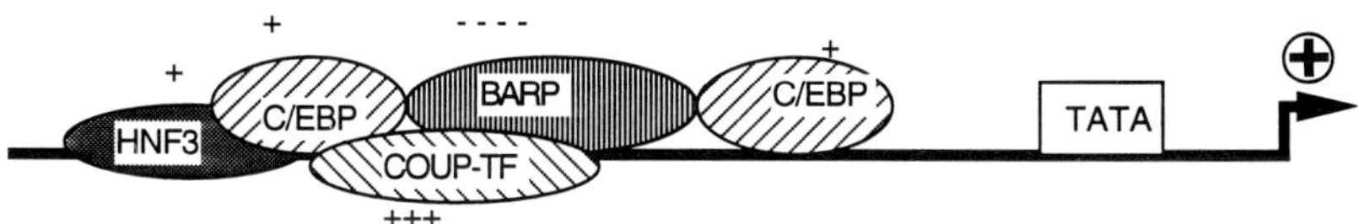

B. Bile Acid Feedback Repression

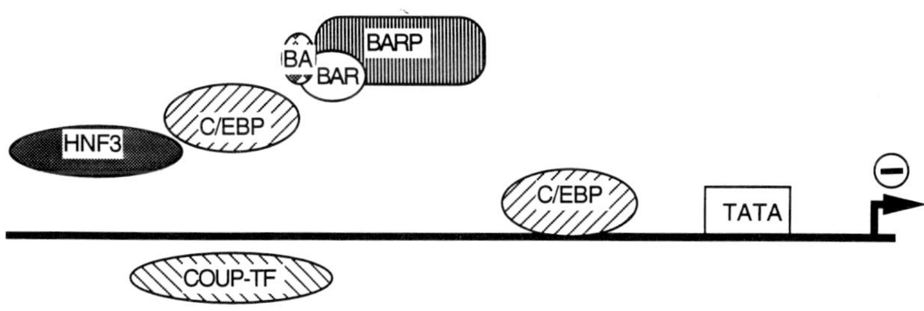

Fig. 6 Model of regulation of the cholesterol 7α-hydroxylase gene. Footprint A contains overlapping sequence motifs for positive transcription factors TGT3/HNF3, C/EBP, and COUP-TFII, and a proposed negative regulator bile acid response protein (BARP) which binds to a direct repeat (DR) sequence. A: Basal transcriptional activation: interactions among HNF3, C/EBP, COUP-TFII and BARP form a regulatory unit which regulates the general transcriptional machinery TFIID complex. B: Bile acid feedback repression: hydrophobic bile acids (BA) may bind to a bile acid receptor (BAR) or binding protein, and prevent the interactions between BARP and other regulatory factors. Without binding of BARP to BARE, positive regulators may not bind to the promoter and the *CYP7* gene expression is thus repressed

CYP7 gene promoter activity. COUP-TF is an orphan receptor of the nuclear receptor superfamily which recognizes a sequence motif GGTCA[11]. The level of expression of these liver-enriched transcription factors and the interactions of these positive transcription factors with the bile acid-regulated repressor BARP may determine the level of the *CYP7* gene expression in hepatocytes.

The observed inhibitory effect of deoxycholate on the binding of a negative regulator to the response element seems to be opposite to what one would expect for the action of a bile acid repressor. Figure 6 is a model illustrating the structure of the *CYP7* proximal promoter and a possible mechanism of gene regulation by bile acids. The basal level of liver-specific gene expression requires the binding and interactions of positive transcription factors, i.e. HNF3, C/EBP, COUP-TF, and a negative regulator, BARP. These transcription factors bind to overlapping sequence motifs in Fp A and form a regulatory unit which interacts with general transcriptional machinery TFIID complex. Hydrophobic bile acids may bind to a receptor or a binding protein BAR and subsequently interrupt the formation of the regulatory unit, thus repressing *CYP7* gene expression. The level of *CYP7* gene expression may be determined by the binding affinity and the amount of positive and negative regulatory factors which are interacting and binding to the BARE.

Acknowledgements

This research was supported by NIH grants GM31584 and DK44442 and a research contract from Hoechst, AG, Germany. D.S. is a recipient of a Postdoctoral Fellowship of the American Heart Association Ohio Affiliate, M.C. is on leave from the Institute of Pharmacological Sciences, University of Milan, Italy.

References

1. Vlahcevic ZR, Heuman DM, Hylemon PB. Regulation of bile acid synthesis. Hepatology. 1991;13:590–600.
2. Pandak WM, Li YC, Chiang JYL *et al*. Regulation of cholesterol 7α-hydroxylase mRNA and transcriptional activity by taurocholate and cholesterol in the chronic biliary diverted rat. J Biol Chem. 1991;266:3416–21.
3. Li YC, Wang DP, Chiang JYL. Regulation of cholesterol 7α-hydroxylase in the liver. Cloning, sequencing and regulation of cholesterol 7α-hydroxylase mRNA. J Biol Chem. 1990;265:12012–19.
4. Hylemon PB, Gurley EC, Stravitz RT *et al*. Hormonal regulation of cholesterol 7α-hydroxylase mRNA levels and transcriptional activity in primary rat hepatocyte cultures. J Biol Chem. 1992;267:16866–71.
5. Lavery DJ, Schibler U. Circadian transcription of the cholesterol 7α-hydroxylase gene may involve the liver enriched bZip protein DBP. Gene Dev. 1993;7:1871–84.
6. Chiang JYL, Wang TP, Wang DP. Cloning and 5'-flanking sequence of a rat cholesterol 7α-hydroxylase gene. Biochim Biophys Acta. 1992;1132:337–9.
7. Crestani M, Galli G, Chiang JYL. Genomic cloning, sequencing and analysis of the hamster cholesterol 7α-hydroxylase gene (*CYP7*). Arch Biochem Biophys. 1993;306:451–60.
8. Chiang JYL, Stroup D. Identification and characterization of a putative bile acid responsive element in cholesterol 7α-hydroxylase gene promoter. J Biol Chem. 1994;269:17502–7.
9. Crestani M, Karam WG, Chiang JYL. Effects of bile acids and steroid/thyroid hormones on the expression of cholesterol 7α-hydroxylase mRNA and the *CYP7* gene in HepG2 cells. Biochem Biophys Res Commun. 1993;198:546–53.
10. Graham FL, Van der Eb AJ. A new technique for the assay of infectivity of human adenovirus 5 DNA. Virology. 1973;52:456–67.
11. Cooney AJ, Tsai SY, O'Malley BW, Tsai M-J. Chicken ovalbumin upstream promoter transcription factor (COUP-TF) dimers bind to different GGTCA response elements, allowing COUP-TF to repress hormonal induction of the vitamin D_3, thyroid hormone, and retinoic acid receptors. Mol Cell Biol. 1992;12:4153–63.

10
Regulation of cholesterol 7α-hydroxylase mRNA and transcriptional activity by protein phosphorylation in primary cultures of rat hepatocytes

R. T. STRAVITZ, Z. R. VLAHCEVIC, E. C. GURLEY and
P. B. HYLEMON

INTRODUCTION

Hepatic microsomal cholesterol 7α-hydroxylase, the rate-determining enzyme of a major pathway of bile acid biosynthesis, is subject to feedback repression by hydrophobic bile acids undergoing enterohepatic recirculation[1]. In primary cultures of rat hepatocytes[2,3] and chronic biliary-diverted rats[4], bile acids concomitantly feedback inhibit cholesterol 7α-hydroxylase specific activity, steady-state mRNA levels, and transcriptional activity, suggesting an effect on the cholesterol 7α-hydroxylase 5'-flanking region. However, the intracellular mechanisms by which the hepatocyte senses the concentration of bile acids and transduces this signal to the hepatocyte nucleus remain obscure.

Two general models might account for the transcriptional repression of cholesterol 7α-hydroxylase by bile acids: a 'direct' model, in which bile acids bind to an intracellular receptor, enter the nucleus, and interact with the cholesterol 7α-hydroxylase promoter region; and an 'indirect' model, in which bile acids generate one or more extranuclear signals. In the indirect model these signals may ultimately result in covalent modification of a *trans*-acting factor required for cholesterol 7α-hydroxylase transcription. To date little scientific evidence strongly supports either model, although bile acids may be excluded from hepatocyte nuclei[5].

During preliminary experiments to identify mechanisms of cholesterol 7α-hydroxylase regulation in cultured rat hepatocytes, we observed a rapid and potent decline in steady-state mRNA levels after adding inhibitors of serine–threonine protein phosphatases. Since transcription factor phosphorylation is

"""

a common mechanism regulating gene transcription[6], we reasoned that bile acids might inhibit cholesterol 7α-hydroxylase transcription by activating a serine–threonine protein kinase. Specific inhibitors of protein kinase C, but not protein kinase A, were found to prevent the suppression of cholesterol 7α-hydroxylase mRNA by taurocholate. This observation prompted us to explore more closely a possible link between the feedback inhibition of cholesterol 7α-hydroxylase by bile acids and protein kinase C.

EXPERIMENTAL PROCEDURES

Primary cultures of adult rat hepatocytes

The isolation of hepatocytes from male Sprague–Dawley rats has been described previously[7]. Briefly, 3.5×10^6 cells were plated on rat-tail collagen and incubated in 3 ml serum-free Williams' E medium containing insulin (0.25 U/ml), thyroxine (1.0 μmol/l), and dexamethasone (0.1 μmol/l). Bile acids, protein kinase inhibitors, protein phosphatase inhibitors, and phorbol esters were added to the culture medium 18 h after plating, except where noted. Hepatocytes were harvested 18–42 h after plating, as indicated.

Cholesterol 7α-hydroxylase mRNA levels and transcriptional activity

Total RNA was isolated using a chloroform/phenol/guanidinium thiocyanate method (TriReagent, Molecular Research Center, Cincinnati, OH). Cholesterol 7α-hydroxylase mRNA was quantitated using the radiolabelled cDNA (kindly provided by Dr J. Y. L. Chiang) by dot and Northern blot hybridization. The hybridization and washing conditions have been described previously[8]; cholesterol 7α-hydroxylase mRNA was normalized for variation of loading to rat cyclophilin mRNA. The isolation of hepatocyte nuclei and nuclear 'run-on' determination of cholesterol 7α-hydroxylase transcriptional activity was performed exactly as described previously[8]. Cholesterol 7α-hydroxylase transcriptional activity was normalized to rat cyclophilin transcriptional activity.

Determination of protein kinase C activity in cultured rat hepatocyte protein fractions

Hepatocytes (eight plates/sample) were washed in ice-cold phosphate-buffered saline and scraped into 1.0 ml homogenization buffer (Tris HCl [20 mmol/l, pH 7.5], disodium EDTA [2 mmol/l], EGTA [5 mmol/l], 2-mercaptoethanol [10 mmol/l], leupeptin [50 μmol/l], and PMSF [1 mmol/l]). Hepatocytes were homogenized and the lysate centrifuged at 100 000 g (1 h at 4°C). The supernatant (cytosol) was removed and pellet resuspended in 1 ml homogenization buffer containing 0.5% Triton X-100. Membrane homogenates were incubated on ice for 30 min, and centrifuged at 10 000 g for

2 min. The supernatant and cytosol were then purified over $400\,\mu l$ DEAE-cellulose columns, and eluted with 300 mmol/l NaCl, as described[9]. Protein kinase C activity in membrane and cytosol extracts was determined using a commercially available assay system (Amersham). Briefly, aliquots of extract were incubated for 15 min at 25°C with a protein kinase C-specific acceptor peptide and $[\gamma^{32}P]$ATP. The terminated reaction mixture was then applied to filter paper, washed, and the extent of acceptor protein phosphorylation determined by liquid scintillation spectrometry. Sample activity was controlled to protein concentration of post-DEAE column extracts.

Statistical analysis

The data are presented as mean ± SE. Significance was determined by the unpaired Student's *t*-test.

RESULTS

Effects of serine – threonine protein phosphatase inhibitors on cholesterol 7α-hydroxylase mRNA

In order to document a possible regulatory role of protein phosphorylation in cholesterol 7α-hydroxylase mRNA expression, two inhibitors of serine – threonine protein phosphatases, okadaic acid and calyculin A, were added to primary cultures of rat hepatocytes. Okadaic acid and calyculin A inhibit protein phosphatase 2A with equimolar potency, but calyculin A inhibits protein phosphatase 1 $10^2 - 10^3$-fold more potently than okadaic acid[10]. As shown in Fig. 1, the addition of both inhibitors for 6 h decreased cholesterol 7α-hydroxylase mRNA with a similar IC_{50} of 10 – 20 nmol/l. In contrast, the addition of 1-*nor*-okadaone (50 nmol/l), an inactive okadaic acid analogue, had no significant effect on cholesterol 7α-hydroxylase mRNA. These data imply that the inhibition of protein phosphatase 2A may decrease cholesterol 7α-hydroxylase transcription.

Regulation of cholesterol 7α-hydroxylase mRNA and transcriptional activity by protein kinase C

In order to identify serine – threonine kinases potentially responsible for phosphorylating the protein phosphatase 2A substrate implicated above, cholesterol 7α-hydroxylase mRNA and transcriptional activity were assessed after the addition of activators of protein kinase C to the culture medium. Figure 2 depicts the response of cholesterol 7α-hydroxylase mRNA to phorbol 12-myristate, 13-acetate (PMA; 100 nmol/l) over a 24-h time-course. Cholesterol 7α-hydroxylase mRNA initially underwent a rapid decline to approximately 30% of no-addition control cultures, followed by a recovery phase beginning 3 – 6 after the addition. Cholesterol 7α-hydroxylase mRNA levels rebounded to, and then exceeded, control levels between 18 and 24 h

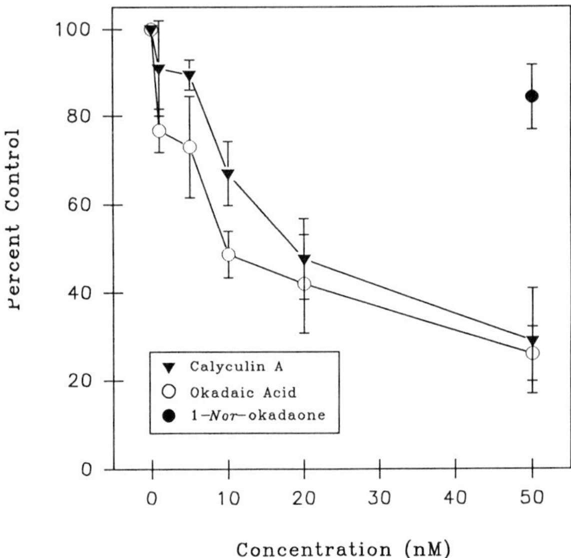

Fig. 1 Effect of serine–threonine protein phosphatase inhibitors on cholesterol 7α-hydroxylase mRNA levels in primary cultures of rat hepatocytes. Okadaic acid (sodium salt) or calyculin A were added to the culture medium in the indicated concentrations 18 h after plating, and hepatocytes were harvested 6 h later. Cholesterol 7α-hydroxylase mRNA was quantitated by dot blot hybridization and controlled to rat cyclophilin mRNA. Mean ± SE of three experiments

after the addition. In contrast, 4α-PMA (100 nmol/l), which does not activate protein kinase C, had no significant effect on cholesterol 7α-hydroxylase mRNA (Fig. 2).

The initial decrease in cholesterol 7α-hydroxylase mRNA in response to PMA resulted from the suppression of cholesterol 7α-hydroxylase transcriptional activity. As shown in Fig. 3, 1.5 h after the addition of PMA (100 nmol/l), cholesterol 7α-hydroxylase transcriptional activity as determined by nuclear 'run-on' assays decreased to $40 \pm 16\%$ of no-addition controls.

Effect of protein kinase inhibitors on the repression of cholesterol 7α-hydroxylase mRNA by taurocholate

We next used specific inhibitors of protein kinase C and A to attempt to abolish the ability of taurocholate to repress cholesterol 7α-hydroxylase mRNA. As shown in Fig. 4, the addition of taurocholate (25 μmol/l) for 6 h to the culture medium decreased cholesterol 7α-hydroxylase mRNA by $64 \pm 3\%$, compared to untreated controls. However, after a 1-h preincubation with the highly specific protein kinase C inhibitor calphostin C (100 nmol/l), a similar addition of taurocholate decreased cholesterol 7α-hydroxylase mRNA by only $1 \pm 2\%$, compared to cultures treated with calphostin C alone. (Calphostin C alone decreased cholesterol 7α-hydroxylase mRNA by $10-20\%$, compared to

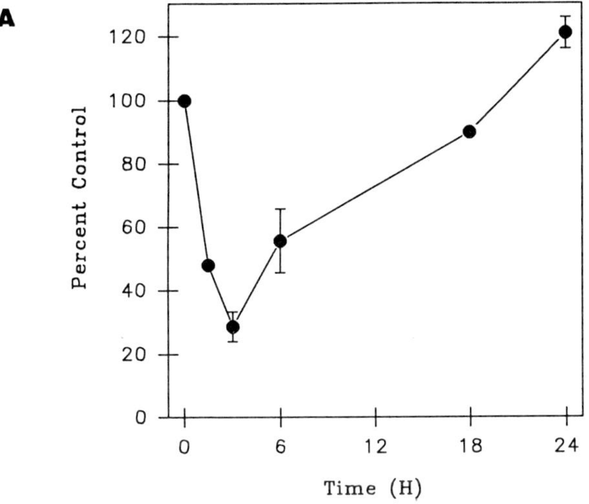

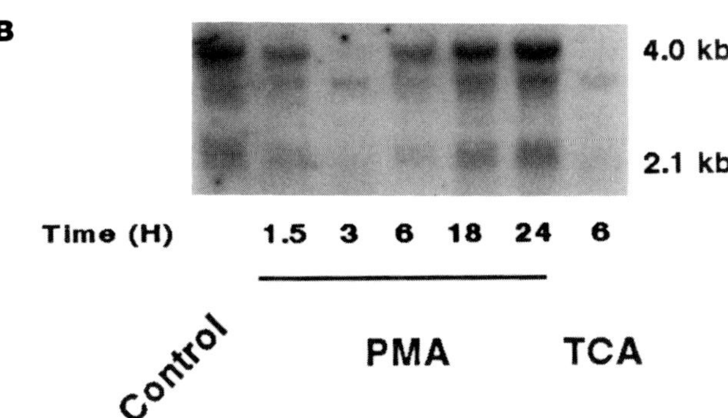

Fig. 2 Effects of phorbol diesters on cholesterol 7α-hydroxylase mRNA levels in primary cultures of rat hepatocytes. Phorbol 12-myristate, 13-acetate (PMA; 100 nmol/l) was added to the culture medium at the indicated times before harvest, beginning 4 h after plating. All cultures were harvested 28 h after plating, and cholesterol 7α-hydroxylase mRNA was quantitated by dot (**A**) or Northern (**B**) blot hybridization, and controlled to rat cyclophilin mRNA. As a negative control, 4α-PMA (100 nmol/l) was added to other cultures and hepatocytes were harvested 3 h later. Mean ± SE of three experiments

untreated cultures.) The ability of calphostin C to block the bile acid effect on cholesterol 7α-hydroxylase mRNA was specific, as pretreatment with R_p-adenosine-3′,5′-cyclic monophosphothioate (Rp-cAMPS; 100 μmol/l), a specific inhibitor of protein kinase A, was unable to prevent the down-regulation of cholesterol 7α-hydroxylase mRNA by taurocholate (decrease of 57%, compared to cultures treated with R_p-cAMPS alone).

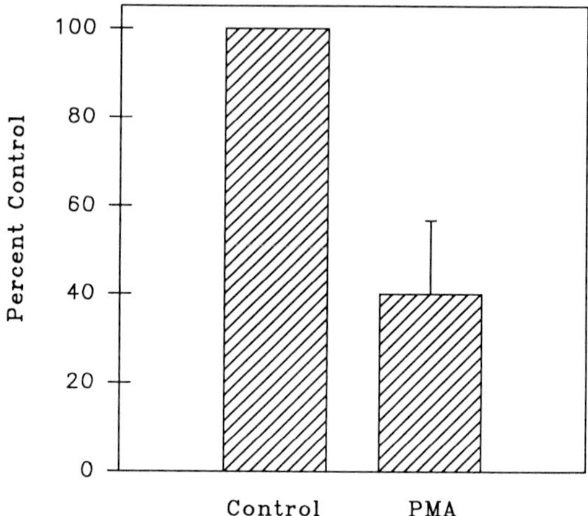

Fig. 3 Cholesterol 7α-hydroxylase transcriptional activity in primary cultures of rat hepatocytes. PMA (100 nmol/l) was added to the culture medium 18 h after plating, and hepatocyte nuclei were harvested 1.5 h later. Nascent cholesterol 7α-hydroxylase and cyclophilin mRNAs were elongated *in vitro* in the presence of [^{32}P]GTP. Cholesterol 7α-hydroxylase transcriptional activity was normalized to rat cyclophilin transcriptional activity in the same nuclei. Mean ± SE of three experiments, expressed as a percentage of untreated control cultures

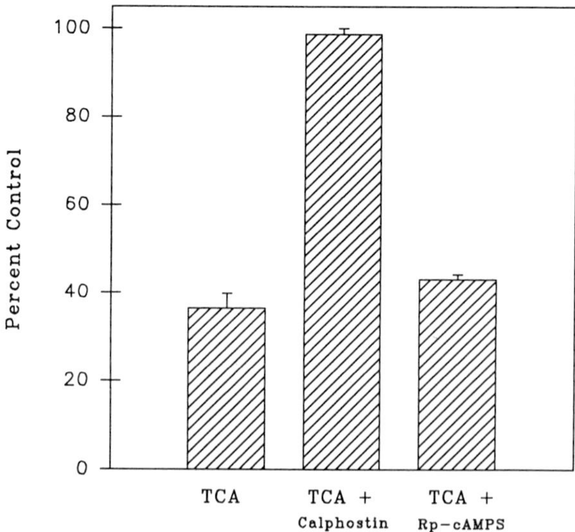

Fig. 4 Effect of protein kinase inhibitors on taurocholate-induced repression of cholesterol 7α-hydroxylase mRNA. Hepatocytes were incubated with taurocholate alone (TCA; 25 μmol/l) for 6 h, or TCA + kinase inhibitor (1 h preincubation with calphostin C [100 nmol/l], or R_p-adenosine-3′,5′-cyclic monophosphothioate [R_p-cAMPS; 100 μmol/l]). Data are expressed as a percentage of untreated controls for TCA, or a percentage of calphostin C-treated or R_p-cAMPS-treated cells for TCA + kinase-treated hepatocytes. Mean ± SE of three experiments

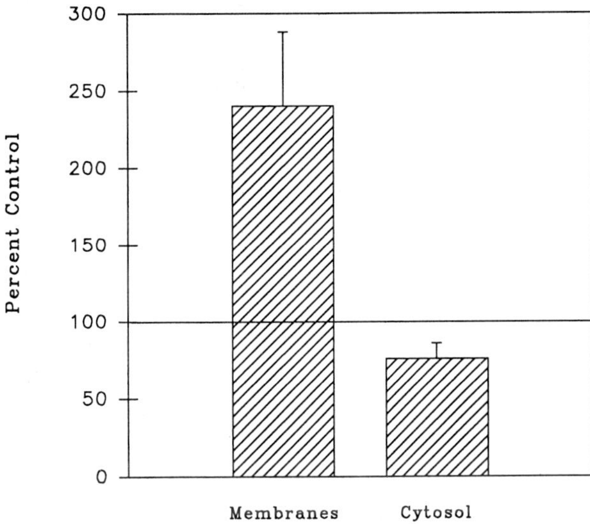

Fig. 5 Effects of taurocholate on protein kinase C activity in primary cultures of rat hepatocytes. Taurocholate (50 μmol/l) was added to hepatocyte culture medium 18 h after plating and cells scraped into iced homogenization buffer 5 min later. Hepatocytes were homogenized, and protein fractions isolated as described in 'Experimental procedures'. Hepatocyte fractions were partially purified over DEAE-cellulose columns, and protein kinase C activity determined using the Protein Kinase C Assay Kit from Amersham. Activity was controlled for protein concentration, and expressed as a percentage of no-addition controls. Mean ± SE of four experiments

Taurocholate induces the translocation and activation of protein kinase C activity in cultured rat hepatocytes

Under resting conditions, most protein kinase C isoforms reside in the cytosol. The activation of protein kinase C involves its translocation to the inner leaflet of plasma membranes, where it phosphorylates protein substrates[11]. As shown in Fig. 5, at 5 min after the addition of taurocholate (50 μmol/l) to cultured rat hepatocytes, membrane-associated protein kinase C activity increased by 240 ± 48% compared to no-addition control cultures ($p < 0.05$). Concomitantly, cytosolic protein kinase C activity decreased by 26 ± 4% ($p < 0.05$ compared to no-addition controls), suggesting bile acid-induced protein kinase C translocation.

DISCUSSION

The data presented strongly suggest that the transcriptional repression of cholesterol 7α-hydroxylase by bile acids is mediated through a protein kinase C-dependent mechanism. First, the activation of protein kinase C with phorbol diesters resulted in a reversible decline in cholesterol 7α-hydroxylase mRNA levels. Decreased gene transcription as assessed by nuclear 'run-on' assays was primarily responsible for this decline. Equimolar concentrations of 4α-PMA, which does not activate protein kinase C, had no effect. Second, the inhibition of protein kinase C with calphostin C prevented the down-regulation of cholesterol 7α-hydroxylase mRNA by taurocholate. A similar preincubation with an inhibitor of protein kinase A, which may also be involved in the regulation of cholesterol 7α-hydroxylase transcription[8], was unable to prevent the bile acid effect. Finally, bile acids in concentrations found in portal serum[12] were shown to increase membrane-associated, and decrease cystosolic, protein kinase C activity. The magnitude of the decline in cytosolic protein kinase C activity was less than the increase in membrane-associated activity, presumably because most protein kinase C in unstimulated cells resides in the cytosol[11]. Interestingly, bile acids have also been reported to increase membrane-associated protein kinase C in colon carcinoma cells and human platelets, leading to phosphorylation of endogenous protein substrates[13].

The biphasic response of cholesterol 7α-hydroxylase mRNA to PMA is compatible with well-recognized effects of phorbol diesters on protein kinase C. Initially, phorbol diesters induce translocation of cytosolic protein kinase C to membranes, where phosphorylation of target proteins occurs[11]. Proteolytic cleavage of membrane-associated protein kinase C ensues (so-called 'down-regulation'), terminating its phosphorylating activity[11,14]. The first phase of cholesterol 7α-hydroxylase mRNA decline may represent phosphorylation of a positive *trans*-acting factor by protein kinase C, decreasing its affinity for specific nucleotides in the cholesterol 7α-hydroxylase 5'-flanking region, or its ability to traverse the nuclear envelope[6]. Subsequent down-regulation of protein kinase C, dephosphorylation of the *trans*-acting factor, and restoration of cholesterol 7α-hydroxylase transcription, may account for the rebound phase. Additional investigation will be required to determine whether the protein kinase C substrate and the protein phosphatase 2A substrate implicated by these studies are the same proteins.

Several laboratories have recently implicated the proximal cholesterol 7α-hydroxylase 5'-flanking region in mediating its transcriptional inhibition by bile acids[15-17]. In DNA mobility shift assays, Chiang and Stroupe[17] have recently observed bile acid-induced changes in protein (putative transcription factor)–nucleotide binding using rat proximal cholesterol 7α-hydroxylase promoter oligonucleotides. These authors have proposed a model in which bile acids bind an intracellular receptor, which then displaces a positive *trans*-acting factor from the proximal cholesterol 7α-hydroxylase promoter. The demonstration that these oligonucleotides also exhibit differential protein binding in response to phorbol diesters would provide additional strong evidence that bile acids repress cholesterol 7α-hydroxylase transcription through a protein kinase C-dependent mechanism. A putative AP-1 consensus sequence, the recognition site for protein kinase C-dependent transcription factors, c-Fos and c-Jun, has been identified in the far upstream cholesterol 7α-hydroxylase 5'-flanking region[18]. The functional significance of this sequence awaits further investigation, but its location argues against it acting as a 'bile acid-responsive element'. Recently, protein kinase C-dependent phosphorylation of the CCAAT-enhancer binding protein (C/EBP), a positive *trans*-acting factor, was shown *in vitro* to decrease its affinity for [^{32}P]CCAAT oligonucleotides[19]. Although a putative C/EBP site exists in the proximal cholesterol 7α-hydroxylase 5′-flanking region[18], it lies 3′ to the oligonucleotides identified by Chiang and Stroupe[17].

Acknowledgements

This work was supported by grants from the Veterans Administration and the National Institutes of Health (grant PO1 DK-38030). RTS is the recipient of the Associate Investigator Career Development Award from the Veterans Administration.

References

1. Russell DW, Setchell KDR. Bile acid biosynthesis. Biochemistry. 1992;31:4737–9.
2. Twisk J, Lehmann EM, Princen HMG. Differential feedback regulation of cholesterol 7α-hydroxylase mRNA and transcriptional activity by rat bile acids in primary monolayer cultures of rat hepatocytes. Biochem J. 1993;290:685–91.
3. Stravitz RT, Hylemon PB, Heuman DM et al. Transcriptional regulation of cholesterol 7α-hydroxylase mRNA by conjugated bile acids in primary cultures of rat hepatocytes. J Biol Chem. 1993,268:13987–93.
4. Pandak WM, Li YC, Chiang JYL et al. Regulation of cholesterol 7α-hydroxylase mRNA and transcriptional activity by taurocholate and cholesterol in the chronic biliary diverted rat. J Biol Chem. 1991;266:3416–21.
5. Lamri Y, Roda A, Dumont M, Feldmann G, Erlinger S. Immunoperoxidase localization of bile salts in rat liver cells. Evidence for a role of the Golgi apparatus in bile salt transport. J Clin Invest. 1988;82:1173–82.
6. Hunter T, Karin M. The regulation of transcription by phosphorylation. Cell. 1992;70:375–87.
7. Bissell DM, Guzelian PS. Phenotypic stability of adult rat hepatocytes in primary monolayer culture. Ann NY Acad Sci. 1980;349:85–98.
8. Hylemon PB, Gurley EC, Stravitz RT et al. Hormonal regulation of cholesterol 7α-hydroxylase mRNA levels and transcriptional activity in primary cultures of rat hepatocytes. J Biol Chem. 1992;267:16866–71.
9. Pittner RA, Fain JN. Activation of membrane protein kinase C by glucagon and Ca^{2+}-mobilizing hormones in cultured rat hepatocytes. Biochem J. 1991;277:371–8.
10. Pugazenthi S, Yu B, Gali RR, Khandelwal RL. Differential effects of calyculin A and okadaic acid on the glucose-induced regulation of glycogen synthase and phosphorylase activities in cultured hepatocytes. Biochim Biophys Acta. 1993;1179:271–6.
11. Hug H, Sarre TF. Protein kinase C isozymes: divergence in signal transduction? Biochem J. 1993;291:329–43.
12. Stange EF, Scheibner J, Ditschuneit H. Role of primary and secondary bile acids as feedback inhibitors of bile acid synthesis in the rat in vivo. J Clin Invest. 1989;84:173–80.
13. Huang XP, Fan XT, Desjeux JF, Castagna M. Bile acids, non-phorbol ester-type tumor promoters, stimulate the phosphorylation of protein kinase C substrates in human platelets and colon cell line HT29. Int J Cancer. 1992;52:444–50.
14. Huang FL, Yoshida Y, Cunha-Melo JR, Beaven MA, Huang KP. Differential down-regulation of protein kinase C isozymes. J Biol Chem. 1989;264:4238–43.
15. Hoekman MFM, Rientjes JMJ, Twisk J, Planta RJ, Princen HMF, Mager WH. Transcriptional regulation of the gene encoding cholesterol 7α-hydroxylase in the rat. Gene. 1993;130:217–23.
16. Ramirez MI, Karaglu D, Haro D, Barillas C, Bashirzadeh R, Gil G. Cholesterol and bile acids regulate cholesterol 7α-hydroxylase expression at the transcriptional level in culture and in transgenic mice. Mol Cell Biol. 1994;14:2809–21.
17. Chiang JYL, Stroupe D. Identification and characterization of a putative bile acid-responsive element in cholesterol 7α-hydroxylase gene promoter. J Biol Chem. 1994;269:17502–7.

18. Chiang JYL, Yang TP, Wang DP. Cloning and 5′-flanking sequence of a rat cholesterol 7α-hydroxylase gene. Biochim Biophys Acta. 1992;1132:337–9.
19. Mahoney CW, Shuman J, McKnight SL, Chen HC, Huang KP. Phosphorylation of CCAAT-enhancer binding protein by protein kinase C attenuates site-selective DNA binding. J Biol Chem. 1992;267:19396–403.

11
Inborn errors of bile acid biosynthesis: update on biochemical aspects

K. D. R. SETCHELL and N. C. O'CONNELL

INTRODUCTION

Hepatic synthesis of the primary bile acids, cholic and chenodeoxycholic acids, is critical to the development and maintenance of the enterohepatic circulation. The pathway for bile acid synthesis from cholesterol is relatively complex[1,2], involving at least 15 reactions that are catalysed by various enzymes located within different subcellular fractions of the hepatocyte (Fig. 1). There is consequently considerable trafficking of the intermediates within the hepatocyte, but presently little is understood about these events. Identified genetic defects involving the reactions catalysed by these enzymes fall into two main categories: (a) defects involving oxidation of the cholesterol side-chain, and this includes the lipid storage disease of cerebrotendinous xanthomatosis (CTX) and a broad spectrum of peroxisomal disorders, which are bile acid defects secondary to abnormal peroxisomal assembly, structure, or function; (b) defects involving the reactions that result in changes to the steroid nucleus, and these include the recently described 3β-hydroxy-C_{27}-steroid dehydrogenase/isomerase deficiency and the Δ^4-3-oxosteroid 5β-reductase deficiency.

Progressive cholestatic liver disease is a striking clinical manifestation of patients presenting with impaired primary bile acid synthesis, and this includes patients with both the steroid nuclear defects and severe peroxisomopathies.

3β-HYDROXY-C_{27}-STEROID DEHYDROGENASE/ISOMERASE DEFICIENCY

The conversion of 7α-hydroxycholesterol to 7α-hydroxy-4-cholesten-3-one is catalysed by a microsomal NAD$^+$-dependent 3β-hydroxy-C_{27}-steroid dehydrogenase/isomerase enzyme. The enzyme has a reported molecular weight of 46 kDa and was thought to have been purified to apparent homogeneity[3]. Recent studies,

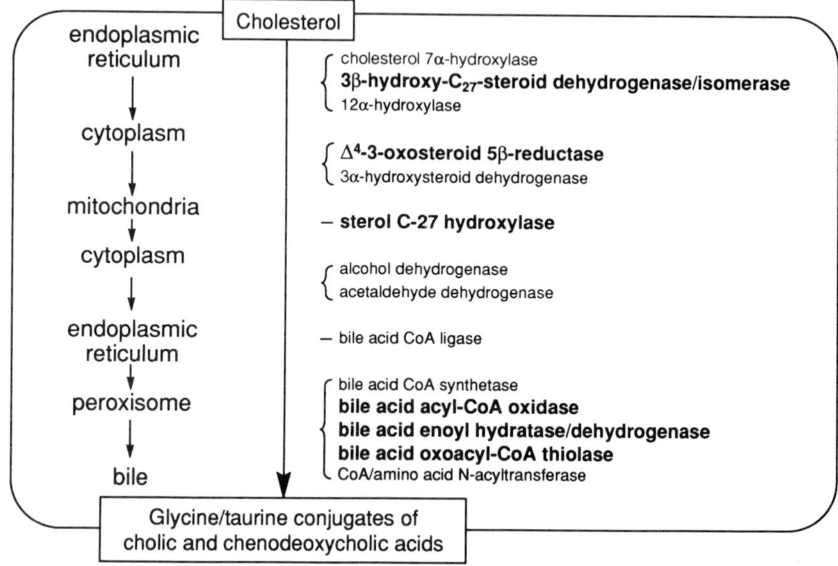

Fig. 1 Enzymes involved in the pathway for primary bile acid synthesis from cholesterol and their location within the hepatocyte. Highlighted are the known defects in bile acid synthesis

however, would suggest that the 46 kDa protein, which was originally shown to catalyse reactions in the C_{19} and C_{21} steroid hormone pathways, differs from the enzyme active in bile acid synthesis[4]. This is supported by the observation that patients lacking the bile acid isozyme have no apparent endocrine abnormalities.

Biochemically, patients with a deficiency of this enzyme lack, or have markedly reduced levels of, cholic and chenodeoxycholic acids in the serum, bile and urine, and elevated concentrations of atypical bile acids and sterols that retain the 3β-hydroxy-Δ^5 structure characteristic of the substrate for the deficient enzyme[5]. These 'signature' metabolites are not detected by routine or classical methods for bile acid measurement; therefore patients with these disorders may be misdiagnosed. Mass spectrometric techniques at present provide the most appropriate means of characterizing defects in bile acid synthesis, and screening procedures using fast atom bombardment ionization and liquid secondary ionization mass spectrometry (FAB-MS and LSIMS) yield unique and diagnostic profiles[6,7].

Conveniently, the 3β-hydroxy-C_{27}-steroid dehydrogenase/isomerase enzyme is expressed in fibroblasts, although its role in this cell line is unknown. Determination of its activity in cultured human fibroblasts[8] can provide confirmatory evidence for a defect initially identified by mass spectrometry. In addition, the parents of patients with this defect show a reduced activity of the enzyme, consistent with the heterozygous phenotype[8].

Since bile acid synthesis is well developed in early gestation[9], prenatal diagnosis of this enzyme defect should in principle be possible from the analysis of the bile acid composition of amniotic fluid. Previous studies have shown that cholic and chenodeoxycholic acids are present in amniotic fluid at concentrations

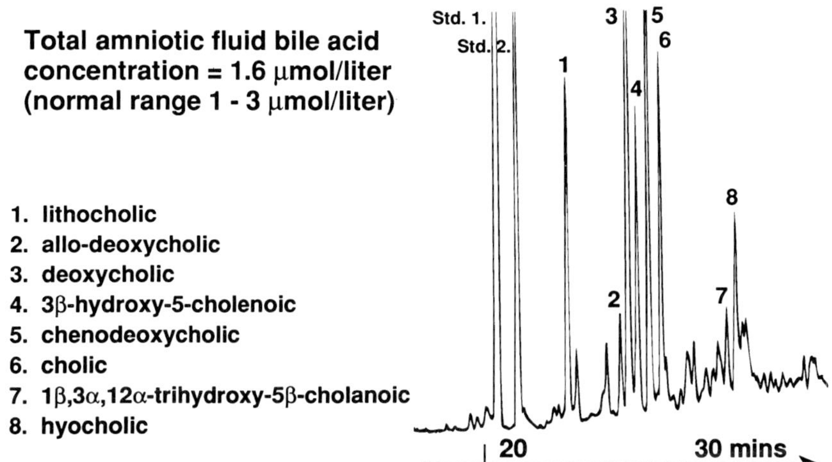

Fig. 2 Gas chromatography/mass spectrometry analysis of the bile acids of amniotic fluid obtained during early gestation from a carrier of the 3β-hydroxy-C_{27}-steroid dehydrogenase/isomerase deficiency

similar to that in serum[10] and, in addition, secondary bile acids of maternal origin are also present. Prenatal diagnosis of this enzyme defect was recently attempted for the first time by analysis of amniotic fluid obtained in early gestation from a woman who had previously given birth to two infants with the 3β-hydroxy-C_{27}-steroid dehydrogenase/isomerase deficiency (Fig. 2). Amniotic fluid bile acid concentration was $1.6\,\mu$mol/l, which is similar to previously published values[10] for normal pregnancies ($1-3\,\mu$mol/l). Qualitatively, both primary and secondary bile acids were found, as well as many other bile acids typical of early life[11], but allylic 3β-hydroxy-Δ^5 bile acids characteristic of the enzyme deficiency were not detected in this sample. The mother subsequently gave birth to an apparently clinically normal child; however, this defect often presents as late-onset chronic cholestasis[12]; and therefore analysis of urine from the infant is necessary to establish biochemical normality. At the time of publication this information was not available.

Clinical presentation of this defect has been variable among patients, but typical biochemical abnormalities include elevations in serum liver enzymes, a conjugated hyperbilirubinaemia and evidence of fat-soluble vitamin malabsorption[12,13]. In the early course of this disease many of the patients had normal serum transaminases and presented with fat-soluble vitamin malabsorption that was correctable with vitamin supplementation. Interestingly, a normal γ-glutamyltranspeptidase has been shown to be highly associated with, although not exclusive to, this inborn error. Thus far, more than 20 cases of the 3β-hydroxy-C_{27}-steroid dehydrogenase/isomerase deficiency have been recognized.

Δ^4-3-OXOSTEROID 5β-REDUCTASE DEFICIENCY

The fourth step in the conventional pathway for bile acid synthesis from cholesterol involves saturation of the steroid ring, a reaction that is catalysed by a cytosolic, NADPH-dependent Δ^4-3-oxosteroid 5β-reductase enzyme[1,2]. This enzyme, which was partially purified from rat liver in 1967 by Berséus[14], was later purified from rat liver cytosol by Okuda and Okuda[15] and monoclonal antibodies have been raised[16,17]. These monoclonal antibodies were found to have cross-reactivity with the human Δ^4-3-oxosteroid 5β-reductase enzyme, and have proven useful in demonstrating an absence of this 38 kDa protein in patients with biochemical evidence of a deficiency of the enzyme[2]. Rat[16,17] and human[18] cDNAs have been isolated and sequenced, and the enzyme activity expressed in COS cells. The cDNA indicated the enzyme to consist of 326 amino acid residues with a $M_r = 37\,376$. The amino acid sequence of the human Δ^4-3-oxosteroid 5β-reductase enzyme was shown to exhibit 79% homology with the rat enzyme, and a 54% identity with the rat 3α-hydroxysteroid dehydrogenase enzyme. The substrate specificity of the human enzyme was shown to be narrower than that of the rat enzyme, and appeared to be more important for bile acid synthesis than for steroid metabolism[18].

A deficiency of the Δ^4-3-oxosteroid 5β-reductase enzyme results in decreased concentrations of the primary bile acids in biological fluids, and elevated concentrations of atypical bile acids having a 3-oxo-Δ^4 structure characteristic of the sterol substrate[19]. Increased urinary excretion of 3-oxo-Δ^4 bile acids is frequently observed in advanced stages of liver disease, and is often a feature of physiological cholestasis in the first weeks of life[11], but in the latter case these metabolites disappear with development. In our experience, significantly elevated levels of 3-oxo-Δ^4 bile acids in the presence of primary bile acids are generally indicative of a poor prognosis. It is apparent that a reduced activity of the Δ^4-3-oxosteroid 5β-reductase, secondary to severe liver disease, can explain this biochemical pattern[20], but why the activity of this enzyme should be selectively reduced in severe hepatocellular damage is unclear. While the enzyme is labile[17], it is likely that the increased excretion of 3-oxo-Δ^4 bile acids is explained by the fact that, in severe cholestasis, an up-regulation in cholesterol 7α-hydroxylase-specific activity[21] will result in an increased synthesis of 3-oxo-Δ^4 sterol precursors that accumulate in concentration, exceeding the V_{max} for the Δ^4-3-oxosteroid 5β-reductase. Under severe cholestasis it is probable that the Δ^4-3-oxosteroid 5β-reductase then becomes the rate-limiting enzyme for bile acid synthesis. This contention is supported by our finding of high proportions of 3-oxo-Δ^4 bile acids in the urine of patients with chronic, profuse diarrhoea (unpublished observation), where excessive faecal bile acid loss will up-regulate the activity of cholesterol 7α-hydroxylase, resulting in an increased supply of substrate for the Δ^4-3-oxosteroid 5β-reductase enzyme.

An example of a urinary profile from an infant born with liver failure that later resolved is shown in Fig. 3. This profile was similar to that of patients with Δ^4-3-oxosteroid 5β-reductase deficiency in revealing high proportions of 3-oxo-Δ^4-(51%) and allo-(20%) bile acids. Interestingly, the elevation in 3-oxo-Δ^4-cholestenoic acids is not typical, and indicates the activation of alternative pathways for bile acid synthesis[22]. In contrast to patients with the primary enzyme

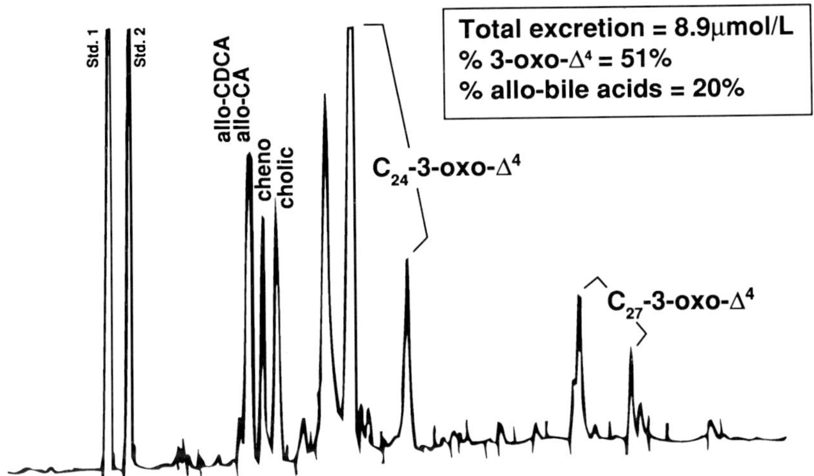

Fig. 3 Gas chromatography/mass spectrometry analysis of urinary bile acids from a neonatal patient born with liver failure that later resolved, showing high proportions of C_{24} and C_{27} bile acids with a 3-oxo-Δ^4 structure

deficiency the total concentration of bile acids in the urine of this patient was in the normal range, and qualitatively normalized with resolution of the hepatic injury.

Several patients diagnosed with neonatal haemochromatosis have been found to exhibit biochemical profiles consistent with a deficiency in Δ^4-3-oxosteroid 5β-reductase[23]. Whether this is a primary enzyme defect causing iron accumulation, or is secondary to severe liver failure, is difficult to establish definitively because, unlike the 3β-hydroxy-C_{27}-steroid dehydrogenase/isomerase deficiency, the Δ^4-3-oxosteroid 5β-reductase enzyme is exclusively hepatic in origin and not expressed in fibroblasts. Western blots performed on liver tissue obtained from several of these patients failed to reveal a 38 kDa protein, typically present in the liver of patients with severe liver disease that synthesize primary bile acids, and in some cases showed a truncated protein, a feature that is more consistent with a primary defect than a non-specific loss of proteins due to hepatocellular injury. The recent sequencing of a human cDNA encoding the Δ^4-3-oxosteroid 5β-reductase[18] will soon permit definitive identification of the defect by molecular genetic techniques. In the meantime, confirmatory evidence of a primary enzyme defect of the Δ^4-3-oxosteroid 5β-reductase can best be established from the observation that an interruption in primary bile acid therapy, after liver function tests have returned to normal, results in a reappearance of 3-oxo-Δ^4 bile acids as major metabolites in the urine.

MECHANISM OF LIVER INJURY IN BILE ACID SYNTHETIC DISORDERS

We previously suggested that the liver injury in patients with these bile acid

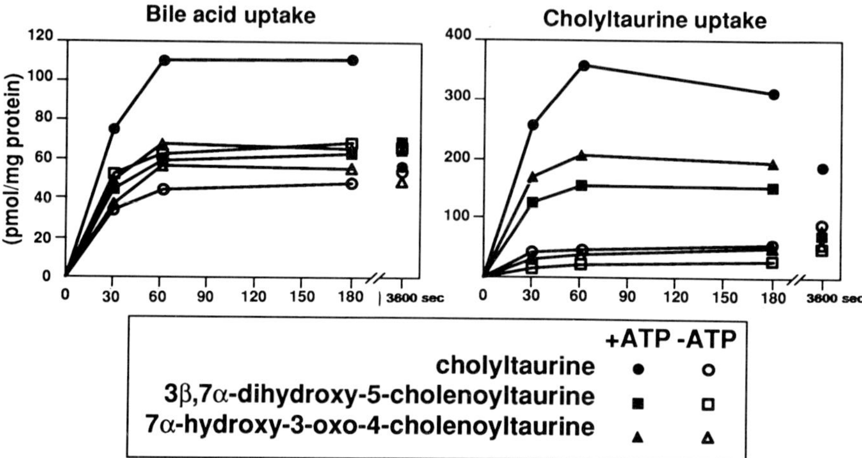

Fig. 4   Rat liver canalicular plasma membrane transport of 3β-hydroxy-Δ^5 and 3-oxo-Δ^4 analogues of taurocholate (left panel) and the competitive inhibition of these bile acids on cholyltaurine uptake (right panel) in canalicular membrane vesicles. Data are redrawn from ref. 24

defects is the result of both the lack of primary bile acids, which are essential for the promotion and secretion of bile, and the accumulation of atypical bile acids which we proposed had cholestatic and cytotoxic properties[5,19]. Recently, radiolabelled taurine-conjugated analogues of the 3β-hydroxy-Δ^5 and 3-oxo-Δ^4-forms of cholic acid were prepared, and their transport characteristics evaluated in rat liver canalicular plasma membrane vesicles[24]. Both synthetic bile acids inhibited ATP-dependent bile acid transport located in the canalicular plasma membrane (Fig. 4), and neither was transported in an ATP-dependent manner into canalicular plasma membrane vesicles, which may explain the cholestatic effects in patients. Furthermore, these findings may explain the failure to find significant amounts of bile acids in the bile of patients with these inborn errors. Canalicular transport of cholic and chenodeoxycholic acids is not defective in these patients, because primary bile acids are secreted in bile when given therapeutically.

Early diagnosis of these inborn errors is important because these patients are responsive to primary bile acid therapy[25,26]. Oral administration of primary bile acids is accompanied by a down-regulation in the synthesis of the atypical bile acids. Our experience to date indicates that, providing cirrhosis is not advanced, a normalization in serum liver enzymes, resolution of jaundice and an improvement in liver histology is attained with primary bile acid therapy, thereby circumventing the need for liver transplantation.

Acknowledgements

We acknowledge the continued and generous support of this work by the Falk Foundation e.V., Freiburg, and the many physicians who have submitted samples for analysis. The sample of amniotic fluid was obtained from a patient of

Professor O. Bernard and Dr E. Jacquemin (Centre Hospitalier Universitaire de Bicêtre, Paris), and the urine from the newborn with liver failure was from a patient of Drs W. F. Balistreri and J. E. Heubi (Children's Hospital Medical Center, Cincinnati).

References

1. Björkhem I. Mechanism of bile acid biosynthesis in mammalian liver. In: Danielsson H, Sjövall J, editors. Sterols and bile acids. Amsterdam: Elsevier; 1985:231–78.
2. Russell DW, Setchell KDR. Bile acid biosynthesis. Biochemistry. 1992;31:4737–49.
3. Wikvall K. Purification and properties of a 3β-hydroxy-Δ^5-C_{27}-steroid oxidoreductase from rabbit liver microsomes. J Biol Chem. 1981;256:3376–80.
4. Doerner KC, Bohdan PM, Vlahcevic ZR, Hylemon PB. Purification and characterization of rat hepatic 3β-hydroxy-Δ^5-C_{27}-steroid dehydrogenase (3β-HSDH). Presented at Falk Symposium 75, Maastricht, Netherlands, 1994.
5. Clayton PT, Leonard JV, Lawson AM *et al.* Familial giant cell hepatitis associated with synthesis of $3\beta,7\alpha$-dihydroxy- and $3\beta,7\alpha,12\alpha$-trihydroxy-5-cholenoic acids. J Clin Invest. 1987;79:1031–8.
6. Setchell KDR. Disorders of bile acid synthesis. In: Walker WA, Durie PR, Hamilton JR, Walker-Smith JA, Watkins JB, editors. Pediatric gastrointestinal disease: pathophysiology, diagnosis, management. Philadelphia: B. C. Decker; 1991:992–1013.
7. Setchell KDR, O'Connell NC. Inborn errors of bile acid metabolism. In: Suchy FJ, editor. Liver disease in children. St Louis: Mosby–Year Book; 1994:835–51.
8. Buchmann MS, Kvittingen EA, Nazer H, Gunasekaran T, Clayton PT, Sjövall J. Lack of 3β-hydroxy-$\Delta5$-C_{27}-steroid dehydrogenase/isomerase in fibroblasts from a child with urinary excretion of 3β-hydroxy-$\Delta5$-bile acids – a new inborn error of metabolism. J Clin Invest. 1990;86:2034–7.
9. Setchell KDR, Dumaswala R, Colombo C, Ronchi M. Hepatic bile acid metabolism during early development revealed from the analysis of human fetal gallbladder bile. J Biol Chem. 1988;263:16637–44.
10. Nakagawa M, Setchell KDR. Bile acid metabolism in early life: studies of amniotic fluid. J Lipid Res. 1990;31:1089–98.
11. Setchell KDR, Russel DW. Ontogenesis of bile acid synthesis and metabolism. In: Suchy FJ, editor. Liver disease in children. St Louis: Mosby–Year Book; 1994:81–104.
12. Jacquemin E, Setchell KDR, O'Connell NC *et al.* A new cause of progressive intrahepatic cholestasis: 3β-hydroxy-C_{27}-steroid dehydrogenase/isomerase deficiency. J Pediatr. 1994;125:379–84.
13. Setchell KDR. Inborn errors of bile acid synthesis: a new category of metabolic liver disease. In: van Berge Henegouwen GP et al., eds. Cholestatic liver diseases: new strategies for prevention and treatment of hepatobiliary and cholestatic liver diseases. Doredrecht: Kluwer Academic Publishers; 1994:164–7.
14. Berséus O. Conversion of cholesterol to bile acids in rat: purification and properties of a Δ^4-3-ketosteroid-5β-reductase and a 3α-hydroxysteroid dehydrogenase. Eur J Biochem. 1967;2:493–502.
15. Okuda A, Okuda K. Purification and characterization of Δ^4-3-ketosteroid 5β-reductase. J Biol Chem. 1984;259:7519–24.
16. Onishi Y, Noshiro M, Shimosato T, Okuda K. Molecular cloning and sequence analysis of cDNA encoding Δ^4-3-ketosteroid 5β-reductase of rat liver. FEBS Lett. 1991;283:215–18.
17. Onishi Y, Noshiro M, Shimosato T, Okuda K. Δ^4-3-oxosteroid 5β-reductase. Structure and function. Biol Chem Hoppe-Seyler. 1991;372:1039–49.
18. Kondo K-H, Kai M-H, Setoguchi Y *et al.* Cloning and expression of cDNA of human Δ^4-3-oxosteroid 5β-reductase and substrate specificity of the expressed enzyme. Eur J Biochem. 1994;219:357–63.
19. Setchell KDR, Suchy FJ, Welsh MB, Zimmer-Nechemias L, Heubi J, Balistreri WF. Δ^4-3-oxosteroid 5β-reductase deficiency described in identical twins with neonatal hepatitis. A new inborn error in bile acid synthesis. J Clin Invest. 1988;82:2148–57.
20. Clayton PT, Patel E, Lawson AM *et al.* 3-oxo-Δ^4 bile acids in liver disease. Lancet. 1988;4:1283–4.

21. Pandak WM, Li YC, Chiang JYL *et al.* Regulation of cholesterol 7α-hydroxylase mRNA and transcriptional activity by taurocholate and cholesterol in the chronic biliary diverted rat. J Biol Chem. 1991;266:3416–21.
22. Axelson M, Sjövall J. Potential bile acid precursors in plasma – possible indicators of biosynthetic pathways to cholic and chenodeoxycholic acids in man. J Steroid Biochem. 1990;36:631–40.
23. Shneider BL, Setchell KDR, Whitington PF, Neilson KA, Suchy FJ. Δ^4-3-oxosteroid 5β-reductase deficiency causing neonatal liver failure and hemochromatosis. J Pediatr. 1994;124:234–8.
24. Stieger B, Zhang J, O'Neill B, Sjövall J, Meier P. Transport of taurine conjugates of 7α-hydroxy-3-oxo-4-cholenoic acid and 3β,7α-dihydroxy-5-cholenoic acid in rat liver plasma membrane vesicles. In: van Berge Henegouwen GP et al., eds. Cholestatic liver diseases: new strategies for prevention and treatment of hepatobiliary and cholestatic liver diseases. Dordrecht: Kluwer Academic Publishers; 1994:82–7.
25. Ichimiya H, Nazer H, Gunasekaran T, Clayton P, Sjövall J. Treatment of chronic liver disease caused by 3β-hydroxy-Δ5-C$_{27}$-steroid dehydrogenase deficiency with chenodeoxycholic acid. Arch Dis Child. 1990;65:1121–4.
26. Setchell KDR, Balistreri WF, Piccoli DA, Clerici C. Oral bile acid therapy in the treatment of inborn errors of bile acid synthesis with liver disease. In: Paumgartner G, Stiehl A, Gerok W, editors. Bile acids as therapeutic agents. From basic science to clinical practice. Dordrecht: Kluwer; 1990:367–73.

Section IV
Bile acid transport: hepatic

12
Properties of two cloned basolateral bile acid uptake proteins of rat and human liver

P. J. MEIER, B. HAGENBUCH and B. STIEGER

INTRODUCTION

The liver efficiently extracts a wide variety of amphipathic organic anions from portal blood plasma. Quantitatively the bile acids represent the major cholephilic organic compounds. Their uptake into hepatocytes is mediated by both Na^+-dependent and Na^+-independent transport systems[1,2]. In contrast, non-bile acid organic anions are predominantly taken up into hepatocytes by Na^+-independent transport systems[3]. Two of these transport systems have been cloned from rat and human liver, namely a Na^+/taurocholate cotransporting polypeptide (rat, ntcp; human, NTCP) and a Na^+-independent sulphobromophthalein (BSP)/bile acid transporting polypeptide (rat, oatp; human OATP)[4-7]. In the following the properties of these two bile acid transport systems are summarized.

Na⁺/TAUROCHOLATE COTRANSPORTING POLYPEPTIDE (Ntcp; NTCP)

Ntcp mediates strictly Na^+-dependent taurocholate uptake and consists of 362 amino acids[4]. It presumably contains seven transmembrane domains (Fig. 1). Using a polyclonal antibody it could be demonstrated that the C-terminal end is localized intracellularly[8]. Consequently, the N-terminal end is localized outside of the cell and is glycosylated at positions 5 and 11 as revealed by recent site-directed mutagenesis experiments (data not shown). The same antibody reacted with a 51 kDa protein in Western blots of isolated rat liver plasma membranes[8]. Deglycosylation of the native Ntcp decreased the molecular weight[8] to 33.5 kDa, which corresponds to the molecular mass of the previously shown *in vitro* translation product in the absence of dog pancreatic microsomes[6]. Ntcp is selectively localized at the basolateral membrane of differentiated hepatocytes[8]. Its functional expression rapidly decreases in primary cultured hepatocytes[9]. It is

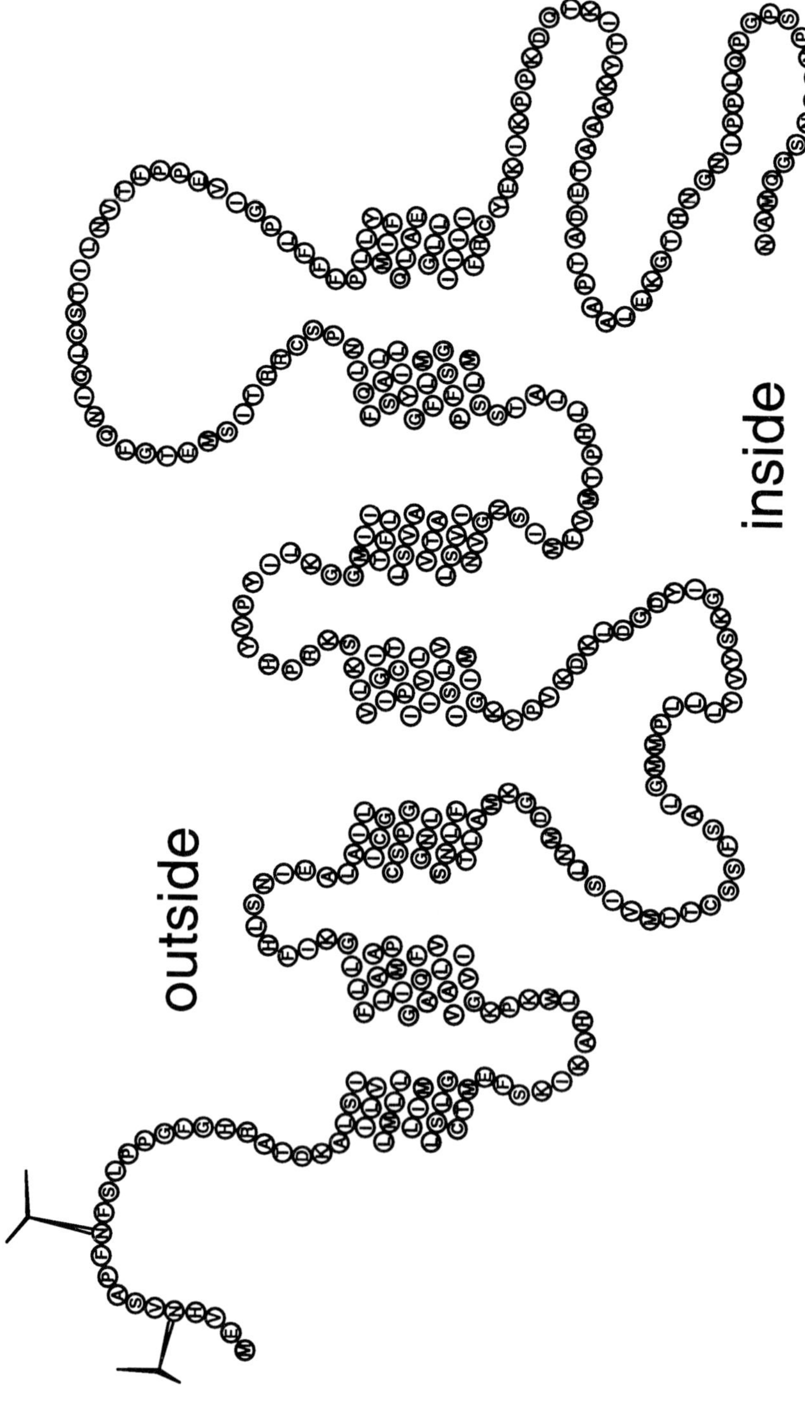

Figure 1   Model of the rat hepatic Na+/bile acid cotransporter

not expressed in hepatoma cell lines (ATC and Hep G2) or in non-mammalian liver[10]. This late phylogenic expression is mirrored by a similar late ontogenic expression in developing rat liver, where it appears during days 18–21 of the prenatal period[10]. ntcp expression also decreases during pregnancy in female rat liver[11] and during ethinyloestradiol treatment of male rats[12]. However, a marked increase of ntcp expression is seen post-partum and after prolactin treatment of ovariectomized rats[11]. These data indicate that ntcp expression is regulated by hormones during pregnancy and in the post-partum period. *Functionally*, ntcp mediates saturable Na^+-dependent uptake of conjugated and unconjugated bile acids both in cRNA-injected *Xenopus laevis* oocytes[4] and in transiently transfected COS[10] or in stably transfected CHO cells[8]. In all systems the apparent K_m values for taurocholate were found to lie between 25 and 42 μmol/l, which is in the same range as the values previously demonstrated in isolated hepatocytes[10]. Although Ntcp transports best conjugated bile acids (e.g. taurocholate, taurochenodeoxycholate, tauroursodeoxycholate), its substrate specificity also extends to non-bile acid organic anions such as oestrone-3-sulphate[13]. However, in stably transfected CHO cells no evidence could be found for ntcp-mediated transport of cyclosporine and bumetanide, both of which have previously been suggested to competitively inhibit Na^+-dependent taurocholate uptake in hepatocytes[13].

The molecular structure of the human liver NTCP is illustrated in Fig. 2. It consists of 349 amino acids and exhibits a 77% amino acid homology with the rat Ntcp[5]. It also mediates Na^+-dependent bile acid uptake, but its affinity for taurocholate ($K_m \sim 6\,\mu$mol/l) is higher than that of the rat protein. Southern blot analysis of genomic DNA from a panel of human/hamster somatic cell hybrids mapped the human NTCP gene to chromosome 14[5].

HEPATOCYTIC Na^+-INDEPENDENT ORGANIC ANION TRANSPORTING POLYPEPTIDE (oatp; OATP)

The rat oatp represents a protein of 670 amino acids with 12 putative transmembrane-spanning domains (Fig. 3). Three of the four possible N-linked glycosylation sites are localized on one side of the membrane, suggesting that both the N- and C-termini of the protein are situated inside the cell (Fig. 3). The same or similar organic anion transporters are also expressed in the kidney and, most importantly, in the brain[6]. Oatp mediates Na^+-independent uptake of BSP (apparent $K_m \sim 1.5\,\mu$mol/l) and of cholate and taurocholate (apparent $K_m \sim 50\,\mu$mol/l)[6,14]. Furthermore, recent experiments indicated that oatp can transport oestrone-3-sulphate, as well as neutral steroids such as ouabain. This latter finding raises the important question as to the physiological mechanism(s) involved in the transport mediation of differently charged cholephilic compounds. The driving force for oatp-mediated substrate transport remains to be elucidated.

The human OATP also represents a 670 amino acid protein with 12 putative transmembrane domains (Fig. 4). Sequence analysis revealed a 67% amino acid homology with the rat liver oatp[7]. OATP also mediates saturable Na^+-independent uptake of BSP ($K_m \sim 20\,\mu$mol/l), taurocholate ($K_m \sim 60\,\mu$mol/l) and

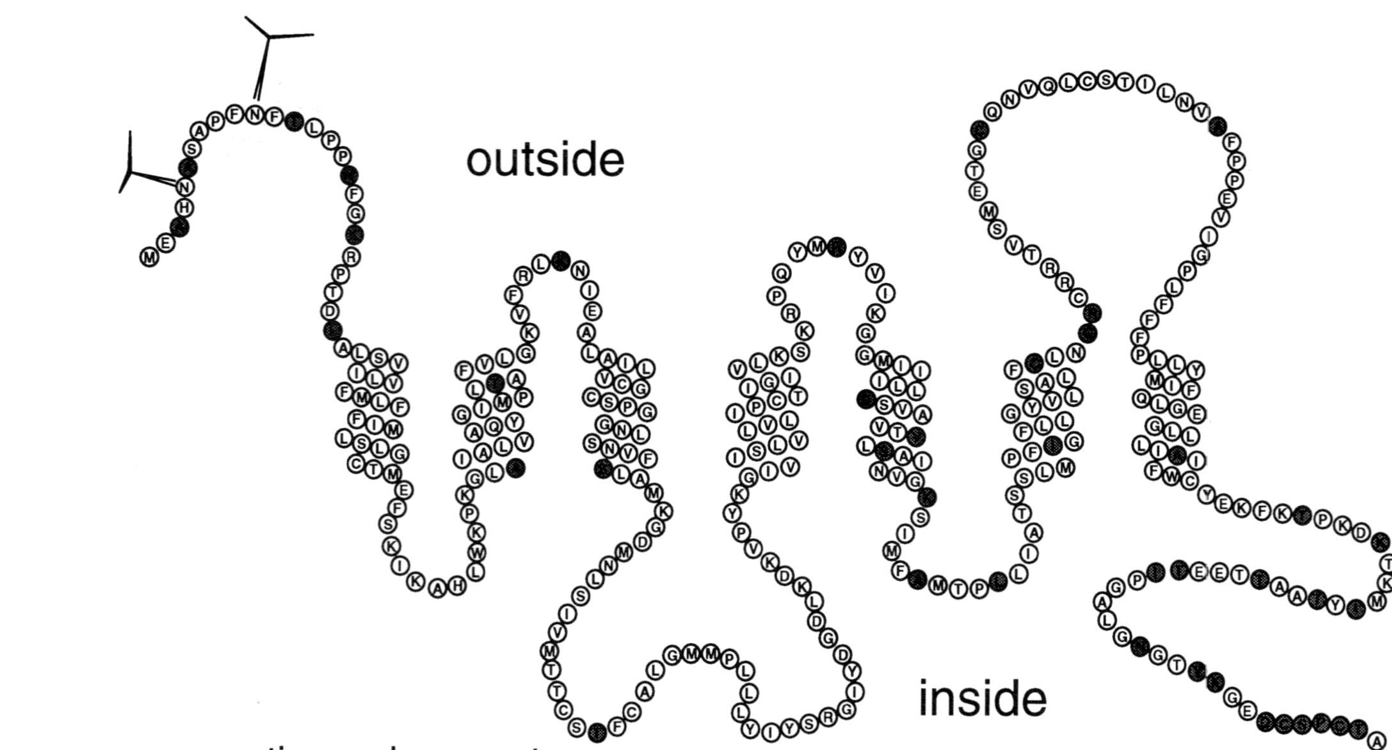

Figure 2 Model of the human hepatic Na$^+$/bile acid cotransporter

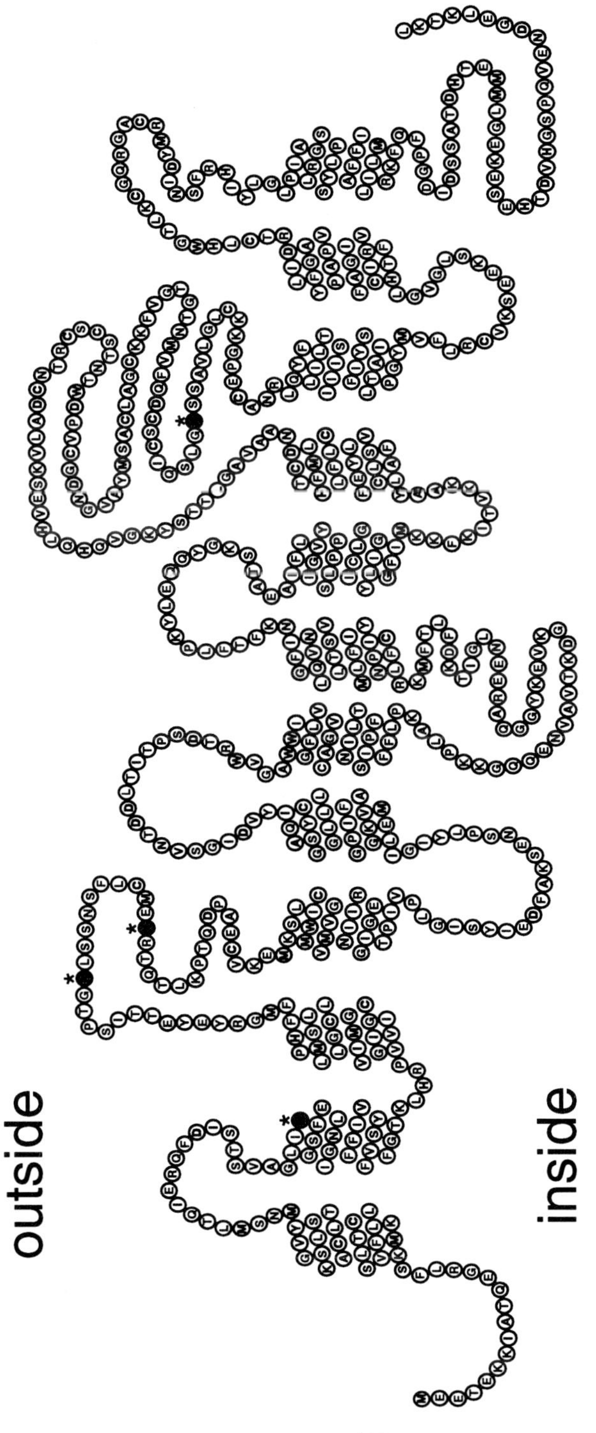

Figure 3 Model of the rat hepatic organic anion transporting polypeptide

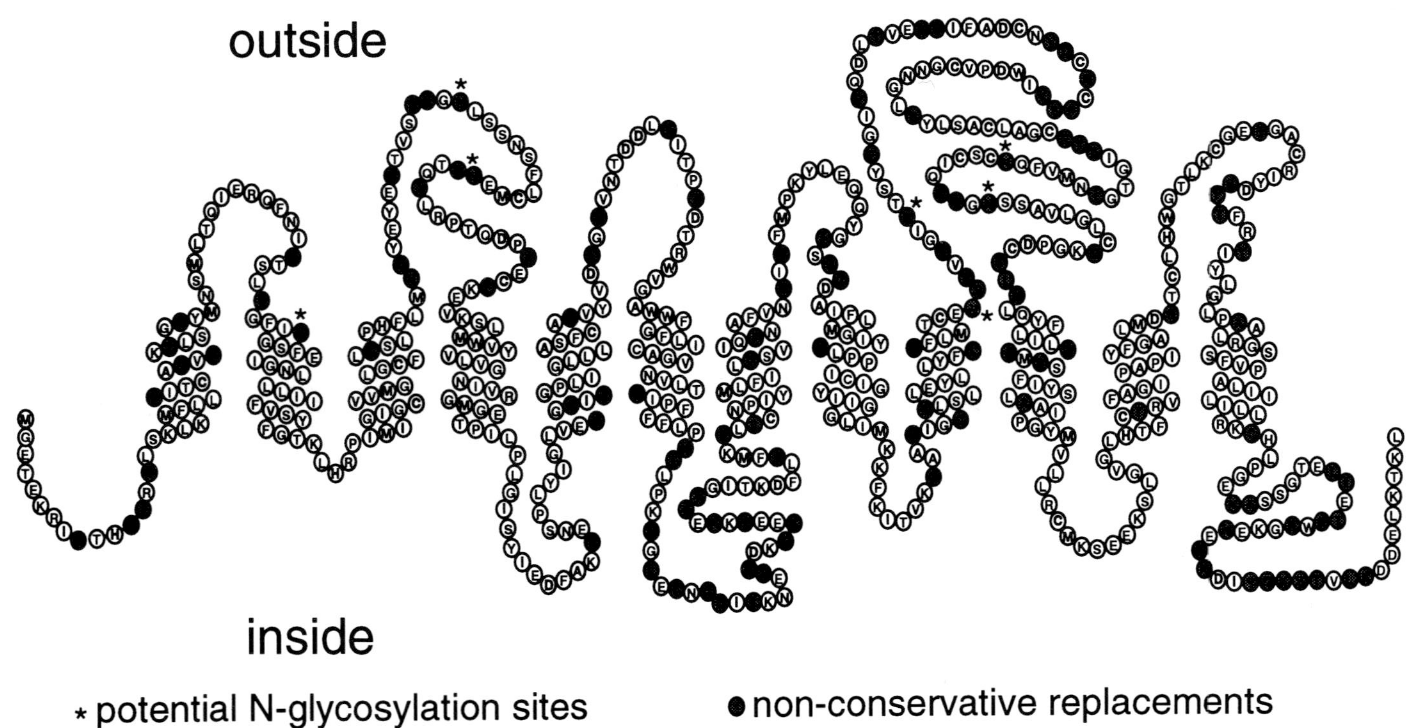

Figure 4 Model of the human hepatic organic anion transporting polypeptide

cholate ($K_m \sim 93\,\mu\text{mol/l}$). Interestingly, OATP transports BSP and bile acids with a lower affinity than the rat oatp, while for Ntcp-mediated (or NTCP-mediated) bile acid transport the opposite is true (see above). PCR analysis of genomic DNA from a panel of human–rodent somatic cell hybrids mapped the human OATP gene to chromosome 12. Northern blot analysis showed cross-reactivity of OATP–cDNA with mRNA species from human liver, brain, lung, kidney and testis. This wide tissue distribution suggests a fundamental role of OATP in transepithelial organic substrate transport of various organs.

CONCLUSIONS

Two basolateral bile acid and organic anion transporting polypeptides have been cloned from rat and human liver. The Na^+-dependent bile acid transporter exerts a higher affinity for conjugated bile acids in human as compared to rat liver. Furthermore, it is absent in the liver of lower vertebrates and represents a differentiation marker of mammalian hepatocytes. In contrast, the human OATP exerts lower affinities for bile acids and BSP as compared to the rat protein. Furthermore, the substrate specificity of oatp is broader than that of Ntcp and oatp-related transporting polypeptides are most probably also present in lower vertebrates. Taken together these transporters may represent phylogenic older transport systems than Ntcp. These assumptions, however, remain to be experimentally validated. The same is true for the elucidation of the driving force of oatp-mediated transport, as well as for the identification and characterization of the hypothetical oatp-related transporting polypeptides.

Acknowledgements

This study was supported by the Swiss National Science Foundation Grant 32-29878.90. Dr Hagenbuch is a recipient of a Cloëtta Foundation fellowship.

References

1. Frimmer M, Ziegler K. The transport of bile acids in liver cells. Biochim Biophys Acta. 1988;947:75–99.
2. Nathanson MH, Boyer JL. Mechanisms and regulation of bile secretion. Hepatology. 1991;14:551–66.
3. Tiribelli C, Lunazzi GC, Sottocasa GL. Biochemical and molecular aspects of the hepatic uptake of organic anions. Biochim Biophys Acta. 1990;1031:261–75.
4. Hagenbuch B, Stieger B, Foguet M, Luebbert H, Meier PJ. Functional expression cloning and characterization of the hepatocyte Na^+/bile acid cotransport system. Proc Natl Acad Sci USA. 191;88:10629–33.
5. Hagenbuch B, Meier PJ. Molecular cloning, chromosomal localization and functional characterization of a human liver Na^+/bile acid cotransporter. J Clin Invest. 1994;93:1326–31.
6. Jacquemin E, Hagenbuch B, Stieger B, Wolkoff AW, Meier PJ. Expression cloning of a rat liver Na^+-independent organic anion transporter. Proc Natl Acad Sci USA. 1994;91:133–7.
7. Kullak-Ublick GA, Hagenbuch B, Stieger B, Schteingart CD, Hofmann AF, Meier PJ. Cloning and functional characterization of a human liver basolateral organic anion transporting polypeptide (OATP). Hepatology. 1994;4:871.
8. Stieger B, Hagenbuch B, Landmann L, Höchli M, Schroeder A, Meier PJ. *In situ* localization of

the hepatocytic Na⁺/taurocholate cotransporting polypeptide (Ntcp) in rat liver. Gastroenterology. 1994 (In press).

9. Liang D, Hagenbuch B, Stieger B, Meier PJ. Parallel decrease of Na⁺/taurocholate (TCA) cotransport and its encoding mRNA in primary cultures of rat hepatocytes. Hepatology. 1993;18:1162-6.
10. Boyer JL, Ng OCh, Ananthanaryanan M *et al*. Expression and characterization of a functional rat hepatocyte sodium bile acid co-transport system in COS-7 cells. Am J Physiol. 1994;266:6382-7.
11. Ganguly TC, Lin Y, Hyde JF, Hagenbuch B, Meier PJ, Vore M. Prolactin increases hepatic Na⁺/taurocholate co-transport activity and mRNA post partum. Biochem J. 1994;303:33-6.
12. Kupferschmidt H, Hagenbuch B, Stieger B, Krähenbühl St, Meier PJ. Ethinylestradiol induces differential effects on various transporter mRNA and protein levels in rat liver. Hepatology. 1994;20:175A.
13. Schroeder A, Hagenbuch B, Stieger B *et al*. The rat hepatocyte Na⁺/taurocholate cotransporting polypeptide (Ntcp) mediates multispecific substrate transport in stably transfected Chinese hamster ovary (CHO) cells. Gastroenterology. 1994;20:A979.
14. Kullak-Ublick GA, Hagenbuch B, Stieger B, Wolkoff AW, Meier PJ. Functional characterization of the basolateral rat liver organic anion transporting polypeptide. Hepatology. 1994;20:411-16.

13
Hepatobiliary transport of sulphated and taurine-conjugated bile salts

W. DIEMINGER, A. DIETRICH, M. FALK, W. GEROK, G. KURZ and D. SCHWAB

INTRODUCTION

Sulphated and taurine-conjugated bile salts are found in enterohepatic circulation[1], though they are final excretion products of mammalian bile salt metabolism[2]. These dianionic bile salts differ from the usual monoanionic bile salts most obviously by the additional negative charge of the sulphatoester at position 3 of the steroid. The changes in physicochemical behaviour this causes make it improbable that dianionic and monoanionic bile salts share the same pathways during their hepatobiliary transport. In order to determine whether sinusoidal transport of sulphated and taurine-conjugated bile salts on the one hand and taurine conjugated bile salts on the other hand, is mediated either by the same or by separate transport systems, we studied uptake of (3α-sulphate-5β-cholan-24-oyl)-$2'$-aminoethanesulphonate (SLCT) and cholyltaurine (Fig. 1) into freshly isolated rat hepatocytes, as well as the mutual inhibition of their uptake. In order to identify the cytosolic proteins involved in intracellular translocation of dianionic and monoanionic bile salts on their path from sinusoidal to canalicular membrane of the hepatocyte, photoaffinity labelling studies were performed with biological material of different levels of organization using [^{3}H]7,7-ASLCT and [^{3}H]7,7-ACT as photolabile derivatives (Fig. 1).

MATERIALS AND METHODS

Materials

[^{3}H]Taurine ([^{3}H(N)]aminoethanesulphonate), with a specific radioactivity of 750–1500 GBq/mmol was obtained from NEN/Du Pont de Nemours GmbH Division (Dreieich, Germany). Heptafluorostearate (2,2,3,3,18,18,18-heptafluorooctadecanoate), and [^{3}H]11,11-azoheptafluorostearate, 11,11-azo-

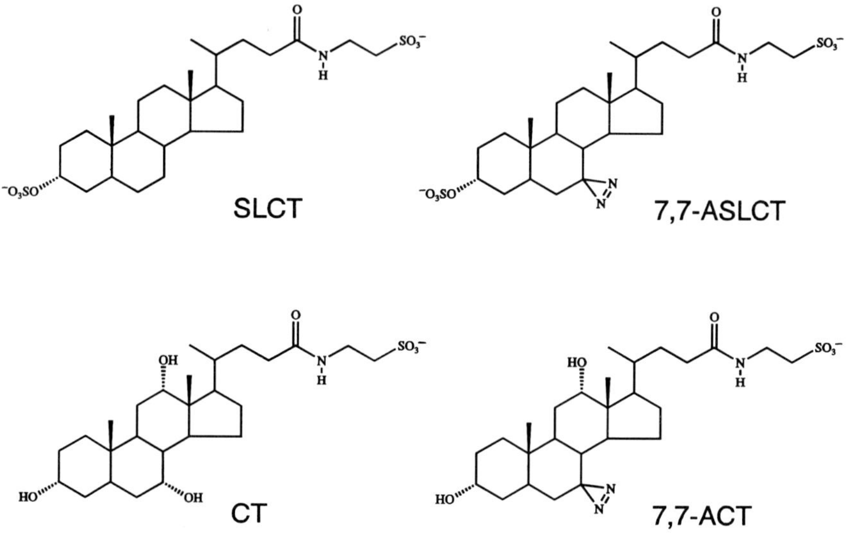

Fig. 1 Structures of SLCT ((3α-sulphato-5β-cholan-24-oyl)-2′-aminoethanesulphonate), CT (cholyltaurine), and of their photolabile derivatives 7,7-ASLCT ((7,7-azo-3α-sulphato-5β-cholan-24-oyl)-2′-aminoethanesulphonate) and 7,7-ACT ((7,7-azo-3α,12α-dihydroxy-5β-cholan-24-oyl)-2′-aminoethanesulphonate)

2,2,3,3,18,18,18-heptafluoro[G-^{3}H]octadecanoate) (2.63 TBq/mmol), SLCT, the [^{3}H]taurine conjugates of cholic acid, 7,7-azo-3α,12α-dihydroxy-5β-cholan-24-oic acid ([^{3}H]7,7-ACT), 7,7-azo-α-sulphato-5β-cholan-24-oic acid ([^{3}H]7,7-ASLCT), 7α-hydroxy-3α-sulphato-5β-cholan-24-oic acid ([^{3}H]SLCT), and 7,7-azo-5β-cholan-24-oic acid ([^{3}H]7,7ALCT), were synthesized and characterized as described[3,4].

Animals

Male Wistar rats (Tierzuchtanstalt Jautz, Hannover, Germany) weighing 200–250 g were used. The animals had free access to food (standard rat diet Altromin 300 R, Altromin GmbH, Lage, Germany) and tap water, and were housed in a constant-temperature environment with natural day–night rhythm.

Methods

Isolation of hepatocytes and uptake studies

Isolation and characterization of hepatocytes, uptake studies of bile salts and data analyses were performed exactly as described[5–7]. Uptake of bile salts was determined in the presence of 143 mmol/l Na$^+$.

Preparation of cytosol, purification of proteins and production of antibodies

Preparation of cytosol from liver snips and isolated hepatocytes, isolation of glutathione transferases 1-1,1-2, H-FABP and production of antibodies against these proteins were carried out as described recently[8].

Photoaffinity labelling

Photoaffinity labelling of liver snips and of isolated hepatocytes was carried out as described[8,9].

Polyacrylamide gel electrophoresis and isoelectric focusing

Discontinuous SDS-PAGE using vertical slab gels ($200 \times 180 \times 2.8$ mm) was performed as described[10]. Isoelectric focusing was carried out on Ampholine gel PAG plates pH 3.5–9.5 (Pharmacia LKB, Freiburg, Germany). The pI values were determined using pI marker proteins (Broad calibration kit, Pharmacia LKB, Freiburg, Germany) and controlled by cutting out zones of the gel, elution with 10 mmol/l KCl and measuring the pH values.

Detection of radioactivity

Either directly after electrophoresis, or after the staining procedure, the lanes of the polyacrylamide gels were cut into discs of 2 mm thickness using a comb for gel slicing. The radioactivity of each gel disc was determined as described[11]. For detection of radioactivity by fluorographic analysis hypersensitized films were used[12,13].

RESULTS AND DISCUSSION

Sinusoidal transport of SLCT

Monoanionic taurine-conjugated as well as unconjugated bile salts are taken up into freshly isolated hepatocytes by two distinct transport systems[5–7]. In order to determine the number of transport systems involved in uptake of SLCT, and their correlation to those for monoanionic bile salts, the dependency of initial influx rates on the extracellular concentration of SLCT and the inhibition of SLCT uptake by cholyltaurine were analysed (Fig. 2). Uptake of SLCT exhibited saturability and competitive inhibition by cholyltaurine. Graphical analysis of SLCT uptake by linear transformation in the J/A-versus-J plot revealed that the experimental data, measured in the presence of cholyltaurine, do not fit a straight line (Fig. 2B). This suggests, in analogy with sinusoidal transport of the monoanionic bile salts, that SLCT uptake is likewise effected by two different transport systems. Kinetic analysis proved that the apparent half-saturation constant of only one of the two transport systems is increased in the presence of cholyltaurine.

In order to examine whether SLCT competes with cholyltaurine as a true alternative substrate during uptake into hepatocytes, or acts simply as a

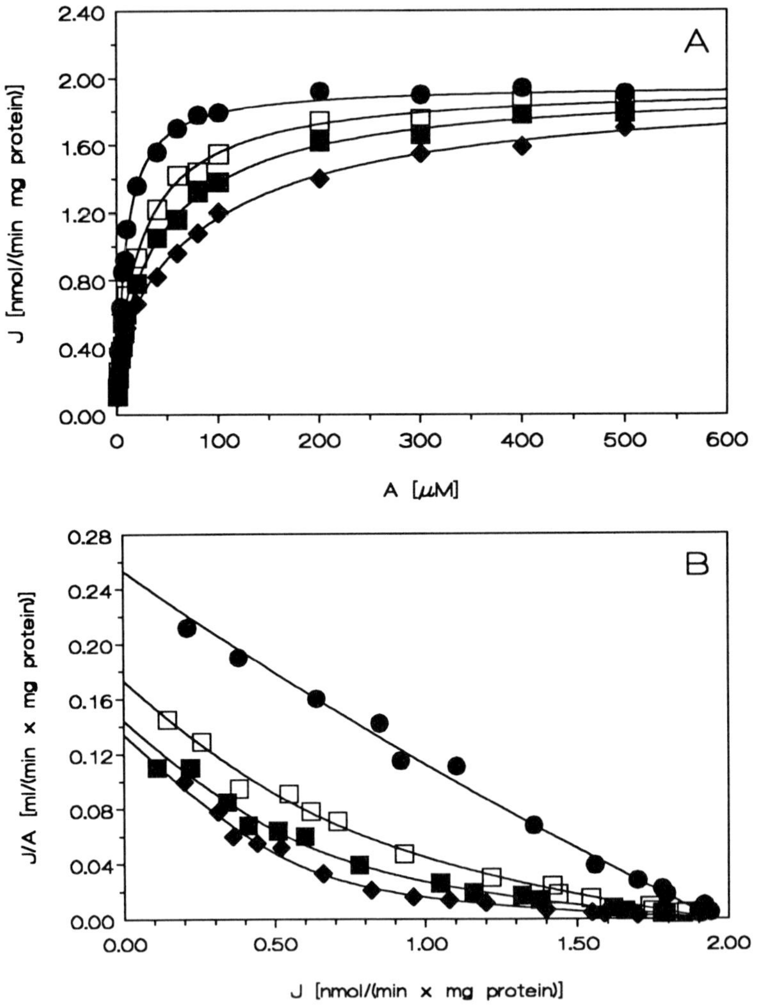

Fig. 2 Effect of different concentrations of cholyltaurine on the dependency of initial flux rates of SLCT into isolated hepatocytes on SLCT concentration in the presence of 143 mmol/l Na⁺. In the absence of cholyltaurine (●), and in the presence of 50 μmol/l (□), 100 μmol/l (■), 200 μmol/l (◆) cholyltaurine. **A**: J-versus-a plot, **B**: J/A-versus-J plot

competitive dead-end inhibitor, the effect of the presence of SLCT on the concentration dependency of initial flux rates of cholyltaurine was investigated (Fig. 3). The presence of SLCT exhibited a clear inhibitory effect on the uptake of cholyltaurine (Fig. 3A) and graphical analysis in J/A-versus-J plot demonstrates that this inhibition is clearly competitive (Fig. 3B). Detailed kinetic analysis revealed that of the two transport systems involved in the uptake of cholyltaurine only one is inhibited by SLCT.

The kinetic parameters for the uptake of SLCT into freshly isolated hepatocytes were calculated to be for transport system 1: $J_1 = 0.55$ nmol/(min/mg

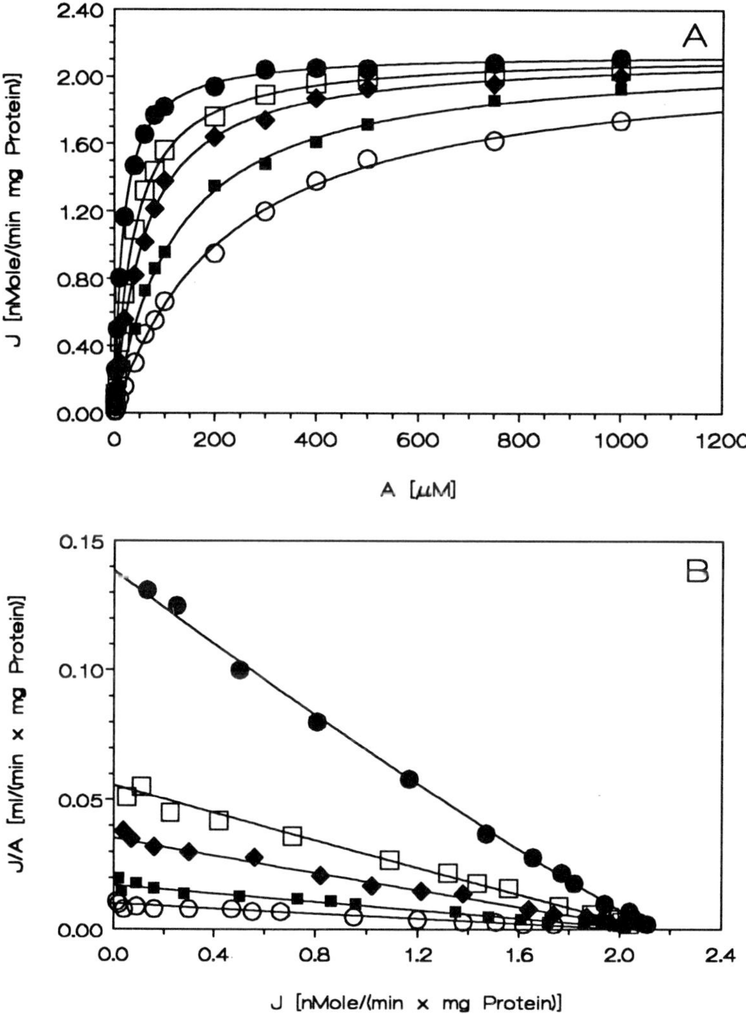

Fig. 3 Effect of different concentrations of SLCT on the dependency of initial flux rates of cholyltaurine into isolated hepatocytes on cholyltaurine concentration in the presence of 143 mmol/l Na^+. In the absence of SLCT (●), and in the presence of 5 μmol/l (□), 10 μmol/l (◆), 25 μmol/l (■), 50 μmol/l ○ SLCT. **A**: *J-versus-A* plot, **B**: *J/A-versus-J* plot

protein) and $K_{T1} = 4.2$ μmol/l and for transport system 2: $J_2 = 1.4$ nmol/(min/mg protein) and $K_{T2} = 11.1$ μmol/l. The K_I value for the uptake of cholyltaurine by transport system 1 has been determined to be $K_{I1} = 2.8$ μmol/l. The satisfactory agreement of the K_I value for the inhibition of cholyltaurine uptake with the K_T value for the uptake of SLCT justifies the assumption that SLCT and cholyltaurine are transported in the presence of Na^+ ions by the same transport system. The kinetic results require the assumption of three different sinusoidal transport systems to adequately explain bile salt transport. One is involved in transport of dianionic bile salts, a second in transport of monoanionic bile salts, and for a third one dianionic and monoanionic bile salts are competing substrates.

Intracellular transport of SLCT

In order to identify the cytosolic polypeptides which interact with SLCT, the soluble fraction obtained from rat liver was submitted to photoaffinity labelling, using [^{3}H]7,7-ASLCT as photolabile derivative. Subsequent analysis by SDS-PAGE revealed a clear incorporation of radioactivity in polypeptides with the apparent M_r values of 26000, 28000, 54000 and 67000 (Fig. 4A). The predominantly labelled polypeptide with the apparent M_r of 26000 was identified by immunoprecipitation with polyclonal antibodies against glutathione transferase 1 – 1 (also designated as $Y_a Y_a$), as well as against glutathione transferase 1–2 (also designated as $Y_a Y_c$) as subunit 1 of glutathione transferase (Fig. 4B). The coprecipitation of the slightly labelled polypeptide with the apparent M_r of 28000 by both antibodies demonstrates that subunit 2 of glutathione transferases also has the capability to interact with [^{3}H]7,7-ASLCT.

In order to compare the SLCT-binding polypeptides of liver cytosol with those interacting with monoanionic bile salts, photoaffinity labelling of the soluble fraction obtained from rat liver was performed using [^{3}H]7,7-ACT as a photolabile derivative of choyltaurine. The pattern of labelled polypeptides obtained after SDS-PAGE (Fig. 5) differs from that resulting from photoaffinity labelling experiments with [^{3}H]7,7-ASLCT. Incorporation of radioactivity occurred into polypeptides with the apparent M_r values of 14000, 26000, 28000, 33000, 38000, 43000, 54000, and 67000. The appearance of the labelled polypeptides with the apparent M_r values of 54000, and 67000 in the soluble fraction was dependent on the method of liver disintegration. The polypeptides with the apparent M_r values of 26000 and 28000 were identified by the immunoprecipitation as subunits 1 and 2 of glutathione transferases. Photoaffinity labelling of the cytosolic fraction of liver resulted in the identification of all bile salt-binding polypeptides which have been identified by binding studies using hepatic cytosol or purified proteins[14].

However, the biological significance of investigations requiring the disruption of the cellular organization is restricted with regard to the native state. Intracellular transport processes should be studied in systems where morphological and functional integrity is preserved[15]. Photoaffinity labelling of isolated cells and intact tissues allows the identification of interactions occurring under physiological conditions because the labelling reactions precede the disintegration of the intact biological systems. Thus, in order to obtain clear information about the interactions occurring *in vivo*, photoaffinity labelling of freshly prepared isolated hepatocytes using $1-10\,\mu$mol/l [^{3}H]7,7-ASLCT was performed. Subsequent analysis of total cell protein (Fig. 6A) and of cytosol from labelled hepatocytes (Fig. 6B) by SDS-PAGE revealed a labelling pattern completely different from that obtained by labelling of isolated cytosol (Fig. 4A). Predominantly a polypeptide with the apparent M_r of 14000 was found labelled. Labelling of subunits of glutathione transferases occurred only to a negligible

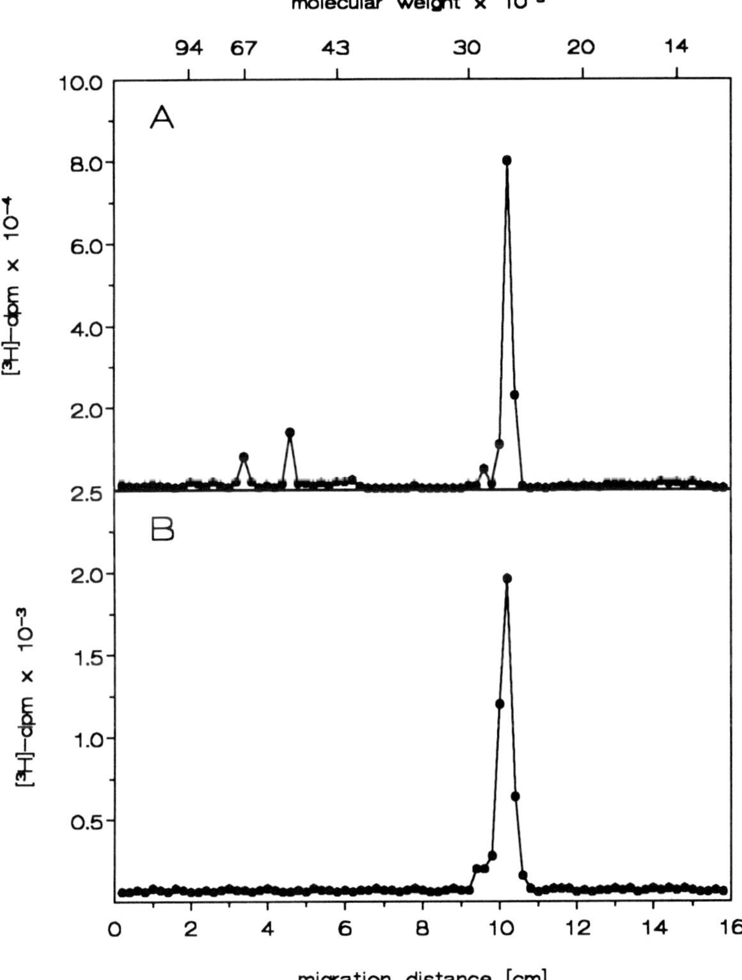

Fig. 4 Identification of ASLCT-binding polypeptides of cytosol from rat liver. Distribution of radioactivity after SDS-PAGE of cytosol. A solution of 400 μg of cytosol in standard medium was incubated with 1 μmol/l [³H]7,7-ASLCT (370 kBq) at 30°C for 5 min and irradiated for 10 min with light having a maximum at 350 nm. Total acrylamide concentration of the gel was 12% at a ratio of acrylamide:bisacrylamide of 97.2:2.8. **A**: Photoaffinity labelling with [³H]7,7-ASLCT. **B**: Distribution of radioactivity of the immunoprecipitate from cytosol labelled by [³H]7,7-ASLCT with antibodies against glutathione transferase 1–2[8]

extent, and may be due to the small amount of non-viable hepatocytes present in all cell preparations.

Results obtained with isolated hepatocytes may not be valid for intact liver, because they have lost their structural polarity and their capability for canalicular bile salt secretion[5,15]. In order to identify the intracellular SLCT-binding polypeptides in hepatocytes having an intact hepatobiliary transport, tiny liver

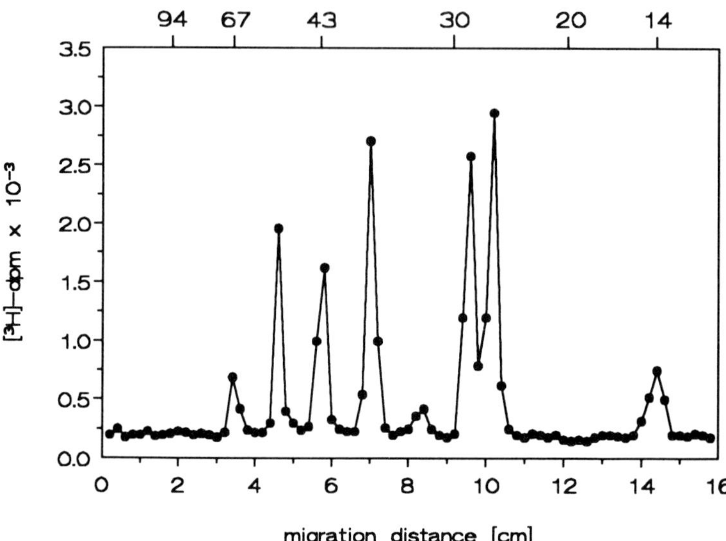

Fig. 5 Identification of ACT-binding polypeptides of cytosol from rat liver. Distribution of radioactivity after SDS-PAGE of cytosol. A solution of 400 μg of cytosol in standard medium was incubated with 1 μmol/l [³H]7,7-ACT (370 kBq). All other conditions were as described in the legend to Fig. 4

snips were submitted to photoaffinity labelling with $1-10\,\mu$mol/l [³H]7,7-ASLCT. The hepatocytes of the outer cell layers of these liver snips exhibit at least qualitatively an intact hepatobiliary transport of bile salts, and are therefore suitable for the identification of transport processes requiring the polarity of the cells. In order to analyse only the results obtained with intact hepatocytes, the impaired cells on the surface of the snips were removed by enzymatic digestion[15]. The pattern of labelled polypeptides obtained from total cell protein (Fig. 7A) and from the cytosolic fraction (Fig. 7B) after photoaffinity labelling showed the highest incorporation of radioactivity into a polypeptide with the apparent M_r of 14 000. The labelling pattern obtained from liver snips subsequent to photoaffinity labelling is similar to that obtained with cytosol from labelled isolated hepatocytes (Fig. 6B). The low labelling of a polypeptide with the apparent M_r of 26 000, resulting once more from the subunit of a glutathione transferase, is probably due to the fact that removal of impaired cells is almost always incomplete.

The photoaffinity labelling studies with [³H]7,7-ASLCT using isolated hepatocytes and intact liver tissue are only consistent with the conclusion that a cytosolic polypeptide with the M_r of 14 000 is involved in intracellular transport of sulphated and taurine-conjugated bile salts. In order to determine whether this polypeptide is identical with H-FABP, or represents another binding protein, comparative results were performed using the photolabile derivative of a metabolically stable long-chain fatty acid salt (Fig. 8)[3]. Photoaffinity labelling of isolated hepatocytes with $0.1-1\,\mu$mol/l of [³H]11,11-azo-heptafluorostearate, and subsequent analysis of the cytosolic fraction by SDS-PAGE, shows that,

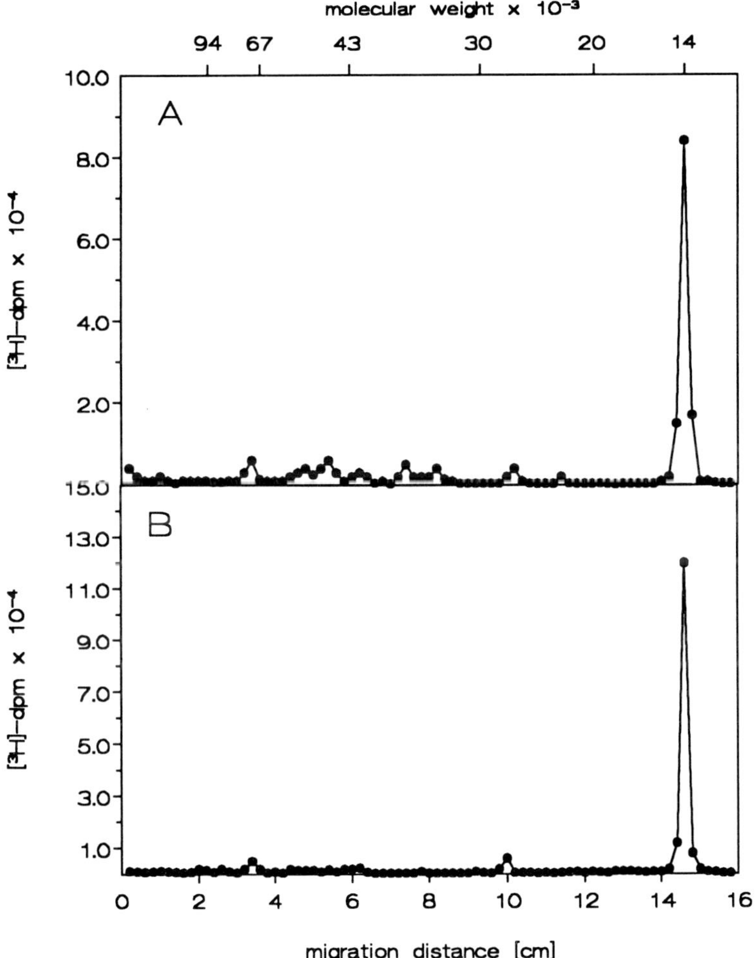

Fig. 6 Identification of SLCT-binding polypeptides in isolated hepatocytes. Distribution of radioactivity after SDS-PAGE of freshly isolated hepatocytes subsequent to photoaffinity labelling. A cell suspension of 1 ml containing about 1×10^6 (2 mg protein) hepatocytes in standard medium was incubated with $1\,\mu$mol/l [³H]7,7-ASLCT (370 kBq) at 37°C for 10 min, and subsequently submitted to photoaffinity labelling. All other conditions were as described in the legend to Fig. 4. **A:** Total cell protein (500 μg). **B:** Cytosolic protein (500 μg)

under the conditions used, incorporation of radioactivity occurred predominantly in a polypeptide with the M_r of 14000 (Fig. 9). In order to examine whether the SLCT-binding polypeptide is identical with H-FABP, isolated H-FABP (Fig. 10A) was submitted to differential photoaffinity labelling. The extent of photoaffinity labelling of H-FABP using [³H]7,7-ASLCT was clearly decreased in the presence of stearate as competing ligand (Fig. 10B) and vice-versa, incorporation of radioactivity by photoaffinity labelling using [³H]11,11-azo-heptafluorostearate was diminished in the presence of SLCT (Fig. 10C). These

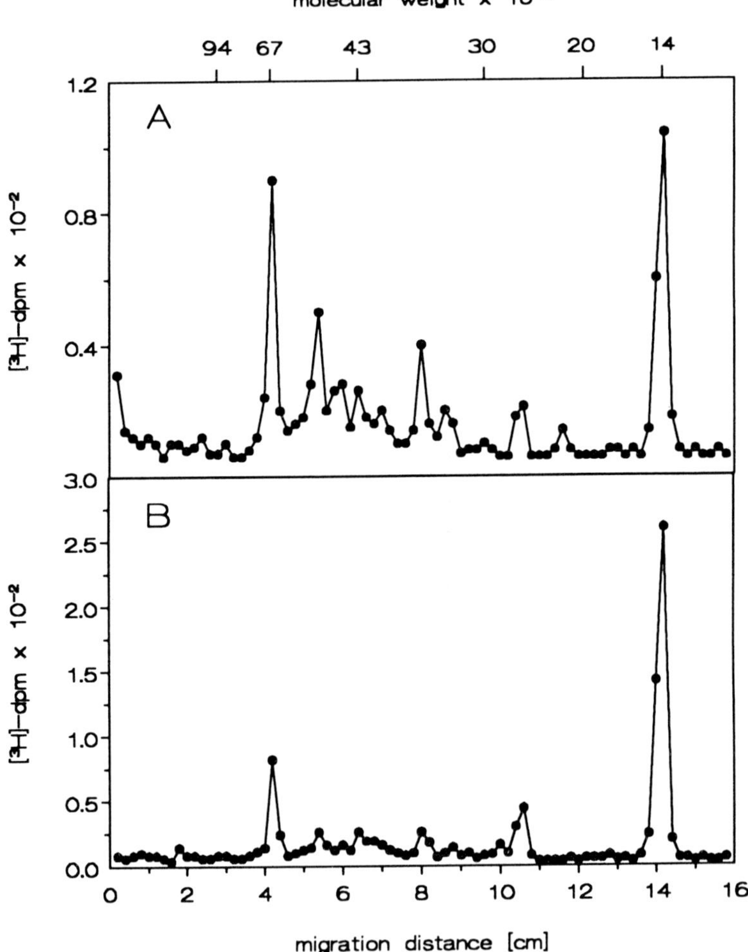

Fig. 7 Identification of SLCT-binding polypeptides in intact liver tissue. Distribution of radioactivity after SDS-PAGE. Ten liver snips were preincubated for 30 min with 4 μmol/l [³H]7,7-ASLCT (1.5 MBq) in standard medium at 37°C and irradiated at 30°C for 15 min. SDS-PAGE was performed using an acrylamide gel gradient from 10% to 15%. **A**: Total protein of liver snips (450 μg) after removal of impaired cells by enzymatic digestion. **B**: Cytosolic protein from liver snips (450 μg)

Fig. 8 Structure of the photolabile derivative of the metabolically stable long-chain fatty acid salt [³H]11,11-azoheptafluorostearate

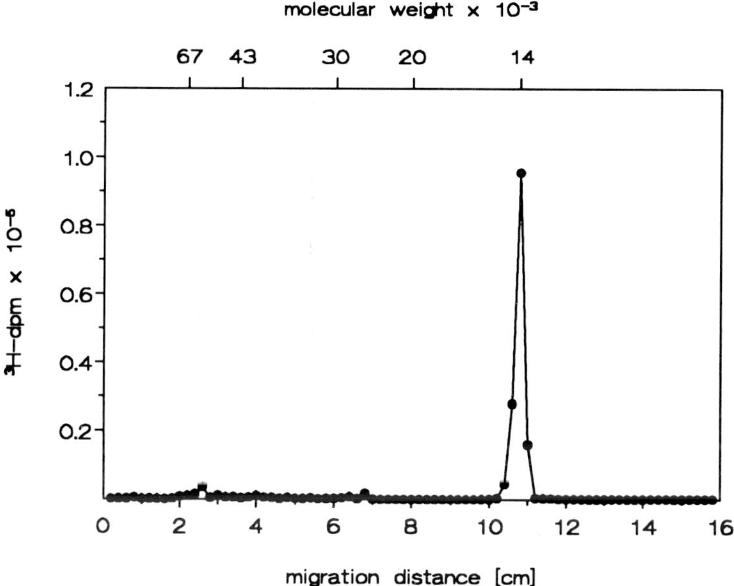

Fig. 9 Identification of H-FABP in cytosol of isolated hepatocytes. Distribution of radioactivity after SDS-PAGE of cytosol obtained from freshly isolated hepatocytes subsequent to photoaffinity labelling with [³H]11,11-azo-heptafluorostearate. A cell suspension of 0.5 ml containing about 1×10^6 (2 mg protein) hepatocytes in standard medium was incubated with 0.2 μmol/l [³H]11,11-azo-heptafluorostearate (280 kBq) at 37°C for 10 min and subsequently irradiated. Total acrylamide concentration of the gel was 15%; 400 μg of cytosolic protein were applied to electrophoresis. All other conditions were as described in the legend to Fig. 4

results demonstrate unequivocally that sulphated and taurine-conjugated bile salts and long-chain fatty acid salts compete for the same binding sites of H-FABP.

The identity of the polypeptide labelled by [³H]7,7-ASLCT with H-FABP has been further demonstrated by immunoprecipitation with monospecific antibodies against the purified H-FABP and by partial amino acid sequence analysis.

Sulphated and taurine-conjugated bile salts interact in the course of their transport from sinusoidal to canalicular membrane practically only with H-FABP, which therefore must have a function in storage and/or transport. To examine whether H-FABP is the main intracellular binding protein not only for the dianionic, but also for the monoanionic, bile salts, comparative photoaffinity labelling studies were carried out, using [³H]7,7-ASLCT as a photolabile derivative of dianionic bile salts and [³H]7,7-ACT, as well as [³H]7,7-ALCT, as derivatives of monoanionic bile salts. Photoaffinity labelling of isolated hepatocytes with these three photolabile derivatives, and subsequent analysis of the cytosolic proteins by SDS-PAGE, revealed clear differences between the labelling patterns obtained with [³H]7,7-ASLCT on the one hand, and those with [³H]7,7-ACT and [³H]7,7-ALCT on the other hand (Fig. 11). Whereas photoaffinity labelling using [³H]7,7-ASLCT caused the predominant labelling of H-FABP (Fig. 11, lane B), the application of [³H]7,7-ACT (Fig. 11, lane A)

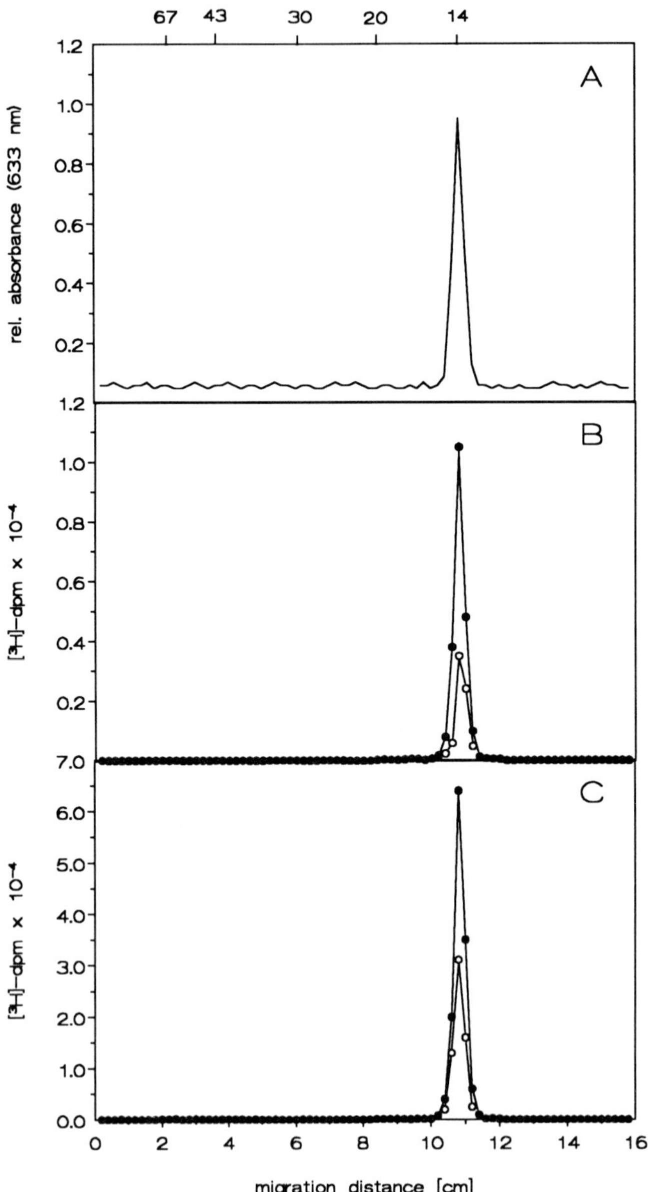

Fig. 10 Differential photoaffinity labelling of isolated H-FABP. Photoaffinity labelling of 30 μg of the purified protein was performed either with 1 μmol/l [³H]7,7-ASLCT (370 kBq) in the absence and in the presence of 50 μmol/l stearate or with 0.4 μmol/l [³H]11,11-azo-heptafluorostearate (110 kBq) in the absence and in the presence of 100 μmol/l SLCT. Total acrylamide concentration of the gel was 15%. All other conditions were as described in the legend to Fig. 4. **A**: Relative absorbance at 633 nm after staining with Coomassie Brilliant Blue R; **B**: Distribution of radioactivity after photoaffinity labelling with [³H]7,7-ASLCT in the absence (●) and in the presence (○) of stearate. **C**: Distribution of radioactivity after photoaffinity labelling with [³H]11,11-azo-hepta-fluorostearate in the absence (●) and in the presence (○) of SLCT

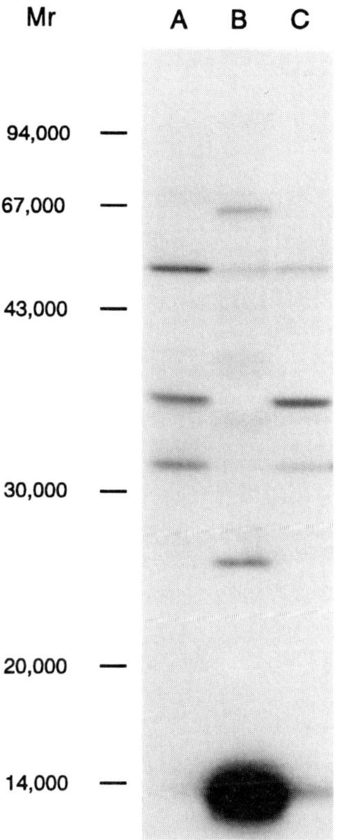

Fig. 11 Fluorographic identification of bile-salt binding polypeptides in the cytosol after photoaffinity labelling of freshly isolated hepatocytes. A cell suspension of 1 ml containing about 2×10^6 (4 mg protein) hepatocytes in standard medium was incubated with 1 μmol/l (370 kBq) of the respective photolabile derivative. All conditions were as described in the legend to Fig. 6. Cytosolic proteins (300 μg) were applied to electrophoresis. Total acrylamide concentration was 12%. Lane **A**: Photoaffinity labelling with [³H]7,7-ACT; lane **B**: photoaffinity labelling with [³H]7,7-ASLCT; lane **C**: photoaffinity labelling with [³H]7,7-ALCT

and [³H]7,7-ALCT (Fig. 11, lane C) resulted in the labelling of polypeptides with the apparent M_r values 33 000, 38 000 and 54 000; H-FABP was found labelled only to an insignificant extent. Common to all three patterns is the insignificant labelling of polypeptides with M_r about 26 000, ruling out the involvement of glutathione transferases in intracellular transport of dianionic as well as monoanionic bile salts. Even the inhibition of their enzymatic activity by bile salts[16–18] is physiologically of no relevance. Whereas the physiological significance of distinct cytosolic proteins for the transport of monoanionic bile salts remains to be established, for sulphated and taurine-conjugated bile salts H-FABP is the essential intracellular binding protein. Photoaffinity labelling studies of intact hepatocytes, and of specimens of intact liver tissue, proved that dianionic and monoanionic bile salts use different paths within the hepatocyte during their hepatobiliary transport. This would also be in accordance with the assumption that in transcellular traffic of monoanionic bile salts a vesicular component may play a distinct role[19-23].

Acknowledgements

This investigation was supported by the Deutsche Forschungsgemeinschaft (SFB 154). One of us (A. Dietrich) is indebted to the Fitz-Thyssen-Stiftung for a scholarship.

References

1. Kuipers F, Heslinga H, Havinga R, Vonk RJ. Intestinal adsorption of lithocholic acid sulfates in the rat: inhibitory effects of calcium. Am J Physiol. 1986;251:G189–94.
2. Hofmann AF. Chemistry and enterohepatic circulation of bile acids. Hepatology. 1984;4:4–14S.
3. Stoll GH, Gerok W, Kurz G. Synthesis of a metabolically stable modified long-chain fatty acid salt and its photolabile derivative. J Lipid Res. 1991;32:843–57.
4. Dietrich A, Dieminger W, Gerok W, Kurz G. Synthesis and applicability of a photolabile 7,7-azo analogue of 3-sulfated taurine conjugated bile salts. J Lipid Res. (Submitted).
5. Schramm U, Fricker G, Buscher H-P, Gerok W, Kurz G. Fluorescent derivatives of bile salts. III. Uptake of 7β-NBD-NCT into isolated hepatocytes by the transport systems for cholyltaurine. J Lipid Res. 1993;34:741–57.
6. Gerok W, Kurz G, Schwab D. Transport of conjugated and unconjugated bile salts across the sinusoidal membrane. In: Keppler D, Jungermann K, editors. Transport in the liver. Dordrecht: Kluwer; 1994:82–94.
7. Schwab D, Gerok W, Kurz G. Sinusoidal transport of unconjugated bile salts. Uptake of norcholansulfonate and cholate into isolated hepatocytes by the transport systems for taurine conjugated bile salts. J Lipid Res. (Submitted).
8. Dietrich A, Dieminger W, Fuchte K et al. Functional significance of interaction of H-FABP with sulfated and nonsulfated taurine conjugated bile salts in rat liver. J Lipid Res. (Submitted).
9. Schramm U, Dietrich A, Schneider S, Buscher H-P, Gerok W, Kurz G. Fluorescent derivatives of bile salts. II. Suitability of NBD-amino derivatives of bile salts for the study of biological transport. J Lipid Res. 1991;32:1769–79.
10. Laemmli UK. Cleavage of structural proteins during the assembly of the head of bacteriophage T4. Nature. 1970;227:680–5.
11. Kramer W, Bickel U, Buscher H-P, Gerok W, Kurz G. Bile-salt-binding polypeptides in plasma membranes of hepatocytes revealed by photoaffinity labelling. Eur J Biochem. 1982;129:13–24.
12. Laskey RA, Mills AD. Quantitative film detection of ^{3}H and ^{14}C in polyacrylamide gels by fluorography. Eur J Biochem. 1975;56:335–41.
13. Chamberlain JP. Fluorographic detection of radioactivity in polyacrylamide gels with the water-soluble fluor, sodium salicylate. Anal Biochem. 1979;98:132–5.
14. Stolz A, Takikawa H, Ookhtens M, Kaplowitz N. The role of cytoplasmic proteins in hepatic bile acid transport. Ann Rev Physiol. 1989;51:161–76.
15. Fricker G, Schneider S, Gerok W, Kurz G. Identification of different transport systems for bile salts in sinusoidal and canalicular membranes of hepatocytes. Biol Chem Hoppe-Seyler. 1987;368:1143–50.
16. Vessey DA, Zakim D. Inhibition of glutathione S-transferase by bile acids. Biochem J. 1981;197:321–5.
17. Hayes JD, Chalmers J. Bile acid inhibition of basic and neutral glutathione S-transferases in rat liver. Biochem J. 1983;215:581–8.
18. Takikawa H, Kaplowitz N. Comparison of the binding sites of GSH S-transferases of the Y_a- and Y_b-subunit classes: effect of glutathione of the binding of bile acids. J Lipid Res. 1988;29:279–86.

19. Suchy FJ, Balistreri WF, Hung J, Miller P, Garfield SA. Intracellular bile acid transport in rat liver as visualized by electron microscope autoradiography using a bile acid analogue. Am J Physiol. 1983;245:G681–9.
20. Simion FA, Fleischer B, Fleischer S. Subcellular distribution of bile acids, bile salts, and taurocholate binding sites in rat liver. Biochemistry. 1984;23:6459–66.
21. Lamri Y, Roda A, Dumont M, Feldmann G, Erlinger S. Immunoperoxidase localization of bile salts in rat liver cells. J Clin Invest. 1988;82:1173–82.
22. Crawford JM, Berken CA, Gollan JL. Role of the hepatocyte microtubular system in the excretion of bile salts and biliary lipid: implications for intracellular vesicular transport. J Lipid Res. 1988;29:144–56.
23. Hayakawa T, Ng OC, Ma A, Boyer JL. Taurocholate stimulates transcytotic vesicular pathways labelled by horseradish peroxidase in the isolated perfused rat liver. Gastroenterology. 1990;99:216–28.

14
Effects of bile acids on signalling mechanisms in the hepatocyte

U. BEUERS, G. PAUMGARTNER and J. L. BOYER

INTRODUCTION

Cholephilic compounds are secreted from blood to bile by the hepatocyte via two major mechanisms: (a) transport across the membranes via carrier proteins; (b) transport from blood to bile via vesicles (for review, see ref. 1). Experimental evidence indicates that carrier proteins are inserted into the membrane via fusion of protein-carrying vesicles with the membrane[2,3]. Thus, vesicle fusion with the membrane, or exocytosis, seems to be of dual importance for maintenance of transport function of the liver cell. However, vesicle fusion is impaired in experimental cholestasis[2,4].

Transport mechanisms in the liver cell are regulated by a number of intracellular messengers, of which cytosolic free Ca^{2+} ($[Ca^{2+}]_i$) and protein kinase C (PKC) may play a key role[1].

Ursodeoxycholic acid (UDCA) improves biliary secretion in cholestatic liver disease by unknown mechanisms[5–7]. Therefore, we studied the effect of UDCA conjugates in comparison to other hydrophilic and hydrophobic bile acids on signalling and secretory mechanisms in isolated rat hepatocytes and the isolated perfused rat liver.

METHODS

$[Ca^{2+}]_i$ was measured in groups of approximately 20 cells in short-term culture loaded with the fluorescent dye indo-1 using microspectrofluorometry[8]. Ca^{2+} influx across the plasma membrane was determined radiochemically in hepatocytes in suspension[9] analysing uptake of $^{45}Ca^{2+}$. Inositol 1,4,5-trisphosphate was measured with a radio-binding assay in cells in short-term culture[8]. PKC isoenzymes were identified and their intracellular distribution studied in hepatocytes in suspension using immunoblotting and immunofluorescence techniques[10]. Vesicular exocytosis was quantified by studying biliary secretion of horseradish peroxidase (HRP) in the perfused rat liver preloaded with HRP[9].

RESULTS AND DISCUSSION

Cytosolic free Ca2+ ([Ca2+]i)

TUDCA induced a marked and sustained increase of $[Ca^{2+}]_i$ in isolated hepatocytes in short-term culture at $1-10\,\mu mol/l$, concentrations well within the physiological range of serum bile acid levels[8]. A maximum effect was observed at $5\,\mu mol/l$ concentrations under the experimental conditions chosen[8]. The sustained $[Ca^{2+}]_i$ increase observed in cells treated with $10\,\mu mol/l$ TUDCA was significantly higher after 15 min than that of any other bile acid (TLCA, TCDCA, TCA, UDCA) tested at equimolar concentrations[8]. This $[Ca^{2+}]_i$ increase was of both intra- and extracellular origin.

Pretreatment of cells with TUDCA inhibited a further $[Ca^{2+}]_i$ increase by the α-adrenergic agonist phenylephrine and the microsomal Ca^{2+}-ATPase inhibitor 2,5-di-(*tert*-butyl)-1,4-benzohydroquinone (tBuBHQ), indicating that TUDCA depletes the same endogenous IP_3-sensitive microsomal Ca^{2+} stores as do phenylephrine and tBuBHQ[8].

TUDCA-induced $[Ca^{2+}]_i$ increase was significantly reduced and only transient when cells were (a) pretreated with the Ca^{2+} channel-blocker Ni^{2+}, (b) superfused with a Ca^{2+}-free medium, or (c) superfused with a medium containing only low Ca^{2+} levels ($<0.2\,mmol/l$)[8,9] avoiding agonist-induced Ca^{2+} influx via Ca^{2+} channels[11] but also Ca^{2+} depletion of the cells. The contribution of extracellular Ca^{2+} in TUDCA-induced $[Ca^{2+}]_i$ increase was confirmed by increased $^{45}Ca^{2+}$ uptake in hepatocytes treated with TUDCA[9].

In cholestatic cells of bile duct-ligated rats, TUDCA-induced $[Ca^{2+}]_i$ increase was markedly diminished, and only transient[9]. The effect was similar to TUDCA-induced $[Ca^{2+}]_i$ increases in the presence of the Ca^{2+} channel blocker Ni^{2+} or low extracellular Ca^{2+} levels ($<0.2\,mmol/l$) in normal hepatocytes. This suggests that Ca^{2+} influx is impaired in cholestatic hepatocytes.

The relatively low concentration of TUDCA necessary to affect $[Ca^{2+}]_i$ in hepatocytes ($1-5\,\mu mol/l$), when compared to the concentration required for similar effects in neutrophils ($500-1000\,\mu mol/l$)[12], suggests that TUDCA exerts its effects on $[Ca^{2+}]_i$ after uptake into the cell, and that Ca^{2+} ionophoresis by TUDCA may be of minor importance under physiological conditions.

Comparisons of these results with those of other studies[13–21] have to be performed cautiously regarding the following differences in the experimental design of the studies: (a) type of bile acid studied (mono- vs di- vs trihydroxy bile acids; conjugated vs unconjugated bile acids); (b) concentration of bile acid studied (low vs high micromolar range); (c) type of cell preparation studied (short-term culture of hepatocytes[8,9,19] vs suspension of hepatocytes[13–18] vs isolated perfused rat liver[20,21]; rat[8–10,13–17,19–21] vs hamster[18]); (d) type of Ca^{2+} indicator used (indo-1[8,9,19] vs quin2[13,15–18] vs Ca^{2+}-sensitive electrode[20,21]).

Experimental evidence[8,9,13–21] indicates that:

1. Mono- and dihydroxy bile acids, but not trihydroxy bile acids increase $[Ca^{2+}]_i$ in hepatocytes at low micromolar concentrations[8,13,15,16,18].
2. Mono- and dihydroxy bile acids deplete IP_3-sensitive microsomal Ca^{2+} stores[8,9,13,15,16,18].
3. Dihydroxy bile acids stimulate Ca^{2+} influx across the plasma

membrane[8,9,18,19], whereas the effect of monohydroxy bile acids on Ca^{2+} influx is not completely clear[13,15–17].

4. Hydrophobic, but not hydrophilic bile acids at high micromolar concentrations induce Ca^{2+} efflux[14,18]; however, monohydroxy bile acids at low micromolar concentrations do not stimulate Ca^{2+} efflux into the hepatic veins[20].

5. Biliary secretion of Ca^{2+} is stimulated by GUDCA, but not by TCDCA[21].

A further insight into the molecular mechanisms and spatial distribution of Ca^{2+} signalling within the hepatocyte[22] is needed to fully understand the differential effects of bile acids on hepatocellular Ca^{2+} homeostasis.

Inositol 1,4,5-trisphosphate (IP$_3$)

TUDCA (10 μmol/l) did not affect levels of IP$_3$ in hepatocytes in short-term culture, whereas the α-adrenergic agonist phenylephrine[8] induced a marked increase of IP$_3$. Similar findings were reported by Combettes *et al.*[15] and Bouscarel *et al.*[18], who did not observe any effect of TLCA or UDCA, respectively, on IP$_3$ levels in hepatocytes. Formation of IP$_3$ from phosphatidylinositolbisphosphate (PIP$_2$) is known to be mediated by phospholipase C. Thus, it may be concluded that the bile acids tested do not affect phospholipase C in hepatocytes at the concentrations used.

Protein kinase C (PKC)

By Western blotting we identified four isoenzymes of PKC in rat hepatocytes: α-, δ-, ε-, and ζ-PKC[10]. TUDCA (10 μmol/l), but not TCA (10 μmol/l) selectively induced translocation of the Ca^{2+}-sensitive α-isoform to the hepatocellular membrane, a key step for the activation of PKC[10]. This finding is of interest because α-PKC was recently shown to mediate stimulation of exocytosis[23,24] and opening of Ca^{2+} channels[25] in different types of cells.

Vesicular exocytosis

A sustained $[Ca^{2+}]_i$ increase and activation of α-PKC are key signals for the stimulation of vesicular exocytosis in different types of cells[23,24,26,27]. We observed that TUDCA, but not TCDCA or TCA at equimolar concentrations, induced a sustained stimulation of biliary exocytosis of HRP, an established marker protein of the vesicular pathway of the liver cell[9]. The effect of TUDCA was observed in the presence of high but not low extracellular Ca^{2+}, indicating that mobilization of extracellular Ca^{2+} by TUDCA is essential for TUDCA-induced stimulation of exocytosis, a mechanism defective in cholestasis[9].

CONCLUSION

The data reported lead us to propose the following mechanism of TUDCA-induced stimulation of hepatocellular exocytosis (Fig. 1): TUDCA, after uptake

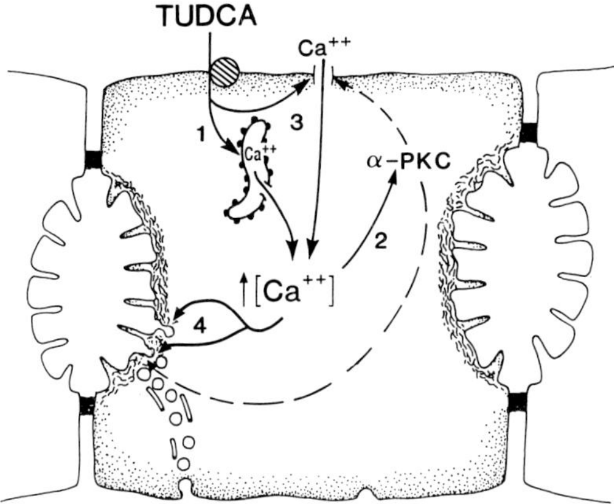

Fig. 1 Proposed mechanism of TUDCA-induced stimulation of hepatocellular exocytosis (for details see 'Conclusion')

into the cell, may induce an increase of $[Ca^{2+}]_i$ by depleting microsomal IP_3-sensitive Ca^{2+} stores independent of IP_3. $[Ca^{2+}]_i$ increase may stimulate translocation of the Ca^{2+}-sensitive α-PKC. α-PKC might play a role in TUDCA-induced Ca^{2+} influx via Ca^{2+} channels of the plasma membrane. The sustained $[Ca^{2+}]_i$ increase due to Ca^{2+} influx, and perhaps α-PKC, may induce a sustained stimulation of biliary exocytosis of the hepatocyte. Regarding the key importance of vesicle fusion for maintenance of transport function of the liver cell, this mechanism may play a role in the beneficial effect of UDCA in chronic cholestatic liver disease.

References

1. Nathanson MH, Boyer JL. Mechanisms and regulation of bile secretion. Hepatology. 1991;14: 551–66.
2. Barr VA, Hubbard AL. Newly synthesized hepatocyte plasma membrane proteins are transported in transcytotic vesicles in the bile duct-ligated rat. Gastroenterology. 1993;105:554–71.
3. Benedetti A, Strazzabosco M, Ng OC, Boyer JL. Regulation of activity and apical targeting of the Cl^-/HCO_3^- exchanger in rat hepatocytes. Proc Natl Acad Sci USA. 1994;91:792–6.
4. Larkin JM, Palade GE. Transcytotic vesicular carriers for polymeric IgA receptors accumulate in rat hepatocytes after bile duct ligation. J Cell Sci. 1991;98:205–16.
5. Poupon RE, Balkau B, Eschwege B, Poupon R, and the PBC–UDCA study group. A multicenter, controlled trial of ursodiol for the treatment of primary biliary cirrhosis. N Engl J Med. 1991;324:1548–54.
6. Leuschner U, Fischer H, Kurtz W et al. Ursodeoxycholic acid in primary biliary cirrhosis: results of a controlled double-blind trial. Gastroenterology. 1989;97:1268–74.
7. Beuers U, Spengler U, Kruis W et al. Ursodeoxycholic acid for treatment of primary sclerosing cholangitis: a placebo-controlled trial. Hepatology. 1992;16:707–14.
8. Beuers U, Nathanson MH, Boyer JL. Effects of tauroursodeoxycholic acid on cytosolic Ca^{++} signals in isolated rat hepatocytes. Gastroenterology. 1993;104:604–12.
9. Beuers U, Nathanson MH, Isales CM, Boyer JL. Tauroursodeoxycholic acid stimulates hepatocellular exocytosis and mobilizes extracellular Ca^{++}, mechanisms defective in cholestasis. J Clin Invest. 1993;93:2984–93.
10. Beuers U, Throckmorton DC, Anderson ML, Isales CM, Boyer JL. Tauroursodeoxycholic acid

induces translocation of α-, but not δ-, ε-, and ζ-protein kinase C in isolated rat hepatocytes. Hepatology. 1993;18:153A.

11. Mauger JP, Poggioli J, Guesdon F, Claret M. Noradrenaline, vasopressin and angiotensin increase Ca^{++} influx by opening a common pool of Ca^{++} channels in isolated rat liver cells. Biochem J. 1984;221:121–7.

12. Beuers U, Thiel M, Bardenheuer H, Paumgartner G. Tauroursodeoxycholic acid inhibits the cytosolic Ca^{++} increase in human neutrophils stimulated by formyl-methionyl-leucyl-phenylalanine. Biochem Biophys Res Commun. 1990;171:1115–21.

13. Anwer MS, Engelking LR, Sullivan D, Zimniak P, Lester P. Hepatotoxic bile acids increase cytosolic Ca^{++} activity of isolated rat hepatocytes. Hepatology. 1988;8:887–91.

14. Anwer MS, Little JM, Oelberg DG, Zimniak P, Lester R. Effect of bile acids on Ca^{++} efflux from isolated rat hepatocytes and perfused rat livers. Proc Soc Exp Biol Med. 1989;191:147–52.

15. Combettes L, Dumont M, Berthon B, Erlinger S, Claret M. Release of calcium from the endoplasmatic reticulum by bile acids in rat liver cells. J Biol Chem. 1988;263:2299–303.

16. Combettes L, Berthon B, Doucet E, Erlinger S, Claret M. Characteristics of bile acid-mediated Ca^{++} release from permeabilized liver cells and liver microsomes. J Biol Chem. 1989;264:157–61.

17. Combettes L, Berthon B, Doucet E, Erlinger S, Claret M. Bile acids mobilise internal Ca^{++} independently of external Ca^{++} in rat hepatocytes. Eur J Biochem. 1990;190:619–23.

18. Bouscarel B, Fromm H, Nussbaum R. Ursodeoxycholate mobilizes intracellular Ca^{++} and activates phosphorylase a in isolated hepatocytes. Am J Physiol. 1993;264:G243–51.

19. Thibault N, Ballet F. Effect of bile acids on intracellular calcium in isolated rat hepatocyte couplets. Biochem Pharmacol. 1993;34:289–93.

20. Farrell GC, Duddy SK, Kass GEN, Llopis J, Gahm A, Orrenius S. Release of Ca^{++} from the endoplasmic reticulum is not the mechanism for bile acid-induced cholestasis and hepatotoxicity in the intact rat liver. J Clin Invest. 1990;85:1255–9.

21. Hamada Y, Karjalainen A, Setchell BA, Millard JE, Bygrave FL. Acute effects of cholestatic and choleretic bile salts on vasopressin- and glucagon-induced hepato-biliary calcium fluxes in the perfused rat liver. Biochem J. 1992;283:575–81.

22. Nathanson MH. Cellular and subcellular calcium signaling in gastrointestinal epithelium. Gastroenterology. 1994;106:1349–64.

23. Ganesan S, Calle R, Zawalich K, Smallwood JI, Zawalich WS, Rasmussen H. Glucose-induced translocation of protein kinase C in rat pancreatic islets. Proc Natl Acad Sci USA. 1990;87:9893–7.

24. Ganesan S, Calle R, Zawalich K $et\ al.$ Immunocytochemical localization of α-protein kinase C in rat pancreatic β-cells during glucose-induced insulin secretion. J Cell Biol. 1992;119:313–24.

25. Riedel H, Parissenti AM, Hansen H, Su L, Shieh HL. Stimulation of calcium uptake in Saccharomyces cerevisiae by bovine protein kinase C α. J Biol Chem. 1993;268:3456–62.

26. Burgoyne RD, Morgan A. Regulated exocytosis. Biochem J. 1993;293:305–16.

27. Tsunoda Y, Stuenkel EL, Williams JA. Characterization of sustained $[Ca^{++}]_i$ increase in pancreatic acinar cells and its relation to amylase secretion. Am J Physiol. 1990;259:G792–801.

15
Molecular characterization of cytosolic rat and human bile acid binding proteins

A. STOLZ, L. HAMMOND and H. LOU

INTRODUCTION

Major advances have provided important new information on the fundamental mechanism of bile acid transport and metabolism in the liver. Previous studies of bile acid transport in enriched hepatocyte plasma membrane domains, isolated cells, couplets and whole organ perfusion are now complemented by the recent molecular identification of membrane spanning bile acid transporters and specific cytosolic binding proteins[1-6]. With these new tools the mechanism of bile acid uptake, efflux and transport within the cell can be examined. We have focused on the molecular characterization of both human and rat cytosolic bile acid binding proteins to define their physiological function. This chapter will review the biochemical characteristic of specific cytosolic bile acid binding proteins in human and rat liver. Molecular cloning of these genes reveals them to be members of a newly emerging family of monomeric reductases suggesting a multifunctional role for this class of proteins.

IDENTIFICATION OF INTRACELLULAR BILE ACID BINDING PROTEINS

Identification of a specific cytosolic bile acid binding protein has been a major goal of our laboratory. We have purified two 37 kDa monomeric bile acid binding proteins in human and rat hepatic cytosol by monitoring binding affinities using equilibrium dialysis during protein purification[7-9]. In rat, this 37 kDa protein migrates with an apparent molecular weight of 33 kDa on SDS-PAGE. Other investigators have utilized chemical and photoaffinity radiolabelled bile acid probes to covalently bind and selectively identify cytosolic and membrane proteins. Using intact, isolated rat hepatocytes with different radiolabelled bile acid photoprobes, Kurz preferentially labelled a 33 kDa protein in SDS-PAGE from rat liver cytosol, whereas a different pattern of labelling was observed when cytosol and bile acid were mixed and irradiated *in vitro*[10,11]. Similar-size bile acid binding protein was identified by Ziegler using a different, radiolabelled bile acid probe[12]. Identification of similar-size bile acid binding protein by different methodology substantiates our approach of identifying specific binding proteins by their *in vitro* binding affinities. In the rat we also demonstrated that the 37 kDa bile acid binding protein co-purified with 3α-hydroxysteroid dehydrogenase activity (3α-HSD).

BIOCHEMICAL CHARACTERISTICS AND cDNA CLONING OF THE RAT AND HUMAN BILE ACID BINDERS

In addition to binding bile salts, human and rat bile acid binders are oxidoreductases that preferentially utilize NADP(H) as a cofactor. In the rat, 3α-HSD metabolizes endogenous steroids as well as xenobiotic compounds. Both primary bile acid precursors and other steroids such as progesterone and adrostenedione are stereospecifically reduced by 3α-HSD[13,14]. In rat liver, 3α-HSD also co-elutes with dihydrodiol dehydrogenase (DDH) activity, which has been shown to reduce the mutagenic potential of benzopyrene metabolites in a bacterial mutagenicity test system[15–17]. DDH prevents the formation of the genotoxic dihydrodiol epoxide metabolites through elimination of the proximal carcinogen by catechol formation. DDH activity is expressed by many enzymes in different tissues[17]. Sensitivity to inhibitors has been used to classify the various subtypes of DDH present in specific organs[18,19]. As more of these proteins are cloned and sequenced, the relationship between these various enzymes can be directly compared among themselves and the human and rat bile acid binders.

cDNA cloning of the rat bile acid binder/3α-HSD gene

We were the first group to report the cDNA cloning of the entire rat hepatic 3α-HSD gene and to characterize its tissue distribution[5]. A 2.4 kB cDNA clone was isolated and found to encode for a 322 amino acids with a predicted weight of 37 022 daltons. The deduced amino acid sequence completely agreed with primary amino acid sequence determined by microsequence analysis. A unique feature of this gene as compared to other gene family members is a large, 1.3 kB 3′-untranslated region. Northern blot analysis of Sprague-Dawley male and female rat organs correlated well with protein distribution determined by a radioimmunoassay[20]. The 3α-HSD mRNA is predominantly expressed in the liver and intestine, with respectively decreasing expression in the stomach, colon and lung. Other tissues containing 3α-HSD activity, such as the kidney, brain and testis, failed to hybridize with the rat hepatic 3α-HSD cDNA, indicating that this activity is encoded by non-related gene(s).

Regulation of rat hepatic 3α-HSD

Alterations in 3α-HSD gene expression were examined in both primary rat hepatocytes and the bile fistulae rat model in response to manipulation of bile acid synthesis, bile acid flux and hormone manipulation[21]. Because 3α-HSD is

Table 1 Biochemical features of human and rat bile acid binding proteins

	Monomer	MW	3α-HSD	DDH	Lithocholate	Chenodeoxycholate	Cholate
Rat	+	37 022	0.55	1.15	1–2	1–2	100
Human	+	37 325	<0.03	2.3	0.5	0.1	1

Enzyme activity: (μmol NADPH mg^{-1} min^{-1}) 3α-HSD determined with chenodeoxycholate (500 μmol/l) and DDH activity utilizing 1-acenaphthenol (0.9 mmol/l). Dissociation constants for bile acids are in micromoles

required for bile acid synthesis, we postulated that coordinate gene expression with other bile acid synthetic enzymes may be occurring. We also sought its regulation by increased bile acid flux in the liver. The effects of a combination of bile acid replacement therapy with and without HMG-CoA reductase inhibitors were determined in a bile acid-depleted rat, and steady-state mRNA levels were compared with a non-inducible gene, cyclophilin[21,22]. No increase in steady-state 3α-HSD was found in bile fistula rats treated with cholesterol, cholestyramine or mevinolin, which all transcriptionally induced expression of the rate-limiting enzyme in bile acid synthesis, cholesterol 7α-hydroxylase. Bile acid replacement treatment with chenodeoxycholate or cholate in a depleted rat inhibited cholesterol 7α-hydroxylase expression but did not alter 3α-HSD gene expression, suggesting that 3α-HSD is not coordinately regulated with cholesterol 7α-hydroxylase. Hormonal requirements for maintenance of 3α-HSD gene expression in primary adult rat hepatocyte tissue culture were also examined. A combination of thyroxine and dexamethasone was able to maintain 3α-HSD expression after 72 h, whereas cells plated without supplemental hormones had minimally detectable mRNA. Cells plated with a single hormone had increased steady-state mRNA levels and protein by both Western blot and activity, but this effect was significantly potentiated when hormones were combined. Thyroxine caused an increase in transcriptional activity, whereas dexamethasone functioned by stabilization of mRNA half-life[21].

Biochemical characterization of human bile acid binder (HBAB)

We purified a 36 kDa human bile acid binder (HBAB) that has a remarkably high bile acid binding affinity using a purification protocol similar to the one we used to purify the rat protein[7,23]. No information is available on other potential human cytosolic bile acid binding proteins using the previously cited bile acid affinity probes as in the rat. Table 1 lists the biochemical features of these two similar proteins. Thus, in contrast to the rat, the HBAB appears unmatched in its ability to bind bile acids, and demonstrates 1 to 2 orders of magnitude lower affinities for bile acids than does the rat.

We sought oxidoreductase activity for HBAB because these activities eluted with the rat protein. In rat liver, only one DDH isoform is present, whereas a complex elution pattern of DDH and 3α-HSD activities was found in human liver cytosol, as reported by us and Drs Hara and Sawada[24,25]. At least six fractions of DDH activity were identified in the chromatofocusing chromatogram of the 30–40 kDa human liver cytosol fraction, using the single hydroxyl substrate,

1-acenaphthenol. Only one of these fractions demonstrated high-affinity bile acid binding. The 3α-HSD activity co-eluted with some other fractions of DDH activity, but was clearly distinct from the high-affinity bile acid binding activity. Thus, unlike the rat, the human protein is unable to utilize bile acid as a substrate for enzymatic activity[25].

cDNA cloning and expression of HBAB

Human bile acid binder was cloned by probing a human Hep-G2 cDNA library with the 5′ Eco R1 proximal fragment of the rat hepatic 3α-HSD cDNA[6]. A 1252 bp cDNA clone was sequenced, and its deduced peptide sequence compared with primary sequence data. In order to confirm the specificity of the clone, and to begin to characterize its structural domains, the human and rat bile acid binders were recombinantly expressed as either a lone protein (Pharmacia pKK 233-2) or as part of a glutathione *S*-transferase (GST) fusion protein, using a Pharmacia pGEX-2T modified plasmid.

Table 1 lists the bile acid binding and enzyme kinetic features of the rat and human bile acid binding protein. Both recombinant rat and human protein expressed the same catalytic rates and substrate specificities as the native protein, indicating that recombinantly expressed proteins are properly folded. We previously demonstrated in the native 3α-HSD that K_d values for bile acids are the same as K_m values, indicating that binding occurs at the substrate site. Bile acid K_m for recombinant protein is the same as the native protein, yet we were unable to determine bile acid binding by equilibrium dialysis because of protein precipitation.

Rat and HBABs are members of a novel monomeric reductase gene family

Comparison of the deduced cDNA sequence for our rat and human proteins identified a new family of highly related oxidoreductases (>50% amino acid homology). These genes share common features of functioning as reductases *in vivo*, preferential utilization of NADP(H), and are composed of monomers. These genes share 50% sequence homology with the evolutionary distant gene, gamma lens crystalline, suggesting evolution from a common ancestral gene with potential conservation of catalytic and nucleotide cofactor binding sites[26–30].

The aldose reductase and other recently cloned NADP(H) oxidoreductases represent a major group of proteins that share 50–80% sequence identity[5,31–35], suggesting that these proteins are members of the newly emerging aldo-keto reductase gene family. Of these proteins the aldose reductase has been extensively analysed because of its hypothesized role in mediating the sorbitol toxicity of diabetes. Recently, the X-ray crystal coordinates for aldose reductase with the $NADP^+$ cofactor were reported by two different groups[36,37]. The aldose reductase protein is an eight-chain, parallel alpha/beta barrel structure that establishes a new motif for the NADP-binding domain of an oxidoreductase. This crystallographic data provide detailed information about the cofactor binding site, the candidate residues involved in the transfer of hydrogen from cofactor to substrate and the dimensions of the catalytic pocket. Figure 1 shows the amino acid sequence homology of some members of this emerging gene family. This is a rapidly progressing field because a majority of these proteins were cloned within the past 2 years.

The greatest sequence divergence among all these genes is at the carboxyl end, which suggests the possibility that catalytic specificity or substrate binding site may reside within this region. Deletion of the 13 residues of the carboxyl terminal end of aldose reductase markedly reduced catalytic rates for uncharged substrates, proving the critical role of the carboxyl terminal end in orientating substrate to the active site[38]. We have recently discovered, by determining HBAB genomic organization, that the carboxyl terminal end of the protein beginning at position 310 and the entire 3′-untranslated region of the gene is contained within the last exon, which is also true for other members of this gene family[39–41]. Conservation of exon domains is a feature of gene family members. As an initial hypothesis the shuffling of the last exon, which may potentially be critical for substrate specificity, would provide a mechanism for the generation of highly related proteins with different substrate specificity. We have identified at least six isoforms of DDII activity in the 30–40 kDa gel filtration fraction in the human liver and other related genes during genomic cloning of HBAB, indicating the existence of a large number of highly related genes. This hypothesis will require additional information about the genomic organization of other potential family members to substantiate this hypothesis.

Preliminary studies to identify substrate specificity of the rat and human bile acid binding proteins

The availability of both the human and rat proteins which are highly related, yet having distinct catalytic activity, will be beneficial for defining the role of specific residues to determine substrate specificity and binding properties of these proteins. Comparing these similar yet different proteins allows us to potentially define the protein domains responsible for these differences. In addition, the availability of the crystal coordinates for the human aldose reductase provides a paradigm for other members of this gene family. Our preliminary strategy for defining substrate and bile acid binding sites on these proteins has been first to generate and express chimeric human–rat proteins and compare catalytic active to wild-type protein.

We first generated and expressed chimeric human and rat bile acid binding proteins to dissect the contributions of adjoining peptide regions, and recognized the limits of this approach because functional protein domains may be constructed from non-contiguous amino acids. Amino terminal (1–63) and carboxyl terminal (285–322(3)) peptide regions of the human and rat monomeric reductases were exchanged at mutual, shared endonuclease restriction sites, which did not disrupt the open-reading frame. Constructs were confirmed by restriction mapping and DNA sequence analysis. Only two of nine chimeric and truncated proteins were expressed, either because of precipitation or inability to be cleaved by thrombin from the GST fusion protein. Table 2 lists preliminary features of these two chimeric proteins that were stably expressed.

```
                10        20        30        40        50        60
HBAB    MDSKYQCVKLNDGHFMPVLGFGTYAPAEVPKSKALEATKLAIEAGFRHIDSAHLYNNEEQ
ORF     ----Q-------------------P---R-----V-------------------------
20 OH   --P-F-R-A-S----I----------E-------M----I--D---------YF-K--KE
HUMCR           ----------P---RNR-V-V---------------Y------
BOVPGF  --P-S-R---------I----------E-----E------F---V---V-----Q----
RH3HSD  ---ISLR-A----N-I-------TV-EK-A-DEVIK---I--DN----F---Y--EV--E
                10        20        30        40        50
MUSMVD    MATF-E-STKAK--PL-L--WKS***SPGQVKEAV-A--D--Y----C-YV-H--NE
HUMALR    MASRLL--N-AK--I--L--WKS***-PGQVTE-V-V--DV-Y----C--V-Q--NE


                70        80        90       100       110       120
HBAB    VGLAIRSKIADGSVKREDIFYTSKLWCNSHRPELVRPALERSLKNLQLDYVDLYLIHFPV
ORF     ------------------------------STF----------N---KA----------HS-M
20 OH   ------------------------------TF--------S--D-------------I----T
HUMCR   ------------------------------TFFQ-QM-Q----S---K----------L---M
BOVPGF  --Q---------T----------------LQ---------K--Q----------I--S--
RH3HSD  --Q------E--T----------------STF-------TC--KT--ST-------I----M
                60        70        80        90       100       110
MUSMVD  --E--QE--KENA-----L-IV----ATFFEKS--KK-FDNT-SD-K---L----V-W-Q
HUMALR  --V--QE-LREQV----EL-IV-----TY-EKG--KG-CQKT-SD-K---L------W-T


               130       140       150       160       170       180
HBAB    SVKPGEEVIPKDENGKILFDTVDLCATWEAVEKCKDAGLAKSIGVSNFNRRQLEMILNKP
ORF     -L-----LS-T-----VI--I----T----M-----------------------------
20 OH   AL---V-I--T--H--AI-----------M-----------------------------
HUMCR   AL----TPL-------VI------S----VM---------------------C-------
BOVPGF  -L---GNKF----E--KL--D----C----L----------TK-------HK---K-----
RATDAH  ALQ--DIFF-R--H--L--E---I-D----M-----------------C----R-----
               120       130       140       150       160       170
MUSMVD  GFQA-NALL---NK--V-LSKSTFLDA---M-ELV-Q--V-AL-I----HF-I-RL----
HUMALR  GF---K-FF-L--S-NVVPSDTNILD--A-M-ELV-E-LV-A--I----HL-V-------


               190       200       210       220       230       240
HBAB    GLKYKPVCNQVECHPYFNQRKLLDFCKSKDIVLVAYSALGSHREEPWVDPNSPVLLEDPV
ORF     ------------------RS-------------------Q-DKR--------------
20 OH   ---------------L--G---E-----G-------------PE---QSA-------L
HUMCR   ---------------L--S---------------H----TQ-HKL------------
BOVPGF  ---------------L--S---E----H-------A---AQLLSE--NS-N--------
RH3HSD  -------------L-L--S-M--Y------I--S-CT---S-DKT---QK-----D---
               180       190       200       210       220       230
MUSMVD  ---H---T--I-S---LT-E--IQY-Q--G-AVT---PLGS*PDR-YAK-ED--VM-I-K
HUMALR  ------AV--I-----LT-E--IQY-Q--G--VT---P---*PDR--AK-ED-S-----R


               250       260       270       280       290       300
HBAB    LCALAKKHKRTPALIALRYQLQRGVVVLAKSYNEQRIRQNVQVFEFQLTSEEMKAIDGLN
ORF     --------------------------------------------------A-D--------
20 OH   IG-------QQ-------------I------FT-K--KE-I--------P-DMKV--S--
HUMCR   ----------------------------------E-I----------D--VL----
BOVPGF  ---I-----Q----V-----V---------F-KK--KE-M---D-E--P-D--------
RH3HSD  ---I---Y-Q----V----------P-IR-F-AK--KELT------A--D---L----
               240       250       260       270       280       290
MUSMVD  IKEIAA---K-V-QVLIRFHV--N---IP--VTPS--QE-L---D---SE-D-A--LSF-
HUMALR  IK-I-A--NK-T-QVLI-FPM--NL--IP--VTPE--AE-FK--D-E-S-QD-TTLLSYN


               310       320
HBAB    RNVRYLTLDIFAGPPNYPFSDEY
ORF     --LH-FNS-S--SH----Y----
20 OH   --F--V-A-FAI-H---------
HUMCR   --Y--VVM-FLMDH-D-------
BOVPGF  --I---YDFQKGI-H-E----E--
RH3HSD  --F--NNAKY-DDH--H--TD-
               300       310
MUSMVD  --W-ACD-LDARTEED---HE--
HUMALR  --W-VCA-LSCTSHKD---HE-F
```

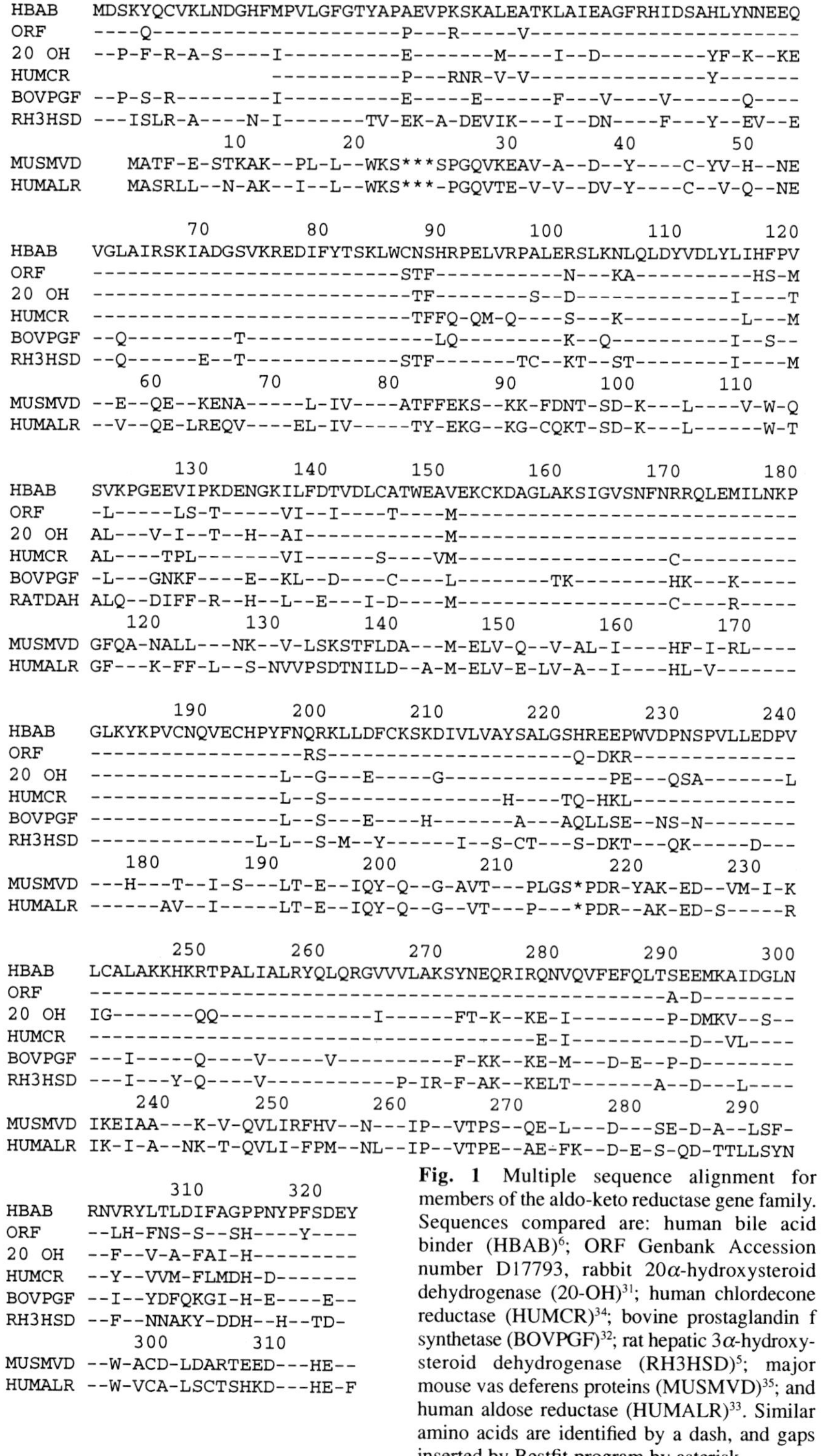

Fig. 1 Multiple sequence alignment for members of the aldo-keto reductase gene family. Sequences compared are: human bile acid binder (HBAB)[6]; ORF Genbank Accession number D17793, rabbit 20α-hydroxysteroid dehydrogenase (20-OH)[31]; human chlordecone reductase (HUMCR)[34]; bovine prostaglandin f synthetase (BOVPGF)[32]; rat hepatic 3α-hydroxy-steroid dehydrogenase (RH3HSD)[5]; major mouse vas deferens proteins (MUSMVD)[35]; and human aldose reductase (HUMALR)[33]. Similar amino acids are identified by a dash, and gaps inserted by Bestfit program by asterisk

172

Table 2 Catalytic activity of recombinant wild-type and chimeric bile acid binding proteins

Enzyme activity	Rat	H1–63/R64–322	Human	H1–285/R286–322
3α-HSD	0.61	1.2	<0.03	0.3
DDH	1.3	0.6	2.3	0.6

Enzyme activity determined as in Table 1

The addition of the rat carboxyl terminal end to the human protein resulted in 3α-HSD activity, although with a lower V_{max} value than the rat protein. These preliminary data support the concept that the carboxyl terminal is a major determinant of substrate specificity. The relationship of binding to substrate site will require additional study.

SUMMARY

In conclusion, human and rat bile acid binding proteins serve an important role in maintaining bile acids within the cytosolic compartment of the hepatcytes so that they may be rapidly and efficiently transported out of the hepatocyte. In addition to binding, these homologous proteins are members of the newly emerging monomeric aldo-keto reductase gene family. Preliminary studies with chimeric protein demonstrate the potential significance of the carboxyl terminal end in dictating substrate specificity. The ability of these proteins both to bind bile acids and to metabolize hydrophobic molecules suggests a new, multifunctional role for these monomeric reductases.

Acknowledgement

These studies were supported in part by National Institute of Health Grant DK-41014.

References

1. Hagenbuch B, Luebbert H, Stieger B, Meier PJ. Expression of the hepatocyte Na$^+$/bile acid cotransporter in *Xenopus laevis* oocytes. J Biol Chem. 1990;265:5357–60.
2. Hagenbuch B, Stieger B, Foguet M, Luebbert H, Meier PJ. Functional expression cloning and characterization of the hepatocyte Na$^+$/bile acid cotransport system. Proc Natl Acad Sci USA. 1991;88:10629–33.
3. Coleman R. Biochemistry of bile secretion. Biochem J. 1987;244:249–61.
4. Nathanson MH, Boyer JL. Mechanisms and regulation of bile secretion. Hepatology. 1991;14:551–66.
5. Stolz A, Rahimi Kiani M, Ameis D, Chan E, Ronk M, Shively JE. Molecular structure of rat hepatic 3 alpha-hydroxysteroid dehydrogenase. A member of the oxidoreductase gene family. J Biol Chem. 1991;266:15253–7.
6. Stolz A, Hammond L, Lou H, Takikawa H, Ronk M, Shively JE. cDNA cloning and expression of the human hepatic bile acid-binding protein. A member of the monomeric reductase gene family. J Biol Chem. 1993;268:10448–57.
7. Stolz A, Sugiyama Y, Kuhlenkamp J, Kaplowitz N. Identification and purification of a 36 kDa bile acid binder in human hepatic cytosol. FEBS Lett. 1984;177:31–5.

8. Stolz A, Takikawa H, Ookhtens M, Kaplowitz N. The role of cytoplasmic proteins in hepatic bile acid transport. Annu Rev Physiol. 1989;161–76.

9. Sugiyama Y, Yamada T, Kaplowitz N. Newly identified bile acid binders in rat liver cytosol. Purification and comparison with glutathione *S*-transferases. J Biol Chem. 1983;258:3602–7.

10. Abberger H, Bickel U, Buscher H-P *et al*. Transport of bile acids: lipoproteins, membrane polypeptides, and cytosolic protein carriers. In: Paumgartner G, Stiehl A, Gerok W, editors. Bile acids and lipids. Lancaster: MTP; 1981:233–46.

11. Abberger H, Buscher H-P, Fuchte K *et al*. Compartmentation of bile salt synthesis and transport revealed by photoaffinity labelling of isolated hepatocytes. In: Paumgartner G, Stiehl A, Gerok W, editors. Bile acids and cholesterol in health and disease. Lancaster: MTP; 1983:77–87.

12. Ziegler K. Further characterization of 3'-isothiocyanatobenamido[^{3}H]cholate binding to hepatocytes. Correlation with bile acid transport inhibition and protection by substrates and inhibitors. Biochim Biophys Acta. 1985;819:37–44.

13. Takikawa H, Stolz A, Kuroki S, Kaplowitz N. Oxidation and reduction of bile acid precursors by rat hepatic 3 alpha-hydroxysteroid dehydrogenase and inhibition by bile acids and indomethacin. Biochim Biophys Acta. 1990;1043:153–6.

14. Stolz A, Takikawa H, Sugiyama Y, Kuhlenkamp J, Kaplowitz N. 3 alpha-hydroxysteroid dehydrogenase activity of the Y' bile acid binders in rat liver cytosol. Identification, kinetics, and physiologic significance. J Clin Invest. 1987;79:427–34.

15. Vogel K, Bentley P, Platt KL, Oesch F. Rat liver cytoplasmic dihydrodiol dehydrogenase. Purification to apparent homogeneity and properties. J Biol Chem. 1980;255:9621–5.

16. Glatt HR, Cooper CS, Grover PL *et al*. Inactivation of a diol epoxide by dihydrodiol dehydrogenase but not by two epoxide hydrolases. Science. 1982;215:1507–9.

17. Woerner W, Oesch F. Identity of dihydrodiol dehydrogenase and 3 alpha-hydroxysteroid dehydrogenase in rat tissues. Biochem Pharmacol. 1985;34:831–5.

19. Smithgall TE, Penning TM. Electrophoretic and immunochemical characterization of 3 alpha-hydroxysteroid/dihydrodiol dehydrogenases of rat tissues. Biochem J. 1988;254:715–21.

20. Stolz A, Sugiyama Y, Kuhlenkamp J *et al*. Cytosolic bile acid binding protein in rat liver: radioimmunoassay, molecular forms, developmental characteristics and organ distribution. Hepatology. 1986;6:433–9.

21. Stravitz RT, Vlahcevic ZR, Pandak WM, Stolz A, Hylemon PB. Regulation of rat hepatic 3 alpha-hydroxysteroid dehydrogenase in vivo and in primary cultures of rat hepatocytes. J Lipid Res. 1994;35:239–47.

22. Pandak WM, Li YC, Chiang JY *et al*. Regulation of cholesterol 7 alpha-hydroxylase mRNA and transcriptional activity by taurocholate and cholesterol in the chronic biliary diverted rat. J Biol Chem. 1991;266:3416–21.

23. Takikawa H, Stolz A, Sugimoto M, Sugiyama Y, Kaplowitz N. Comparison of the affinities of newly identified human bile acid binder and cationic glutathione *S*-transferase for bile acids. J Lipid Res. 1986;27:652–7.

24. Hara A, Taniguchi H, Nakayama T, Sawada H. Purification and properties of multiple forms of dihydrodiol dehydrogenase from human liver. J Biochem Tokyo. 1990;108:250–4.

25. Takikawa H, Stolz A, Sugiyama Y, Yoshida H, Yamanaka M, Kaplowitz N. Relationship between the newly identified bile acid binder and bile acid oxidoreductases in human liver. J Biol Chem. 1990;265:2132–6.

26. Baker ME. a common ancestor for human placental 17 beta-hydroxysteroid dehydrogenase, *Streptomyces coelicolor* actIII protein, and *Drosophila melanogaster* alcohol dehydrogenase. FASEB J. 1990;4:222–6.

27. Baker ME. Human placental 17 beta-hydroxysteroid dehydrogenase is homologous to NodG protein of *Rhizobium meliloti*. Mol Endocrinol. 1989;3:881–4.

28. Borras T, Persson B, Joernvall H. Eye lens zeta-crystallin relationships to the family of 'long-chain' alcohol/polyol dehydrogenases. Protein trimming and conservation of stable parts. Biochemistry. 1989;28:6133–9.

29. Wistow G, Piatigorsky J. Recruitment of enzymes as lens structural proteins. Science. 1987;236:1554–6.

30. Joernvall H, Persson M, Jeffery J. Alcohol and polyol dehydrogenases are both divided into two protein types, and structural properties cross-relate the different enzyme activities within each type. Proc Natl Acad Sci USA. 1981;78:4226–30.

31. Lacy WR, Washenick KJ, Cook RG, Dunbar BS. Molecular cloning and expression of an

abundant rabbit ovarian protein with 20 alpha-hydroxysteroid dehydrogenase activity. Mol Endocrinol. 1993;7:58–66.

32. Watanabe K, Fujii Y, Nakayama K *et al*. Structural similarity of bovine lung prostaglandin F synthase to lens epsilon-crystallin of the European common frog. Proc Natl Acad Sci USA. 1988;85:11–15.

33. Bohren KM, Bullock B, Wermuth B, Gabbay KH. The aldo-keto reductase superfamily. cDNAs and deduced amino acid sequences of human aldehyde and aldose reductases. J Biol Chem. 1989;264:9547–51.

34. Winters CJ, Molowa DT, Guzelian PS. Isolation and characterization of cloned cDNAs encoding human liver chlordecone reductase. Biochemistry. 1990;29:1080–7.

35. Pailhoux EA, Martinez A, Veyssiere GM, Jean CG. Androgen-dependent protein from mouse vas deferens. cDNA cloning and protein homology with the aldo-keto reductase superfamily. J Biol Chem. 1990;265:19932–6.

36. Wilson DK, Bohren KM, Gabbay KH, Quiocho FA. An unlikely sugar substrate site in the 1.65 A structure of the human aldose reductase holoenzyme implicated in diabetic complications. Science. 1992;257:81–4.

37. Rondeau JM, Tete Favier F, Podjarny A *et al*. Novel NADPH-binding domain revealed by the crystal structure of aldose reductase. Nature. 1992;355:469–72.

38. Bohren KM, Grimshaw CE, Gabbay KH. Catalytic effectiveness of human aldose reductase. Critical role of C-terminal domain. J Biol Chem. 1992;267:20965–70.

39. Pailhoux E, Veyssiere G, Fabre S, Tournaire C, Jean C. The genomic organization and DNA sequence of the mouse vas deferens androgen-regulated protein gene. J Steroid Biochem Mol Biol. 1992;42:561–8.

40. Graham A, Brown L, Hedge PJ, Gammack AJ, Markham AF. Structure of the human aldose reductase gene. J Biol Chem. 1991;266:6872–7.

41. Lou H, Hammond L, Sharma V, Sparkes RS, Lusis AJ, Stolz A. Genomic organization and chromosomal localization of a novel human hepatic dihydrodiol dehydrogenase with high affinity bile acid binding. J Biol Chem. 1994;269:8416–22.

16
The role of vesicle targeting in hepatic bile acid transport

J. L. BOYER and C. J. SOROKA

It is becoming increasingly clear from studies in a variety of cell systems that membrane transport activity can be modified by the rapid insertion and removal of transport proteins from their functional site in the plasma membrane. This process occurs by exocytosis and endocytosis, and is highly regulated. It occurs independently from events that alter the kinetic activity of the transport protein directly, such as phosphorylation, and involves instead a change in the number of transport proteins that reside at the functional site[1]. There are a growing number of examples of transporters that can be regulated by their turnover rate in the membrane, including the insulin-responsive GLUT-4 glucose transporter in adipocytes[2], the CFTR chloride channel in T84 and HT29 colonocytes which responds to VIP and forskolin[3,4], and the renal collecting tubule water channel which is stimulated by ADH[5].

Little is known about the regulation of transport activity in hepatocyte membranes, although the general view has held that changes in transport activity would be primarily a function of modifications in the transport protein itself. For example, bile acid uptake can be stimulated by cAMP/protein kinase-A-mediated mechanisms presumed to occur by direct phosphorylation of the transporter[6]. Protein kinase-C agonists stimulate canalicular excretion of organic anions[7], and studies of bile acid transport in COS cells transfected with the canalicular Ca^{2+}, Mg^{2+}-ecto-ATPase demonstrate phosphorylation on specific serine and threonine residues that are required to both sustain and modify membrane-translocating properties of this putative canalicular membrane bile acid carrier[8,9].

Nevertheless, there is increasing evidence that transport activity in hepatocytes, particularly canalicular excretion, may also be regulated by recruitment of vesicles containing transporters as an integral component of their membranes. Fusion of vesicles containing canalicular transporters (exocytosis) with the apical plasma membrane should up-regulate transport activity, while vesicle retrieval (endocytosis) should result in down-regulation.

It is generally accepted that most, if not all, apical membrane proteins in hepatocytes traffic to this domain after their synthesis, by an indirect pathway via the basolateral membrane[10,11]. Canalicular transporters are then sorted from resident proteins in the basolateral membrane by a process of vesicular budding, which may also involve early endosomes[12]. These vesicles then move to the canalicular membrane attached to microtubules. This microtubule-dependent transcytotic vesicle pathway is the final determinant for the targeting of transport proteins to the canalicular domain, and establishes both the cell's polarity and its excretory capacity.

The most widely studied example of this process is the trafficking of the polymeric immunoglobulin receptor[13-15]. After targeting this protein to the basolateral membrane in hepatocytes, clatherin-coated vesicles containing this protein bud off the plasma membrane, lose their clatherin coat and fuse with the early endosomal compartment. Following acidification within the endosomes, vesicles containing the IgA receptor as an integral membrane protein and its attached ligand, bud off and move on microtubules to the subapical region of the cell, where the vesicles fuse with the canalicular membrane. The receptor is proteolytically cleaved, discharging an 80 kDa fragment and polymeric IgA into the biliary lumen[14].

The contribution of canalicular membrane vesicle-mediated fusion events to the formation of bile, and to the biliary excretion of organic solutes such as bile acids, is less well understood. Earlier studies suggested that inhibitors of microtubule function had little effect on endogenous rates of bile acid excretion, although they clearly inhibited bile acid excretion when higher rates of bile acid infusions were administered or when the bile acid pool was first drained and then readministered[16,17]. In contrast, more hydrophobic biliary solutes associate with membrane vesicles en route to excretion in bile[18,19]. However, recent evidence suggests that the activity of the Cl^-/HCO_3^- exchange in rat hepatocytes may be regulated by apical targeting of a subpopulation of vesicles containing this transport activity[20]. The anion exchange-2 protein, a Cl^-/HCO_3^- exchanger, has been characterized in purified canalicular membrane vesicles from rat liver[21] and localized immunocytochemically to the canalicular membrane in human liver[22]. When hepatocytes are cultured in the presence of HCO_3^- or DBcAMP, the activity of this exchanger is significantly stimulated, an effect that can be blocked by either microtubule inhibitors (colchicine) or by phorbol esters[20]. This apparent recruitment of transporters can be reproduced in the isolated perfused rat liver, where manoeuvres that acutely alkalinize the cell, immediately stimulate both bile flow and excretion of horseradish peroxidase (HRP), a fluid-phase marker, while simultaneously increasing the biliary excretion of bicarbonate[23]. These effects are also prevented by pretreatment with the stilbene, DIDS or a microtubule inhibitor, suggesting that the increase in bicarbonate and HRP excretion is mediated by microtubule-dependent insertion of vesicles containing the Cl^-/HCO_3^- exchanger into the canalicular domain[23].

The possibility that other canalicular membrane transporters, particularly bile acid transporters, might also be recruited from populations of cytoplasmic vesicles has received support from several different independent observations.

First when the canalicular membrane Ca^{2+},Mg^{2+}-ecto-ATPase was localized with immunocytochemical techniques in hepatocyte couplets incubated in the presence of HCO_3^- or DBcAMP, ratios of canalicular membrane/cytoplasmic fluorescence increased[20]. This ecto-ATPase has been transfected into COS cells, and has been proposed as a candidate for an ATP-dependent canalicular membrane bile acid transporter[8,24].

Bile acid transport can also be stimulated by cell swelling in the isolated perfused rat liver, a manoeuvre that stimulates vesicle targeting to the canalicular domain and the transient stimulation of bile flow and biliary excretion of HRP, a fluid-phase marker[25]. Here again, these effects can be blocked by colchicine, but are not affected by lumicolchicine, an analogue that does not affect microtubule function[25]. If bile acids are infused into the perfusate of isolated perfused rat livers at rates that exceed the excretory transport maximum, and the liver is exposed to hypotonic media, the transport maximum for taurocholate increases during the period during which volume regulation and fusion of vesicles with the canalicular domain also occur[26,27]. This process is also inhibited by colchicine pretreatment or exposure to hypertonic media, which diminishes the bile acid transport maximum[27]. These experiments suggest that it is possible to regulate fusion of vesicles with the canalicular membrane by several different manoeuvres, and that, irrespective of the stimulus, this phenomenon also results in a change in the capacity for canalicular membrane transport, presumably because of the simultaneous insertion or retrieval of transport proteins.

More recently we have obtained additional evidence to support this hypothesis[28]. Studies in the isolated perfused rat liver had demonstrated that infusions of DBcAMP could stimulate vesicle movement to the pericanalicular region of the hepatocyte in association with an increase in excretion of HRP into bile[29]. Using this observation as background, isolated hepatocyte couplets were incubated in the presence or absence of DBcAMP/IBMX or nocodazole, an inhibitor of microtubule function, for a period of 4h. The functional status of this primary bile secretory unit was then assessed by exposing the cells to 1 μmol/l FITC-glycocholate for 5min, washing the cells and incubating them for an additional 15min before examining their ability to excrete the fluorescent bile acid into the canalicular lumen using confocal fluorescent microscopy[28]. The circumference of the canalicular space was measured, and changes in this parameter were assumed to represent differences in insertion and/or retrieval of cytoplasmic vesicles into the apical domain. DBcAMP/IBMX treatment stimulated the percentage of FITC glycocholate taken up by the couplets that was excreted into the canalicular lumen, while inhibition of microtubule function resulted in a marked impairment of the percentage of FITC glycocholate excreted. None of the treatments significantly affected the total fluorescent uptake when expressed as a function of the area of the two cells. When the circumference of the canalicular lumen was plotted as a function of the ability of the couplets to excrete the bile acid, a direct relationship was observed. Fluorescent microscopic studies of the putative bile acid transporter, canalicular membrane ecto-ATPase, in control vs DBcAMP-stimulated cells provided morphological evidence for translocation of vesicle containing this transport protein to the canalicular domain, a finding consistent with the functional changes observed in the canalicular excretion of this fluorescent bile acid.

In summary, hepatocytes, like many other transporting epithelia, appear to be able to regulate the activity of apical membrane transporters by recruitment of cytoplasmic vesicles, or through the inhibition of vesicle-mediated transcytosis. Transport proteins which are associated with vesicle membranes become incorporated in the apical membrane through fusion events which result in exocytosis, or are removed by endocytic events. Present evidence suggests that canalicular bile acid transporters can be regulated in this manner. Future work will need to be directed to the molecular events that control this process.

Acknowledgements

This work was supported by grants DK 25636 and DK34989.

References

1. Bradbury NA, Bridges RJ. Role of membrane trafficking in plasma membrane solute transport. Am J Physiol. 1994;267:C1–24.
2. Lienhard GE. Regulation of cellular membrane transport by exocytic insertion and endocytic retrieval of transporters. Trends Biochem Sci. 1983;8:125–7.
3. Bradbury NA, Jilling T, Berta G, Sorscher EJ, Bridges RJ, Kirk KL. Regulation of plasma membrane recycling by CFTR. Science Wash DC. 1992;256:444–5.
4. Morris AP, Cunningham SA, Tousson A, Benos DJ, Frizzell RA. Polarization-dependent apical membrane CFTR targeting underlies cAMP-stimulated Cl^- secretion in epithelial cells. Am J Physiol. 1994;266:C254–68.
5. Handler JS. Antidiuretic hormone moves membranes. Am J Physiol. 1988;25:F375–82.
6. Grune S, Engelking LR, Anwer MS. Role of intracellular calcium and protein kinases in the activation of hepatic Na^+/taurocholate cotransport by cyclic AMP. J Biol Chem. 1993;268:17734–41.
7. Roelofsen H, Ottenhoff R, Elferink RPJO, Jansen PLM. Hepatocanalicular organic-anion transport is regulated by protein kinase-C. Biochem J. 1991;278:637.
8. Sippel CJ, McCollum MJ, Perlmutter DH. Bile acid transport by the rat liver canalicular bile acid transport/ecto-ATPase protein is dependent on ATP but not on its own ecto-ATPase activity. J Biol Chem. 1994;269:2820–6.
9. Sippel CJ, Fallon RJ, Perlmutter DH. Bile acid efflux mediated by the rat liver canalicular bile acid transport/ecto-ATPase protein requires serine 503 phosphorylation and is regulated by tyrosine 488 phosphorylation. J Biol Chem. 1994;26:19539–45.
10. Bartles JR, Feracci HM, Stieger B, Hubbard AL. Biogenesis of the rat hepatocyte plasma membrane *in vivo*: comparison of the pathways taken by apical and basolateral proteins using sub-cellular fractionation. J Cell Biol. 1987;105:1241–51.
11. Hubbard AL, Stieger B, Bartles JR. Biogenesis of endogenous plasma membrane proteins in epithelial cells. Annu Rev Physiol. 1989;51:755–70.
12. Geuze HJ, Slot JW, Strous Ger JAM *et al*. Intracellular receptor sorting during endocytosis: comparative immunoelectron microscopy of multiple receptors in rat liver. Cell. 1984;37:195–204.
13. Hoppe CA, Connolly TP, Hubbard AL. Transcellular transport of polymeric IgA in the rat hepatocyte: biochemical and morphological characterization of the transport pathway. J Cell Biol. 1985;101:2113–23.
14. Musil LS, Baenziger JU. Proteolytic processing of rat liver membrane secretory component. J Biol Chem. 1988;263:15799–808.
15. Goldman IS, Jones AL, Hradek CT, Huling S. Hepatocyte handling of immunoglobulin A in the rat: the role of microtubules. Gastroenterology. 1983;85:30–40.
16. Crawford JM, Berken CA, Gollan JL. Role of the hepatocyte microtubular system in the excretion of bile salts and biliary lipid: implications for intracellular vesicular transport. J Lipid Res. 1988;29:144–56.
17. Crawford JM, Gollan JL. Hepatocyte cotransport of taurocholate and bilirubin glucuronides: role

of microtubules. Am J Physiol. 1988;255:G121–31.

18. Crawford JM, Gollan JL. Transcellular transport of organic anions in hepatocytes. Hepatology. 1991;14:192–7.

19. Aoyama N, Tokamo H, Ohya T, Chandler K, Holzbach RT. A novel transcellular transport pathway for non-bile salt cholephilic organic anions. Am J Physiol. 1991;261:G305–11.

20. Benedetti A, Strazzabosco M, Ng OC, Boyer JL. Regulation of activity and apical targeting of the Cl^-/HCO_3^- exchanger in rat hepatocytes. Proc Natl Acad Sci USA. 1994;91:792–6.

21. Meier PJ, Knickelbein RG, Moseley RH, Dobbins JW, Boyer JL. Evidence for carrier-mediated chloride/bicarbonate exchange in canalicular rat liver plasma membrane vesicles. J Clin Invest. 1985;75:1256–63.

22. Martinez-Anso E, Castillo JE, Diez J, Medina JF, Prieto J. Immunohistochemical detection of chloride/bicarbonate anion exchangers in human liver. Hepatology. 1994;19:1400–6.

23. Bruck R, Benedetti A, Strazzabosco M, Boyer JL. Intracellular alkalinization stimulates bile flow and vesicular-mediated exocytosis in IPRL. Am J Physiol. 1993;265:G347–53.

24. Sippel CJ, Suchy FJ, Ananthanarayanan M, Perlmutter DH. The rat liver ecto-ATPase is also a canalicular bile acid transport protein. J Biol Chem. 1993;268:2083–91.

25. Bruck R, Haddad P, Graf J, Boyer JL. Regulatory volume decrease stimulates bile flow, bile acid excretion, and exocytosis in isolated perfused rat liver. Am J Physiol. 1992;262:G806–12.

26. Haussinger D, Hallbrucker C, Saha N, Lang, Gerok W. Cell volume and bile acid excretion. Biochem J. 1992;288:681–90.

27. Haussinger D, Saha N, Hallbrucker C, Lang F, Gerok W. Involvement of microtubules in the swelling-induced stimulation of transcellular taurocholate transport in perfused rat liver. Biochem J. 1993;291:355–60.

28. Boyer JL, McGrath JW, Ng OC. Microtubule dependent targeting of transporters to the apical membrane determines the canalicular excretion of bile acids in hepatocyte couplets. Hepatology. 1993;18:107A.

29. Hayakawa T, Bruck R, Ng OC, Boyer JL. DBcAMP stimulates vesicle transport and HRP excretion in isolated perfused rat liver. Am J Physiol. 1990;25:G727–35.

17
Adenosine triphosphate-dependent canalicular transport of bile salts and intrahepatic cholestasis

D. KEPPLER, M. BÖHME, M. BÜCHLER, R. MAYER, I. LEIER and G. JEDLITSCHKY

INTRODUCTION

The primary-active adenosine triphosphate (ATP)-driven bile salt export pump in the hepatocyte canalicular membrane was first described in 1991, and provides a sufficient explanation for the steep bile salt gradient from the hepatocyte into bile[1-4]. This discovery has raised the question of whether the potential-driven bile salt transporter[5-7], previously considered to be decisive for canalicular bile salt secretion[8], is a distinct and physiologically relevant transporter in this membrane domain. Two lines of evidence support the concept that canalicular bile salt secretion is ATP-driven and not potential-dependent: (a) selective inhibition of the ATP-dependent transporter by cyclosporins[9-11] inhibits taurocholate secretion *in vivo* and causes cholestasis[11]; and (b) potential-dependent and ATP-dependent taurocholate transport in rat liver have distinct subcellular localizations in the endoplasmic reticulum and the canalicular membrane, respectively[12].

Inhibition or down-regulation of the canalicular ATP-dependent bile salt transporter may be a key mechanism of intrahepatic cholestasis[11]. However, the contribution to bile flow of additional ATP-dependent export pumps in the canalicular membrane should also be considered (Fig. 1). These additional transport systems include

1. The conjugate export pump which secretes the glutathione conjugate leukotriene C_4 and structurally related amphiphilic anionic conjugates[13-15]. This export pump was recently identified as a 190 kDa membrane glycoprotein encoded by the multidrug resistance-associated gene[16,17].
2. The phospholipid export pump identified by means of gene knock-out in mice as the product of the *mdr 2* (*mdr* = multidrug resistance) gene[18,19].
3. The multidrug export pump encoded by the *MDR1* gene in humans and the *mdr1a* and *mdr1b* genes in rodents[20].

No evidence exists suggesting that the multidrug export pump or the *mdr2* gene

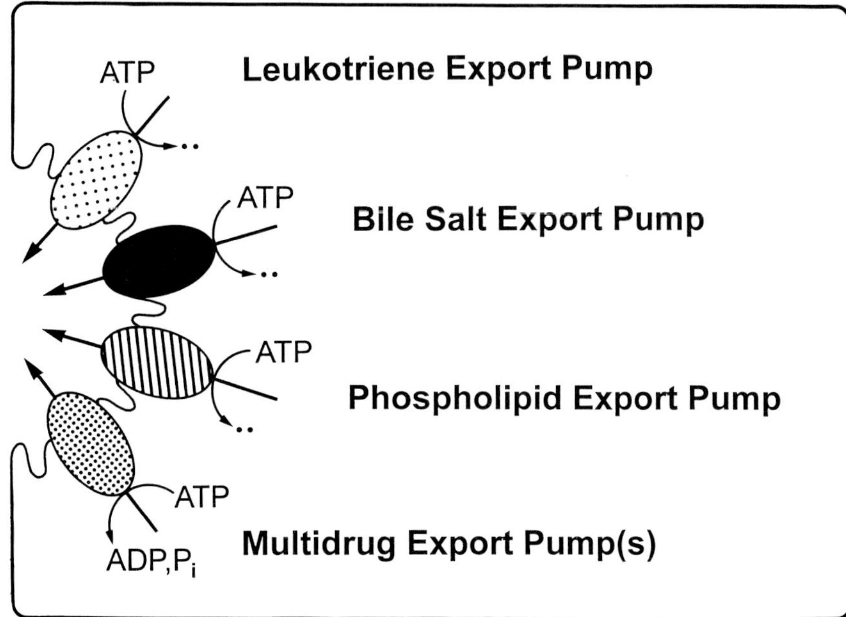

Fig. 1 ATP-dependent export pumps in the hepatocyte canalicular membrane. The leukotriene or conjugate export pump excretes a number of amphiphilic anions structurally related to the high-affinity endogenous substrate leukotriene C_4[13–17]. Recent work in human non-hepatic cell lines has established that this export pump is encoded by the multidrug resistance-associated gene *(MRP)*[16,17]. The ATP-dependent bile salt export pump has been functionally well characterized[1–4,10,11], but the molecular composition and identity of the transport system is still under investigation[22]. The phospholipid export system is now known as the *mdr2* gene product[18,19]. Furthermore, there is one multidrug export pump in humans[20] and Mdr1a and Mdr1b pumps in rats and mice[19,20,23,24]

product contribute significantly to bile flow. On the contrary, *mdr2* gene knock-out mice exhibit a significant increase in bile flow associated with ductular proliferation and portal inflammation[18].

Comparison of the presently known ATP-driven export pumps in the hepatocyte canalicular membrane (Fig. 1) suggests that the major contribution to bile flow is provided by the ATP-dependent bile salt export pump and an additional significant contribution from the ATP-dependent glutathione *S*-conjugate (leukotriene) export pump[11]. The latter conclusion is consistent with the reduction in bile flow in the TR⁻ (TR⁻ rats are Wistar rats deficient in the canalicular transport of leukotriene C_4 and related glutathione, glucuronate and sulphate conjugates) or GY (GY, Groningen yellow rats, are the same as TR⁻ rats[15]) mutant rats[13,15,21].

RESULTS AND DISCUSSION

The relative importance of the different hepatocyte membrane transport systems for bile salts for the physiology and pathophysiology of bile flow has been extensively discussed on the basis of the concept of sinusoidal Na⁺-dependent

Table 1 Kinetic constants and inhibitor efficiency of cyclosporin A, calculated by the K_m/K_i ratio, for the three different taurocholate (TC) transport systems in liver plasma membrane subfractions. K_m and K_i values are micromolar concentrations. For experimental conditions see Böhme *et al.*[11]

TC transport system	K_m	K_i	K_m/K_i
Na⁺-dependent	45	5	9
Potential-dependent	45	70	0.6
ATP-dependent	6	0.2	30

Table 2 Distribution of [¹⁴C]taurocholate in normal (TR⁺) and mutant (TR⁻) Wistar rats with and without cyclosporin A (CsA) 20 min after i.v. injection. For experimental details see Böhme *et al.*[11]

	Percentage of injected dose		
	Liver	*Bile*	*Liver/Bile*
TR⁺	3	85	0.04
TR⁺ with CsA	39	47	0.8
TR⁻	6	85	0.07
TR⁻ with CsA	61	26	2.3

bile salt uptake and canalicular potential-driven bile salt secretion[5–8]. Potential-dependent taurocholate (TC) transport into preparations of canalicular membrane vesicles is inhibited by relatively high cyclosporin A (CsA) concentrations (Table 1). CsA also inhibits TC uptake into sinusoidal membrane vesicles and into isolated hepatocytes[26]. However, comparison of the kinetic data for the sinusoidal Na⁺-dependent TC transport and for the canalicular ATP-dependent transport reveals that ATP-dependent transport is much more susceptible to inhibition (Table 1). The kinetic constants K_m and K_i (inhibition constant), which are not affected by the orientation of the membrane vesicles, identify the ATP-dependent transport as the most sensitive to inhibition by CsA and its non-immunosuppressive analogue PSC-833 ((3′-oxo-4-butenyl-4-methyl threonine¹)-(val²)-cyclosporin). This is consistent with our results from the *in vivo* distribution of ¹⁴C-labelled TC indicating an accumulation of the bile salt in hepatocytes and a block in the secretion across the canalicular membrane (Table 2). TC radioactivity in blood was not significantly different under the conditions used in the *in vivo* experiments shown in Table 2.

In the rat about 50% of total bile flow is independent of bile salt secretion[27]. The bile salt-independent flow includes the fraction related to secretion of amphiphilic anions such as conjugates with glutathione, glucuronate and sulphate. These substances are secreted by a canalicular hepatocyte transport system different from the bile salt transporter in the canalicular membrane (Fig. 1). The relative contribution of transport systems in the canalicular membrane to total bile flow may be elucidated further when selective inhibitors for distinct transport systems are available, as exemplified by the cyclosporins as a novel

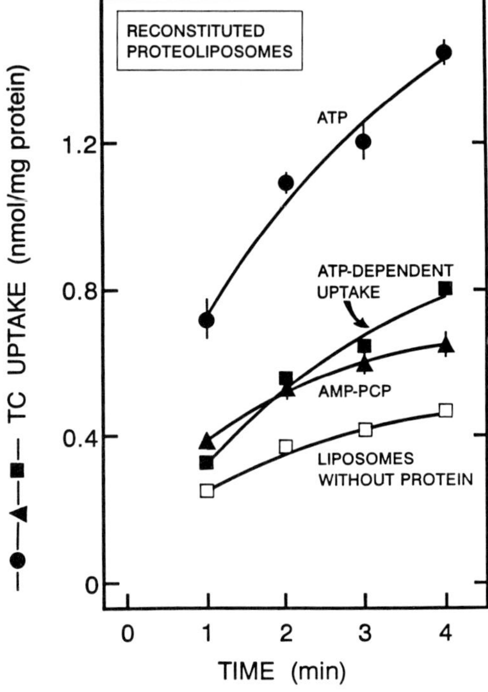

Fig. 2 ATP-dependent transport of taurocholate into reconstituted proteoliposomes. [³H]TC transport was determined in proteoliposomes reconstituted with solubilized canalicular membrane of rat liver in the presence of either ATP and a regenerating system (●) or the non-hydrolysable ATP analogue AMP-PCP (▲). The TC concentration was 5 μmol/l. Liposomes without protein showed background levels of uptake (□). Reproduced with permission from Büchler *et al.*[22]

tool[9–11]. CsA did not inhibit the ATP-dependent transport of the glutathione conjugate LTC$_4$ (leukotriene C$_4$) as potently as the TC transport[10,11]. Our *in vivo* and *in vitro* data allow for a better characterization of the cyclosporin action on bile flow with preferential inhibition of bile salt secretion. The reduction of bile flow to 14% of the control TR⁻ group with a complete block of [¹⁴C]TC secretion for 5 min[11] has two implications: on one hand, in the absence of ATP-dependent transport of glutathione, glucuronate and sulphate conjugates, bile flow is largely maintained by the ATP-dependent bile salt transporter: on the other hand, the nearly complete cessation of bile flow in TR⁻ rats after administration of CsA suggests that bile flow in normal animals is generated largely (by more than 80%) by ATP-dependent transport of bile salts and glucuronate, sulphate, and glutathione *S*-conjugates[11,15]. In normal TR⁺ rats (normal transport-competent Wistar rats) bile flow is lowered to about 50% by CsA, and bile flow in TR⁻ rats is 50% of the normal TR⁺ value. This suggests that both the aforementioned transporters contribute equally to bile flow in the rat.

The potent inhibition of the ATP-dependent bile salt export pump by CsA provides an important tool for elucidation of at least one molecular mechanism of intrahepatic cholestasis. ATP-dependent bile salt transport was not only

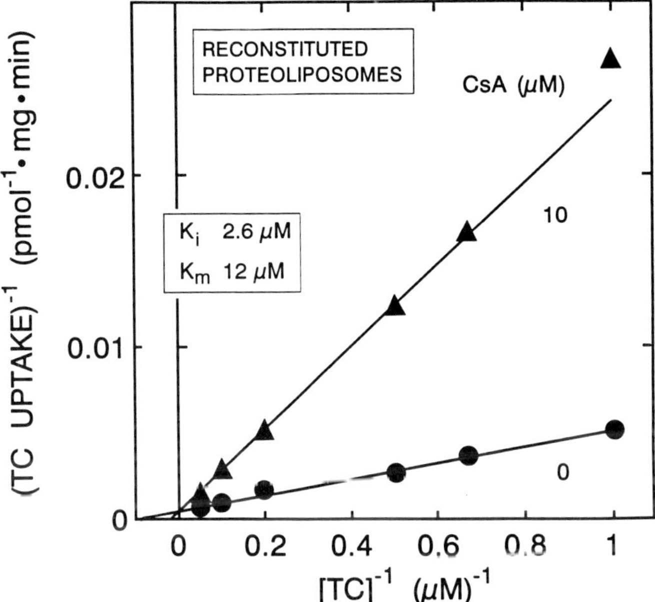

Fig. 3 Inhibition by cyclosporin A (CsA) of the ATP-dependent bile salt export pump from the canalicular membrane reconstituted in proteoliposomes. [³H]TC uptake was measured in the presence or absence of 10 μmol/l CsA for 2 min at 37°C. ATP-dependent uptake is calculated from the difference between measurements in the presence of ATP and AMP-PCP (see legend to Fig. 2). Reproduced with permission from Büchler *et al.*[22]

sensitive to cyclosporins in the membrane vesicle transport system but also in reconstituted proteoliposome vesicles (Figs. 2 and 3). The functional reconstitution of the canalicular ATP-dependent bile salt export pump will serve to isolate and further characterize this transporter protein. In addition, this system enables the identification of components of the export pump by means of their selective removal by immunodepletion[22].

CONCLUSIONS

The comparison of different bile salt transport systems in rat hepatocyte membrane vesicles demonstrates that the ATP-dependent bile salt export pump is by far the most sensitive to inhibition by CsA as well as its non-immunosuppressive analogue PSC-833.

The molecular composition of the ATP-driven bile salt export pump in the canalicular membrane has not been fully elucidated. Progress has been made by the functional reconstitution of the solubilized transport system in proteoliposomes. CsA is also a potent inhibitor of the solubilized and reconstituted pump.

Selective inhibition of the ATP-dependent bile salt export pump results in intrahepatic cholestasis, as evidenced by the action of cyclosporins used as tools.

Potential-dependent transport of bile salts across the canalicular membrane of hepatocytes plays a negligible role in the secretion of bile salts into bile.

References

1. Müller M, Ishikawa T, Berger U *et al.* ATP-dependent transport of taurocholate across the hepatocyte canalicular membrane mediated by a 110-kDa glycoprotein binding ATP and bile salt. J Biol Chem. 1991;266:18920–6.
2. Adachi Y, Kobayashi H, Kurumi Y, Shouji M, Kitano M, Yamamoto T. ATP-dependent taurocholate transport by rat liver canalicular membrane vesicles. Hepatology. 1991;14:655–9.
3. Nishida T, Gatmaitan Z, Che M, Arias IM. Rat liver canalicular membrane vesicles contain an ATP-dependent bile acid transport system. Proc Natl Acad Sci USA. 1991;88:6590–4.
4. Stieger B, O'Neill B, Meier PJ. ATP-dependent bile-salt transport in canalicular rat liver plasma-membrane vesicles. Biochem J. 1992;284:67–73.
5. Inoue M, Kinne R, Tran T, Arias IM. Taurocholate transport by rat liver canalicular membrane vesicles. J Clin Invest. 1984;73:659–63.
6. Meier PJ, Meier-Abt AS, Barrett C, Boyer JL. Mechanisms of taurocholate transport in canalicular and basolateral rat liver plasma membrane vesicles. J Biol Chem. 1984;259:10614–22.
7. Ruetz S, Hugentobler G, Meier PJ. Functional reconstitution of the canalicular bile salt transport system of rat liver. Proc Natl Acad Sci USA. 1988;85:6147–51.
8. Boyer JL, Graf J, Meier PJ. Hepatic transport systems regulating pH$_i$, cell volume, and bile secretion. Annu Rev Physiol. 1992;54:415–38.
9. Kadmon M, Klünemann C, Böhme M *et al.* Inhibition by cyclosporin A of adenosine triphosphate-dependent transport from the hepatocyte into bile. Gastroenterology. 1993;104:1507–14.
10. Böhme M, Büchler M, Müller M, Keppler D. Differential inhibition by cyclosporins of primary-active ATP-dependent transporters in the hepatocyte canalicular membrane. FEBS Lett. 1993;333:193–6.
11. Böhme M, Müller M, Leier I, Jedlitschky G, Keppler D. Cholestasis caused by inhibition of the adenosine triphosphate-dependent bile salt transport in rat liver. Gastroenterology. 1994;107:255–65.
12. Kast C, Stieger B, Winterhalter K II, Meier PJ. Evidence for distinct subcellular localizations of electrogenic and ATP-dependent taurocholate transport in rat hepatocytes. J Biol Chem. 1994;269:5179–86.
13. Ishikawa T, Müller M, Klünemann C, Schaub T, Keppler D. ATP-dependent primary active transport of cysteinyl leukotrienes across liver canalicular membrane. Role of the ATP-dependent transport system for glutathione S-conjugates. J Biol Chem. 1990;265:19279–86.
14. Keppler D. Leukotrienes: biosynthesis, transport, inactivation, and analysis. Rev Physiol Biochem Pharmacol. 1992;121:1–30.
15. Jansen PLM, Oude Elferink RPJ. Defective hepatic anion secretion in mutant TR⁻ rats. In: Tavoloni N, Berk PD, editors. Hepatic transport and bile secretion: physiology and pathophysiology. New York: Raven, 1993:721–31.
16. Jedlitschky G, Leier I, Buchholz U, Center M, Keppler D. ATP-dependent transport of glutathione *S*-conjugates by the multidrug resistance-associated protein. Cancer Res. 1994;54:4833–6.
17. Leier I, Jedlitschky G, Buchholz U, Cole SPC, Deeley RG, Keppler D. The *MRP* gene encodes an ATP-dependent export pump for leukotriene C$_4$ and structurally related conjugates. J Biol Chem. 1994;269:27807–10.
18. Smit JJM, Schinkel AH, Oude Elferink RPJ *et al.* Homozygous disruption of the murine *mdr2* P-glycoprotein gene leads to complete absence of phospholipids from bile and to liver disease. Cell. 1993;75:451–62.
19. Oude Elferink RPJ, Smit JJM, Schinkel AH *et al.* The physiological role of *mdr2* P-glycoprotein in hepatobiliary phospholipid transport. In: Keppler D, Jungermann K, editors. Transport in the liver. Dordrecht: Kluwer; 1994:204–13.
20. Gottesman MM, Pastan I. Biochemistry of multidrug resistance mediated by the multidrug transporter. Annu Rev Biochem. 1993;62:385–427.
21. Huber M, Guhlmann A, Jansen PLM, Keppler D. Hereditary defect of hepatobiliary cysteinyl leukotriene elimination in mutant rats with defective hepatic anion excretion. Hepatology. 1987;7:224–8.

22. Büchler M, Böhme M, Ortlepp H, Keppler D. Functional reconstitution of ATP-dependent transporters from the solubilized hepatocyte canalicular membrane. Eur J Biochem. 1994;224:345–52.
23. Schinkel AH, Smit JJM, Van Tellingen O *et al.* Disruption of the mouse *mdr1a* P-glycoprotein gene leads to a deficiency in the blood–brain barrier and to increased sensitivity to drugs. Cell. 1994;77:491–502.
24. Silverman JA, Raunio H, Gant TW, Thorgeirsson SS. Cloning and characterization of a member of the rat multidrug resistance (mdr) gene family. Gene. 1991;106:229–36.
25. Moseley RH, Johnson TR, Morrissette JM. Inhibition of bile acid transport by cyclosporine A in rat liver plasma membrane vesicles. J Pharmacol Exp Ther. 1990;253:974–80.
26. Ziegler K, Frimmer M. Cyclosporin A and a diaziridine derivative inhibit the hepatocellular uptake of cholate, phalloidin and rifampicin. Biochim Biophys Acta. 1986;855:136–42.
27. Erlinger S. Bile flow. In: Arias IM, et al. editors. The liver: biology and pathobiology, 3rd edn. New York: Raven, 1994:769–86.

Section V
Bile acid transport: biliary and intestinal

18
Serial quantitative image analysis of uptake and transport of fluorescent bile acids in polarized biliary epithelial cells

A. BENEDETTI, L. MARUCCI, A. DI SARIO, G. SVEGLIATI BARONI,
C. D. SCHTEINGART, H-T. TON-NU and A. F. HOFMANN

INTRODUCTION

The recent development of techniques for isolation of biliary epithelial cells or polarized intrahepatic bile duct units[1] as shown in Fig. 1 has provided a new tool for the study of hepatic physiopathology. It has been suggested that the morphological and functional properties of biliary epithelial cells are not identical along the whole biliary tree but vary according to the size of the ducts[2], thus suggesting a different role played by various segments of the ductular wall in the elaboration of bile and the necessity to well define the section of bile ducts in any physiopathological study. We have recently developed a technique of isolation and culture of intrahepatic bile ducts[1]. This technique briefly requires the enzymatic digestion and gentle combing of the biliary tree. Isolated bile ducts present a good preservation of the morphological appearance, of the tight junctions and of the basal membranes (Fig. 1). This isolation technique permits the obtaining of bile ducts of different diameter.

The biliary ductular epithelium is known to absorb glucose and other solutes from canalicular bile[3]. Conjugated bile acids pass down the biliary tree and are either stored in the gallbladder or secreted into the gut. Under some circumstances, unconjugated bile acids may also be secreted into bile in appreciable amounts. Lipophilic unconjugated mono- and dihydroxy bile acids may be absorbed passively by cholangiocytes, seem to be conjugated during cellular transport and finally return to the sinusoid via the periductular capillary plexus as suggested by the hypothesis of the cholehepatic shunt[4]. The morphological and anatomical organization of the liver tissue suggests in fact a tight relationship between biliary ductular cells and the capillary plexus. According to the theory of the cholehepatic shunt, the end point of the transport of bile acids through the

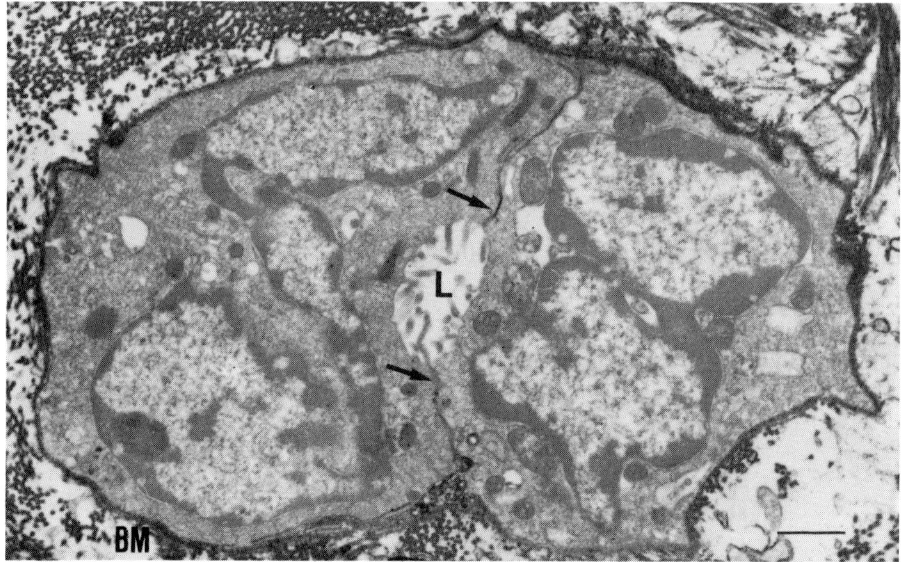

Fig. 1 A well preserved isolated bile duct with intact basement membrane (BM) and tight junctions (large arrows). L = lumen. Bar = 1 μm. (Figure from Hepatology. 1993;18:422–32, with permission)

biliary epithelium should be the secretion of conjugated bile acid anions from the basolateral membranes of cholangiocytes. This step should be mediated by a carrier mechanism because conjugated bile acids do not traverse membranes passively. Such a carrier is present in ileal enterocytes, but nothing is known regarding bile ducts.

Therefore different experiments have been performed to test in vitro for the presence of an active transport of conjugated bile acid anions in polarized biliary epithelial cells of intrahepatic bile ductules isolated from rat liver.

MATERIALS AND METHODS

Intrahepatic bile ductules with a mean ductular diameter between 15 and 25 μm were used after isolation from parenchymal tissue and cultured up to 24 hours on glass cover slips precoated with the extracellular matrix (Matrigel) in a medium containing bicarbonate (alfa-MEM medium).

Sequential morphological and morphometrical studies have been performed to evaluate the time course of uptake and cellular localization of the fluorescent conjugated bile acids, cholyl-*N*-NBD-lysine (C-NBD-Lys) and chenodeoxy-cholyl-*N*-NBD-lysine (CDC-NBD-Lys).

Isolated bile ductules were incubated at 37°C in alfa-MEM medium containing up to 3 μmol/L of fluorescent bile acids for different progressive time intervals (0, 1, 3, 5, 10, 15, 20 and 60 min) and the fluorescent signal was analysed under a fluorescent microscope by a quantitative image analysis system (CUE-3 image analyser system by Olympus) in different culture conditions.

Similar fluorescent studies have been performed in isolated fibroblasts obtained from calvaria of newborn rats.

The fluorescent studies were performed in control samples, in samples preincubated at 15° and 4°C, in samples incubated in the absence of Na^+ or Cl^-, in samples preincubated with DIDS (0.1 or 1 mmol/l) or finally in samples incubated in the presence of taurocholic acid (TCA, 10 μmol/l) or probenecid (1 mmol/l).

RESULTS

In control samples, the serial quantitative image analysis of uptake and cellular localization of fluorescent conjugated bile acids did not show significant differences between C-NBD-Lys and CDC-NBD-Lys at any time intervals. At 1 and 3 min, fluorescence was distributed at the periphery of the cytoplasm with a preferential localization in the basolateral area. In contrast, the staining in the apical region of the biliary epithelium occurred later, between 10 and 20 min.

The basolateral uptake of both fluorescent conjugated bile acids was temperature-dependent; in fact, it was decreased by 70% and 80%, at 15 and 4°C respectively as compared to samples incubated at 37°C.

The basolateral uptake (at 1 and 3 min) of fluorescent conjugated bile acids was uninfluenced by the absence of Na^+ in the perfusate, while it was significantly inhibited by 35% in samples preincubated for 2 h with 1 mmol/L DIDS as compared to control samples. Moreover, it was inhibited by 50% in the absence of Cl^- in the perfusate.

Finally, the basolateral uptake of fluorescent conjugated bile acids was partially inhibited by incubation of samples in the presence of 1 mmol/L probenecid while it was not significantly modified by the presence of TCA-concentrations up to 10 μmol/L in the medium.

Morphological studies in isolated rat fibroblasts incubated with fluorescent conjugated bile acids showed no evaluable uptake with both bile acids at 37°C or at 4°C.

SUMMARY AND DISCUSSION

In summary, in isolated polarized bile ductules with a mean diameter of 15–25 μm, the uptake and the cellular localization of cholyl and chenodeoxycholyl-NBD-lysine did not appear significantly different. Fluorescent bile acids were preferentially localized in the basolateral area after 1–3 min of incubation, while the apical staining occurred later. This basolateral uptake appeared temperature-dependent and Na^+-independent. It was decreased by preincubation with 1 mmol/L DIDS, by the absence of Cl^- in the perfusate or finally by incubation in the presence of probenecid.

In contrast, isolated rat fibroblasts did not show any significant uptake of fluorescent conjugated bile acids.

All these data suggest an active transport of di- and trihydroxy bile acids through the basolateral membrane of the biliary epithelium. This active transport could be involved in the cholehepatic circulation of the bile acids but this implication has to be confirmed by further studies.

Acknowledgements

We would like to express our most sincere thanks to Prof F. Orlandi and to Prof Anne Marie Jezequel for helpful discussions and to Luciano Trozzi and Antonella Fava for their excellent technical assistance.

This work was supported by CNR 94.0278CT04, MPI (Progetto Nazionale Cirrosi) and CNR (Progetto Finalizzato FATMA, 94.00516PF41 and 94.00527PF41).

References

1. Benedetti A, Marucci L, Bassotti C, Mancini R, Contucci S, Jezequel AM, Orlandi F. Tubulovescicular transcytotic pathway in rat biliary epithelium. A study in perfused liver and in isolated intrahepatic bile ducts. Hepatology. 1993;18:422–32.
2. Alpini G, Roberts S, Podila P, Yano M, La Russo NF. Molecular and functional characterization of specific cholangiocyte subpopulation involved in somastostatin-regulated ductal bile secretion. Hepatology. 1994;20:267A (abstract).
3. Lira M, Schteingart CD, Steinbach JH, Lambert K, McRoberts JA, Hofmann AF. Sugar absorption by the biliary ductular epithelium of the rat: evidence for two transport systems. Gastroenterology. 1992;102:563–71.
4. Yoon YB, Hagey LR, Hofmann AF, Gurantz D, Michelotti EL, Steinbach JH. Effect of side-chain shortening on the physiologic properties of bile acids: hepatic transport and effect on biliary secretion of 23-nor-ursodeoxycholate in rodents. Gastroenterology. 1986;90:837–52.

19
Carrier-mediated absorption of conjugated bile acids in the jejunum of guinea pigs

A. AMELSBERG, C. D. SCHTEINGART and A. F. HOFMANN

The role of the ileal sodium-dependent bile acid cotransporter is well established[1]. Less is known about the mechanisms of jejunal bile acid absorption, for which there is considerable evidence in animals including humans[2,3]. It has been suggested that jejunal absorption is an important, and in some animals the most important, pathway of intestinal bile acid absorption[4-7]. Several lines of evidence indicate that the transport system prefers conjugated dihydroxy- over trihydroxy-bile acids[8-11].

We have carried out experiments to test the hypothesis that at least some jejunal absorption involves carrier-mediated transport. To characterize such transport, jejunal perfusion experiments and experiments with isolated jejunal guinea pig cells were performed. ^{3}H- or ^{14}C-taurine conjugated bile acids with and without the addition of bile acid-based transport inhibitors were used. In perfusion experiments the apparent permeability (P_{app}; cm/s) and in experiments with isolated cells the initial rate of uptake (nmol/mg protein per minute) were calculated.

The P_{app} of cholyltaurine in perfusion experiments was significantly lower than for either taurine-conjugated ursodeoxycholic acid, chenodeoxycholic acid or deoxycholic acid. The P_{app} for glycine-conjugated bile acids was comparable, with the exception of glycine-conjugated ursodeoxycholic acid which was not significantly different from cholyltaurine. Co-perfusion of ursodeoxycholyltaurine with chenodeoxycholyltaurine or deoxycholyltaurine, but not with taurine, showed a significant competitive inhibition in P_{app}. Perfusions of ursodeoxycholyltaurine in various concentrations below the CMC gave a saturation kinetics.

Incubation of isolated cells yielded a significantly lower initial rate of uptake for cholyltaurine compared to chenodeoxycholyltaurine and ursodeoxycholyltaurine. Addition of unlabelled chenodeoxycholyltaurine decreased the initial rate of uptake for ursodeoxycholyltaurine significantly by 43%. Incubation of isolated cells in ice-cold medium decreased the initial rate of uptake for ursodeoxycholyltaurine significantly by 53%. Initial rate of uptake was independent of sodium gradient.

In the jejunum of guinea pigs a Na^+-independent carrier mechanism that transports taurine-conjugated bile acid anions is present. The mechanism could be either facilitated diffusion or an anion exchange process. The presence of this carrier, together with non-ionic diffusion of protonated glycine-conjugated dihydroxy bile acids, can account for the jejunal uptake of bile acids.

References

1. Wilson FA. Intestinal transport of bile acids. In: Schultz SG, Field M, Frizzell RA, Rauner BB, editors. Handbook of physiology. The gastrointestinal system, Vol. IV. Bethesda: American Physiological Society; 1991:389–404.
2. McClintock C, Shiau YF. Jejunum is more important than terminal ileum for taurocholate absorption in rats. Am J Physiol. 1983;244:G507–14.
3. Lewis MC, Root C. *In vivo* transport kinetics and distribution of taurocholate by rat ileum and jejunum. Am J Physiol. 1990;259:G233–8.
4. Hurwitz S, Bar A, Katz M, Sklan D, Budowski P. Absorption and secretion of fatty acids and bile acids in the intestine of the laying fowl. J Nutr. 1973;103:543–7.
5. Sklan D, Budowski P, Hurwitz S. Site of bile acid absorption in the rat. Lipids. 1976;11:467–71.
6. Spittell D, Vongroven LK, Subbiah MT. Concentration changes of bile acids in sequential segments of pigeon intestine and their relation to bile acid absorption. Biochim Biophys Acta. 1976;441:32–7.
7. Sklan D. Site of digestion and absorption of lipids and bile acids in the rat and turkey. Comp Biochem Physiol [A]. 1980;65A:91–5.
8. Barbara L, Roda A, Roda E *et al*. Diurnal variations of serum primary bile acids in healthy subjects and hepatobiliary disease patients. Rendic Gastroenterol. 1976;8:194–8.
9. Schalm SW, LaRusso NF, Hofmann AF *et al*. Diurnal serum levels of primary conjugated bile acids. Assessment by specific radioimmunoassays for conjugates of cholic and chenodeoxycholic acid. Gut. 1978;19:1006–14.
10. Ponz De Leon M, Murphy GM, Dowling RH. Physiological factors influencing serum bile acid levels. Gut. 1978;19:32–9.
11. Angelin B, Einarsson K, Hellstrom K. Evidence for the absorption of bile acids in the proximal small intestine of normo- and hyperlipidaemic subjects. Gut. 176;17:420–5.

20
The apical membrane bile acid transporter of the ileal enterocyte

P. A. DAWSON and M. H. WONG

INTRODUCTION

Bile acids are acidic sterols synthesized from cholesterol in the liver and secreted into bile[1]. Following secretion, the bile acids enter the lumen of the small intestine and facilitate absorption of cholesterol and fat-soluble vitamins. Greater than 90% of bile acids are reabsorbed from the intestine and returned to the liver via the portal venous circulation. At the sinusoidal membrane of the liver, bile acids are quantitatively extracted and resecreted into bile[2]. This hepatic extraction of bile acids from the portal circulation is extremely efficient, and allows only a small fraction of bile acids to enter the systemic circulation. Of this fraction, very little bile acid is eliminated in the urine. Bile acids in the circulation escape urinary excretion by several mechanisms. First, bile acids are bound to serum proteins, thereby preventing glomerular filtration. Second, bile acids are actively absorbed from the proximal renal tubules and returned to the liver for uptake[3]. The amount of bile acid filtered through the renal tubules therefore exceeds the amount excreted in urine[4]. The presence of an active bile acid uptake mechanism also explains why bile acid concentrations in peripheral blood may climb precipitously in obstructive liver disease[5].

In the small intestine, bile acids are absorbed by both passive and active mechanisms[6]. Whereas passive absorption may occur down the length of the small intestine, active absorption of bile acids in humans and in experimental animals is believed to be restricted to the ileum[7-9]. The active uptake of bile acids is first mediated by a Na+ gradient-driven transporter located at the brush-border (apical) membrane of the ileocyte[10]. After entering the ileocyte, bile acids are delivered to the basolateral membrane and secreted into the portal circulation via a Na+-independent organic anion exchange system[11]. The transport kinetics and specificity of this Na+/bile acid cotransport system have been studied using a variety of experimental systems, including everted gut sacs[8,9], isolated ileocytes[12,13] and ileal brush-border membranes[14,15]. However, despite extensive study of the properties of ileal bile acid transport, very little was known about the protein(s) involved. Recently, we have employed an expression cloning strategy to identify and isolate a hamster ileal Na[+]/bile acid cotransporter (ISBT)[16]. This cDNA was subsequently used to isolate the human ISBT cDNA[17]. In this chapter we review the cloning and general properties of the bile acid transporter of the apical membrane of the ileal enterocyte.

RESULTS AND DISCUSSION

We have recently reported the expression cloning and characterization of the hamster ileal Na[+]/bile acid cotransporter[16]. In those studies the isolated hamster cDNA produced a protein that stimulated taurocholate uptake almost 1000-fold following transfection into COS cells. As a first step towards elucidating the role of the ileal bile acid transporter in the pathogenesis of human intestinal disorders, the hamster ISBT cDNA was used to identify the human ISBT. For those experiments, oligonucleotide primers were synthesized corresponding to amino acid sequences conserved between the hamster ISBT and rat liver Na[+]/bile acid cotransporter (LSBT)[18]. PCR amplification was performed using human ileal cDNA and oligonucleotides corresponding to amino acids 75–81 and 261–266 of the hamster ISBT. The human PCR product was isolated and labelled with ^{32}P for use as a hybridization probe. This product was used to screen an ileal λgt10 cDNA library to isolate a human ISBT cDNA clone[17]. The deduced amino acid sequences of the hamster and human ISBTs are compared in Fig. 1. The hamster and human ISBT cDNAs encode 348 amino acid proteins with three and two potential N-linked glycosylation sites, respectively. Overall, the hamster ISBT protein shares 84% identity with the human ISBT. Comparison of their amino acid sequences revealed that the majority of non-conservative amino acid substitutions are restricted to the amino and carboxyl termini, whereas the putative transmembrane domains and intracellular and extracellular loops are highly conserved (Fig. 1). The Kyte–Doolittle hydropathy profile[20] of the hamster ISBT is almost identical to both the human ISBT and human LSBT[19], indicating similar membrane topologies. This analysis suggested a topology with an extracellular amino terminus, seven transmembrane domains and a cytosolic carboxyl terminus. The ileal and liver bile acid transporters do not exhibit sequence identity with the Na[+]/glucose cotransporter or other members of the large family of 12 transmembrane domain Na[+] cotransport proteins[21]. Rather, the bile acid transporters appear to constitute a new family of sodium cotransport proteins, exhibiting considerable structural similarity to the seven transmembrane domain proteins such as rhodopsin and the G protein coupled receptors[22].

Na[+]-dependent bile acid uptake has been demonstrated in the sinusoidal membranes of the liver[23] and the brush-border membranes of the kidney[10]. In the small intestine, active bile acid uptake is found in the ileum but absent from the duodenum and proximal jejunum[10]. Northern blot analysis was performed with poly(A)[+] RNA from hamster kidney, liver, duodenum, jejunum and ileum to compare the mRNA expression for ISBT with the known tissue distribution of bile acid transport activity, and with other proteins believed to be involved in bile acid transport. As shown in Fig. 2, the ISBT probe hybridized to a single 4.0kb message that was readily detectable in hamster ileum and kidney, weakly

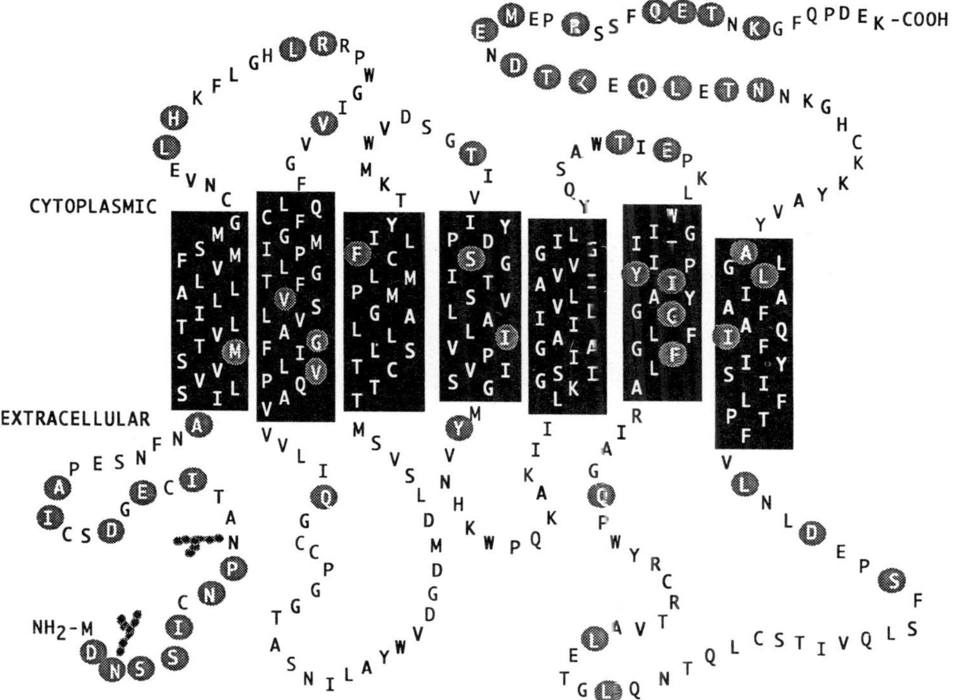

Fig. 1 Sequence and proposed membrane topology of the hamster ileal Na$^+$/bile acid cotransporter; comparison to the human ileal Na$^+$/bile acid cotransporter. The predicted topology was determined by Kyte–Doolittle hydropathy analysis over a sliding window of 11 amino acids[20], and topogenic signals were assigned as described by von Heijne and Manoil[31]. The proposed transmembrane domains appear as black boxes. Glycosylation at Asn 3 and Asn 10 is indicated by the small circles. The encircled amino acids are not conserved between the hamster and human ileal Na$^+$/bile acid cotransporters

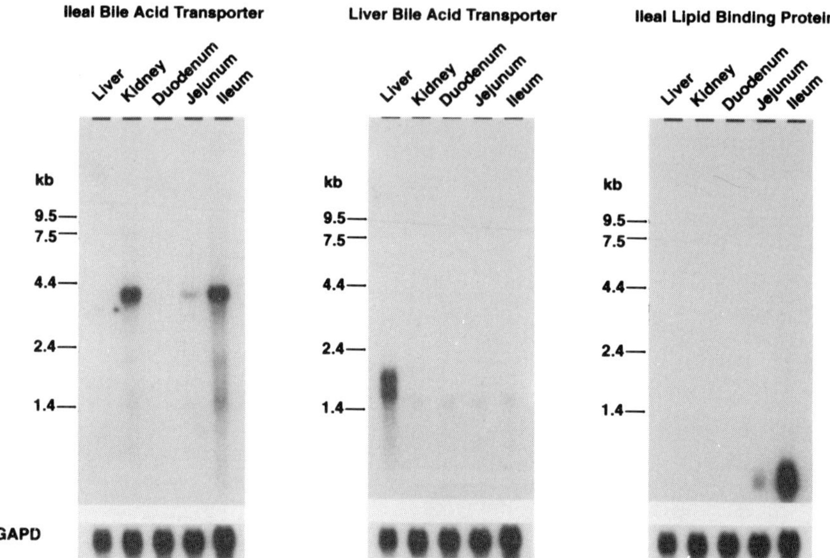

Fig. 2 Northern blot hybridization of mRNA from hamster tissues with ISBT, LSBT and ILBP probes. Poly(A)$^+$ RNA (5 μg) from the indicated hamster tissues was subjected to electrophoresis on a 1.2% agarose gel containing 2.2 mol/l formaldehyde and blotted onto GeneScreen membrane (DuPont-NEN). *Upper panels:* hybridization was performed in 50% formamide buffer at 42°C with the indicated ^{32}P-labelled probes. The filter was washed in 0.2×SSC containing 0.1% SSC at 65°C for 30 min and exposed to Amersham Hyperfilm with an intensifying screen at −70°C. The migration of RNA standards run in an adjacent lane is indicated. *Lower panels:* the filter was stripped and rehybridized with a uniformly ^{32}P-labelled human glyceraldehyde-3-phosphate dehydrogenase probe, washed and exposed to Amersham Hyperfilm

detectable in jejunum, and absent from duodenum and liver. In contrast, hybridization with a rat LSBT probe detected two liver transcripts of 1.5 and 1.8 kb and no hybridization to kidney or intestinal RNAs. The nature of the multiple LSBT transcripts is unknown, but may represent alternate splicing or differential termination–polyadenylation site usage. In contrast to previous reports in the rat[18], LSBT mRNA was not detectable in hamster kidney. This difference may be due to the stringency employed for the hybridization, or may represent a species difference between the rat and hamster. In addition to the transporters, the Northern blot was hybridized with a mouse ileal lipid binding protein (ILBP) probe. ILBP (also called bile acid binding protein: BABP) is a 14 kDa protein thought to be involved in the transcellular transort of bile acids in the intestine[24,25]. For ILBP, a 0.6 kb message was readily detected in ileum; weakly detected in jejunum; and absent from duodenum, kidney and liver. These results are similar to previous studies in the mouse[24] and rat[25].

To examine expression of the ISBT protein, polyclonal antiserum was raised against a C-terminal peptide corresponding to amino acids 335–348 of the hamster ISBT (SFQETNKGFQPDEK). Since this sequence is identical in the hamster and rat ISBT[30], rat ileal and jejunal brush-border membranes were examined by immunoblotting. Approximately 100 μg of brush-border membrane

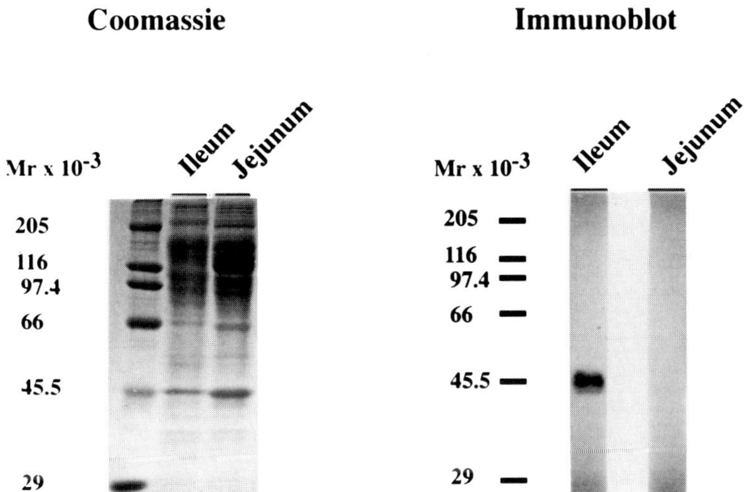

Fig. 3 Immunoblot analysis of the ileal bile acid transporter. 100 μg of rat jejunal or ileal brush-border membrane protein was denatured and reduced in Laemmli sample buffer containing 2% (w/v) SDS and 2.5% (v/v) β-mercaptoethanol. The protein was subjected to electrophoresis on a 10% SDS-polyacrylamide gel and either stained with Coomassie blue (*Coomassie*) or transferred to a nitrocellulose filter (*Immunoblot*). The nitrocellulose filter was incubated with 1.8 μg/ml of rabbit antipeptide IgG directed against the carboxyl terminus of the hamster ileal bile acid transporter. To visualize the primary antibody the filter was incubated with alkaline phosphatase-conjugated goat anti-rabbit IgG (1:2500 dilution). The positions of molecular weight markers run in adjacent lanes were determined by staining the nitrocellulose filter with Ponceau S prior to blocking the filter

protein was subjected to polyacrylamide gel electrophoresis under denaturing and reducing conditions. Duplicate lanes were either stained with Coomassie blue or transferred to nitrocellulose and probed with the anti-ISBT peptide antibody. As shown in Fig. 3, a 46 kDa protein was readily detected in ileum but absent from jejunum. Although no additional higher molecular weight forms of the transporter were observed in this study, an apparent dimer of 92 kDa, as well as higher molecular weight forms, have been observed in other experiments[30]. The relationship between the higher molecular weight proteins observed on the immunoblots and ISBT is not clear at this time.

A critical property of the ileal bile acid transporter is its dependence on an external Na^+ gradient[9]. To examine the Na^+-dependence of ISBT, hamster and human ISB-transfected COS cells were incubated in a modified Hanks buffer containing either 100 mmol/l Na^+ or equal concentrations of tetraethyl-ammonium (TEA) or K^+. As shown in Fig. 4, [^{3}H]taurocholate uptake was stimulated in the presence of Na^+, whereas small cations such as K^+ or organic cations such as TEA were unable to support [^{3}H]taurocholate uptake. In the transfected COS cells the activity of the human ISBT cDNA was consistently less than that of the hamster ISBT. This may represent lower catalytic efficiency

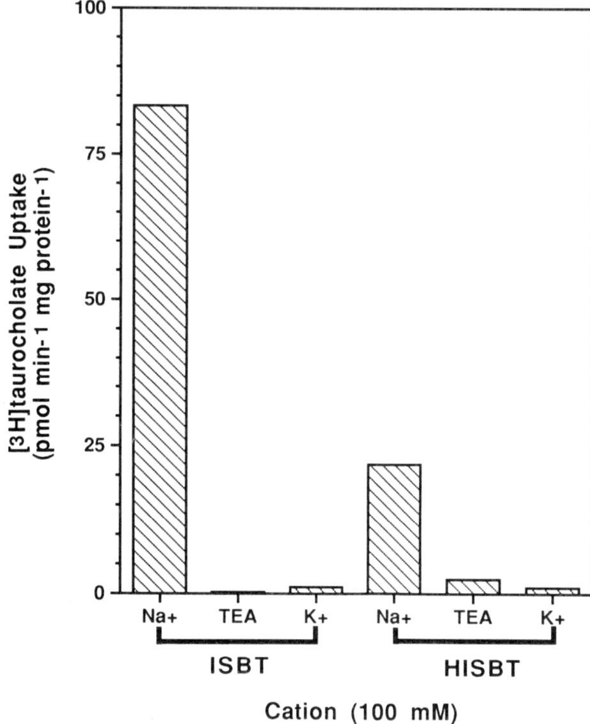

Fig. 4 Na⁺-dependence of bile acid uptake by human and hamster ileal bile acid transporters. On day 0, 1.5×10^5 COS cells per 100 mm dish were plated in Dulbecco's modified Eagle's medium containing 4500 mg/l D-glucose, 10% (v/v) fetal calf serum, 100 units/ml penicillin, and 100 μg/ml streptomycin. On day 1 the cells were transfected with 5 μg of hamster ISBT, human ISBT, or β-galactosidase expression vector plasmid by the DEAE-dextran method. On day 2 each group of transfected cells was treated with trypsin, pooled, and replated in 24-well culture plates at 7×10^4 cells/well. On day 4 the cells were incubated with Hanks' buffered salt solution supplemented with 5 μmol/l [³H]taurocholate (2.0 Ci/mmol) and containing 100 mmol/l sodium or equal concentrations of tetraethylammonium (TEA) or potassium. After 15 min at 37°C the medium was removed, and each cell monolayer was washed and processed to determine cell-associated protein and radioactivity. Each value represents the mean of three independent transfections performed in duplicate ($n=6$)

for the human ISBT, or differences in transfection efficiency or promoter strength. Interestingly, a lower activity was also noted in *Xenopus* oocytes for the expressed human liver Na⁺/bile acid cotransporter when compared to the rat liver transporter[18,19].

The properties and tissue-specificity of mRNA expression strongly argue that the ISBT cDNAs identified in these studies encode the Na⁺/bile acid cotransporter described previously in the ileum. The isolated cDNAs encoded proteins of 348 amino acids with an approximate mass of 38 kDa and two (human) or three (hamster) potential N-linked glycosylation sites. By immunoblotting, the rodent ISBT exhibited a molecular weight of approximately 46 kDa that is consistent with the monomer plus the addition of N-linked carbohydrate chains. This mass clearly differs from the 93 and 99 kDa proteins identified previously by affinity labelling using photolabile derivatives of taurocholate[26,27], and the nature of the relationship between ISBT and the photoaffinity-labelled proteins is unclear. Most likely the 90–99 kDa proteins represent a dimer of the 46 kDa Na^+/bile acid cotransporter that is poorly dissociated by SDS-polyacrylamide gel electrophoresis. There is precedence for this phenomenon with other seven transmembrane domain proteins. For example, rhodoposin is known to form dimers and oligomers under the denaturing and reducing conditions used for SDS-polyacrylamide gel electrophoresis[28,29]. With the availability of cDNA and antibody probes for the hamster and human ISBTs it should be possible to begin detailed studies of the structure of the transporter, as well as the molecular mechanism of ileal bile acid transport.

Acknowledgements

This work was supported by the National Institutes of Health (grant DK47987) to P. A. Dawson and an American Heart Association Grant-In-Aid (North Carolina Affiliate; NC92GS15). M. H. Wong is a recipient of a Predoctoral Fellowship from the National Institutes of Health (grant DK08718). P. A. Dawson is an American Gastroenterology Association/Janssen Pharmaceutical Research Scholar.

References

1. Russell DW, Setchell KDR. Bile acid biosynthesis. Biochemistry. 1992;31:4737–49.
2. Hofmann AF. The enterohepatic circulation of bile acids in health and disease. In: Sleisenger MH, Fordtran S, editors. Gastrointestinal disease. Pathophysiology/diagnosis/management. Philadelphia: Saunders; 1993:127–50.
3. Weiner IM, Glasser JE, Lack L. Renal excretion of bile acids: taurocholate, glycocholate, and cholic acids. Am J Physiol. 1964;207:964–70.
4. Rudman D, Kendall FE. Bile acid content of human serum. I. Serum bile acids in patients with hepatic disease. J Clin Invest. 1957;36:530–7.
5. Javitt NB. Diagnostic value of serum bile acids. Clin Gastroenterol. 1977;6:219–26.
6. Dietschy J. Mechanisms for the intestinal absorption of bile acids. J Lipid Res. 1968;9:297–309.
7. Krag E, Phillips SF. Active and passive bile acid absorption in man. J Clin Invest. 1974;53: 1686–4.
8. Schiff ER, Small NC, Dietschy JM. Characterization of the kinetics of the passive and active transport mechanisms for bile acid absorption in the small intestine and colon of the rat. J Clin Invest. 1972;51:1351–62.
9. Lack L. Properties and biological significance of the ileal bile salt transport system. Environ Health Perspect. 1979;33:79–90.
10. Wilson FA. Intestinal transport of bile acids. In: Schultz, Stanley, editors. Handbook of physiology. The gastrointestinal system, Vol. IV. Baltimore: Waverly Press; 1991:389–404.
11. Weinberg SL, Burckhardt G, Wilson FA. Taurocholate transport by rat intestinal basolateral membrane vesicles. Evidence for the presence of an anion exchange transport system. J Clin Invest. 1986;78:44–50.
12. Wilson FA, Treanor LL. Glycodeoxycholate transport in brush border membrane vesicles isolated from rat jejunum and ileum. Biochim Biophys Acta. 1979;554:430–40.
13. Schwenk ME, Hegazy E, Lopez del Pino V. Kinetics of taurocholate uptake by isolated ileal cells of guinea pig. Eur J Biochem. 1983;131:387–91.
14. Barnard JA, Ghishan FK. Taurocholate transport by human ileal brush border membrane vesicles. Gastroenterology. 1987;93:925–33.

15. Kramer W, Nichol S-B, Girbig F, Gutjahr U, Kowalewski S, Fasold H. Characterization and chemical modification of the Na⁺-dependent bile-acid transport system in brush-border membrane vesicles from rabbit ileum. Biochim Biophys Acta. 1992;111:93–102.
16. Wong MH, Oelkers P, Craddock AL, Dawson PA. Expression cloning and characterization of the hamster ileal sodium-dependent bile acid transporter. J Biol Chem. 1994;269:1340–7.
17. Wong MH, Dawson PA. Cloning and chromosomal localization of the ileal sodium-dependent bile acid transporter. J Clin Invest. 1994(Submitted).
18. Hagenbuch B, Stieger B, Foguet M, Lubbert H, Meier PJ. Functional expression cloning and characterization of the hepatocyte Na⁺/bile acid cotransport system. Proc Natl Acad Sci USA. 1991;8:10629–33.
19. Hagenbuch B, Meier PJ. Molecular cloning, chromosomal localization and functional characterization of a human liver Na⁺/bile acid cotransporter. J Clin Invest. 1994;93:1326–31.
20. Kyte J, Doolittle RF. A simple method for displaying the hydrophobic character of a protein. J Mol Biol. 1982;157:105–32.
21. Wright EM, Hager KM, Turk E. Sodium cotransport proteins. Curr Opinion Cell Biol. 1992;4:696–702.
22. Baldwin JM. The probable arrangement of the helices in G protein-coupled receptors. EMBO J. 1993;12:1693–70.
23. Boyer JL, Graf J, Meier PJ. Hepatic transport systems regulating pH_i, cell volume, and bile secretion. Annu Rev Physiol. 1992;54:415–38.
24. Sacchettini JC, Hauft SM, Van Camp SL, Cistola DP, Gordon JI. Developmental and structural studies of an intracellular lipid binding protein expressed in the ileal epithelium. J Biol Chem. 1990;265:19199–207.
25. Gong Y-Z, Everett ET, Schwartz DA, Norris JS, Wilson FA. Molecular cloning, tissue distribution, and expression of a 14-kDa bile acid binding protein from rat ileal cytosol. Proc Natl Acad Sci USA. 1994;91:4741–5.
26. Kramer W, Girbig F, Gutjahr U et al. Intestinal bile acid absorption. J Biol Chem. 1993;268:18035–46.
27. Lin MC, Kramer W, Wilson FA. Identification of cytosolic and microsomal bile acid-binding proteins in rat ileal enterocytes. J Biol Chem. 1990;265:14986–95.
28. De Grip WJ. Purification of bovine rhodoposin over concanavalin A–sepharose. Methods Enzymol. 1982;81:197–207.
29. Fliesler SJ, Basinger SF. Tunicamycin blocks the incorporation of opsin into retinal rod outer segment membranes. Proc Natl Acad Sci USA. 1985;82:1116–20.
30. Shneider BL, Dawson PA, Christie D-M, Hardikar W, Wong MH, Suchy FJ. Cloning and molecular characterization of the ontogeny of a rat ileal sodium-dependent bile acid transporter. J Clin Invest. 1995 (Submitted).
31. von Heijne G, Manoil C. Membrane proteins: from sequence to structure. Protein Eng. 1990;4:109–12.

21
Design and properties of ileal bile acid transport inhibitors

W. KRAMER, G. WESS, K.-H. BARINGHAUS, G. BÖGER,
A. ENHSEN, E. FALK, M. FRIEDRICH, H. GLOMBIK,
A. F. HOFMANN, G. NECKERMANN, C. PITTIUS, H.-L. SCHÄFER
and M. URMANN

INTRODUCTION

Hypercholesterolaemia is a primary risk factor for arteriosclerosis and coronary heart disease, which are major causes of death in Western countries[1]. A major therapeutic goal to prevent arteriosclerosis is the decrease of serum LDL-cholesterol levels. Methods of decreasing serum cholesterol levels include inhibition of cholesterol biosynthesis, as with the HMG-CoA reductase inhibitors, which today represent the standard therapy for the treatment of hypercholesterolaemia[2], or the inhibition of intestinal cholesterol absorption. Interruption of the enterohepatic circulation of bile acids with polymeric bile acid sequestrants is a well-established and safe therapy for elevated serum cholesterol levels[3]. The interruption of bile acid enterohepatic circulation balances the feedback inhibition of hepatic cholesterol-7α-hydroxylase by bile acids recirculating with portal blood. The resulting stimulation of bile acid synthesis leads, via increased hepatic LDL receptor expression, to a dramatic decrease of serum cholesterol levels. The efficacy of interruption of the enterohepatic circulation of bile acids to decrease serum cholesterol levels and slow down the progression of arteriosclerosis was convincingly demonstrated by the POSCH-study[4,5]. The main disadvantages of bile acid sequestrants are the high dosages of 15–30 g/day, causing obstipation, maldigestion and malabsorption syndromes, and compliance problems. A more effective way to interrupt the enterohepatic circulation of bile acids would be the development of highly specific non-absorbable inhibitors for the transport systems responsible for the reabsorption of bile acids in the small intestine – bile acid reabsorption inhibitors (BARIs)

Specific inhibitors of the ileal bile acid transporter would have a variety of putative advantages compared to sequestrants.

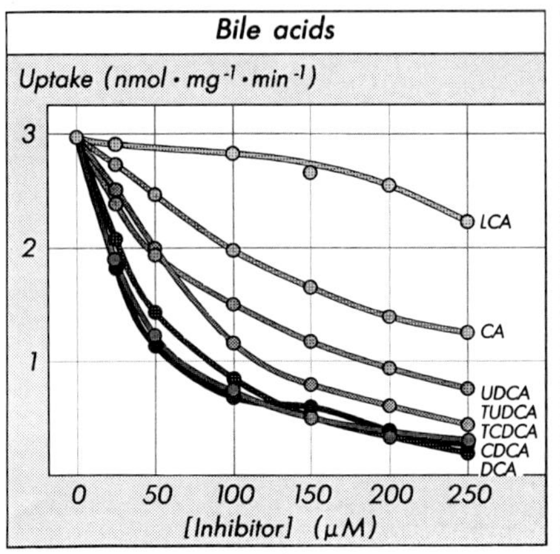
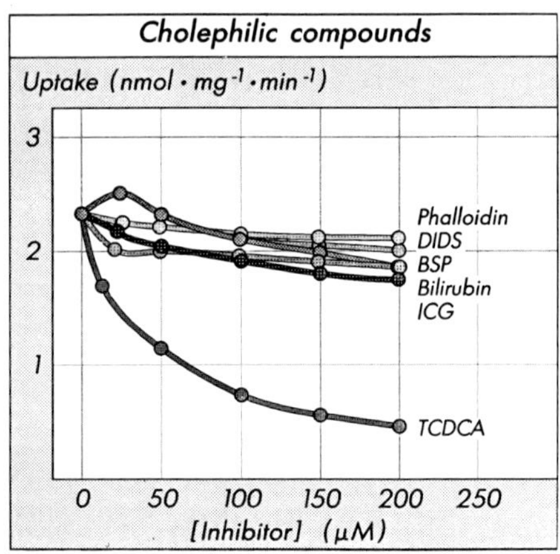

Fig. 1 Effect of natural bile acids (*left panel*) and cholephilic compounds (*right panel*) on Na⁺-dependent [³H]taurocholate uptake by rabbit ileal brush-border membrane vesicles. The uptake of 50 μmol/l [³H]taurocholate in 10 mmol/l Tris/HEPES buffer (pH 7.4)/100 mmol/l NaCl, 100 mmol/l mannitol into rabbit brush-border membrane vesicles (100 μg of protein) was measured for 60 s at 30°C in the absence and presence of the indicated concentration of bile acids and cholephilic compounds: LCA: lithocholate; DCA: deoxycholate; CA: cholate; TCDCA: taurochenodeoxycholate; UDCA: ursodeoxycholate, CDCA: chenodeoxycholate, TUDCA: tauroursodeoxycholate, BSP: bromosulphophthalein, ICG: indocyanine green; DIDS: 4,4′-diisocyanostilbenedisulfonate, PHD: phalloidin

1. A high specific mode of action.
2. No systemic drug load and consequently no systemic toxicity.
3. No malabsorption and maldigestion syndromes.
4. Low dosage and high compliance.

The intestinal uptake of bile acids occurs by a Na⁺-dependent active transport system in the terminal ileum[6–10] and by passive mechanisms in the upper small intestine[10,11]. Protein candidates for these transporters have been identified by expression cloning in the hamster[12] and by photoaffinity labelling techniques in the rat[13–16] and rabbit[9,17]. The ileal Na⁺/bile acid cotransporter is highly specific for bile acids which leads to a concentration-dependent inhibition of [³H]taurocholate uptake into ileal brush-border membrane vesicles. Cholephilic compounds such as BSP, bilirubin, ICG, DIDS or phalloidin, which all inhibit hepatic bile acid transport[18–20], are not recognized by the ileal bile acid transporter and have no effect on ileal bile acid transport (Fig. 1).

For the design of specific transport inhibitors the structure/activity relationships of bile acids for recognition by the ileal Na⁺/bile acid cotransport system[7,13,17] need to be thoroughly considered (Fig. 2):

1. a negatively charged side-chain of the bile acid at carbon C-24,
2. a *cis* configuration of rings A and B of the steroid nucleus,
3. at least one axial hydroxyl group on the steroid nucleus at positions 3, 7 or 12.

However, to date it is not known whether bile acids are transported head-ahead or tail-ahead across the ileal brush-border membrane.

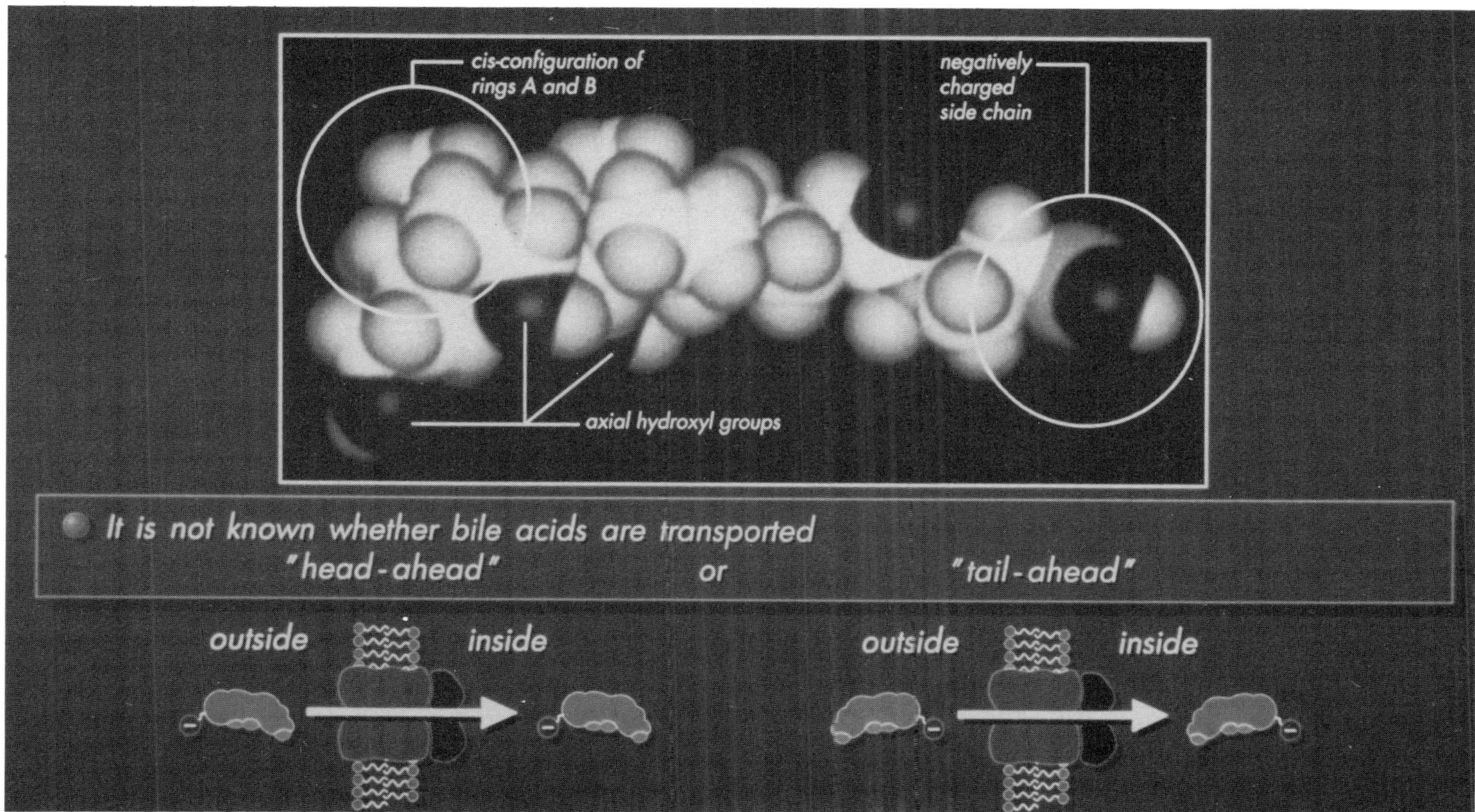

Fig. 2 Structural requirement of a bile acid for recognition by the ileal Na$^+$/bile acid cotransport system

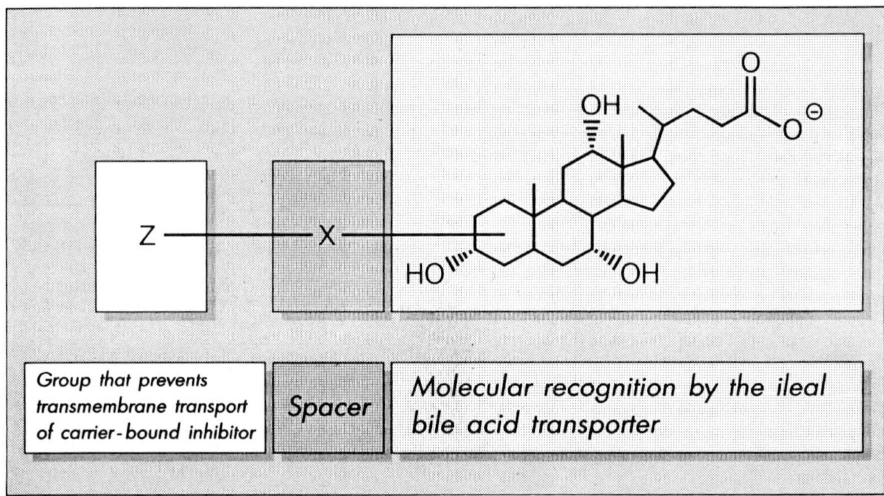

Fig. 3 Concept for the design of specific ileal bile acid transport inhibitors

DESIGN OF BILE ACID TRANSPORT INHIBITORS

According to the hitherto known structure–activity relationships of compounds for recognition by the active ileal bile acid transport system only molecules with bile acid structure interact with the ileal bile acid transporter. Therefore we decided to use modified bile acids as putative inhibitors. The bile acid structure in these molecules should allow a specific and high-affinity binding to the transporter, and the attachment of bulky groups linked via spacers of different length and structure to the bile acid moiety should prevent transmembrane transport of the inhibitor across the ileal brush-border membrane (Fig. 3).

In the rabbit, photoaffinity labelling of ileal brush-border membrane vesicles revealed a specific Na^+-dependent labelling of an integral 93 kDa and a peripheral 14 kDa membrane bile acid binding protein[17]. Target-size analysis with high-energy electrons revealed a functional molecular mass of 451 ± 35 kDa for the rabbit ileal bile acid transporter, suggesting a protein complex composed of four transmembrane 93 kDa and four cytoplasmic peripheral 14 kDa membrane protein subunits[21,22] (Fig. 4). According to this complex structure, with more than one transporter site in the functional ileal Na^+/bile acid cotransporter, it seems possible that the covalent coupling of two bile acid molecules via a spacer should allow simultaneous binding of the bile acid moieties to more than one transporter site. As a result high-affinity binding of such an inhibitor to the ileal bile acid transporter should occur, but the resorption and transmembrane transport of such a dimeric bile acid derivative should be very low, owing to the simultaneous occupation of two bile acid binding sites in the transporter complex. Since the molecular requirements for optimal molecular recognition of such bile acid dimers by the ileal transporter are not known, we have synthesized a large number of bile acid dimers where the individual bile acid moieties are linked together via the steroid rings A, B, C or the side-chain

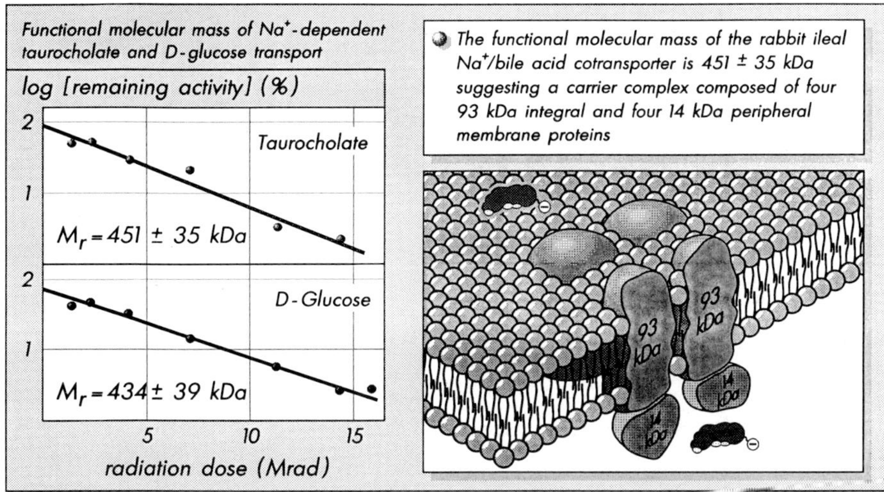

Fig. 4 Target size analysis of the rabbit ileal Na⁺/bile acid cotransporter. Rabbit ileal brush-border membrane vesicles frozen in cryoprotectant buffer were irradiated with high-energy electrons (0–25 MeV) from a linear accelerator at -80 to $-130°C$. Afterwards, the Na⁺-dependent uptake of $50\,\mu mol/l$ [³H]taurocholate and $19\,\mu mol/l$ D [¹⁴C]glucose was measured. Linearization by plotting of the logarithm of residual Na⁺-dependent transport activity against radiation dose revealed a functional molecular mass of $451 \pm 35\,kDa$ for the Na⁺/bile acid cotransport system and $434 \pm 39\,kDa$ for the Na⁺/D-glucose transporter. This functional molecular size for the Na⁺/bile acid cotransporter suggests a protein complex composed of four 93 kDa integral membrane and four 14 kDa peripheral membrane bile acid binding proteins

at carbon C-24 (Fig. 5). A prerequisite for such a synthetic programme was the availability of bile acid building blocks with different protecting groups at the side-chain and the individual hydroxyl groups, as well as of spacers of defined stereochemistry, length and terminal functional groups at position 3, 7 and 12 (Fig. 6). For example, the dimer S 1178 can be viewed in a retrosynthetic approach composed of two building blocks G_1 and G_2 connected via a spacer X (Fig. 7A). G_1 is synthesized from cholic acid by esterification, acetylation and selective deacetylation at position 3, followed by diphenylmethylation. After deprotection of hydroxyls 7 and 12 the monoamide with propyldiamine was formed (Fig. 7B). Bile acid building block G_2 is synthesized starting from cholic acid by selective mesylation in position 3 followed by ether formation with ethylene glycol. After esterification of the bile acid side-chain the hydroxyethyl linker was mesylated, and after reaction with sodium azide the azidoethyl function was catalytically reduced to the aminoethylether linker (Fig. 7C).

INTERACTION OF BILE ACID REABSORPTION INHIBITORS (BARI) WITH ILEAL BILE ACID UPTAKE

At first we investigated whether such dimeric bile acids are still recognized by the ileal bile acid transporter and are competitive inhibitors of ileal bile acid

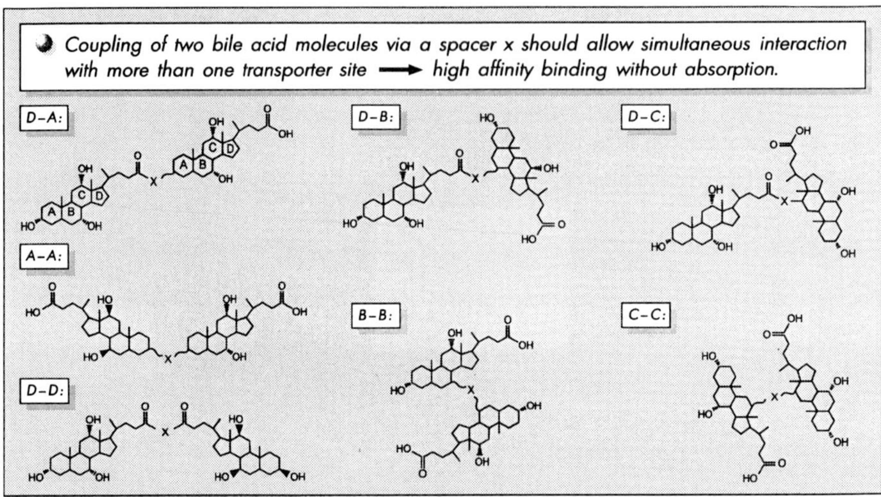

Fig. 5 Structures of possible bile acid dimers

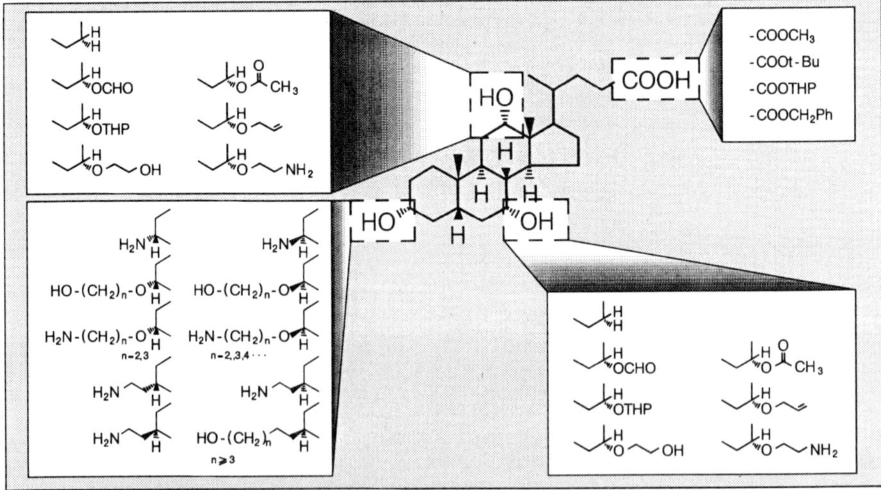

Fig. 6 Diagram for the synthesis of bile acid building blocks with linker structures and protecting groups

Fig. 7 Opposite: Synthesis of the dimeric bile acid reabsorption inhibitor S 1178. **A**: retrosynthetic approach, **B**: synthesis of building block G1, **C**: synthesis of building block G2

transport. The uptake of [³H]taurocholate into rabbit ileal brush-border membrane vesicles was concentration-dependently inhibited by the dimeric bile acid analogues (Fig. 8). The inhibitory potency depended strongly on the

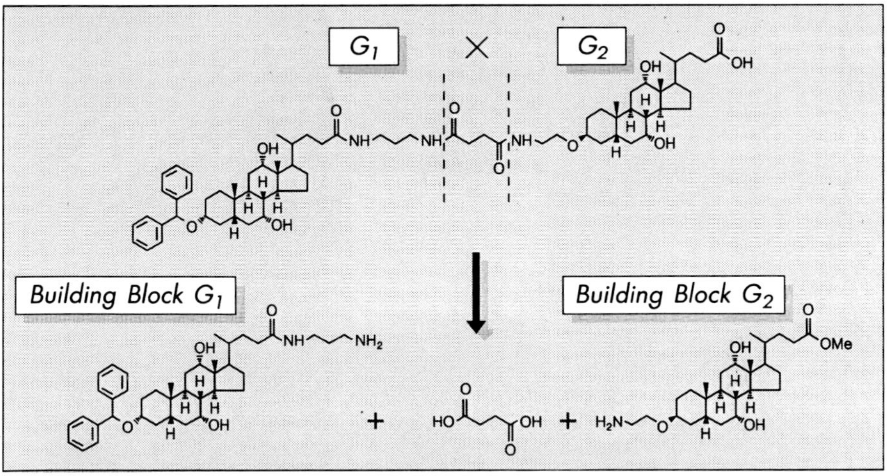
G1
G2
Building Block G1
Building Block G2
NH
NH2
OMe
OH
HO
H2N

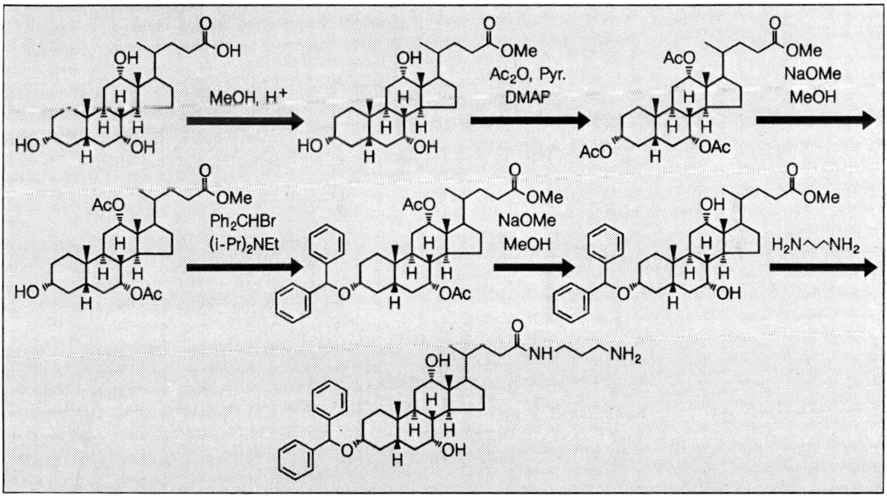
MeOH, H+
Ac2O, Pyr.
DMAP
NaOMe
MeOH
Ph2CHBr
(i-Pr)2NEt
NaOMe
MeOH
H2N NH2

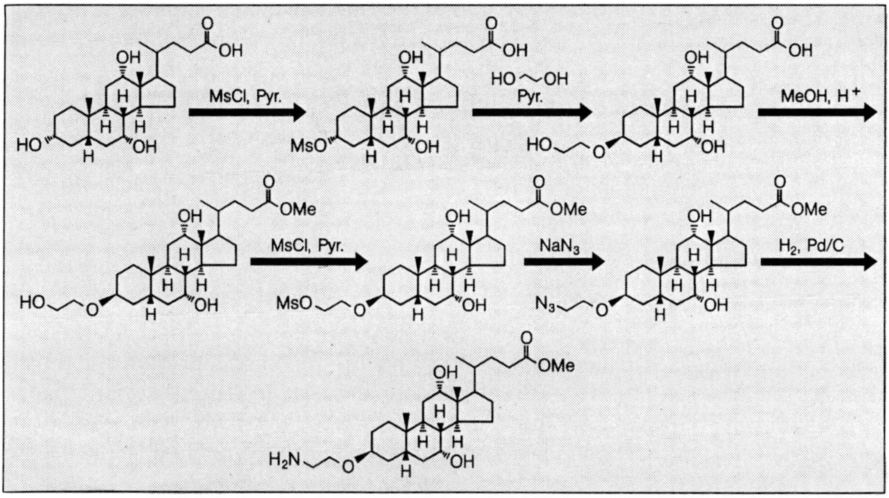
MsCl, Pyr.
HO OH
Pyr.
MeOH, H+
MsCl, Pyr.
NaN3
H2, Pd/C

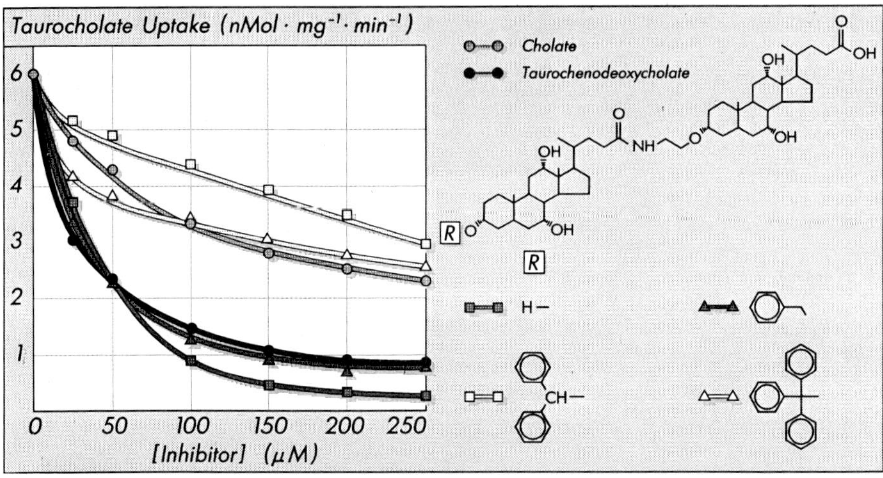

Fig. 8 Inhibition of [³H]taurocholate uptake into rabbit ileal brush-border membrane vesicles by BARI. The uptake of 50 μmol/l [³H]taurocholate dissolved in 10 mmol/l Tris/HEPES buffer (pH 7.4)/100 mmol/l NaCl/100 mmol/l mannitol into rabbit ileal brush-border membrane vesicles (50 μg of protein) was measured for 60 s at 30°C in the absence and presence of the indicated concentrations of BARI

position, number and functionality of the hydroxyl groups in both bile acid moieties. The specific interaction of BARI with the ileal bile acid transporter is also evident from photoaffinity labelling studies. Photoaffinity labelling of the 93 kDa and 14 kDa subunits of the rabbit ileal bile acid transporter by 3 and 7-azi-derivatives of taurocholate was concentration-dependently inhibited by these inhibitors (Fig. 9). The inhibitory potency of dimeric BARI *in vivo* was evaluated in an *in vivo* ileal perfusion model. Since the intestinal absorption of bile acids across the ileocyte brush-border membrane is the rate-limiting step of bile acid enterohepatic circulation, the secretion of [³H]taurocholate into bile after ileum perfusion with [³H]taurocholate in the absence or presence of BARI was measured as an indicator for the inhibition of ileal bile acid absorption. The intestinal absorption of 3 mmol/l taurocholate at a flow rate of 1 ml/min was very efficiently and concentration-dependently inhibited by the dimeric bile acid analogues in the micromolar-range (Fig. 10). Thus, the bile acid transport inhibitors specifically reach their primary target, the Na⁺-dependent ileal bile acid transporter.

As new non-systemic hypolipidaemic drugs the BARI should not be intestinally absorbed. Therefore we investigated the ileal absorption of radiolabelled bile acid transport inhibitors in comparison to [³H]taurocholate in the closed-loop *in vivo* ileum perfusion model. After instillation of 50 μmol/l concentrations either of [³H]taurocholate or the [³H]taurine-conjugated inhibitors, taurocholate was secreted into bile showing the typical secretion profile (Fig. 11). In contrast, almost no radiolabelled BARI could be detected in bile. In the perfusion medium the taurocholate concentration decreased

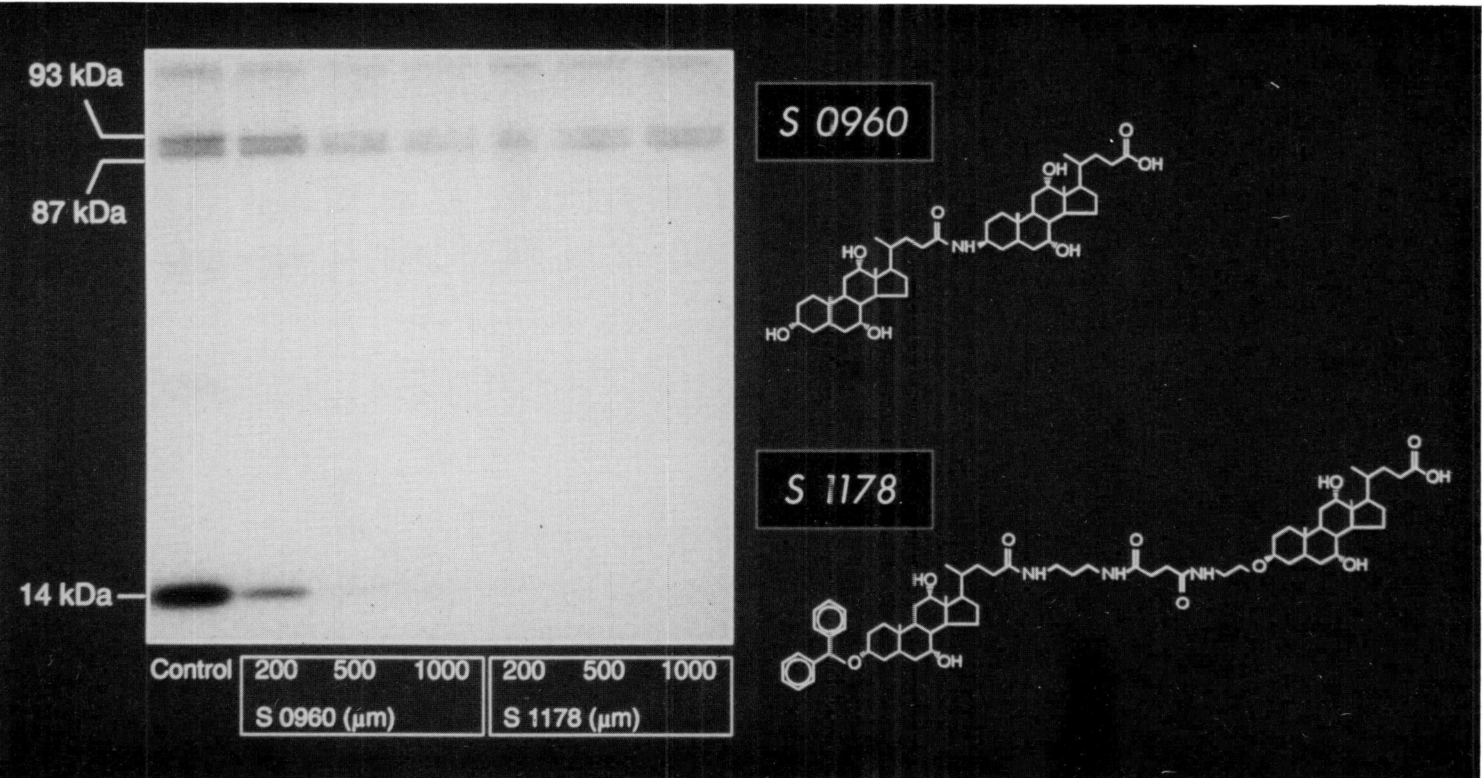

Fig. 9 Effect of BARI on photoaffinity labelling of the bile acid binding proteins in rabbit ileal brush-border membrane vesicles. Rabbit ileal brush-border membrane vesicles (150 µg of protein) were photolabelled for 10 min at 350 nm with 0.2 µmol.l (1 µCi) (7,7-azo-3α,12α-dihydroxy-5β[3β-^{3}H]cholan-24-oyl)-2-aminoethanesulphonic acid in the absence or presence of the indicated concentrations of the bile acid transport inhibitors S 0960 and S 1178. Subsequently, brush-border membrane proteins were separated by SDS-PAGE and radioactivity was detected by fluorography

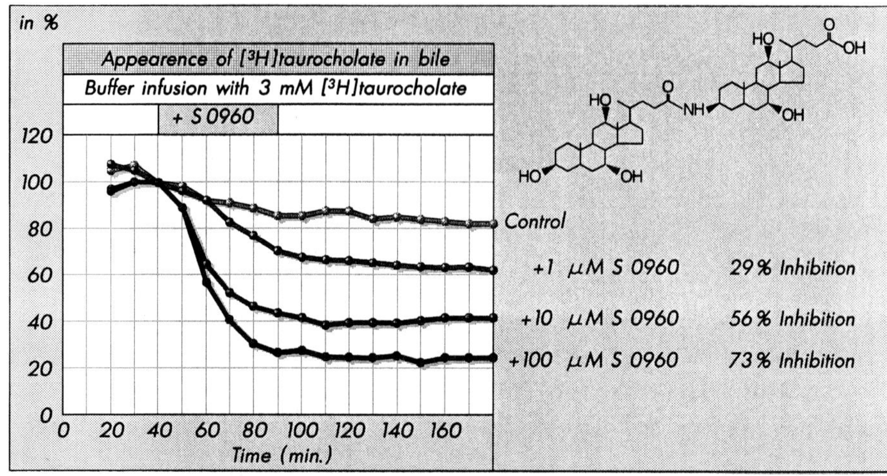

Fig. 10 Effect of BARI on ileal absorption of [³H]taurocholate. A solution of 3 mmol/l [³H]taurocholate was perfused at a flow rate of 1 ml/min through an 8 cm ileal segment of anaesthetized rats and the time-dependent secretion of [³H]taurocholate into bile was measured prior to, during and after addition of the indicated concentrations of compound S 0960

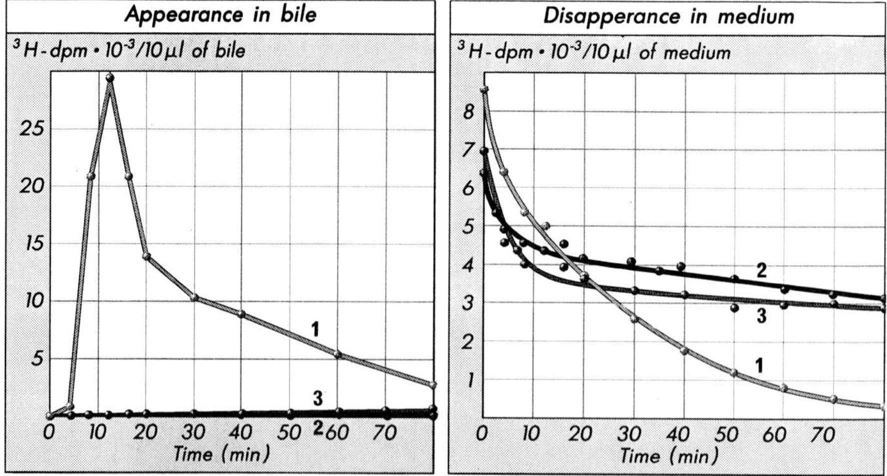

Fig. 11 Intestinal absorption of [³H]taurocholate and [³H]labelled BARI. A 50 μmol/l solution of [³H]taurocholate or the tritium-labelled BARI shown was instilled into an ileal segment of an anaesthetized rat and recirculated at a flow rate of 0.25 ml/min. Bile was collected after the indicated time points and analysed by liquid scintillation counting. The left panel shows the secretion profiles into bile, the right panel the concentration dependence in the perfusion medium. 1: [³H]Taurocholate. 2: Photolabile [³H]taurine conjugate of BARI S 1178 with a 7-diazirinofunction in G1. 3: Photolabile [³H]taurine conjugate of BARI S 1178 with a 7-diazirinofunction in G2

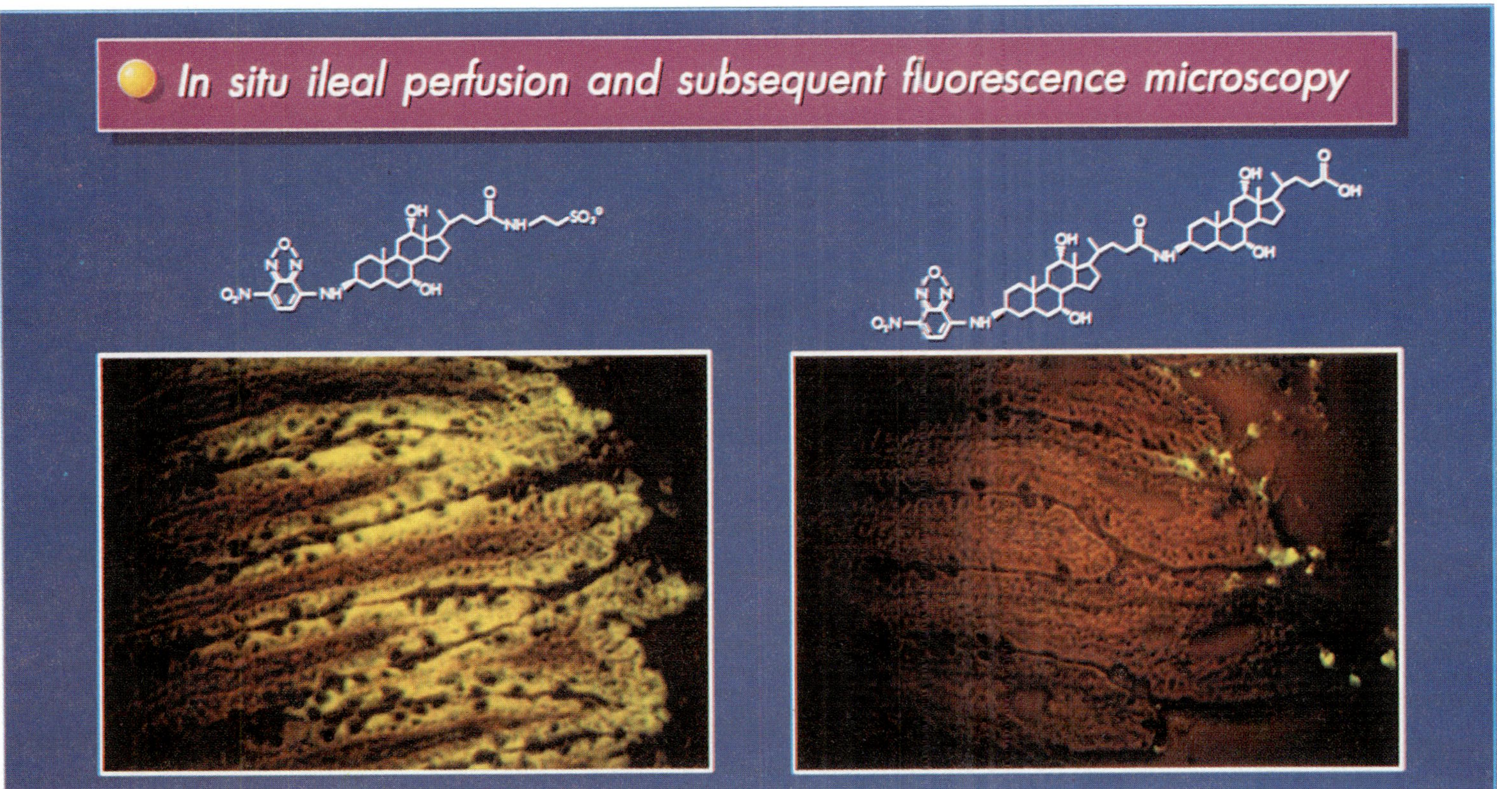

Fig. 12 Fluorescence microscopy of rat ileal segments after perfusion with fluorescent bile acids and fluorescent BARI. Solutions of 3β-NBD-taurocholate ($50\,\mu$mol/l) or the fluorescent BARI 3β-NBD-S 0960 ($100\,\mu$mol/l) were instilled for 15 min into the ileum of anaesthetized rats. The ileum was removed, fixed with Entelan and shock-frozen in liquid nitrogen. Sections of $6\,\mu$m thickness were analysed by combined fluorescence and phase-contrast microscopy

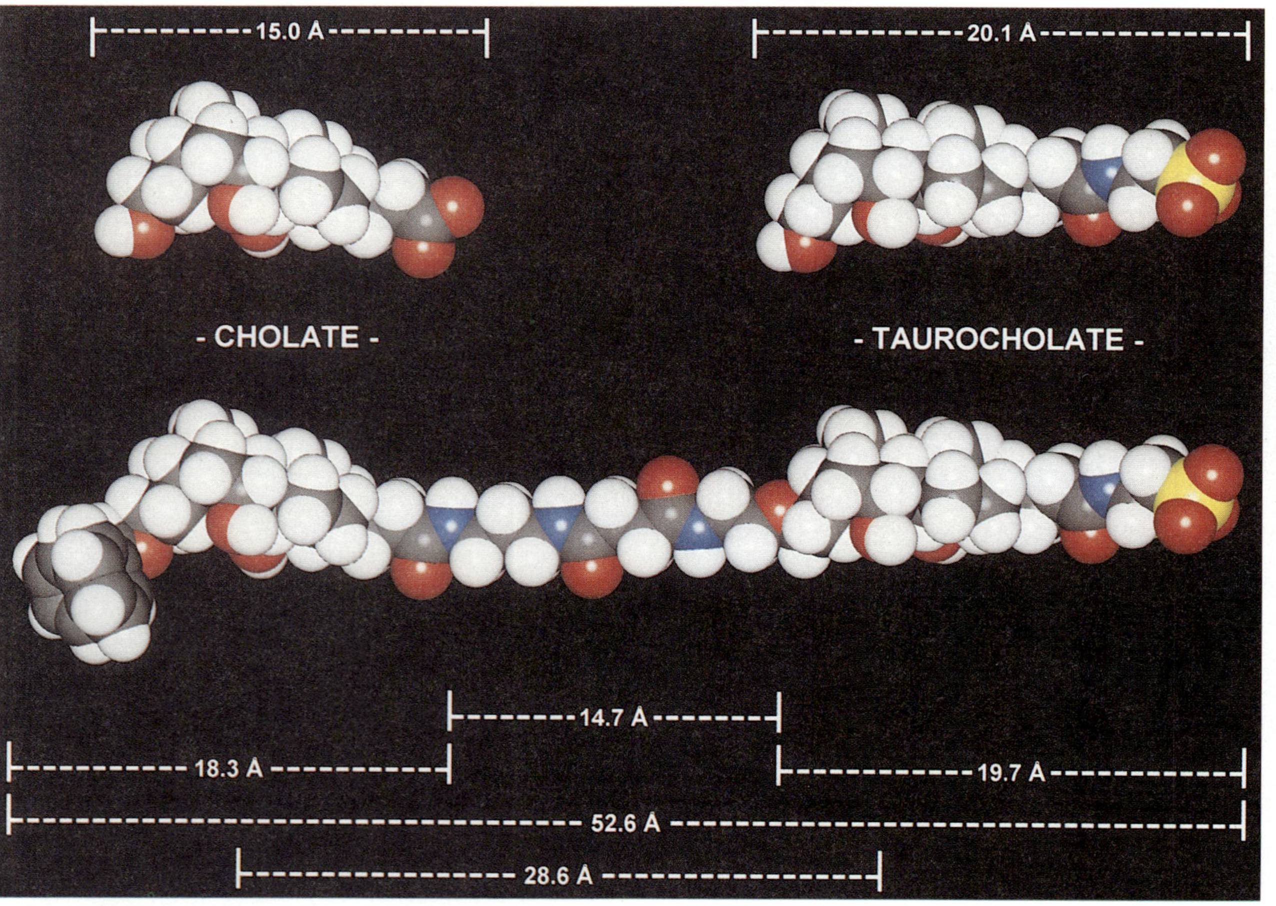

Fig. 13   Space-filling molecular modelling of the dimeric BARI S 1179

exponentially owing to intestinal absorption, whereas the BARI rapidly bound to the ileal brush-border membrane and afterwards no significant further decrease of the luminal concentration of the inhibitors occurred (Fig. 11, right panel). The non-absorbability of BARI was also visualized by fluorescence microscopy. Whereas fluorescent 3β-NBD-analogues of cholate and taurocholate are taken up like natural bile acids by the ileocytes (Fig. 12, left panel), no significant absorption of a NBD-labelled BARI could be detected after *in situ* ileum perfusion and subsequent fluorescence microscopy of frozen ileal sections. The fluorescent regions seen after perfusion with the NBD-labelled BARI (Fig. 12, right panel) are caused by binding of the compound to dead cells.

First hints for a pharmacological action of non-absorbable BARI were obtained by measuring faecal bile acid output. For this the endogenous bile acid pool in hamsters or rats was radiolabelled by oral or i.v. administration of [^{14}C]taurocholate. Subsequently, the inhibitors or cholestyramine were administered either by feeding or by gavage, and faecal bile acid output was determined by measuring daily faecal excretion of radioactively labelled bile acids. Dimeric BARI led to an increase of faecal bile acid output, the equipotent drug amounts being more than one order of magnitude less than with cholestyramine. Since BARI of the structure described above are impermeable to the brush border membrane of the ileocyte it should be possible with these compounds to clarify whether bile acids enter the ileocyte head-ahead or tail-ahead. For this we have chosen bile acid dimers with long spacers with a linear length of more than $50\,\text{Å}$ – a distance greater than the thickness of the lipid bilayer of a biological membrane – and have introduced photolabile diazirino-functions into the left or right bile acid moiety (Fig. 13). Since such compounds strongly inhibited the ileal bile acid transporter without being taken up, and since a 14kDa peripheral membrane protein located at the cytoplasmic site of the brush-border membrane is involved in ileal bile acid uptake[17], we have performed topographic photoaffinity labelling with such impermeable photolabile BARI. Photoaffinity labelling with a set of photolabile BARI demonstrates that the 14kDa protein was labelled to a measurable extent only if the photoreactive diazirino group was located in the left bile acid moiety of the bile acid dimers (Fig. 14). This means that in these bile acid dimers only the 'left' bile acid moiety gets access to the cytoplasmic site of the ileocyte brush-border membrane. From these and other findings it can be hypothesized that bile acids enter the ileocyte head-ahead.

CONCLUSIONS

The experimental data demonstrate that, by covalent coupling of two bile acid molecules via spacers, dimeric bile acid analogues can be obtained which are potent inhibitors of the Na^+-dependent ileal bile acid transport system.

1. These inhibitors (BARI) specifically inhibit active ileal bile acid uptake concentration-dependently, both *in vitro* and *in vivo*.
2. The inhibitory efficacy depends strongly on the length of the spacers, as well as on the number and position of hydroxyl groups in both bile acid moieties.

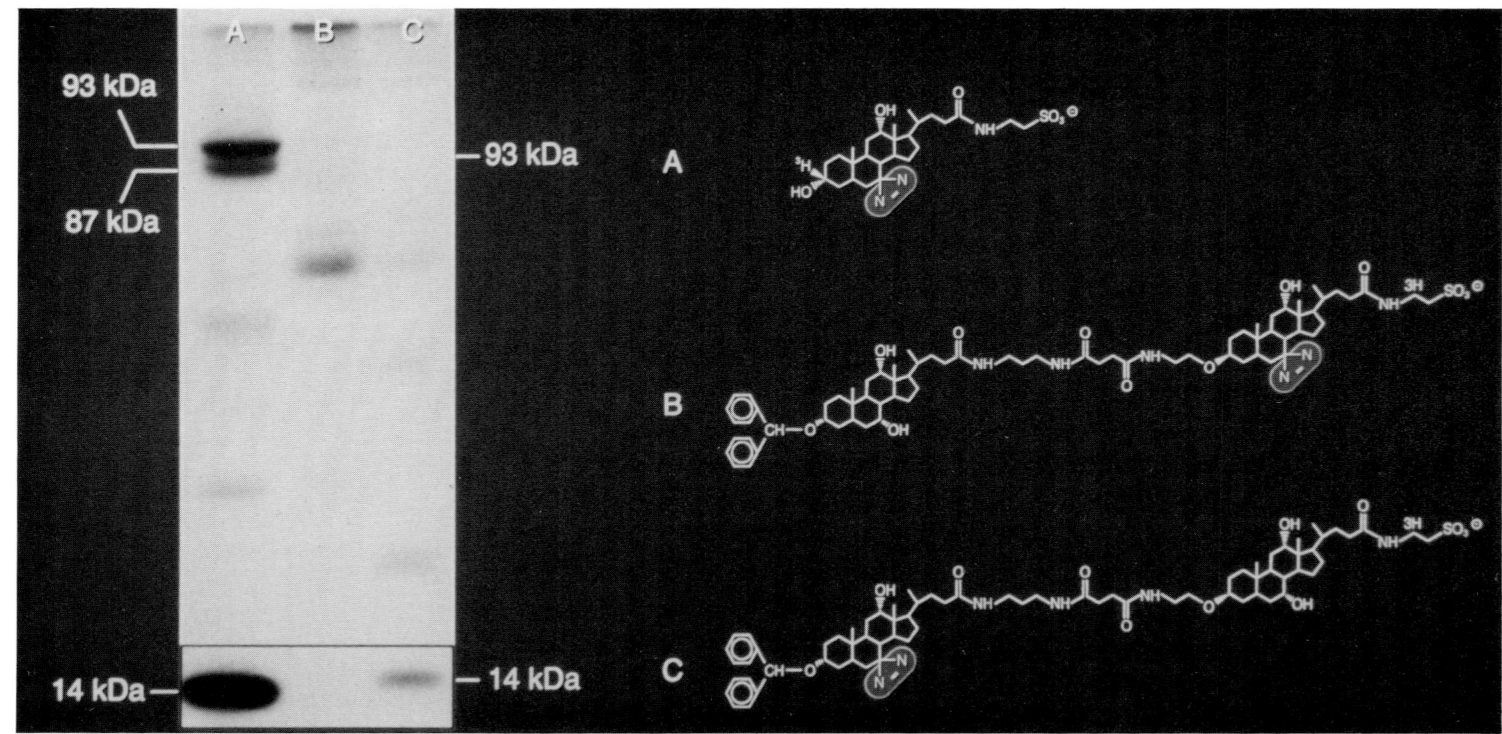

Fig. 14 Topographic photoaffinity labelling of rabbit ileal brush-border membrane vesicles with photolabile impermeable bile acid transport inhibitors. Rabbit ileal brush-border membrane vesicles (150 µg of protein) were incubated for 5 min at 30°C in the dark with 0.2 µmol/l (1 µCi) of the indicated bile acid derivatives. After irradiation at 350 nm for 10 min, membrane proteins were separated by SDS-PAGE on 12% gels and radioactivity was detected by fluorography

218

3. Dimeric BARI are recognized by the ileal Na$^+$/bile acid cotransporter with high affinity, but are not transported across the ileal brush border membrane to a significant extent.

Acknowledgements

For their assistance in synthesis and biological experiments the authors are greatly indebted to: J. Bauer, M. Bauer, K. Benstein, K. Bock, T. Brand, H.-J. Dumke, W. Gerlach, F. Girbig, R.-N. Gottwald, S. Granata, P. Günther, U. Gutjahr, T. Hennig, R. Hofmann, B. Karbe-Thönges, R. Kaulfuß v. d. Heyden, H. Kleine, S. Kowalewski, C. Kremer, A. Labestin, M. Meyer, U. Pfeifer, M. Schmalz, K. Szünder, H.-J. Thönges, R.-M. Victor, R. Watkowiak, B. Worzischek. We thank Mrs Susanne Winkler for excellent secretarial assistance.

References

1. Endo AJ. Compactin (ML-236 B) and related compounds as potential cholesterol-lowing agents that inhibit HMG-CoA reductase. J Med Chem. 1985;28:401–5.
2. Grundy SM. HMG-CoA reductase inhibitors for treatment of hypercholesterolemia. N Engl J Med. 1988;319:24–32.
3. Benson GM, Hickey DMB. Bile acid sequestrants: past and future. Current Drugs: Anti-atherosclerotic Agents. 1991;B43–59.
4. Buchwald H, Varco RL, Matts JP *et al.* and the POSCH Group. Effect of partial ileal bypass surgery on mortality and morbidity from coronary heart disease in patients with hypercholesterolemia. N Engl J Med. 1990;323:946–55.
5. Buchwald H, Matts JP, Fitch LL *et al* and the POSCH Group. Changes in sequential coronary arteriograms and subsequent coronary events: program on surgical control of the hyperlipidemias (POSCH) group. JAMA. 1992;268:1429–33.
6. Wilson FA. Intestinal transport of bile acids. Am J Physiol. 1981;241:683–92.
7. Lack L. Properties and biological significance of the ileal bile salt transport system. Environ Health Perspect. 1979;33:79–90.
8. Burckhardt G, Kramer W, Kurz G, Wilson FA. Inhibition of bile salt transport in brush-border membrane vesicles from rat small intestine by photoaffinity labelling. J Biol Chem. 1983;258:3618–22.
9. Kramer W, Nicol S-B, Girbig F, Gutjahr U, Kowalewski S, Fasold H. Characterization and chemical modification of the Na$^+$-dependent bile acid transport system in brush-border membrane vesicles from rabbit ileum. Biochim Biophys Acta. 1992;1111:93–102.
10. Lewis MC, Root C. *In vivo* transport kinetics and distribution of taurocholate by rat ileum and jejunum. Am J Physiol. 1990;259:G233–8.
11. McClintock C, Shiau Y-F. Jejunum is more important than terminal ileum for taurocholate absorption in rats. Am J Physiol. 1983;244:G507–14.
12. Wong MH, Oelkers P, Craddock AL, Dawson PA. Expression cloning and characterization of the hamster ileal sodium-dependent bile acid transporter. J Biol Chem. 1994;269:1340–7.
13. Kramer W, Burckhardt G, Wilson FA, Kurz G. Identification of components of the bile salt transport system in small intestine by photoaffinity labeling. Hoppe-Seylers Z Physiol Chem. 1982;363:901.
14. Kramer W, Burckhardt G, Wilson FA, Kurz G. Bile salt-binding polypeptides in brush-border membrane vesicles from rat small intestine revealed by photoaffinity labeling. J Biol Chem. 1983;258:3623–7.
15. Lin MC, Weinberg SL, Kramer W, Burckhardt G, Wilson FA. Identification and comparison of bile acid-binding polypeptides in ileal basolateral membrane. J Membr Biol. 1994;106:1–11.
16. Gong Y-Z, Zwarych PP, Lin MC, Wilson FA. Effect of antiserum to a 99 kDa polypeptide on the

uptake of taurocholic acid by rat ileal brush border membrane vesicles. Biochem Biophys Res Commun. 1991;179:204–9.

17. Kramer W, Girbig F, Gutjahr U *et al*. Intestinal bile acid absorption: Na$^+$-dependent bile acid transport activity in rabbit small intestine correlates with the coexpression of an integral 93 kDa and a peripheral 14 kDa bile acid-binding membrane protein along the duodenum–ileum axis. J Biol Chem. 1993;268:18035–46.

18. Wieland T, Nassal M, Kramer W, Fricker G, Bickel U, Kurz G. Identity of hepatic transport systems for bile salts, phalloidin and antamanide. Proc Natl Acad Sci USA. 1984;81:5232–6.

19. Abberger H, Bickel U, Buscher H-P *et al*. Transport of bile acids: lipoprotein, membrane polypeptides and cytosolic proteins as carriers. In: Paumgartner G, Stiehl A, Gerok W, editors. Bile acids and lipids. Lancaster; MTP; 1982:233–46.

20. Frimmer M, Ziegler K. The transport of bile acids in liver cells. Biochim Biophys Acta. 1988;947:75–99.

21. Kramer W, Girbig F, Gutjahr U, Kowalewski S. Radiation inactivation analysis of the Na$^+$/bile acid cotransport system from rabbit ileum. Biochem J. 1994;306:241–6.

22. Kramer W, Girbig F, Gutjahr U *et al*. Subunit composition of the Na$^+$/bile acid cotransport system from rabbit ileum. Hepatology. 1993;18:299A.

Section VI
Physiological actions of bile acids

22
Stimulation of phosphatidylcholine transfer protein activity by submicellar bile salts in model systems: implications for hepatocellular selection and transport of biliary phosphatidylcholines

D. E. COHEN, M. R. LEONARD and M. C. CAREY

INTRODUCTION

Wirtz and Zilversmit made the observation over 25 years ago[1] that rat liver cytosol stimulated phospholipid exchange between membranes. This led to the demonstration that hepatocytes are particularly rich ($\sim 300\,\text{ng/mg}$ of cytosolic protein)[2] in a transfer protein specific for intracellular shuttling of phosphatidylcholines. It is now known that purified phosphatidylcholine transfer protein (PC-TP) catalyses both intermembrane exchange and net transfer of phosphatidylcholines, but not of other phospholipid classes[3], and displays high affinities for species with sn-1 palmitoyl chains[3]. Although postulated to participate in intracellular phosphatidylcholine synthesis[4] and trafficking[3], the physiological function of hepatocellular PC-TP has remained unknown[3]. Biliary phospholipids ($> 95\%$ phosphatidylcholines) promote cholesterol solubilization in bile and dietary fat assimilation from the proximal small intestine, and are highly enriched ($> 80\%$) in sn-1 palmitoyl phosphatidylcholines[5]. We have shown recently that *in vitro* activity of PC-TP is stimulated markedly by submicellar concentrations of common bile salts[6]. A strong positive correlation between PC-TP activity and biliary phosphatidylcholine secretion rates *in vivo* implies that a physiological function of hepatic PC-TP may be the selection and transport of specific biliary phosphatidylcholines intracellularly for biliary secretion.

We modelled the native hepatocyte system by using submicellar bile salt concentrations to stimulate net transfer of phosphatidylcholines via PC-TP from model smooth endoplasmic reticulum (site of synthesis) to model

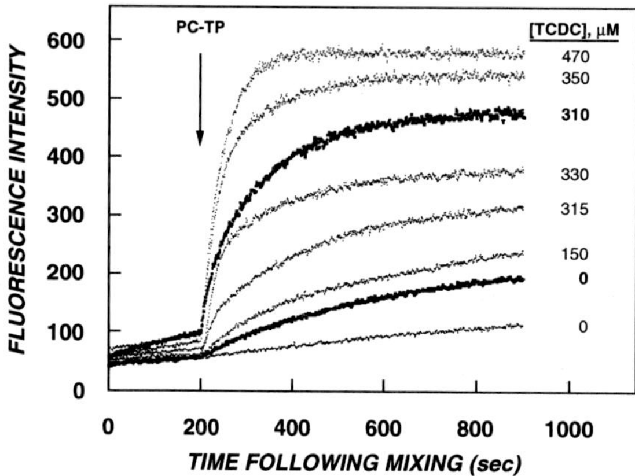

Fig. 1 Bile salt stimulation of phosphatidylcholine transfer protein (PC-TP) activity. Fluorescence intensity is plotted in arbitrary units as functions of time following mixing of donor and acceptor unilamellar vesicles. Submicellar concentrations of added taurochenodeoxycholate (TCDC) are shown by inscribed micromolar values. The arrow indicates 200 s when PC-TP (final concentration 65 nmol/l) was added to the reaction mixture. The lightly stippled lines indicate net phosphatidylcholine *transfer* to acceptor vesicles devoid of phosphatidylcholine (phosphatidylethanolamine : sphingomyelin : phosphatidylserine : phosphatidylinositol : cholesterol, molar ratio 22 : 22 : 8 : 10 : 38). Dark stippling denotes phosphatidylcholine *exchange* with acceptor vesicles containing phosphatidylcholine as the sole phospholipid (egg phosphatidylcholine : cholesterol, molar ratio 62 : 38) (not shown in this experiment are incremental TCDC concentrations). Phosphatidylcholine transfer/exchange rates were measured using the intrinsic fluorescence of sn-1 palmitoyl, sn-2 parinaroyl phosphatidylcholine which was self-quenched in donor vesicles where membrane contents exceeded 50 mol%[9]. Donor unilamellar vesicles were prepared by ethanol injection[9,10] (5.5 nmol in 7.5 μl of sn-1 palmitoyl, sn-2 parinaroyl phosphatidylcholine : egg phosphatidylcholine, molar ratio 75 : 25) into a cuvette designed for fluorescence containing submicellar concentrations of TCDC dissolved in 2.0 ml of 150 mmol/l NaCl, 20 mmol/l Tris-HCl, 5 mmol/l EDTA, 3 mmol/l NaN_3, pH 7.4 at 37°C with continuous stirring. At time zero, 1.0 ml of acceptor small unilamellar vesicles containing 100-fold excess of phospholipid (550 nmol) prepared by sonication in the same buffer[11] was added. Following 200 s equilibration, 5 μg of purified bovine PC-TP[12] in 0.2 ml of buffer (final concentration = 65 nmol/l) was added to the cuvette. Fluorescence intensity was monitored with excitation wavelength of 324 nm and emission wavelength of 420 nm. At the highest bile salt concentrations, phosphatidylcholine transfer rates were determined by fitting fluorescence intensities $F(t)$ to the function $F(t) = A\exp(-kt) + C$ where k is the first-order rate constant, A is the amplitude and C is a constant[13]. (Reprinted from ref. 6 with permission from the American Chemical Society)

canalicular plasma membranes (site of secretion)[7]. We compared net transfer of phosphatidylcholine to phosphatidylcholine-deficient vesicles modelling canalicular plasma membranes[8] with exchange of phosphatidylcholine between phosphatidylcholine-rich vesicles (Fig. 1). Prior to addition of PC-TP, micromolar concentrations of the primary bile salt taurochenodeoxycholate (TCDC)[7] induced very slow phosphatidylcholine movement between vesicles. In agreement with other observations[3], purified bovine PC-TP promoted exchange of phosphatidylcholine (Fig. 1, bold curves) at a rate $(0.2 \times 10^{-2}\,s^{-1})$ that was an order of magnitude faster than net transfer (Fig. 1, light curves). All increments in bile salt concentration activated both PC-TP mediated net transfer and exchange (Fig. 1). However, maximal net transfer

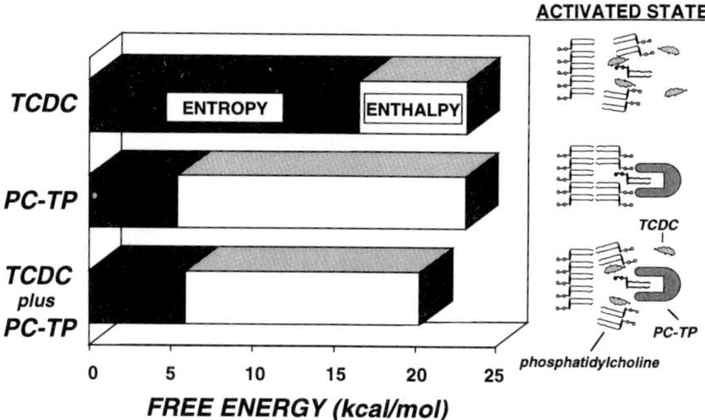

Fig. 2 Energy changes during facilitated phosphatidylcholine transfer. The length of each column represents free energy change for activation ($\Delta G^{\ddagger}$) which equals the sum of the changes in enthalpy ($\Delta H^{\ddagger}$ values represented by open area) and entropy ($T\Delta S^{\ddagger}$ values represented by shaded areas). First-order net transfer rates of phosphatidylcholine were determined in the presence of taurochenodeoxycholate (TCDC, 470 μmol/l) and/or purified bovine PC-TP (65 nmol/l) as functions of temperature (13–41°C) as described in Fig. 1. Activation energies E_a were calculated by fitting transfer rates to the Arrhenius equation: $\ln(\text{transfer rate}) = -E_a/RT + C$, where T is temperature (°K), R is the gas constant, and C is a constant. Free energy change for activation, as well as changes in enthalpy and entropy, were calculated from experimentally determined values of E_a at 31°C[13]. On the right are schematics of likely mechanisms of phosphatidylcholine transfer; see text for details. (Modified from ref. 6 with permission from the American Chemical Society)

($2.2 \times 10^{-2}\,\text{s}^{-1}$) which occurred at 470 μmol/l TCDC was three-fold faster than maximal exchange ($0.8 \times 10^{-2}\,\text{s}^{-1}$), which occurred at 310 μmol/l TCDC. This indicates that although PC-TP alone promotes intermembrane exchange of phosphatidylcholine molecules, the addition of micromolar bile salt concentrations greatly enhances net transfer.

Arrhenius plots were constructed by employing the influence of a range of experimental temperatures (13–41°C) on transfer rates, and thermodynamic constants for activation of phosphatidylcholine transfer were calculated. Figure 2 demonstrates that the change in free energy of activation ($\Delta G^{\ddagger}$) for TCDC-induced phosphatidylcholine transfer without PC-TP was the result of a small increase in enthalpy ($\Delta H^{\ddagger}$) and a large decrease in entropy ($T\Delta S^{\ddagger}$). The high entropic term was most likely due to the low water solubility of desorbed phosphatidylcholine monomers ($\sim 10^{-12}$ mol/l) in water[14]. With added PC-TP but no bile salt (Fig. 2), the relatively large enthalpy change represents the energy required to form a tight complex between phosphatidylcholine and PC-TP[15] and the smaller entropy decrease reflects the higher water-solubility of the complex compared with phosphatidylcholine alone. The combination of TCDC plus PC-TP stimulated phosphatidylcholine transfer (free energy change was ~3 kcal/mol less, Fig. 2) by lowering enthalpy substantially, but not by influencing the entropy term. These results imply that bile salts facilitate PC-TP capture of phosphatidylcholines from donor membranes without exposing the phospholipid molecules to water.

We varied both absolute and relative concentrations of donor and acceptor membranes to determine how bile salts influence PC-TP kinetics (Fig. 3A). It is known that membrane incorporation (2–20 mol%) of negatively charged

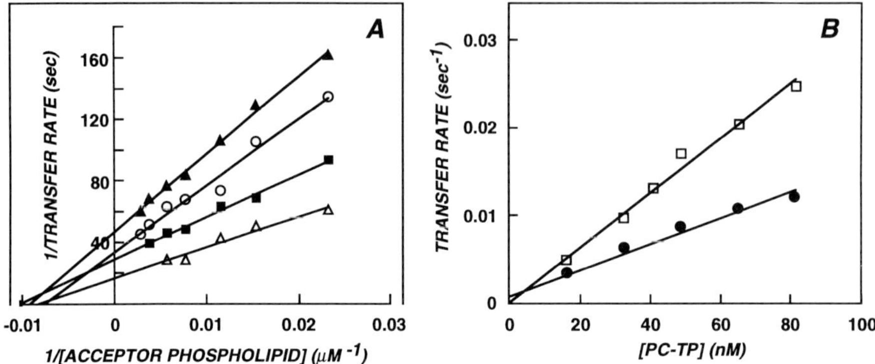

Fig. 3 **A**: Lineweaver-Burk plots demonstrating non-competitive inhibition of PC-TP net transfer of phosphatidylcholines in presence of TCDC (470 μmol/l) which maximally stimulated PC-TP activity. (see Fig. 1). Total phospholipid concentrations of acceptor membranes (composition as in legend to Fig. 1) were 43–347 μmol/l and donor membranes (composition as in legend to Fig. 1) had phosphatidylcholine concentrations of 0.9 μmol/l ($\triangle$), 1.8 μmol/l (■), 2.2 μmol/l (O) and 3.4 μmol/l (▲). **B**: PC transfer rates were linear functions of PC-TP concentrations at constant concentrations of TCDC (470 μmol/l) and acceptor membrane phospholipid (86 μmol/l). Donor PC concentrations were 0.9 μmol/l (□) and 1.8 μmol/l (●). Sizes of symbols in Fig. 3A and 3B represent ± 1 SD. (Reprinted from ref. 6 with permission from the American Chemical Society)

phospholipids (e.g. phosphatidic acid) increases PC-TP binding to vesicles and thereby inhibits phosphatidylcholine transfer[16,17]. We anticipated that anionic bile salts might have similar effects, since they preferentially partition into membranes[18]. The great excess of acceptor membranes (13–281-fold) in the current experiments competed for aqueous bile salt molecules and, at the same time, decreased the mole fraction of bile salts bound to donor membranes. Figure 3A shows that, as a consequence of this competition, added acceptor vesicles increased net transfer by decreasing binding of PC-TP to donor membranes. Conversely, increased donor vesicle concentrations, by binding PC-TP, slowed phosphatidylcholine transfer rates appreciably (Fig. 3A). Figure 3B confirms this hypothesis by demonstrating that phosphatidylcholine transfer rates vary linearly in proportion to total concentration of PC-TP. When we doubled the donor concentration this decreased the slope of the line by a factor of two, reflecting the decrease in the unbound fraction of PC-TP. Therefore, depending upon experimental conditions, phosphatidylcholine vesicles can serve both as donors and as non-competitive inhibitors of PC-TP activity.

The influence of molecular species of bile salts and other detergents on PC-TP transfer activity was studied with eight glycine and taurine conjugated bile salt species representing a wide range of hydrophobicities[19] as well as with other detergents of varied structure and molecular properties. Submicellar concentrations of all detergents stimulated PC-TP transfer activity 40–115-fold. Phosphatidylcholine transfer rates increased linearly in proportion to bile salt hydrophobicity[19], from $0.9 \times 10^{-2}\,\text{s}^{-1}$ with tauroursocholate (most hydrophilic) to $2.5 \times 10^{-2}\,\text{s}^{-1}$ with taurodeoxycholate (most hydrophobic).

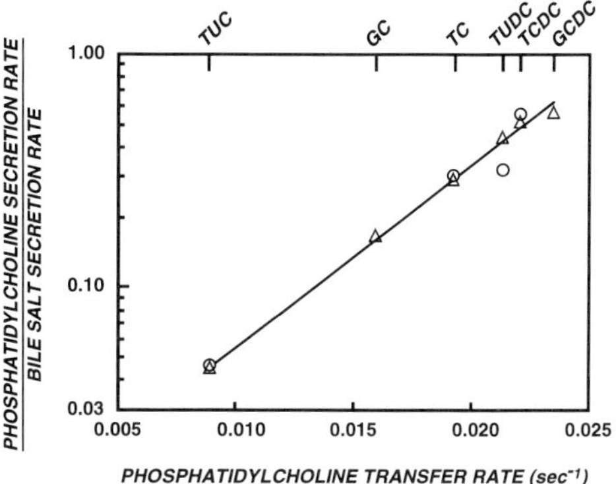

Fig. 4 Positive correlation (fitted by linear least-squares analysis) between PC-TP net transfer rates of phosphatidylcholine *in vitro* as stimulated by individual bile salt molecular species (top abscissa) and *in vivo* biliary phosphatidylcholine secretion rates in bile fistula hamsters[22] ($\triangle$) and prairie dogs[23] (o) normalized for bile salt secretion rate (kg⁻¹ body weight). Maximum phosphatidylcholine transfer rates were determined as described in legend to Fig. 1. Bile salts were taurine (T) and/or glycine (G) conjugates of chenodeoxycholate (CDC), cholate (C), ursodeoxycholate (UDC) and ursocholate (UC). Biliary phosphatidylcholine secretion rates in bile fistula hamsters[22] and prairie dogs[23] were measured following interruption of the enterohepatic circulation, drainage of the endogenous bile salt pool and stimulation of biliary phosphatidylcholine secretion by either intraduodenal (hamster) or intravenous (prairie dog) infusions of pure bile salts. (Modified from ref. 6 with permission from the American Chemical Society)

Submicellar concentrations of taurofusidate (an anionic non-bile salt steroid detergent[20]), sodium dodecyl sulphate (an anionic straight-chain detergent) and octyl glucoside (a non-ionic straight-chain detergent) each stimulated PC-TP activity under the same experimental conditions. However, their maximum effects on PC-TP activities $(0.9 - 1.2 \times 10^{-2}\,\mathrm{s}^{-1})$ were appreciably lower than observed with the common bile salts $(1.6 - 2.5 \times 10^{-2}\,\mathrm{s}^{-1})$. These observations suggest that substituted cholanoic acid salts of humans[21] are especially well designed to optimize hepatic PC-TP transfer activity.

Under physiological conditions, bile salt hydrophobicity is known to have a major influence on biliary phosphatidylcholine secretion rates[22,23]. To test the relevance of the current *in vitro* work to physiological function, Fig. 4 displays a tightly correlated plot of PC-TP transfer rates *in vitro* (this work) versus bile salt-stimulated phosphatidylcholine secretion rates in bile fistula hamsters[22] and prairie dogs[23]. This highly significant relationship supports a physiological role of PC-TP activity in bile formation, and appropriate confirmatory experiments should now be done. Because no precursor phosphatidylcholine pool can be defined physically within hepatocytes[24], and because the molecular species of biliary phosphatidylcholines are conserved among animal species, our results suggest that bile salt regulation of hepatic PC-TP activity could provide a selection and transport mechanism for delivery of the least hydrophobic membrane phosphatidylcholines to the canalicular plasma membrane. Clearly, cellular, molecular biological and physical – chemical experiments of the future will be required to elucidate the putative roles of PC-TP in vertebrate bile formation.

Acknowledgements

Support is acknowledged from the National Institutes of Health (Grant Nos. DK 36588, AM34854, and GM07258) (M.C.C.), the Medical Foundation of Boston and the American Liver Foundation (D.E.C.).

References

1. Wirtz KWA, Zilversmit DB. Exchange of phospholipids between liver mitochondria and microsomes *in vitro*. J Biol Chem. 1968;243:3596–602.
2. Teerlink T, van der Krift TP, Post M, Wirtz KWA. Tissue distribution and subcellular localization of phosphatidylcholine transfer protein in rats as determined by radio-immunoassay. Biochim Biophys Acta. 1982;713:61–7.
3. Wirtz KWA. Phospholipid transfer proteins. Annu Rev Biochem. 1991;60:73–99.
4. Khan ZU, Helmkamp GM. Stimulation of cholinephosphotransferase activity by phosphatidylcholine transfer protein. J Biol Chem. 1990;265:700–5.
5. Hay DW, Carey MC. Chemical species of lipids in bile. Hepatology. 1990;12:6S–16S.
6. Cohen DE, Leonard MR, Carey MC. *In vitro* evidence that phospholipid secretion into bile may be coordinated intracellularly by the combined actions of bile salts and the specific phosphatidylcholine transfer protein of liver. Biochemistry. 1994;33:9975–80.
7. Carey MC, LaMont JT. Cholesterol gallstone formation. 1. Physical-chemistry of bile and biliary lipid secretion. Prog Liver Dis. 1992;10:136–63.
8. Evans WH, Kremmer T, Culvenor JG. Role of membranes in bile formation. Comparison of the composition of bile and a liver bile-canalicular plasma-membrane fraction. Biochem J. 1976;154:589–95.
9. Somerharju P, Brockerhoff H, Wirtz KWA. A new fluorimetric method to measure protein-catalyzed phospholipid transfer using 1-acyl-2-parinaroylphosphatidylcholine. Biochim Biophys Acta. 1981;649:521–8.
10. Batzri S, Korn ED. Single bilayer liposomes prepared without sonication. Biochim Biophys Acta. 1973;298:1015–19.
11. DiCorleto PE, Zilversmit DB. Protein-catalyzed exchange of phosphatidylcholine between sonicated liposomes and multilamellar vesicles. Biochemistry. 1977;16:2145–50.
12. Westerman J, Kamp HH, Wirtz KWA. Phosphatidylcholine transfer protein from bovine liver. Methods Enzymol. 1983;98:581–6.
13. Zucker SD, Storch J, Zeidel ML, Gollan JL. Mechanism of the spontaneous transfer of unconjugated bilirubin between small unilamellar phosphatidylcholine vesicles. Biochemistry. 1992;31:3184–92.
14. Nichols JW. Low concentrations of bile salts increase spontaneous phospholipid transfer between vesicles. Biochemistry. 1986;25:4596–601.
15. Devaux PF, Moonen P, Bienvenue A, Wirtz KWA. Lipid – protein interaction in the phosphatidylcholine exchange protein. Proc Natl Acad Sci USA. 1977;74:1807–10.
16. Berkhout TA, van den Bergh C, Mos H, de Kruijff B, Wirtz KWA. Regulation of the activity of phosphatidylcholine transfer protein by vesicle phosphatidic acid and membrane curvature: a fluorescence study using 2-parinaroylphosphatidylcholine. Biochemistry. 1984;23:6894–900.
17. van den Besselaar AMHP, Helmkamp GM, Wirtz KWA. Kinetic model of the protein-mediated phosphatidylcholine exchange between single bilayer liposomes. Biochemistry. 1975;14:1852–8.
18. Cohen DE, Angelico M, Carey MC. Structural alterations in lecithin – cholesterol vesicles following interactions with monomeric and micellar bile salts: physical – chemical basis for subselection of biliary lecithin species and aggregative states of biliary lipids during bile formation. J Lipid Res. 1990;31:55–70.

19. Heuman DM. Quantitative estimation of the hydrophilic–hydrophobic balance of mixed bile salt solutions. J Lipid Res. 1989;30:719–30.
20. Carey MC, Small DM. Solution properties of taurine and glycine conjugates of fusidic acid and its derivatives. Biochim Biophys Acta. 1973;306:51–7.
21. Carey MC. Physical–chemical properties of bile acids and their salts. In: Danielsson H, Sjövall J, editors. New comprehensive biochemistry. Amsterdam: Elsevier, 1985:345–403.
22. Gurantz D, Hofmann AF. Influence of bile acid structure on bile flow and biliary lipid secretion in the hamster. Am J Physiol. 1984;247:G736–48.
23. Cohen DE, Leighton LS, Carey MC. Bile salt hydrophobicity controls biliary vesicle secretion rates and transformations in native bile. Am J Physiol. 1992;263:G386–95.
24. Curstedt T, Sjövall J. Biosynthetic pathways and turnover of individual biliary phosphatidylcholines during metabolism of [1,1-^{2}H$_2$]ethanol in the rat. Biochim Biophys Acta. 1974;369:173–95.

23
Mechanism of biliary lipid secretion

H. J. VERKADE, R. HAVINGA, F. KUIPERS and R. J. VONK

INTRODUCTION

It has been known for almost four decades that bile acids stimulate the secretion into bile of phospholipids and cholesterol[1,2]. Since the original observation by Kay and Entenman[2] that taurocholic acid induces the secretion of lecithin in the isolated perfused rat liver, stimulation of biliary lipid secretion has been demonstrated for a variety of bile acids in different animal species[1,3–6]. Biliary lipid secretion serves an important physiological role in the homeostasis of cholesterol. Partial malabsorption of bile-derived cholesterol from the intestine constitutes the major excretory pathway from the body for this sterol (see ref. 85 for recent review). In addition, biliary phospholipids play a role in the intestinal absorption of dietary lipids[7–9]. Finally, a defective secretory process for biliary lipids has been implied as playing a role in the aetiology of certain diseases, such as hypercholesterolaemia and gallstone disease[10–12].

Despite significant progress in our understanding of the mechanism of (patho)physiological biliary lipid secretion, a fundamental issue that has so far remained basically unclear is at which hepatocytic level bile acids actually induce the secretion of biliary lipids into the bile. In other words, where is the process quantitatively regulated? In essence two major hypotheses have been put forward in this respect, namely the 'intracellular' and 'intracanalicular' hypotheses (Figs 1 and 2, respectively), which in simple terms, refer to the bile acid action as a matter of 'pushing' and of 'pulling' respectively. These two hypotheses will be discussed below.

THE INTRACELLULAR HYPOTHESIS

The intracellular hypothesis has several variants, but all of them imply that bile acids, en route from their site of uptake at the basolateral membrane of the hepatocyte to their site of secretion at the canalicular membrane, somehow and somewhere exert an intracellular signal. This signal or trigger would lead to bile-directed transport of 'biliary' lipids to the canalicular membrane, and to subsequent secretion of the lipids into the canaliculus[13–16]. Originally it was

230

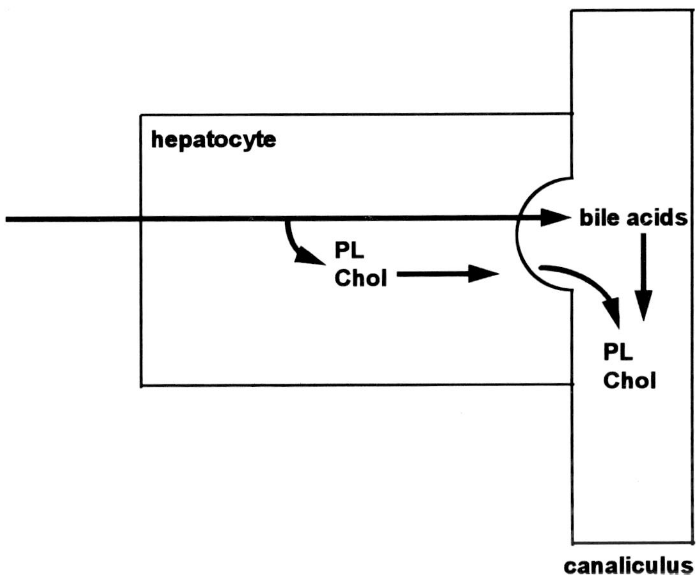

Fig. 1 The intracellular hypothesis of bile acid-induced biliary lipid secretion. Bile acids, en route from their site of uptake at the basolateral membrane of the hepatocyte towards their site of secretion into the bile at the bile canalicular membrane, exert somehow, at some intracellular level, a signal which leads to bile-directed transport of biliary lipids and their subsequent secretion into the bile canaliculus

proposed that intracellular bile acid–phospholipid–cholesterol mixed micelles were formed and targeted to the canaliculus[17,18]. Carey and Mazer[13] speculated about the existence of a functional compartment in the 'smooth' endoplasmic reticulum from which phospholipid and cholesterol molecules would be released by the transcellular flux of bile acids. The intracellular hypothesis was further popularized by the studies of Barnwell *et al.*[20,21] and Gregory *et al.*[16]. These scientists observed that antimicrotubule drugs, such as colchicine, inhibited the biliary secretion of lipids but not that of bile acids, if the latter were administered in a relatively low dose. Other groups reported inhibitory effects of colchicine not only on secretion of lipids but also on the secretion of cholyltaurine, when the bile acid was administered in relatively high doses[14,22,23]. These data were interpreted to suggest that intracellular bile acids induced microtubule-dependent vesicular transport of biliary lipids. However, recent studies by Katagiri and colleagues[24,25] demonstrate that the effects of colchicine on bile acid-induced lipid secretion do not allow a general conclusion on intracellular transport of the bile-destined lipids in the form of vesicles, but may relate to a different process, relatively specific for cholyltaurine. In these studies the induction of biliary lipid secretion by β-muricholate, β-muricholyltaurine or ursodeoxycholyltaurine was not affected in colchicine-treated rat liver, when compared to controls. Furthermore, the colchicine-induced inhibition of biliary lipid secretion after administration of cholyltaurine could be prevented by a simultaneous injection of either of these three bile acids[24,25]. In addition, interpretation of studies employing colchicine should take into account the multitude of its actions[23,26–28],

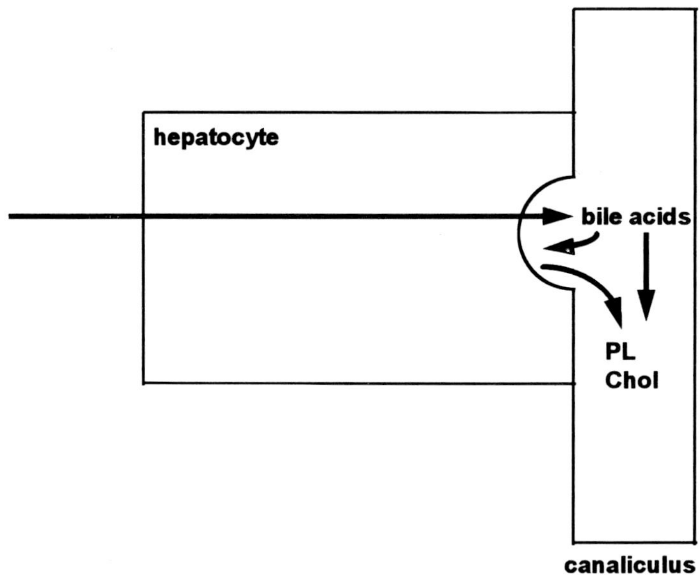

Fig. 2   The intracanalicular hypothesis of bile acid-induced biliary lipid secretion. Bile acids are transported through the hepatocyte and secreted into the bile canaliculus, after which the now *intracanalicular* bile acids interact with the luminal side of the bile canalicular membrane, leading to the segregation from the membrane into the canaliculus of phospholipids and cholesterol

implying that observed effects are not necessarily related to interference with microtubule-dependent transport[19].

Studies which do not support the intracellular hypothesis include those of Reynier *et al.*[19] in the isolated perfused rat liver, which indicate that the Na^+ ionophore monensin inhibits the vesicular transport of horseradish peroxidase, without affecting the biliary output of bile acids or lipids. Finally, preliminary data from Berr *et al.*[29] indicate that inhibition of vesicular transport between endoplasmic reticulum and Golgi complex by brefeldin A does not affect biliary phospholipid secretion. In conclusion, the intracellular hypothesis had been based predominantly on circumstantial evidence, and several recent reports in the literature are clearly not supportive.

THE INTRACANALICULAR HYPOTHESIS

The intracanalicular hypothesis goes back to 1970, when Small hypothesized that the biliary lipids actually are solubilized (canalicular) membrane constituents[30], implying initial secretion into the canaliculus of bile acids alone, followed by induction of lipid secretion by their (solubilizing) activity towards the bile canalicular membrane. Support for this hypothesis has been put forward by Wheeler and King's classical studies in dogs[67], on the relationship between bile acid and lecithin–cholesterol secretion, and by Hardison and Apter[31], who studied this process in bile-fistula rats. Yousef and Fisher[32] incubated bile canalicular membranes, isolated from rat liver, with different concentrations of bile acids. In agreement with the intracanalicular hypothesis, a relatively specific solubilization of cholesterol and 'bile-type' phospholipids was observed[32]. Similarly, Graham and Northfield[33] demonstrated lipid solubilization from hamster bile canalicular membranes by bile acids *in vitro* in an analogous manner as found *in vivo*, depending on bile acid concentration and species. Using the technique of retrograde intrabiliary injection, Coleman *et al.*[34] reported that the biliary secretion of bile-type lipid could be induced by cholyltaurine, but not by the aspecific detergent CHAPS. These latter data, however, are difficult to interpret, as the technique used may be destructive at the level of the bile ducts, ductuli and canaliculi. Cohen *et al.*[35] recently reported on *in vitro* studies on model membranes, which indicate that bile acids selectively solubilize those phosphatidylcholine species which are found in bile *in vivo*.

Since 1983 it has become clear that biliary lipids are not (only) present in the form of mixed micelles, but (also) in the form of phospholipid–cholesterol vesicles[36–45]. Subsequent studies indicated that these lipid vesicles are present not only in supersaturated bile, but also in unsaturated rat bile, either transiently at the early stages of bile formation or during a prolonged period after production[45–48]. As early as 1978, Billington and Coleman reported *in vitro* studies which indicated that bile acids are able to induce the pinching-off of vesicles from erythrocytes[49]. These vesicles were released at lower bile acid concentrations than those inducing lysis of the erythrocytes. No specificity in phospholipid composition could be demonstrated in the vesicles compared to the original erythrocyte membrane. Based on this lack of specificity, the authors concluded (in 1978, before the 'vesicular' era) that the solubilization of membrane outer leaflet components into mixed micelles was probably more important for biliary output of phospholipid than a microvesicular mechanism[49]. Their conclusion has been supported by a number of *in vitro* studies, showing a relative efficacy of *micellar* bile acids to extract lipids from isolated liver plasma, erythrocyte, or model membranes[32,50–54]. However, it should be realized that the intracanalicular hypothesis should not necessarily be regarded as implying *micellar* solubilization of bile canalicular membrane lipids[54,55], but rather as bile acid-induced micellization *and/or* vesiculization[56].

Until recently no conclusive evidence in favour of either the intracellular or the intracanalicular hypothesis has been provided. Yet recent data from our laboratory strongly indicate that the intracanalicular hypothesis describes the actual physiological progress. In our opinion these indications can be appreciated at best using a step-by-step discussion of the various factors which, up till now, have been demonstrated to influence the amount of phospholipids and cholesterol secreted into the bile.

FACTORS DEMONSTRATED TO INFLUENCE THE AMOUNT OF LIPIDS SECRETED INTO THE BILE

Biliary bile acid concentration

The first determinant of the amount of lipids secreted into bile relates to the amount of secreted biliary bile acids[1,2]. A curvilinear relationship between the

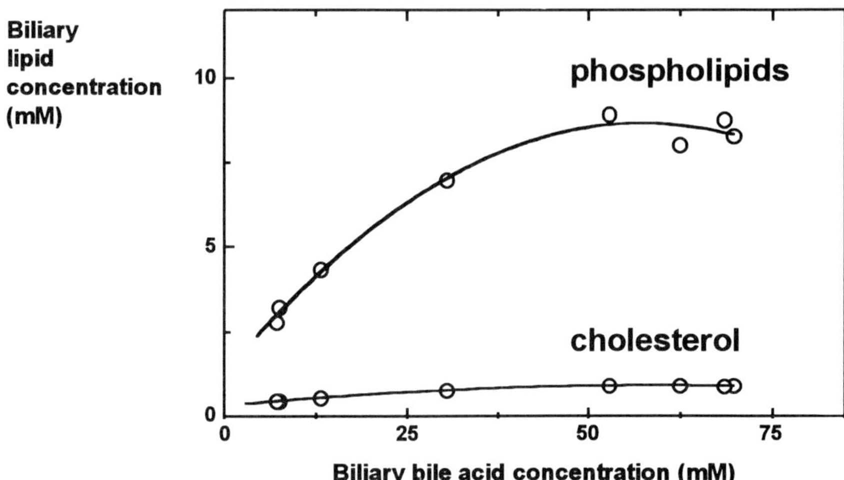

Fig. 3 The relationship between biliary bile acid concentration and biliary phospholipid or cholesterol concentration. A curvilinear relationship exists between biliary bile acid and biliary lipid concentration in a number of different species (see text). Above a certain bile acid concentration, phospholipid concentration tends to decrease, in parallel to the development of cholestasis[21,57,58]. Present data were derived from the acute interruption of the enterohepatic circulation of unanaesthetized Wistar rats (details described in ref. 106)

biliary secretion rates of bile acids on the one hand and phospholipids and/or cholesterol on the other hand have been demonstrated by various researchers in a number of animal species[3,4–6,57,58]. Secretory rates are the product of bile flow and bile concentration and, as the variable 'bile flow' is equally included in the secretory rates of bile acids and lipids, the relationship between bile acid and lipid secretion can be narrowed to a relationship between their biliary concentrations (Fig. 3). At present no definitive explanation for the curvilinearity of the relationship is available, but circumstantial indications strongly favour a rate-limiting role of phospholipid supply towards the (outer leaflet of the) bile canalicular membrane at consistently high intracanalicular bile acid concentrations[57–60] (see also chapter 24 in this volume).

Composition of biliary bile acids

The second factor influencing the amount of biliary lipids is the composition of the bile acids present in the canaliculus. As a general rule it can be stated that the capacity of a certain bile acid to induce biliary lipid secretion is a function of its hydrophobicity, as reflected for example by its critical micellar concentration (Fig. 4)[5,61–66]. Obviously, this positive relationship could be interpreted as supportive for the intracanalicular hypothesis, i.e. by micellization of lipids at the bile canalicular membrane, but this cannot be regarded as conclusive evidence. It should be kept in mind that the process of biliary lipid secretion may be more complex than merely a micellar solubilization phenomenon (see discussion above). As a consequence, an interpretation of the observed relationship between

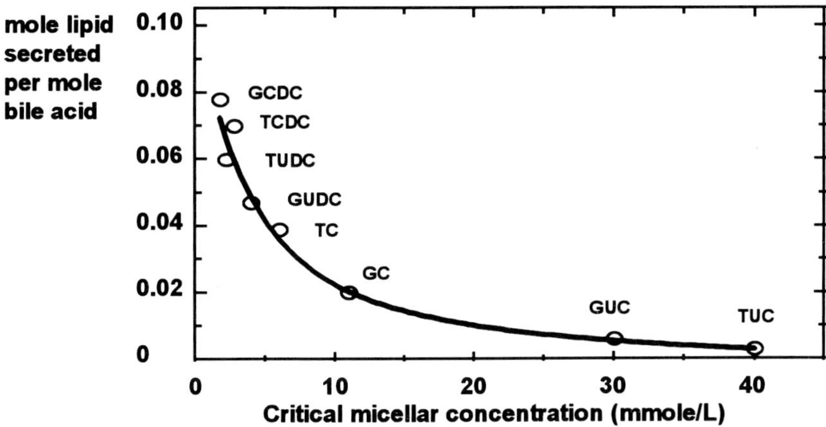

Fig. 4 The relationship between the critical micellar concentration of a bile acid and its potency to induce biliary lipid secretion. An inverse relationship exists between the hydrophobicity of a certain bile acid, as quantified by its critical micellar concentration, and its potency to induce biliary secretion of phospholipids and cholesterol (not shown). Presented data are derived from studies in hamsters by Gurantz and Hofmann[62]. Abbreviations: GCDC, glycochenodeoxycholic acid; TCDC, taurochenodeoxycholic acid; TUDC, tauroursodeoxycholic acid; GUDC, glycoursodeoxycholic acid; TC, taurocholic acid; GC, glycocholic acid; GUC, glycoursocholic acid; TUC, tauroursocholic acid

bile hydrophobicity and amount of biliary lipid secretion according to the intracanalicular hypothesis may not necessarily imply a direct effect of bile acid molecules on phospholipid/cholesterol molecules. An indirect relationship between the two, mediated by interaction with other bile or canalicular membrane constituents, cannot be excluded.

Biliary concentration of hydrophilic organic anions

The third factor influencing the amount of phospholipids and cholesterol secreted into the bile is the biliary concentration of hydrophilic, non-bile acid organic anions. An effect of organic anions on biliary lipid secretion was described first by Wheeler and King[67] and Erlinger[68]. It was observed that some hydrophilic organic anions inhibited biliary lipid secretion in a dose-dependent fashion, without interference with biliary bile acid secretion. Studies from Apstein *et al.* subsequently provided partial insight into the localization of this organic effect[69,70]. These authors observed a dose-dependent decrease in the biliary secretion of phospholipids and cholesterol in Gunn rats during infusion of the conjugated bilirubin analogue bilirubin ditaurate, but not during infusion of unconjugated bilirubin[69]. Gunn rats are genetically deficient in hepatic bilirubin glucuronidation. As bilirubin ditaurate does not require intrahepatic conjugation for its secretion into bile, Apstein's studies concluded that the inhibitory effect of bilirubin on biliary lipid secretion was localized *after* the microsomal conjugation process leading to the formation of bilirubin diglucuronide[69]. Although a partial localization of the 'uncoupling' phenomenon had been achieved, at least for bilirubin, it still remained unclear whether it was mediated by an organic anion effect at some intracellular, intracanalicular or canalicular membrane level. Bellringer and colleagues[71,72] provided indications to suggest that two organic anions, ampicillin and valproic acid, inhibited intracellular vesicle-mediated secretion from hepatocytes. These authors suggested that inhibition of vesicular lipid transport towards the bile canalicular membrane was responsible for the reduction of biliary lipid secretion induced by these organic anions. However, the organic anion concentrations needed to obtain inhibition of vesicular transport were considerably higher than those required to obtain inhibition of biliary lipid secretion[55,71,72]. Furthermore, in subsequent studies by the same group[73] and others[74] it was found that the organic anion cyclobuterol, even at high concentrations, did not affect intracellular vesicle transport, although it did inhibit biliary lipid secretion. This finding indicated that disturbance of vesicular transport processes was not a general observation during organic anion-induced inhibition of biliary lipid secretion.

We performed studies on the 'uncoupling' of biliary lipid secretion by comparing the effects of intravenously injected organic anions in normal Wistar rats with those in the congenitally hyperbilirubinaemic GY rat strain[75]. GY rats, which appear to have an identical phenotype to the TR⁻ Wistar rat strain described by Jansen *et al*[76] and the EBHR Sprague-Dawley rat strain described by Takikawa *et al.*[77], express an autosomal recessive defect in the biliary secretion of several organic anions, but not in their hepatic uptake. Available data indicate that the defect involves ATP-dependent transport of organic anions across the bile canalicular membrane[75,76,78–83]. We reasoned that the GY rat model would allow discrimination between an intracellular versus an intracanalicular mechanism involved in the inhibition of biliary lipid secretion by organic anions. Since the uptake of organic anions into the liver is not affected in the mutant animals, a similar inhibition of lipid secretion by organic anions was to be expected in GY rats when compared to controls if the organic anion effect was based on an intracellular mechanism. Alternatively, when the organic anions were to exert their inhibitory effect on biliary lipid secretion after their (own) secretion into the bile canaliculus, uncoupling of lipid from bile acid secretion should be less pronounced or even absent in the GY rats. As described in detail elsewhere[55,84], the latter situation appeared to occur: after injection of a number of differently structured, non-metabolizing organic anions, (such as ampicillin, sulphated lithocholyltaurine, sulphated lithocholylglycine, dibromosulphophthalein (DBSP), bilirubin ditaurate, cefoperazone, ceftriaxone and valproic acid (details on the last two from unpublished data, Verkade and Kuipers 1993), either no uncoupling or a much less pronounced uncoupling was observed in GY rats when compared to controls. In accordance with a secretory defect at the level of the canalicular membrane, hepatic concentrations of the organic anions injected were similar or higher in the GY than in control livers, whereas bile concentrations were several-fold lower in the mutants[55]. These observations were compatible with a mechanism of organic anion-mediated inhibition of biliary lipid secretion at the level of either the bile canalicular membrane or the bile canalicular lumen. In accordance with an intracanalicular mechanism it was observed that the degree of inhibition of biliary lipid secretion highly correlated with the concentration of the injected organic anion in the bile[55] ($r=0.993$). Still, it could not be excluded that organic anion transport across the bile canalicular

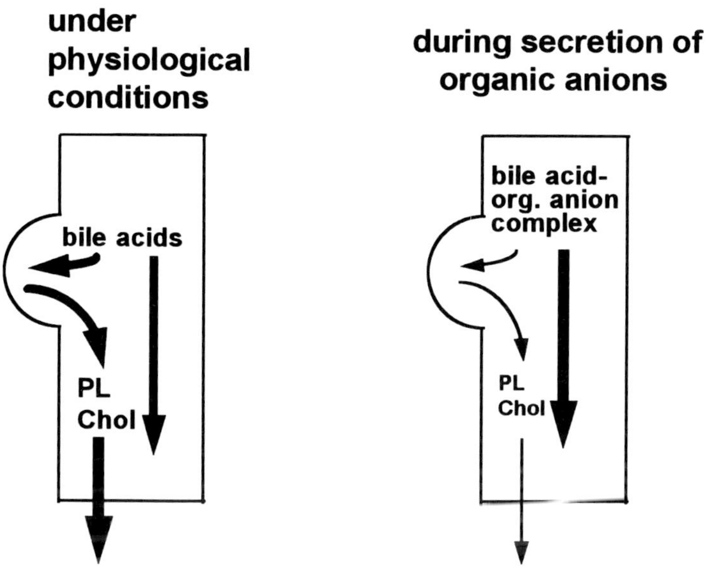

Fig. 5   The mechanism of inhibition of biliary lipid secretion by hydrophilic organic anions. The physiological process of bile acid-induced lipid secretion (left), by which intracanalicular bile acids interact with the luminal side of the canalicular membrane, is interrupted during the secretion of hydrophilic organic anions (right). Hydrophilic organic anions interact with biliary bile acids, leading to the formation of bile acid–organic anion complexes[55,84,91,92]. It is hypothesized that, mediated by this interaction, the bile acids are then inhibited in their capacity to induce biliary lipid secretion[56,84]

membrane in itself would be sufficient to inhibit biliary lipid secretion. Additional studies, however, demonstrated that a number of organic anions, including indocyanine green and rose bengal, do not inhibit biliary lipid secretion either in GY or in control rats[55], notwithstanding their sharing of the same translocation route across the bile canalicular membrane. We interpreted this to mean that a mechanism for 'uncoupling' at the level of bile canalicular membrane translocation of organic anions was therefore unlikely in comparison to an intracanalicular mechanism[55]. A theoretical explanation, put forward by Erlinger et al.[69], would be the dilution of canalicular bile acids by organic anion-induced choleresis. Yet several organic anions (such as sulphated lithocholyltaurine, sulphated lithocholylglycine or bilirubin ditaurate) did inhibit biliary lipid secretion, but did not induce bile flow[55,84]. Partial insight into the presumable mechanism could be derived from gel filtration studies on native rat biles obtained after injection of the various organic anions[55]. The capacity of an organic anion to inhibit biliary lipid secretion *in vivo* was found to coincide with a relatively high affinity for biliary bile acids[55,84]. Organic anions which did not interfere with biliary lipid secretion *in vivo* showed a high affinity for biliary phospholipid and cholesterol vesicles[55]. Based on data from the literature[70,71,86–92] as well as on our own observations[55,85,93], it was concluded that only relatively hydrophilic organic anions have the capacity to uncouple biliary lipid from bile acid secretion, presumably by means of a physicochemical interaction with bile acids inside the bile canaliculus[84] (see Fig. 5).

Composition of the bile canalicular membrane

The fourth factor involved is the composition of the bile canalicular membrane, with respect to its lipid as well as to its protein composition. (Indirect) indications for a role of the lipid composition stems from the work of Yousef and colleagues on bile acid-mediated cholestasis in rats[21,57,58,94,95]. Upon infusion of either lithocholic acid or increasing doses of unconjugated bile acids, cholestasis occurs in parallel to changes in the amount and profile of biliary lipid secretion, and in parallel to alterations in the composition of the bile canalicular membrane. For example, infusion of increasing amounts of deoxycholic acid eventually leads, after an initial increase, to a decrease in the phospholipid secretion rate[21]. During this decrease in phospholipid secretion, the composition of the secreted phospholipids also alters, with increasing amounts of phosphatidylethanolamine and sphingomyelin at the expense of the contribution of phosphatidylcholine[21]. In another study by the same researchers it was found that, in parallel to the changes found in biliary lipids, the lipid composition of the bile canalicular membrane also changed under these conditions, leading to an increased cholesterol to phospholipid ratio[58]. In analogy to these data, lithocholic acid-induced cholestasis is also accompanied by an increase in the cholesterol to phospholipid ratio of the bile canalicular membrane and a decrease in the biliary secretion rate of phospholipids[94,95].

More direct indications that bile canalicular membrane composition influences the amount of biliary lipids can be derived from the recent studies on the physiological role of P-glycoproteins. It had been appreciated for several years that murine P-glycoprotein genes *mdr1* and *mdr3* encode for membrane proteins, capable of pumping hydrophobic compounds out of cells[96]. The physiological function of a homologous gene, *mdr2*, was not understood until the recent gene knock-out studies by Smit *et al.*[97]. These authors observed that mice homozygous for the disruption of the *mdr2* gene did not secrete phospholipids into bile under 'physiological' conditions, and only approximately 6% of the normal amount of cholesterol[97]. Some associated abnormalities in bile and liver physiology in the homozygotes were not present in heterozygous mice, which only showed a 40–50% decrease in phospholipid secretion rate[97]. Based on these observations the authors concluded that the primary defect in the homozygously *mdr2* disrupted mice involves one of the rate-limiting steps in biliary lipid secretion. Initial experiments using this mouse model for biliary lipid secretion have been performed by Oude Elferink and colleagues, who report on their results elsewhere in chapter 24 of this volume.

Magnitude of the bile acid-independent fraction of the bile flow

The fifth and most recently recognized factor which influences the amount of phospholipids secreted into the bile is the magnitude of the bile acid-independent bile flow. The indications for the contribution of the bile acid-independent flow were derived from reviewing the literature on bile formation in different animal species. It was already known that animal species differ in their responsiveness to bile acids with respect to biliary lipid secretion[1,8,98–102]. It became apparent that,

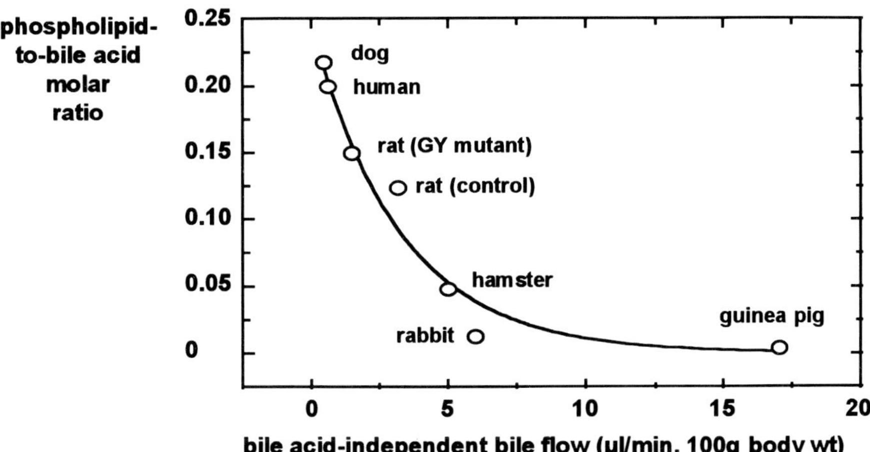

Fig. 6 The relationship between the bile acid-independent bile flow and the biliary lipid-to-bile acid molar ratio in different species. The bile acid-independent fraction of the bile flow of a certain species is inversely related to the efficacy of bile acid-induced lipid secretion, as reflected by the biliary phospholipid-to-bile acid molar ratio. Experimental data used in this figure are derived from the literature. (For experimental details see refs 56, 80, 84, 98–102, 106, 107)

in general, animal species with a relatively large bile acid-independent fraction of bile flow show a relatively inefficient bile acid-induced biliary lipid secretion, quantified for example by the amount of lipids secreted per amount of bile acid (Fig. 6). In addition, in certain forms of experimentally induced cholestasis (e.g. after ethinyloestradiol[102] or during streptozotocin-induced diabetes[104,105]), reduction of the bile acid-independent bile flow appeared to be accompanied by an increased efficacy of bile acids to induce biliary lipid secretion. The hypothesis that bile acid-independent bile flow is an independent regulatory factor in bile acid-induced biliary lipid secretion was tested in the already-mentioned mutant GY rats[106]. It was rationalized that the GY rat strain would be a very suitable model, as in this strain bile acid-independent bile flow is reduced by 50% when compared to normal Wistar rats. By interruption of the enterohepatic circulation of unanaesthetized GY and control rats[85,107] a wide range of bile acid output rates could be obtained without interference of stress or of anaesthetics. For both strains, hyperbolic relationships were found between biliary concentrations of phospholipid or cholesterol and concentration of bile acids (see Fig. 7; data for cholesterol not shown), in accordance with available literature. However, a consistently higher concentration of both phospholipids and cholesterol was found in GY rats, compared to controls, over the whole range of bile acid concentrations studied. After excluding differences in the factors previously mentioned (e.g. bile acid concentration and composition, lipid composition of the bile canalicular membranes), the data were interpreted as showing that a high bile acid-independent bile flow limits the time of exposure of the bile canalicular membrane to bile acids (schematically shown in Fig. 8). This inhibits the efficacy of the bile acids to induce the secretion of lipids into the bile ('exposure time' or 'ET' hypothesis). Comparisons of the magnitude of

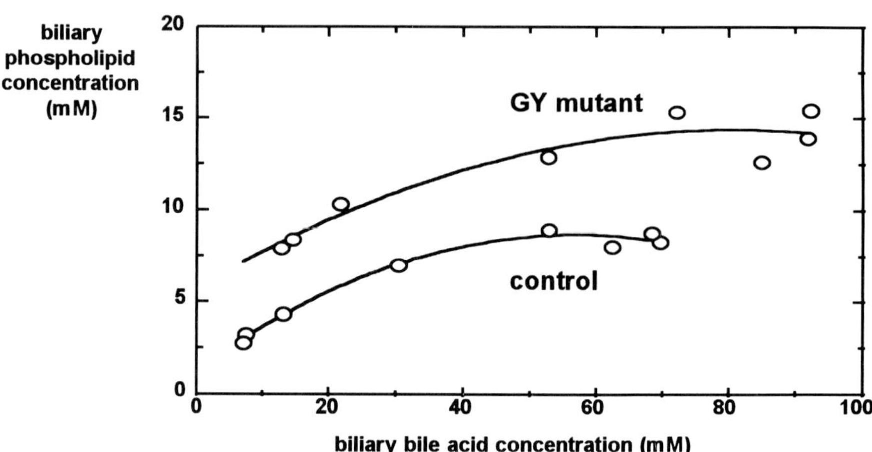

Fig. 7 The relationship between biliary bile acid concentration and biliary phospholipid concentration in GY mutant and control Wistar rats. Both in control and mutant GY Wistar rats a curvilinear relationship exists between biliary bile acid and biliary lipid concentration. However, over the whole range of bile acid concentrations studied, a certain bile acid concentration in GY rats is associated with a significantly higher phospholipid concentration, compared to control rats. GY Wistar rats express an autosomal recessive defect in the biliary secretion of several organic anions[75,80]. GY rats show a decrease in their bile acid-independent bile flow by approximately 50%, which is presumably related to the virtual absence of glutathione in GY rat bile[56,80,107]. Present data were derived from the acute interruption of the enterohepatic circulation of unanaesthetized control and GY Wistar rats (details described in ref. 106)

the bile acid-independent bile flow and the corresponding biliary phospholipid-to-bile acid molar ratio in various species (Fig. 6) strongly suggest that species-dependent quantitative differences in bile acid-induced lipid secretion may, at least partly, be explained by the 'exposure time' hypothesis.

CONCLUSION

At this moment, five factors are known to influence the amount of lipid secretion into the bile: (1) biliary bile acid concentration; (2) species composition of biliary bile acids; (3) biliary concentration of hydrophilic organic anions; (4) composition of the bile canalicular membrane; and (5) magnitude of the bile acid-independent fraction of the bile flow. Available data indicate that each of these factors can act *independently* from the other four. The hypothesized mechanisms by which these five factors regulate biliary lipid secretion share the proposed localization of their actions, namely inside the canaliculus and/or at the canalicular side of the bile canalicular membrane (see for example Figs 5 and 8). The presently available data therefore indicate, in our opinion, that bile acids stimulate biliary lipid secretion only after their secretion into the canalicular lumen. After the translocation step the intracanalicular bile acids interact with the canalicular membrane from the lumenal side (Fig. 2).

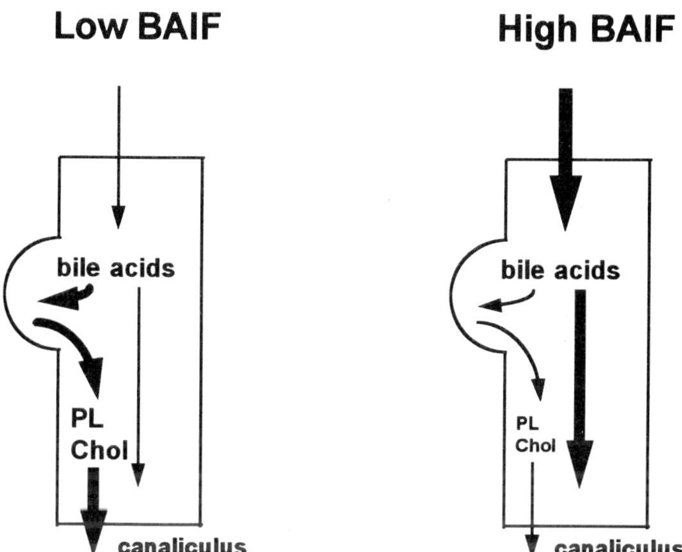

Fig. 8 The exposure time hypothesis. The exposure time or ('ET') hypothesis describes the proposed mechanism for the observed inverse relationship between the bile acid-independent bile flow (BAIF) and the efficacy by which intracanalicular bile acids induce biliary lipid secretion. Under conditions of a low BAIF (left), the bile canalicular membrane is exposed to the intracanalicular bile acids for a relatively long period, when compared with the situation of a high BAIF (right). At a high BAIF, canalicular bile acids are more readily flushed from the canalicular environment, which limits their efficacy to induce biliary lipid secretion. It should be realized that the mechanism is independent of a dilutive effect on bile concentration, as can be derived from the data shown in Fig. 7. Conceptually, it may therefore be best hypothesized that the efficacy of an *individual* bile acid molecule to stimulate lipid secretion is related to the amount of BAIF

Acknowledgement

Our studies were supported by grants from the Dutch Organization for Scientific Research (NWO), the Netherlands Heart Foundation, the Academic Hospital Groningen, and the Royal Netherlands Academy of Arts and Sciences.

References

1. Eriksson S. Biliary excretion of bile acids and cholesterol in bile fistula rats. Proc Soc Exp Biol Med. 1957;94:578–82.
2. Kay RE, Entenman C. Stimulation of taurocholic acid synthesis and biliary excretion of lipids. Am J Physiol. 1961;200:855–9.
3. Kuroki S, Mosbach EH, Stenger RJ, Cohen BI, McSherry CK. Comparative effects of deoxycholate and 7-methyl-deoxycholate in the hamster. Hepatology. 1987;7:229–34.
4. Scherstén T, Nilsson S, Chalin E, Filipson M, Brodin-Persson G. Relationship between the biliary excretion of bile acids and the excretion of water, lecithin, and cholesterol in man. Eur J Clin Invest. 1971;1:242–7.
5. Danzinger RG, Nakagaki M, Hofmann AF, Ljungwe EB. Differing effects of hydroxy-7-oxotaurine-conjugated bile acids on bile flow and biliary lipid secretion in dogs. Am J Physiol. 1984;246:G166–72.

6. Wagner CI, Trotman BW, Soloway RD. Kinetic analysis of biliary lipid excretion in man and dog. J Clin Invest. 1976;57:473–7.

7. Carey MC, Hernell O. Digestion and absorption of fat. Semin Gastroint Dis. 1992;3:189–208.

8. Staggers JE, Hernell O, Stafford RJ, Carey MC. Physical–chemical behaviour of dietary and biliary lipids during intestinal digestion and absorption. 1. Phase behaviour and aggregation states of model lipid systems patterned after aqueous duodenal contents of healthy adult human beings. Biochemistry. 1990;29:2028–40.

9. Hernell O, Staggers JE, Carey MC. Physical–chemical behaviour of dietary and biliary lipids during intestinal digestion and absorption. 2. Phase analysis and aggregation states of luminal lipids during duodenal fat digestion in healthy adult human beings. Biochemistry. 1990;29:2041–56.

10. Harvey PRC, Sömjen G, Gilat T, Gallinger S, Strasberg SM. Vesicular cholesterol in bile. Relationship to protein concentration and nucleation time. Biochim Biophys Acta. 1988;958:10–18.

11. Carey MC. Formation of gallstones: the new paradigms. In: Paumgartner G, Stiehl A, Gerok W, editors. Trends in bile acid research. Dordrecht: Kluwer; 1989:259–81.

12. Hay R, Carey MC. Pathophysiology and pathogenesis of cholesterol gallstone formation. Semin Liver Dis. 1990;10:159–70.

13. Carey MC, Mazer NA. Biliary lipid secretion in health and in cholesterol gallstone disease. Hepatology. 1984;4:31S–37S.

14. Crawford JM, Berken CA, Gollan JL. Role of the hepatocyte microtubular system in the excretion of bile salts and biliary lipid: implications for intracellular vesicular transport. J Lipid Res. 1988;29:144–56.

15. Graham J, Ahmed H, Northfield TC. Unidirectional pathway for vesicular cholesterol transport. In: Paumgartner G, Stiehl A, Gerok W, editors. Trends in bile acid research. Dordrecht: Kluwer; 1989:177–87.

16. Gregory DH, Vlahcevic ZR, Prugh MR, Swell L. Mechanism of secretion of biliary lipids: role of a microtubular system in hepatocellular transport of biliary lipids in the rat. Gastroenterology. 1978;74:93–100.

17. Entenman C, Holloway RJ, Albright ML, Leong GF. Bile acids and lipid metabolism. II. Essential role of bile acids in bile phospholipid excretion. Arch Biochem Biophys. 1969;130:253–6.

18. Reuben A, Allen RM. Intrahepatic sources of biliary-like micelles. Biochim Biophys Acta. 1986;876:1–12.

19. Reynier MO, Hashieh IA, Crotte C, Carbuccia N, Richard B, Gérolami A. Monensin action on the Golgi complex in perfused rat liver: evidence against bile salt vesicular transport. Gastroenterology. 1992;102:2024–32.

20. Barnwell SG, Godfrey PP, Lowe PJ, Coleman R. Biliary protein output by isolated perfused rat livers. Effects of bile salts. Biochem J. 1993;210:549–57.

21. Barnwell SG, Yousef IM, Tuchweber B. The effect of colchicine on the development of lithocholic acid-induced cholestasis. A study of the role of microtubules in intracellular cholesterol transport. Biochem J. 1986;236:345–50.

22. Crawford JM, Gollan JL. Hepatocyte cotransport of taurocholate and bilirubin glucuronides: role of microtubules. Am J Physiol. 1988;255:G121–31.

23. Dubin M, Maurice M, Feldmann G, Erlinger S. Influence of colchicine and phalloidin on bile secretion and hepatic ultrastructure in the rat. Possible interaction between microtubules and microfilaments. Gastroenterology. 1980;79:646–54.

24. Katagiri K, Nakai T, Hoshino M et al. Tauro-β-muricholate preserves choleresis and prevents taurocholate-induced cholestasis in cholchicine-treated rat liver. Gastroenterology. 1992;102:1660–7.

25. Nakai T, Katagiri K, Hoskino M, Hayakawa T, Ohiwa T. Microtubule-independent choleresis and anti-cholestatic action of tauroursodeoxycholate in colchicine-treated rat liver. Biochem J. 1992;288:613–17.

26. Azhar S, Hwang SF, Reaven E. Effects of antimicrotubule agents on phospholipid metabolism in rat hepatic subcellular membranes. Biochem Pharmacol. 1985;34:3153–9.

27. Benedetti A, Marucci L, Ferretti G, Curatola G, Jézéquel AM, Orlandi F. Evidence that plasma membrane fluidity of isolated hepatocytes is modified by exposure to microtubule-depolymerizing drug. J Hepatol. 1990;10:144–8.

28. Sakisaka S, Oi Cheng N, Boyer JL. Tubulovesicular transcytotic pathway in isolated rat hepatocyte couplets in culture. Effect of colchicine and taurocholate. Gastroenterology. 1988;95:793–804.

29. Berr F, Jaeger H, Walli A, Bitterle Th, Wilcox H. Biliary secretion of phospholipids and apolipoprotein A-I: evidence for intracellular supply of phospholipids by a non-vesicular transport route [abstract]. Hepatology. 1993;18:179A.
30. Small DM. The formation of gallstones. Adv Intern Med. 1970;16:243–64.
31. Hardison WGM, Apter JT. Micellar theory of biliary cholesterol excretion. Am J Physiol. 1972;222:61–7.
32. Yousef IM, Fisher MM. *In vitro* effect of free bile acids on the bile canalicular membrane phospholipids in the cat. Can J Biochem. 1976;54:1040–6.
33. Graham JM, Northfield TM. Solubilization of lipids from hamster bile canalicular and contiguous membranes and from human erythrocyte membranes by conjugated bile salts. Biochem J. 1987;242:825–34.
34. Coleman R, Rahman K, Kan K, Parslow RA. Retrograde intrabiliary injection of amphipathic materials causes phospholipid secretion into bile. Taurocholate causes phosphatidylcholine secretion, 3-[(3-cholamidopropyl)dimethylammonio]-propane-1-sulphonate (CHAPS) causes mixed phospholipid secretion. Biochem J. 1989;258:17–22.
35. Cohen DE, Angelico M, Carey MC. Structural alterations in lecithin–cholesterol vesicles following interactions with monomeric and micellar bile salts: physical–chemical basis for subselection of biliary lecithin species and aggregate states of biliary lipids during bile formation. J Lipid Res. 1990;31:55–70.
36. Mazer NA, Carey MC. Quasi-elastic light-scattering studies of aqueous biliary lipid systems. Cholesterol solubilization and precipitation in model bile solutions. Biochemistry. 1983,22:426–42.
37. Mazer NA, Schurtenberger P, Carey MC, Preisig R, Weigand K, Känzig W. Quasi-elastic light scattering studies of native hepatic bile from the dog: comparison with aggregative behavior of model biliary lipid systems. Biochemistry. 1984;23:1994–2005.
38. Pattinson NR. Solubilisation of cholesterol in human bile. FEBS Lett. 1985;181:339–42.
39. Sömjen GJ, Gilat T. A non-micellar mode of cholesterol transport in human bile. FEBS Lett. 1983;156:265–8.
40. Sömjen GJ, Gilat T. Contribution of vesicular and micellar carriers to cholesterol transport in human bile. J Lipid Res. 1985;26:699–704.
41. Pattinson NR, Chapman BA. Distribution of biliary cholesterol between mixed micelles and nonmicelles in relation to fasting and feeding in humans. Gastroenterology. 1986;91:697–702.
42. Sömjen GJ, Gilat T. Changing concepts of cholesterol solubility in bile [editorial]. Gastroenterology. 1986;91:772–5.
43. Sömjen GJ, Harvey PRC, Rosenberg R, Werbin N, Strasberg SM, Gilat T. Quantitation of phospholipid vesicles and their cholesterol content in human bile by quasi-elastic light scattering. Biochim Biophys Acta. 1988;963:265–70.
44. Sömjen GJ, Marikovsky Y, Lelkes P, Gilat T. Cholesterol–phospholipid vesicles in human bile: an ultrastructural study. Biochim Biophys Acta. 1986;879:14–21.
45. Ulloa N, Garrido J, Nervi F. Ultracentrifugal isolation of vesicular carriers of biliary cholesterol in native human and rat bile. Hepatology. 1987;7:235–44.
46. Cohen DE, Angelico M, Carey MC. Quasielastic light scattering evidence for vesicular secretion of biliary lipids. Am J Physiol. 1989;257:G1–8.
47. Lee SP, Park HZ, Madani H, Kaler EW. Partial characterization of a nonmicellar system of cholesterol solubilization in bile. Am J Physiol. 1987;252:G374–83.
48. Little TE, Lee SP, Madani H, Kaler EW, Chinn K. Interconversions of lipid aggregates in rat and model bile. Am J Physiol. 1991;260:G70–9.
49. Billington D, Coleman R. Effects of bile salts on human erythrocytes. Plasma membrane vesiculation, phospholipid solubilization, and their possible relationships to bile secretion. Biochim Biophys Acta. 1978;509:33–47.
50. Puglielli L, Amigo L, Arrese M *et al.* Protective role of biliary cholesterol and phospholipid lamellae against bile acid-induced cell damage. Gastroenterology. 1994;107:244–54.
51. Lapré JA, Termont DSML, Groen AK, Van der Meer R. Lytic effects of mixed micelles of fatty acids and bile acids. Am J Physiol. 1992;263:G333–7.
52. Van der Meer R, Termont DMSL, De Vries HT. Differential effects of calcium ions and calcium phosphate on cytotoxicity of bile acids. Am J Physiol. 1991;260:G142–7.
53. Velardi ALM, Groen AK, Oude Elferink RPJ, Van der Meer R, Palasciano G, Tytgat GNJ. Cell type-dependent effect of phospholipid and cholesterol on bile salt toxicity. Gastroenterology. 1991;101:457–64.

54. Verkade HJ, Kuipers F, De Bruijn MAC, Groen B. *In vitro* interactions of organic anions with biliary vesicles and micelles [abstract]. Gastroenterology. 1992;102:A906.
55. Verkade HJ, Wolbers MJ, Havinga R, Uges DRA, Vonk RJ, Kuipers F. The uncoupling of biliary lipid from bile acid secretion by organic anions in the rat. Gastroenterology. 1990;99: 1485–92.
56. Verkade HJ, Vonk RJ, Kuipers F. New insights in the mechanism of bile acid-induced biliary lipid secretion. Hepatology. 1995, in press.
57. Barnwell SG, Tuchweber B, Yousef IM. Biliary lipid secretion in the rat during infusion of increasing doses of unconjugated bile acids. Biochim Biophys Acta. 1987;922:221–33.
58. Yousef IM, Barnwell S, Gratton F, Tuchweber B, Weber AM, Roy CC. Liver cell membrane solubilization may control maximum secretory rate of cholic acid in the rat. Am J Physiol. 1987;252:G84–91.
59. Coleman R, Rahman K, Bellringer ME, Kan K, Hamlin S. Secretion of biliary lipids and its control. In: Paumgartner G, Stiehl A, Gerok W, editors. Trends in bile acid research. Dordrecht: Kluwer; 1989:161–73.
60. Oude Elferink RPJ, Ottenhof R, Wijland M van, Smit JJM, Schinkel AH, Groen AK. Regulation of biliary lipid secretion by mdr2 P-glycoprotein in the mouse. J Clin Invest. 1995 (in press).
61. Gurantz D, Hofmann AF. Influence of bile acid structure on bile flow and biliary lipid secretion in the hamster. Am J Physiol. 1984;247:G736–48.
62. Hofmann AF. Bile acid secretion, bile flow and biliary lipid secretion in humans. Hepatology. 1990;12:17S–25S.
63. Borgström B, Barrowman J, Krabisch L, Lindström M, Lillienau J. Effects of cholic acid 7β-hydroxy- and 12β-hydroxy-isocholic acid on bile flow, lipid secretion and bile acid synthesis in the rat. Scand J Clin Lab Invest. 1986;46:167–75.
64. Coleman R, Rahman K. Lipid flow in bile formation. Biochim Biophys Acta. 1992;1125: 113–33.
65. Loria P, Carulli N, Medici G et al. Effect of ursodeoxycholic acid on bile lipid secretion and composition. Gastroenterology. 1986;90:865–74.
66. Parquet M, Legrand-Defretin V, Riottot M, Karpouza A, Lutton C. Metabolism and effects on biliary lipid secretion of murocholic acid in the hamster. J Hepatol. 1990;11:111–19.
67. Wheeler HO, King KK. Biliary excretion of lecithin and cholesterol in the dog. J Clin Invest. 1972;51:1337–50.
68. Erlinger S, Bienfait D, Poupon D, Bumont M, Duval M. Effect of lysine acetyl salicylate on biliary lipid secretion in dogs. Clin Sci Mol Med. 1975;49:253–6.
69. Apstein MD. Inhibition of biliary phospholipid and cholesterol secretion by bilirubin in the Sprague-Dawley and Gunn rat. Gastroenterology. 1984;87:634–8.
70. Apstein MD, Robins SJ. Effect of organic anions on biliary lipids in the rat. Gastroenterology. 1982;83:1120–6.
71. Bellringer ME, Rahman K, Coleman R. Sodium valproate inhibits the movement of secretory vesicles in rat hepatocytes. Biochem J. 1988;249:513–19.
72. Bellringer ME, Steele NJ, Rahman K, Coleman R. Ampicillin inhibits the movement of biliary secretory vesicles in rat hepatocytes. Biochem J. 1988;941:71–5.
73. Monte MJ, Parslow RA, Coleman R. Inhibitory action of cyclobuterol on the secretion of biliary cholesterol and phospholipids. Biochem J. 1990;266:165–71.
74. Monte MJ, Cava F, Esteller A, Jimenez R. Inhibition of biliary cholesterol and phospholipid secretion during cyclobuterol-induced choleresis. Biochem J. 1989;263:513–18.
75. Kuipers F, Ensering M, Havinga R et al. Separate transport systems for biliary secretion of sulfated and unsulfated bile acids in the rat. J Clin Invest. 1988;81:1593–9.
76. Jansen PLM, Peters WH, Lamers WH. Hereditary chronic conjugated hyperbilirubinemia in mutant rats caused by defective hepatic anion transport. Hepatology. 1985;5:573–9.
77. Takikawa H, Sano N, Narita T et al. Biliary excretion of bile acid conjugates in a hyperbilirubinemic mutant Sprague-Dawley rat. Hepatology. 1991;14:352–60.
78. Zimniak P, Awashti YC. ATP-dependent transport systems for organic anions. Hepatology. 1993;17:330–9.
79. Kitamura T, Jansen P, Hardenbrook C, Kamimoto Y, Gatmaitan Z, Arias IM. Defective ATP-dependent bile canalicular transport of organic anions in mutant (TR⁻) rats with conjugated hyperbilirubinemia. Proc Natl Acad Sci USA. 1990;87:3557–61.

80. Kuipers F, Ensering M, Havinga R *et al*. Separate transport systems for biliary secretion of sulphated and unsulphated bile acids. In: Paumgartner G, Stiehl A, Gerok W, editors. Trends in bile acid research. Dordrecht: Kluwer; 1989:143–52.

81. Nishida T, Hardenbrook C, Gatmaitan Z, Arias IM. ATP-dependent organic anion transport system in normal and TR⁻ rat liver canalicular membranes. Am J Physiol. 1992;262:G629–35.

82. Pikula S, Hayden JB, Awashti YC, Zimniak P. Organic anion-transporting ATPase of rat liver. I. Purification, photoaffinity labeling, and regulation by phosphorylation. J Biol Chem. 1995 (In press).

83. Pikula S, Hayden JB, Awashti YC, Zimniak P. Organic anion-transporting ATPase of rat liver. II. Functional reconstitution of active transport and regulation by phosphorylation. J Biol Chem. 1995 (In press).

84. Verkade HJ, Havinga R, Gerding A, Vonk RJ, Kuipers F. The mechanism of bile acid-induced biliary lipid secretion in the rat. Effect of conjugated bilirubin. Am J Physiol. 1993;264: G462–9.

85. Wilson MD, Rudel LL. Review of cholesterol absorption with emphasis on dietary and biliary cholesterol. J Lipid Res. 1994;35:943–55.

86. Apsein MD, Russo AR. Ampicillin inhibits biliary cholesterol secretion. Dig Dis Sci. 1985;30:253–6.

87. Arvidsson A, Leijd B, Nord CE, Angelin B. Interindividual variability in biliary excretion of ceftriaxone: effects on biliary lipid metabolism and on intestinal microflora. Eur J Clin Invest. 1988;18:261–6.

88. Bellringer ME, Rahman K, Coleman R. Sodium valproate inhibits the movement of secretory vesicles in rat hepatocytes. Biochem J. 1988;249:513–19.

89. Shaffer EA, Preshaw RM. Effects of sulfobromophthalein excretion on biliary lipid secretion in humans and dogs. Am J Physiol. 1981;240:G85–9.

90. Xia Y, Lambert KJ, Schteingart CD, Gu JJ, Hofmann AF. Concentrative biliary secretion of ceftriaxone. Inhibition of lipid secretion and precipitation of calcium ceftriaxone in bile. Gastroenterology. 1990;99:454–65.

91. Tazuma S, Barnhardt RL, Reeve LE, Tokumo H, Holzbach RT. Biliary secretion of organic anions in the dog: association with defined lipid particles. Am J Physiol. 1988;255:G745–51.

92. Tazuma S, Holzbach RT. Transport of conjugated bilirubin and other organic anions in bile: relation to biliary lipid structures. Proc Natl Acad Sci USA. 1987;84:2052–6.

93. Kuipers F, Derksen JTP, Gerding A, Scherphof GL, Vonk RJ. Biliary lipid secretion in the rat. The uncoupling of biliary cholesterol and phospholipid secretion from bile acid secretion by sulfated glycolithocholic acid. Biochim Biophys Acta. 1987;922:136–44.

94. Kakis G, Phillipis MJ, Yousef IM. The respective roles of membrane cholesterol and of sodium potassium adenosine triphosphate in the pathogenesis of lithocholate-induced cholestasis. Lab Invest. 1980;43:73–81.

95. Kakis G, Yousef IM. Mechanism of cholic acid protection in lithocholate-induced intrahepatic cholestasis in rats. Gastroenterology. 1980;78:1402–11.

96. Devault A, Gros P. Two members of the mouse *mdr* family confer multidrug resistance with overlapping but distinct drug specificity. Mol Cell Biol. 1990;10:1652–63.

97. Smit JJM, Schinkel AH, Oude Elferink RPJ *et al*. Homozygous disruption of the murine *mdr2* P-glycoprotein gene leads to a complete absence of phospholipid from bile and to liver disease. Cell. 1993;75:451–62.

98. Dowling RH, Mack E, Small DM. Biliary lipid secretion and bile composition after acute and chronic interruption of the enterohepatic circulation in the Rhesus monkey. IV. Primary biliary physiology. J Clin Invest. 1971;50:1917–26.

99. Wheeler HO. Secretion of bile acids by the liver and their role in the formation of hepatic bile. Arch Intern Med. 1972;30:533–41.

100. Scheibner J, Fuchs M, Hörmann E, Tauber G, Stange EF. Biliary cholesterol secretion and bile acid formation in the hamster: the role of newly synthesized cholesterol. J Lipid Res. 1994;35:690–7.

101. Cummings SA, Hofmann AF. Physiological determinants of biliary calcium secretion in the dog. Gastroenterology. 1984;87:664–73.

102. Coleman R, Iqbal S, Godfrey PP, Billington D. Membranes and bile formation. Composition of several mammalian biles and their membrane-damaging properties. Biochem J. 1979;178: 201–8.

103. Kern Jr F, Eriksson H, Curstedt T, Sjövall J. Effect of ethinylestradiol on biliary excretion of bile acids, phosphatidylcholines, and cholesterol in the bile fistula rat. J Lipid Res. 1977;18: 623–34.
104. Villanueva GR, Herreros M, Perez-Barriocanal F, Bolanos JP, Bravo P, Marin JJG. Enhancement of bile acid-induced biliary lipid secretion by streptozotocin in rats: role of insulin deficiency. J Lab Clin Med. 1990;115:441–8.
105. Villanueva GR, Herreros M, Perez-Barriocanal F, Fernandez E, Marin JJG. Effect of acute insulin administration on biliary lipid secretion by the diabetic rat. J Exp Pathol. 1990;71: 89–94.
106. Verkade HJ, Wolters H, Gerding A et al. Mechanism of biliary lipid secretion in the rat. A role for bile acid-independent bile flow? Hepatology. 1993;17:1074–80.
107. Kuipers F, Havinga R, Bosschieter H, Toorop GP, Hindriks FR, Vonk RJ. Enterohepatic circulation in the rat. Gastroenterology. 1985;88:403–11.

24
Regulation of biliary lipid secretion by bile salts and *mdr2* P-glycoprotein

R. P. J. OUDE ELFERINK, R. OTTENHOFF, M. VAN WIJLAND, C. M. G. FRIJTERS and A. K. GROEN

INTRODUCTION

P-glycoproteins have been characterized as integral plasma membrane proteins that function as ATP-dependent pumps. The mammalian P-glycoproteins (PgP) are encoded by small families of genes; two in man (*MDR1* and *MDR3*) and three in rodents (*mdr1a, mdr1b* and *mdr2*). High homology is observed between the *mdr1a/b* in rodents and *MDR1* in humans and between *mdr2* and *MDR3*. Overexpression of the *mdr1* (*MDR1*) in tumour cells renders these cells resistant to a diverse group of drugs, e.g. vincristine, doxorubicin, colchicine and many others. Although these compounds have quite different molecular structures they all have an amphipathic character and readily insert into and diffuse across biomembranes. It was demonstrated that the overexpression of these Pgp leads to a decreased cellular content of these compounds, and more recently several studies have shown that Pgp mediate the ATP-dependent extrusion of these compounds out of the cell[1]. Apart from overexpression in resistant tumour cells the Pgp are also expressed in various normal tissues, albeit at much lower levels.

In contrast to *mdr1*, transfection of cells with *mdr2* or the highly homologous *MDR3* Pgp does not confer resistance towards the above-mentioned drugs. It was shown that the expression level of mouse *mdr2*, as well as human *MDR3*, is particularly high in normal liver, and immunological studies indicated that the protein is exclusively present in the canalicular membrane[2,3]. In some other tissues such as spleen and muscle *mdr2* is also expressed, albeit at a much lower level.

To obtain more information about the function of the *mdr2* Pgp, the gene for this protein was disrupted in mouse embryonic stem (ES) cells by homologous recombination[4]. Bile was sampled from mice that were homozygous for *mdr2* gene disruption; (−/−) mice, heterozygotes; (+/−) mice and homozygous normal animals; (+/+) mice. Table 1 shows the composition of bile samples that were

Table 1   Excretion rate of the main bile constituents in *mdr2* knock-out mice

	+/+	+/−	−/−
Bile salts (nmol/min per 100 g)	287±59	702±240*	470±213
Bilirubin (nmol/min per 100 g)	1.07±0.35	2.33±1.30	1.45±0.61
Phospholipid (nmol/min per 100 g)	26.2±6.1	14.2±1.9***	<0.5***
Cholesterol (nmol/min per 100 g)	4.20±1.6	4.43±2.60	0.29±0.16***
Glutathione (nmol/min per 100 g)	90±45	142±35	13±7**
Bile flow (µl/min per 100 g)	8.3±2.3	10.1±1.9	15.7±2.7***

Bile was collected for 15 min directly after canulation of the gallbladder. Data represent means±SD of at least five animals of each strain. Data of (+/−) and (−/−) were compared with controls (+/+) in a Student's *t*-test: *$p<0.05$; **$p<0.01$; ***$p<0.001$

collected within the first 15 min after canulation of the gallbladder. Bile flow was significantly increased in the homozygous knock-outs. There was no significant effect of *mdr2* gene disruption on the secretion of bilirubin and, if anything, bile salt secretion appeared to be increased in the knock-outs. The latter phenomenon can be attributed to an enlarged bile salt pool in (−/−) as compared to (+/+) mice. The most striking change in bile composition concerned the lipids: cholesterol secretion was almost 15-fold decreased while the phospholipid content was below the detection limit. Finally glutathione secretion was strongly decreased in (−/−) mice. Thus, the secretion of several of the main components of bile was affected by the absence of a functional *mdr2* Pgp. In order to resolve which of these changes represented the primary defect we also analysed the bile composition of (+/−) mice. In Table 1 it can be seen that none of the components is significantly different in heterozygotes except phospholipid secretion, which was decreased to 60% of the control level[4]. These results suggested, quite unexpectedly, that *mdr2* Pgp plays an important role in the secretion of phospholipids into bile. It is our hypothesis that *mdr2* Pgp functions as a primary active flippase in the translocation of phosphatidylcholine from the inner to the outer leaflet of the canalicular membrane. Very recently, Ruetz and Gros provided evidence which supports this hypothesis[5]. They transfected the *mdr2* gene into a yeast mutant which has a defect in the secretory apparatus. This mutation leads to the accumulation of plasma membrane proteins in secretory vesicles. After isolation these vesicles were used to demonstrate translocation of fluorescent NBD-PC. They, indeed, observed mdr2 Pgp mediated translocation which was ATP-dependent.

RELATION BETWEEN BILE SALT AND PHOSPHOLIPID SECRETION

Thus far it has been generally accepted that phospholipid secretion is predominantly if not exclusively regulated by the secretion of bile salts. In many studies a clear-cut correlation has been observed between the secretion rate of bile salts and biliary lipids[6]. Because of the detergent activity of the micellar bile salt concentrations in the canaliculus it is generally assumed that bile salts exert their main regulatory function at this level. We have investigated the relation between bile salt and phospholipid secretion in normal (+/+), heterozygous (+/−)

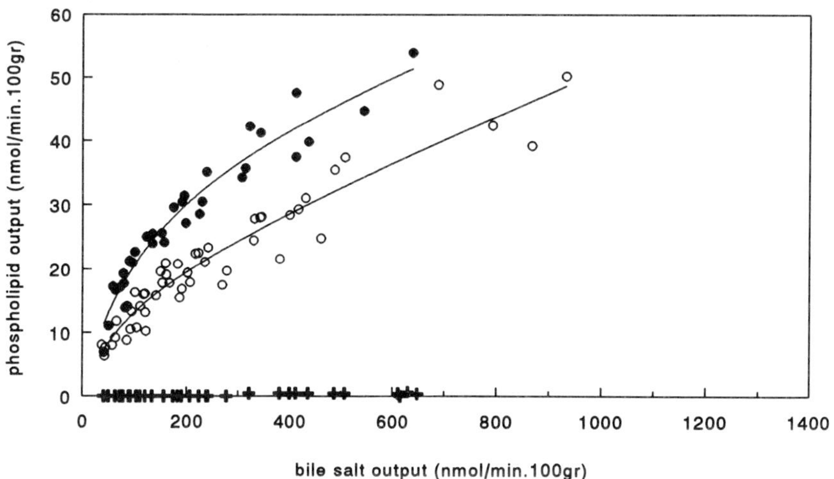

Fig. 1 Relation between phospholipid and bile salt secretion in various mouse genotypes. Mice were canulated in the gallbladder and bile was collected at 10 min periods for 2 h. Due to interruption of the enterohepatic cycling bile salt and phospholipid secretion displayed a time-dependent decrease. For each sample phospholipid secretion was plotted against bile salt secretion. Data represent all separate measurements from six animals of each strain. ●, (+/+) mice; ○, (+/−) mice; +, (−/−) mice

and homozygous (−/−) *mdr2* knock-out mice in order to further delineate the role of *mdr2* Pgp. To this end the gallbladder of the different mice was canulated and bile was collected during different time intervals. Because after canulation the enterohepatic circulation has been interrupted, a time-dependent depletion of the bile salt pool is achieved and lipid secretion can be monitored at different, decreasing, bile salt secretion rates. Figure 1 shows the relation between bile salt secretion and phospholipid secretion that was obtained in these experiments. It is clear that both in the (+/+) and the (+/−) mice a typical curvilinear relation was found, similar to that reported in other species such as the rat, dog and humans[6]. However, at all bile salt output rates phospholipid secretion in (+/−) was lower than in (+/+) mice. At low bile salt secretion rates phospholipid secretion was about 50% of normal, while at the higher rates phospholipid secretion relatively increased to 80% of (+/+). At all bile salt output rates phospholipid secretion in the (−/−) mice was extremely low or absent (<0.5 nmol/min per 100 g). Both in (+/+) and (+/−) mice a linear increase in phospholipid secretion was observed at higher bile salt secretion rates. Curve-fitting of these data using an equation with a hyperbolic term and a linear term produced a good fit with the maximum of the hyperbolic term in (+/−) mice that was 50% of the maximum in (+/+) mice. The fit predicted, however, that the slope of the linear fraction, which becomes particularly relevant at higher bile salt secretion rates, is identical in (+/+) and (+/−) mice. This suggests that at high bile salt secretion rates part of the phospholipid secretion is *mdr2* Pgp-independent. In addition, this fraction of phospholipid secretion does seem to be linearly dependent on the bile salt secretion rate. Therefore, it might represent phospholipids that are directly extracted from the canalicular membrane by the action of bile salt micelles. In contrast with this model stands the observation that phospholipid secretion is completely absent in (–/–) mice, including the linear fraction. This indicates that extraction by bile salt micelles directly from the canalicular membrane does not occur in (–/–) animals. We have analysed the endogenous bile salt composition in all three mouse genotypes and this was identical. This analysis revealed that the majority of the bile salts in mice consists of muricholate (60–70%), the remainder being almost exclusively taurocholate. Since muricholate is a very hydrophilic bile salt, possible aspecific extraction of phospholipid may be relatively unimportant.

In order to test this model we have infused bile salts of different hydrophobicity into mice of the three genotypes and analysed the dependence of phospholipid secretion on bile salt secretion. Figure 2A shows such an experiment in which taurocholate was infused at increasing rates. After an initial decline, both bile salt and phospholipid secretion increase due to the infusion of taurocholate. At high infusion rates a stable bile salt secretion rate was obtained which was considerably lower than the infusion rate, suggesting that the maximum secretion rate for this bile salt was reached. When maximal taurocholate secretion is reached, phospholipid secretion starts to decline both in (+/+) and (+/–) mice. At all bile salt secretion rates phospholipid secretion remained lower in (+/–) mice than in (+/+) mice and was almost completely absent in (–/–) mice. Analysis of the bile salt composition at the end of the infusion demonstrated that >95% of the bile salts consisted of taurocholate in all genotypes. In Fig. 2B phospholipid secretion was plotted against bile salt secretion. The maximum in (+/–) was 65% of that in (+/+). These data suggest that when phospholipid secretion is driven by taurocholate there is little, if any, Pgp-independent phospholipid secretion, which argues against aspecific extraction of phospholipid from the membrane by bile salt micelles. The typical curve in this figure is caused by the induction of cholestasis due to supramaximal infusion rates of taurocholate. When maximal taurocholate secretion is reached both bile salt and phospholipid secretion start to decline.

In a subsequent experiment the more hydrophobic taurochenodeoxycholate (TCDC) was infused at increasing rates. Figure 3 shows that in both (+/+) and (+/–) mice cholestasis sets in fairly rapidly upon infusion of this bile salt. Surprisingly, the decrease of bile salt secretion was similar in (+/+) and (–/–) mice, indicating that (–/–) mice are not more sensitive for hydrophobic bile salt than (+/+) mice. Importantly, infusion of TCDC did not lead to any significant secretion of phospholipids in (–/–) mice. At the end of the infusion period >45% of the secreted bile salts consisted of TCDC, the remainder being muricholate (45%) and cholate (10%). Because TCDC led to the rapid development of cholestasis, plotting phospholipid against bile salts did not create a clear picture. Figure 3, however, clearly shows that with TCDC infusion maximal phospholipid in (+/–) was still substantially reduced compared to (+/+). In this experiment the difference was, however, not significant, due to the large variation in both genotypes. The latter phenomenon was largely caused by the fact that some animals developed cholestasis rapidly, while others demonstrated a prolonged secretion of bile. The absence of phospholipid secretion in (–/–) and the reduction in (+/–) also strongly suggests that TCDC is not capable of aspecific extraction of phospholipids from the canalicular membrane.

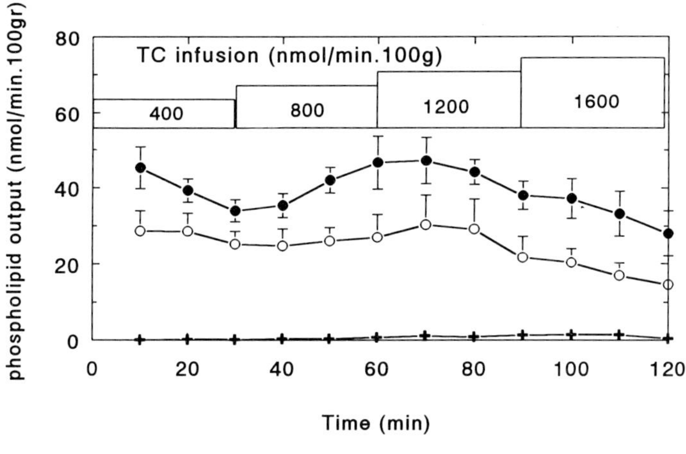

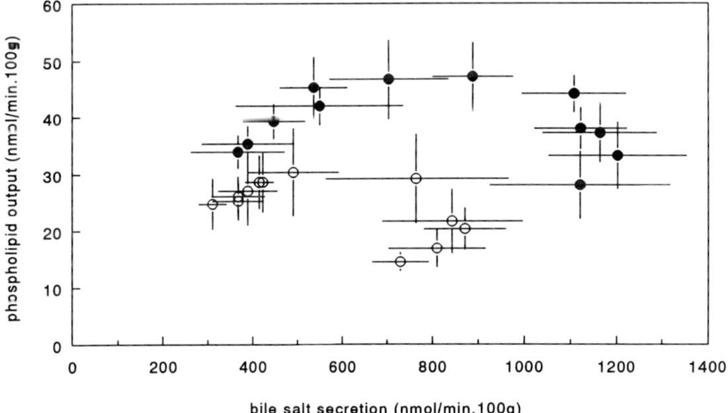

Fig. 2 Phospholipid secretion during i.v. infusion of increasing doses of taurocholate. Mice were canulated in the gallbladder and, directly after starting bile collection, taurocholate was infused into the tail vein at the indicated rate. ●, (+/+) mice; ○, (+/−) mice; +, (−/−) mice. Panel A: phospholipid secretion in time; panel B: relation between phospholipid and bile salt secretion. Data represent averages ± SD from three mice of each strain

In conclusion, our results demonstrate that in the absence of *mdr2* Pgp expression no significant phospholipid secretion can be observed, even when the secreted bile salts are of a hydrophobic type. This suggests that there is little, if any, aspecific extraction of phospholipids from the canalicular membrane by bile salt micelles. It is our hypothesis that the outer leaflet of the canalicular membrane is highly resistant towards bile salt micelles, and that *mdr2* Pgp-mediated translocation of phosphatidylcholine is an obligatory step in the overall process of phospholipid secretion. After translocation of phosphatidylcholine to the outer leaflet, bile salt (micelles) may act to catalyse the release of this phospholipid into the canalicular lumen. The mechanism of this latter step is still poorly understood.

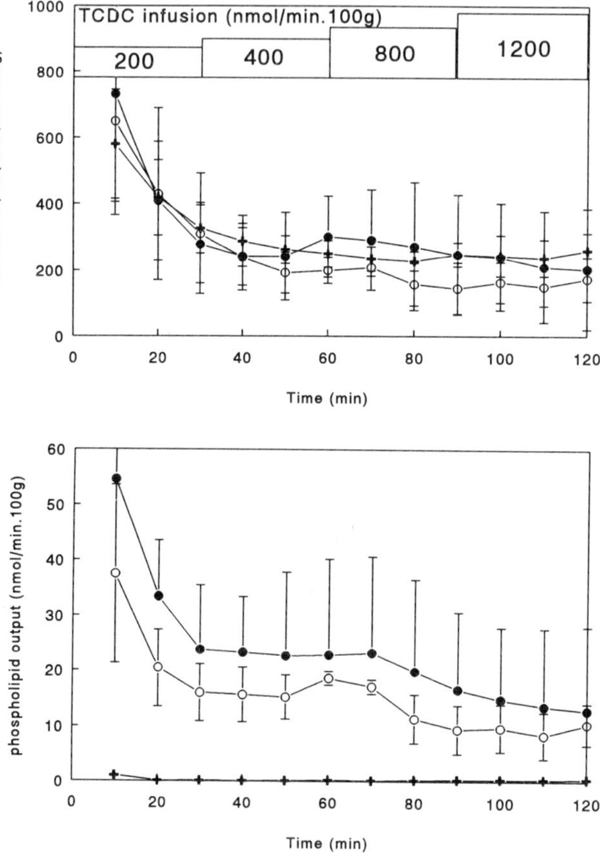

Fig. 3 Bile salt and phospholipid secretion during i.v. infusion of increasing amounts of taurochenodeoxycholate. Mice were canulated in the gallbladder, and directly after starting bile collection taurocholate was infused into the tail vein at the indicated rate. ●, (+/+) mice; ○, (+/−); mice +, (−/−) mice. Panel A: bile salt secretion in time; panel B: phospholipid secretion in time. Data represent averages ± SD from three mice of each strain

References

1. Gottesman MM, Pastan I. Biochemistry of multidrug resistance mediated by the multidrug transporter. Annu Rev Biochem. 1993;284:278–84.
2. van der Bliek AM, Baas F, ten Houte de Lange T, Kooiman PM, van der Velde Koerts T, Borst P. The human MDR3 gene encodes a novel P-glycoprotein homologue and gives rise to alternative spliced mRNAs in liver. EMBO J. 1987;6:3325–31.
3. Buschman E, Arceci RJ, Croop JM, Che MX, Arias IM, Housman DE, Gros P. mdr2 encodes P-glycoprotein expressed in the bile canalicular membrane as determined by isoform-specific antibodies. J Biol Chem. 1992;267:18093–9.
4. Smit JJM, Schinkel AH, Oude Elferink RPJ, Groen AK, Wagenaar E, Van Deemter L, Mol CAAM, Ottenhoff R, Van der Lugt NMT, van Roon MA, Van der Valk MA, Offerhaus GJA, Berns AJM, Borst P. Homozygous disruption of the murine mdr2 P-glycoprotein gene leads to a complete absence of phospholipid from bile and to liver disease. Cell. 1993;75:451–62.
5. Ruetz S, Gros P. Phosphatidylcholine translocase: a physiological role for the mdr2 gene. Cell. 1994;77:1071–82.
6. Mazer NA, Carey MC. Mathematical model of biliary lipid secretion: a quantitative analysis of physiological and biochemical data from man and other species. J Lipid Res. 1984;25:932–53.

25
Hepatocellular secretion of biliary lipid: bile salt-induced vesiculation of the canalicular membrane outer leaflet

J. M. CRAWFORD, A. R. CRAWFORD, V. C. HATCH,
R. C. STEARNS, S. BARNES and J. J. GODLESKI

INTRODUCTION

Previous physical studies of bile suggest that biliary lipid is secreted as vesicles into the bile canalicular lumen[1,2]. Direct visualization of this process has not been achieved, and the mechanism by which vesicles enter bile from hepatocytes remains unknown. In this study, ultrarapid cryofixation of rat liver tissue *in situ* was performed to evaluate whether biliary lipid is secreted from the hepatocyte canalicular plasma membrane as vesicles.

METHODS

Adult male Sprague-Dawley rats (268 ± 7 g, $\pm$SD; $n=8$) were allowed access to rat chow and water *ad libitum* up to the time of sacrifice. A control rat was used without experimental manipulation. A bile salt-depleted rat was prepared[3] by overnight biliary diversion, following surgical placement of biliary and intravenous catheters and maintenance of hydration with an intravenous infusion of saline at 1.5 ml/h. Six other bile salt-depleted animals were reinfused 1 h with 200 nmol/min per 100 g of selected bile salts, listed in order of increasing hydrophobicity: taurodehydrocholate (TDHC), tauroursocholate (TUC), tauromuricholate (TMC, α/β mixture), tauroursodeoxycholate (TUDC), taurocholate (TC), and taurochenodeoxycholate (TCDC).

Animals were anaesthetized with sodium pentobarbital (50 mg/kg i.p.). The abdomen of each rat was opened, and *in situ* cryofixation of a freshly cut liver surface was performed using the DDK PS1000™ device (Delaware Diamond Knives, Inc., Newark, DE). In this manner, an ~3 mm diameter area by 30 μm deep portion of liver parenchyma was brought to $-185°$C with sufficient rapidity

"

to enable vitrification of the liver tissue. Cryofixed liver tissue was freeze-dried and stabilized with paraformaldehyde and osmium tetroxide vapour, using the LifeCell® MDD-C Molecular Distillation Dryer[4]. Following permeation with degassed Araldite 502 resin and polymerization, 50 nm thin sections were cut and examined in the Zeiss CEM902 electron microscope.

RESULTS AND DISCUSSION

On average, 27 ± 7 well-preserved bile canaliculi were observed in liver tissue from each rat ($\pm$SD, $n=216$ total). All structural profiles within the canaliculi were measured morphometrically ($n=2650$ total). A distinct population of vesicles with electron-lucent interiors ($n=318$) was observed, adherent to the outer leaflet of the canalicular membrane ($n=234$) or free within the canalicular lumen ($n=84$). Vesicles were 67 ± 13 nm in mean diameter ($\pm$SD), with no significant differences in size between animals or between adherent and free groups. Their size matched that predicted by light-scattering[5], and average vesicle numbers (one to three per bile canaliculus in those animals secreting physiological bile salts) roughly matched those predicted by phospholipid secretion rates. The percentage area occupied by vesicles in each set of bile canaliculi was measured morphometrically. In depleted and TDHC rats, which exhibited low rates of phospholipid secretion, the percentage area was $0.1 \pm 0.1\%$ and $0.2 \pm 0.1\%$, respectively. Vesicular percentage area was over 10-fold greater ($p < 0.02$) in animals secreting phospholipid at physiological rates: namely control ($2.4 \pm 0.9\%$), TUC ($1.8 \pm 0.6\%$), TMC ($2.5 \pm 0.6\%$), TUDC ($1.7 \pm 0.8\%$), TC ($2.4 \pm .6\%$), and TCDC ($1.9 \pm 0.4\%$) infused rats.

Microvilli ($n - 1944$) were identified as elongated structures having a delimiting membrane in continuity with the canalicular plasma membrane, and a faint electron-dense core in continuity with the cytoplasm. Microvilli measured 73 ± 20 nm in width by 151 ± 72 nm in length. A third group of profiles was designated as uncertain ($n=388$), since it was not clear whether they represented microvilli cut in cross-section or true vesicles. Among the eight animals the numbers of uncertain structures generally paralleled the numbers of microvilli, suggesting that the predominant structures in this group were microvilli cut in cross-section.

Our findings demonstrate that lipid is secreted into the bile canaliculus as vesicles ~67 nm in diameter. Vesicles are largely absent from animals with low phospholipid secretion rates (bile salt-depleted and TDHC), and are more abundant in control animals and those infused with bile salts that promote phospholipid secretion (TUC, TMC, TUDC, TC and TCDC). Our data suggest that biliary lipid is secreted from hepatocytes via vesiculation of the exoplasmic hemileaflet of the canalicular plasma membrane, and that this secretion mechanism is sufficient to account for all phospholipid present in bile.

Acknowledgements

Thanks are given to Rebecca C. Stearns and Caroline Snowman for their expert technical assistance. Special acknowledgement is given to the late Dr Gotthold-

Matthias Möckel, whose unpublished work with Drs Susan J. Hagen and Martin C. Carey provided the initial impetus for these ultrastructural studies. These experiments were supported by NIH grants DK-44981 and DK-39512 (J.M.C.). Experiments were conducted according to the principles set forth in the 'Guide for the Care and Use of Laboratory Animals', Institute of Animal Resources, National Research Council.

References

1. Möckel G-M, Gorti S, Tanaka T, Carey MC. Microscope laser light scattering of bile formation [abstract]. Hepatology. 1988;8:1367A.
2. Cohen DE, Angelico M, Carey MC. Quasielastic light scattering evidence for vesicular secretion of biliary lipids. Am J Physiol. 1989;257:G1–8.
3. Crawford JM, Crawford AR, Strahs DCJ. Microtubule-dependent transport of bile salts through hepatocytes: cholic vs. taurocholic acid. Hepatology. 1993;18:903–11.
4. Crawford JM, Barnes S, Stearns RC, Hastings CL, Godleski JJ. Ultrastructural localization of a fluorinated bile salt in hepatocytes. Lab Invest. 1994;71:42–51.
5. Cohen DE, Leighton LS, Carey MC. Bile salt hydrophobicity controls vesicle secretion rates and transformations in native bile. Am J Physiol. 1992;263:G386–95.

26
Antroduodenal and gallbladder motility in primary sclerosing cholangitis: effect of ursodeoxycholic acid

P. C. VAN DE MEEBERG, F. H. J. WOLFHAGEN, P. PORTINCASA,
M. F. J. STOLK, L. M. A. AKKERMANS, A. J. P. M. SMOUT,
K. J. VAN ERPECUM and G. P. VAN BERGE HENEGOUWEN

INTRODUCTION

The motility of the digestive tract can be divided into a postprandial and an interdigestive pattern. The interdigestive motility, characterized by the 'migrating motor complex' (MMC), consists of three phases: phase I or total motor quiescence; phase II showing a pattern of irregular motor activity; and phase III, a short period of maximal activity, followed by phase I again. In humans the mean MMC cycle length is about 90 min[1]. Several studies suggest an important role for bile in the maintenance of normal interdigestive motility[2]. Diversion of the bile flow leads to a disruption of the MMC in animals, leading to an irregular (phase II-like) pattern[3-6] and a tendency to bacterial overgrowth[7]. Recently we showed a similar disrupted MMC pattern in patients with obstructive jaundice due to pancreatic head cancer[8].

Other studies have shown the existence of a negative feedback mechanism between intraduodenal bile salts and the release of cholecystokinin (CCK)[9]. Furthermore, a combined study with the bile salt resin cholestyramine and the CCK antagonist loxiglumide has shown that this mechanism also affects gallbladder motility[10]. Therefore, interruption of the enterohepatic circulation may lead to changes in gallbladder motility.

Although the enterohepatic circulation is not interrupted it may be expected that patients with primary sclerosing cholangitis (PSC) have an impaired secretion of bile and a subsequent decreased availability of intraduodenal bile salts. This in turn may alter the gallbladder and interdigestive intestinal motility. We therefore decided to study antroduodenal and gallbladder motility and the effect of bile salt repletion with ursodeoxycholic acid (UDCA) in patients with PSC.

MATERIAL AND METHODS

Ambulatory antroduodenal manometry was performed in eight PSC patients (mean age 37.2 ± 11.9 (years $\pm$ SEM), M/F ratio 6/2) and in 10 age- and sex-matched healthy controls. Liver biopsy revealed early-stage disease (stage I–II) in four and late stage disease (stage III–IV) in the other four patients. Endoscopic retrograde cholangiopancreatography (ERCP) showed intrahepatic lesions in four and both intra- and extrahepatic lesions in the other four patients. Patients who had biliary surgery or a colectomy, and patients being classified as Child C according to the Child–Pugh classification, were not included in this part of the study.

Manometry was performed using a six-channel solid-state catheter (Gaeltec, Scotland) being connected to a portable data logger (MMS, The Netherlands). Three transducers were placed in the duodenum and three in the antrum. After ingestion of a standard hot meal all patients remained fasting for the following 18 h. The position of the catheter was verified with fluoroscopy at the beginning and end of the study. The experiment was repeated after 1 month treatment with UDCA ($10 \ \mathrm{mg \, kg^{-1} \, day^{-1}}$).

Twenty-six patients were available for measurement of gallbladder motility. Patients who had thickening of the gallbladder wall of more than 3 mm ($n=3$) or a shrunk (volume <10 ml) gallbladder ($n=1$) were excluded. In three other patients measurement of the gallbladder volume was impossible because the gallbladder could not be entirely visualized. Fasting and postprandial gallbladder volumes were measured in 19 PSC patients (mean age 34.7 ± 8.5 (years $\pm$ SEM), M/F ratio 12/7) and in 20 age- and sex-matched healthy controls. Nine patients with PBC with biochemical cholestasis and eight patients with liver cirrhosis due to other causes (alcohol abuse, autoimmune hepatitis) served as a separate control group. Fasting gallbladder volumes were measured ultrasonographically using the sum of cylinders method[11]. All patients received a standard meal (2800 kJ) containing an egg, cheese, a slice of bread, butter, and sweetened yogurt. Postprandial volumes were measured for a period of 2 h every 10 min. The experiment was repeated after 1 month treatment with UDCA ($10 \ \mathrm{mg \, kg^{-1} \, day^{-1}}$).

RESULTS

The results of the antroduodenal motility study are shown in Table 1. Cycle length was 102.6 ± 8.2 min in the PSC group compared to a mean cycle length of 85.7 ± 7.7 min in the control group ($p=$ n.s.). At the level of the proximal duodenum phase I, II and III accounted for 37.5 ± 5.6 min, 60.1 ± 9.8 min and 5.0 ± 0.4 min in the PSC patients and 46.6 ± 5.7 min, 33.3 ± 5.4 min and 5.8 ± 0.5 min in the control group. An increase in cycle length in the PSC group was due to a significantly longer phase II ($p<0.05$). We were not able to show a difference between early-stage disease and late-stage disease patients. All parameters remained in the same range during treatment with UDCA.

The results of the gallbladder motility study are shown in Table 2. The fasting gallbladder volume in the PSC patients, 82.1 ± 16.4 ml, was much larger than in any of the three control groups: healthy controls: 26.3 ± 1.9 ml, PBC: 29.8 ± 4.8 ml, liver cirrhosis: 20.6 ± 1.6 ml ($p<0.02$). Two patients had a gallbladder volume

Table 1 Studies on antroduodenal motility

Parameter	PSC without UDCA	PSC during UDCA	Control
MMC cycle length (min)	102.0±8.2	108.2±5.8	85.7±7.7
Phase I (min)	37.5±5.6	47.0±5.8	46.6±5.7
Phase II (min)	60.1±9.8*	55.7±4.7	33.3±5.4
Phase II (min)	5.0±0.4	5.3±0.3	5.8±0.5

*$p<0.05$ vs. control (unpaired t-test)

Table 2 Studies on gallbladder motility

Parameter	PSC without UDCA	PSC during UDCA	Controls	PBC	Cirrhosis
Number of patients	19	12	19	9	8
Fasting volume (ml)	82.1±16.4*	92.5±13.2*	26.3±1.9	29.8±4.8	20.6±1.6
Residual volume (ml)	14.0±4.4**	22.3±6.2	3.4±0.7	6.3±2.0	Not measured
Ejection fraction (%)	82.9	75.9	87.1	78.9	Not measured

*$p<0.02$ vs controls, PBC and cirrhotic patients (ANOVA); **$p<0.05$ vs controls (ANOVA)

larger than 200 ml. All patients showed a rapid emptying of the gallbladder in response to the meal. The residual gallbladder volume in PSC patients (14.0±4.4 ml) was significantly enlarged compared to healthy controls (3.4±0.7 ml, $p<0.05$), but not compared to PBC patients (6.3±2.0 ml). Paired measurements of fasting and residual gallbladder volume before and during UDCA treatment was done in 12 patients. No significant changes were seen in either fasting or residual volume. There appeared to be no significant relation between gallbladder volume and disease stage or the extent of common bile duct (CBD) lesions.

DISCUSSION

Although it can be expected that PSC patients have a decreased bile secretion we were not able to demonstrate major disturbances of interdigestive motility at the antroduodenal level. The MMC cycle length was slightly longer in PSC patients due to a significantly longer phase II. No relation was found in our data with the stage of the disease. However, since patients with a Child C classification were excluded, it cannot be ruled out that the motility pattern is further disrupted during end-stage disease. UDCA therapy did not influence MMC cycle length or the length of the different phases.

PSC patients appeared to have larger gallbladders than patients with PBC, liver cirrhosis due to other causes or healthy controls. Although some studies have been performed on gallbladder abnormalities in PSC, to our knowledge this finding has never been reported before[12–15]. Three patients were excluded because they had a thickened gallbladder wall without the presence of gallstones or portal hypertension. This finding has been reported previously to be associated with PSC, and might be the result of a PSC-like inflammation of the gallbladder itself[12].

The residual gallbladder volume also appeared to be significantly enlarged if compared with healthy controls. However, PSC patients and healthy controls had a similar ejection fraction (83% vs. 87% of fasting gallbladder volume) indicating normal gallbladder emptying in PSC patients. Although treatment with UDCA increased the fasting gallbladder volume in PSC patients, as has been reported previously in gallstone patients[16], this did not reach significance.

A clear explanation for gallbladder enlargement in PSC cannot be derived from our data. An outlet obstruction due to strictures in the CBD seems not to be the reason, since we were not able to show a relation between gallbladder volume and the presence of lesions in the CBD. For example the patient with the largest gallbladder has no strictures in the CBD distally from the cystic duct on ERCP. Another patient with a very large gallbladder and a distal CBD stenosis appeared to have the same gallbladder volume after an endoprosthesis had been inserted. A strong argument against the hypothesis of mechanical obstruction is the fact that virtually all patients are capable of emptying the gallbladder rapidly in response to a meal. Other possible explanations are currently being studied by our group.

Ultrasonography of the biliary tract is a common and easy procedure in the work-up of cholestatic liver disease. Since gallbladder volume can be reliably calculated, we believe that gallbladder ultrasound might be a useful tool for screening purposes, especially in patients with ulcerative colitis who are at risk for PSC.

References

1. Rees WDW, Malagelada J, Miller LJ, Go VLW. Human interdigestive and postprandial gastrointestinal motor and gastrointestinal hormone patterns. Dig Dis Sci. 1982;27:321−9.
2. Peeters TL. Bile acids and small intestinal motility during fasting. Acta Gastroenterol Belg. 1988;51:509−15.
3. Nilsson I, Svenberg T, Wallin B, Hedenborg G, Hellström PM. Activity fronts of migrating myoelectric complex: initiation by luminal bile acids in rat small intestine. J Gastroenterol Motil. 1991;3:84−91.
4. Plourde V, Trudel L, Poitras P. Interdigestive intestinal motility in dogs with chronic exclusion of bile from the digestive tract. Can J Physiol Pharmacol. 1987;65:2493−6.
5. Li YF, Newton TJ, Weisbrodt NW, Moody FG. Intestinal migrating myoelectric complexes in rats with acute pancreatitis and bile duct ligation. J Surg Res. 1993;55:182−7.
6. Ozeki K, Sarna SK, Condon RE, Chey WY, Koch TR. Enterohepatic circulation is essential for regular cycling of duodenal migrating motor complexes in dogs. Gastroenterology. 1992;103:759−67.
7. Haagh WAJJM, Verheem A, Akkermans LMA, Visser MR, Obertop H. Does disturbed gastrointestinal motility play a role in the pathophysiology of infective complications in biliary obstruction? Gastroenterology. 1994;106:A340.
8. Haagh WAJJM, Akkermans LMA, Stolk MFJ, Van Erpecum KJ, Obertop H. Disturbed gastric emptying and interdigestive motility in pancreatic and periampullary cancer patients is associated with biliary obstruction. Gastroenterology. 1993;104:A362.
9. Green GM. Feedback inhibition of cholecystokinin secretion by bile acids and pancreatic proteases. Ann NY Acad Sci. 1994;713:167−79.
10. Palasciano G, Portincasa P, Belfiore A, Baldassarre G, Albano O. Opposite effects of cholestyramine and loxiglumide on gallbladder dynamics in humans. Gastroenterology. 1992;102:633−9.
11. Everson GT, Breverman DZ, Johnson ML, Kern F. A critical evaluation for the study of gallbladder volume and contraction. Gastroenterology. 1980;79:40−6.

12. Brandt DJ, MacCarty RL, Charboneau JW, Larusso NF, Wiesner RH, Ludwig J. Gallbladder disease in patients with primary sclerosing cholangitis. AJR. 1988;150:572–4.
13. MacCarty RL, Larusso NF, Wiesner RH, Ludwig J. Primary sclerosing cholangitis: findings on cholangiography and pancreatography. Radiology. 1983;149:39–44.
14. Doyle TC, Roberts-Thomson IC. Radiologic features of sclerosing cholangitis. Australas Radiol. 1983;27:163–6.
15. LaRusso NF. Sclerosing cholangitis and gallstones. Contemp Issues Gastroenterol. 1985;4:231–6.
16. Festi D, Frabboni R, Bazzoli F *et al*. Gallbladder motility in cholesterol gallstone disease: effect of ursodeoxycholic acid administration and gallstone dissolution. Gastroenterology. 1990;99:1779–85.

27
Ursodeoxycholylsarcosine inhibits intestinal cholesterol absorption in rats with intact enterohepatic circulation

XIAO-LIN WANG, QI CHEN, A. F. HOFMANN and P. TSO

INTRODUCTION

Ursodeoxycholic acid is used to treat cholesterol gallstone disease because it decreases cholesterol secretion in bile[1-4]. Cholylsarcosine (the synthetic N-acyl conjugate of cholic acid with sarcosine [N-methylglycine]) is a synthetic conjugate of cholic acid and sarcosine, and has properties similar to natural bile acid conjugates, but is resistant to deconjugation and dehydroxylation. Cholylsarcosine has been demonstrated to be useful for the treatment of fat malabsorption caused by severe bile acid malabsorption in the dog[5]. Ursodeoxycholylsarcosine (UDC-sar) is a synthetic conjugate of ursodeoxycholic acid and sarcosine. In bile fistula rats we demonstrated previously that UDC-sar significantly inhibits the intestinal uptake and lymphatic transport of cholesterol, but not of fatty acids[6]. Since bile was diverted in these rats, we did not know if UDC-sar would still inhibit the intestinal uptake and lymphatic transport of cholesterol in rats with intact enterohepatic circulation of bile salts. The aim of this study was to compare the effect of UDC-sar with that of taurocholate (cholyltaurine, C-tau) on the absorption and transport of triglyceride and cholesterol by the rat small intestine.

METHODS

Surgery

Male Sprague–Dawley rats (300–350 g), fed normal Purina rat chow were used. These animals were fasted overnight before the operation. Under halothane anaesthesia the major intestinal lymph duct lying just superior to the superior mesenteric artery was canulated according to the procedures described by

Bollman *et al.*[7], except that the canula was secured by the application of a drop of Eastman Kodak 910 glue, instead of a suture. The lymph canula was primed with a heparin sodium solution (1000 units/ml) to prevent clotting. A silicone tube (2.2 mm o.d.) was then passed through the fundus of the stomach and extended 2.0 cm into the duodenum. The fundal incision was closed using a purse-string suture. Postoperatively, the animals were infused with a 5% dextrose saline solution (145 mmol/l NaCl, 4 mmol/l KCl, and 0.28 mol/l dextrose) at a constant rate of 3.0 ml/h. The animals were allowed to recover for at least 36 h in restraining cages maintained at a temperature of approximately 30°C before lipid infusion.

Experimental plan

Two groups of lymph fistula rats ($n=6$ in each group) were used in this experiment. On the day of infusion the saline–glucose infusion in the UDC-sar animals was replaced by a lipid emulsion infused at a rate of 3.0 ml/h for 8 h. The emulsion consisted of 40 μmol of glycerol trioleate (labelled with glyceryl [^{3}H]trioleate), 7.8 μmol of phosphatidylcholine (PC), 7.8 μmol of cholesterol (labelled with [^{14}C]cholesterol) and 45 μmol of UDC-sar in 3.0 ml of phosphate-buffered saline (PBS). The PBS (pH 6.4) was composed of 6.75 mmol/l Na$_2$HPO$_4$, 16.5 mmol/l NaH$_2$PO$_4$, 115 mmol/l NaCl, and 5 mmol/l KCl. The C-tau animals were infused with a different lipid emulsion of the same composition but the UDC-sar was replaced by C-tau. Lymph was collected for 1 h prior to lipid infusion and served as the fasting lymph. At the onset of lipid infusion, lymph was collected every 2 h during the first 4 h and then hourly for the remaining 4 h. After the lymph volume was determined, the samples were centrifuged for 15 min at 1500 rpm at room temperature to remove blood cells. Aliquots of lymph were also taken for radioactivity determination by scintillation spectrometry.

Collection of luminal contents

At the termination of lipid infusion, at which time there was a steady lipid output, the rats were anaesthetized with ethrane and sacrificed by exanguination. The small intestine was removed, placed over ice, and divided into four equal segments. Each segment was washed thoroughly with three separate washings of 3.0 ml each of 10 mmol/l sodium taurocholate in normal saline, and the washings combined in preweighed conical test tubes. The caecum and large intestine were extracted, opened longitudinally, and washed three times with 10 mmol/l sodium taurocholate. These washings, along with any faeces passed during the infusion period, were combined. The volumes were recorded for all the separate collections of washings. The samples were then homogenized briefly with a Polytron homogenizer, and two aliquots from each luminal sample were taken for radioactivity determination and the values averaged.

Materials

Glyceryl[^{3}H]trioleate and [^{14}C]cholesterol were purchased from New England Nuclear Research Products, Boston, MA. Glycerol trioleate and cholesterol were

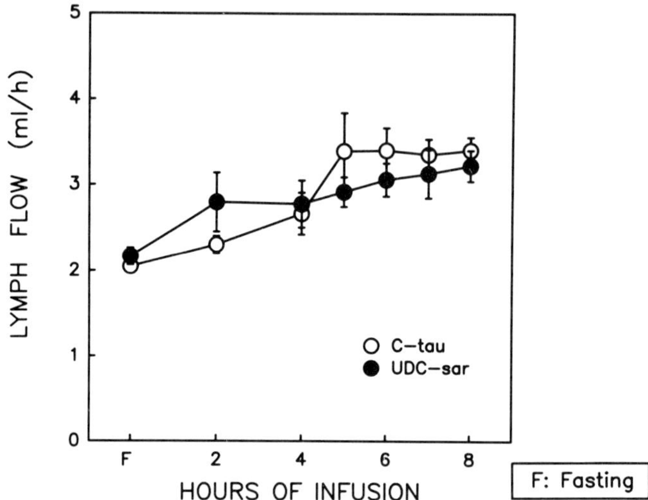

Fig. 1 Intestinal lymph flow. Intestinal lymph flow was measured in ml/h before lipid infusion (fasting), then every 2 h during the first 4 h of lipid infusion and then hourly for the subsequent 4 h of lipid infusion. Each group consisted of six animals, and the values are expressed as mean ± SE

supplied by Sigma Chemical Co. (St Louis, MO) and were used without further purification. UDC-sar was synthesized by the method of Tserng et al.[8]. Egg PC and sodium taurocholate were purchased from Sigma Chemical Co. and were used without further purification. All solvents and reagents used were of analytical grade.

RESULTS

Lymph flow

The fasting lymph flow of both the UDC-sar and C-tau animals was between 2.0 and 2.2 ml/h (Fig. 1). After lipid infusion the lymph flow increased to between 3.3 and 3.7 ml/ by the 7th hour of lipid infusion in both groups of rats. None of the differences in lymph flow rates among the two groups was statistically significant.

Lymphatic radioactive triglyceride output

As shown in Fig. 2, the lymphatic radioactive triglyceride output was expressed as a percentage of the hourly infused dose. Both groups reached a steady lymph radioactive lipid output by the 6th hour of lipid infusion, with both the UDC-sar and C-tau rats transporting about 85% of the hourly infused dose into lymph.

Luminal recovery of radioactive triglyceride

Since labelled triolein was used in this study, the amount of the infused radioactive lipid remaining in the luminal content at the end of 8 h of lipid

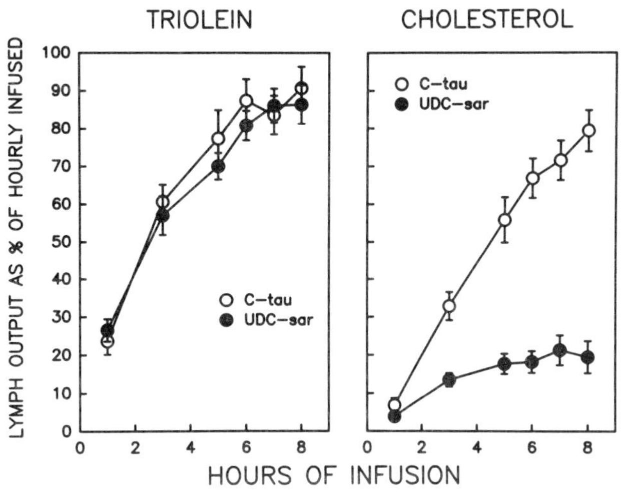

Fig. 2 Lymph radioactive lipid output. Lymph radioactive lipid output is expressed as a percentage of the radioactive lipid infused per hour. On the left is the radioactive triolein output and on the right is cholesterol output. Six animals were used for each group and the values are expressed as mean ± SE

infusion could be determined. There was no significant difference (about 5% of total infused dose) in the amount of radioactive triolein remaining in the gastrointestinal tract of the two groups of rats at the end of 8 h of lipid infusion.

Lymphatic radioactive cholesterol output

As shown in Fig. 2, there was a significant difference in the amount of radioactive cholesterol transported into lymph between the two groups of rats. The lymphatic radioactive cholesterol output was significantly lower in the UDC-sar rats than the C-tau rats during the entire 8 h of lipid infusion ($p < 0.05$) with the exception of the first 2 h.

Luminal recovery of radioactive cholesterol

The markedly suppressed lymphatic cholesterol transport in the UDC-sar rats was accompanied by a significant increase in the luminal recovery of radioactive cholesterol than the C-tau rats. Most of the radioactive cholesterol infused in the UDC-sar rats was recovered in the lumen of the gastrointestinal tract, indicating that the uptake of cholesterol was markedly inhibited by the presence of UDC-sar.

DISCUSSION

This study clearly demonstrates that UDC-sar and C-tau are equally effective in promoting the uptake and lymphatic transport of the fatty acids from triolein. In contrast, the uptake and lymphatic transport of cholesterol are markedly inhibited by UDC-sar as compared to C-tau. This is an important observation, because the animals had intact enterohepatic circulation of endogenous bile salts and yet UDC-sar still managed to inhibit the uptake and the lymphatic transport of cholesterol. Although not tested in this study, we have demonstrated previously that this unique property of UDC-sar is related to the UDC moiety because glycine or taurine conjugates of UDC were equally effective in inhibiting cholesterol absorption[6].

The findings from this study have two important implications. First, the fact that UDC-sar can inhibit cholesterol absorption in animals with intact enterohepatic circulation of bile salts would imply that UDC-sar can potentially be used therapeutically to inhibit cholesterol absorption in humans. Kuipers *et al.*[9] reported a bile acid secretion rate of about $5\,\mu$mol/min per kg body weight in the rat. We are infusing about $2.5\,\mu$mol/min per kg body weight of exogenous bile acids. This would mean that, if one-third of the bile acid pool is replaced by ursodeoxycholic acid, there should be a reduction in intestinal cholesterol absorption. Second, it is tempting to speculate that there may exist a critical ratio of UDC-sar to C-tau above which UDC-sar can inhibit cholesterol absorption. If this is true it may explain why clinical studies have not yielded a definitive effect of UDC therapy on the intestinal absorption of cholesterol in humans. Depending on the experimental protocol and the dose of UDC given, the ratio of UDC conjugates to other bile salts may not have reached the critical ratio for the UDC conjugate to inhibit cholesterol absorption in some previous studies. To test this concept we will perform uptake and lymphatic transport of cholesterol in bile fistula rats using emulsions containing different ratios of UDC-sar or UDC-tau or C-tau.

In summary, we conclude that UDC-sar inhibits intestinal uptake and lymphatic transport of cholesterol even in rats with intact enterohepatic circulation. The fact that UDC does not alter hepatic cholesterol synthesis means that its inhibition of cholesterol absorption is likely to be the mechanism responsible for decreased biliary cholesterol secretion in humans.

Acknowledgements

We are extremely grateful to Ms Laura Gray for her skilful technical assistance. This study was supported by National Institutes of Health grant DK 32288.

References

1. Hofmann AF. Medical dissolution of gallstones by oral bile acid therapy. Am J Surg. 1989;158:198–204.
2. Mazzella G, Bazzoli F, Festi D *et al.* Comparative evaluation of chenodeoxycholic and ursodeoxycholic acids in obese patients. Effects on biliary lipid metabolism during weight maintenance and weight reduction. Gastroenterology. 1991;101:490–6.
3. Salen G, Tint GS, Shefer S. Treatment of cholesterol gallstones with litholytic bile acids. Gastroenterol Clin N Am. 1991;20:171–82.
4. Maudgal DP, Northfield TC. A practical guide to the nonsurgical treatment of gallstones. Drugs. 1991;41:185–92.

5. Longmire-Cook SJ, Lillienau J, Kim YS *et al*. Effect of replacement therapy with cholylsarcosine on fat malabsorption associated with severe bile acid malabsorption. Studies in dogs with ileal resection. Dig Dis Sci. 1992;37:1217–27.
6. Tso P, Fukagawa K, Lillienau J, Hofmann AF. Ursodeoxycholyl sarcosine inhibits intestinal cholesterol (CHOL) absorption but not triglyceride (TG) absorption [abstract]. Gastroenterology. 1993;104:286.
7. Bollman JL, Cain C, Grindlay JH. Techniques for the collection of lymph from liver, small intestine or thoracic duct of the rat. J Lab Clin Med. 1948;33:1349–52.
8. Tserng KY, Hachey DK, Klein PD. An improved procedure for the synthesis of glycine and taurine conjugates of bile acids. J Lipid Res. 1977;18:404–7.
9. Kuipers F, Havinga R, Bosschieter H, Toorop GP, Hindriks FR, Vonk RJ. Enterohepatic circulation in the rat. Gastroenterology. 1985;88:403–11.

28
Effects of bile acids on hepatic cholesterol metabolism in humans

K. EINARSSON, M. RUDLING, E. REIHNÉR, S. SAHLIN,
I. BJÖRKHEM and B. ANGELIN

The liver is a key organ in the metabolism of cholesterol and bile acids[1]. Cholesterol is excreted from the body mainly by the liver into the bile, either directly as free cholesterol or after conversion of cholesterol to bile acids, the rate-determining enzyme being cholesterol 7α-hydroxylase. About 50% of the endogenous cholesterol synthesis occurs in the liver, HMG CoA reductase being a rate-limiting enzyme. The liver is also supplied by plasma lipoprotein cholesterol. In the liver cholesterol may be stored as cholesteryl esters, the esterification process being catalysed by ACAT.

Bile acids may influence hepatic cholesterol metabolism in different ways. We have previously shown that treatment with chenodeoxycholic acid in a daily dose of 15 mg/kg body weight suppresses the activities of the hepatic cholesterol 7α-hydroxylase and HMG CoA reductase[2-4]. Ursodeoxycholic acid, on the other hand, may slightly stimulate bile acid synthesis and hepatic HMG CoA reductase activity[2,4-6]. The hepatic ACAT activity is not affected, and the hepatic content of free and esterified cholesterol is not significantly changed by bile acid treatment[4].

We have now extended our studies on the effect of chenodeoxycholic acid and ursodeoxycholic acid on human hepatic cholesterol metabolism. mRNA levels for cholesterol 7α-hydroxylase and HMG CoA reductase have been quantitated by a solution hybridization technique, mRNA abundancy being expressed as copies of mRNA molecules per cell (unpublished results). The mRNA level of cholesterol 7α-hydroxylase was lower in chenodeoxycholic acid-treated gallstone patients compared with untreated patients. The mRNA level of HMG CoA reductase also tended to be decreased in chenodeoxycholic acid-treated patients compared with controls, but the difference did not reach statistical significance. Corresponding mRNA levels in ursodeoxycholic acid-treated gallstone patients were not significantly different from those of untreated patients.

In conclusion, chenodeoxycholic acid and ursodeoxycholic acid have different effects on hepatic cholesterol metabolism. Chenodeoxycholic acid suppresses both mRNA level and expressed activity of cholesterol 7α-hydroxylase and HMG CoA reductase, whereas ursodeoxycholic acid does not.

Acknowledgement

The study was supported by grants from the Swedish Medical Research Council (Project 03X-04793).

References

1. Turley SD, Dietschy JM. The metabolism and excretion of cholesterol by the liver. In: Arias I, Jacoby W, Popper H, Schachter D, Shafritz D, editors. The liver: biology and pathobiology, 2nd edn. New York: Raven Press; 1988:617–41.
2. Reihnér E, Björkhem I, Angelin B, Ewerth S, Einarsson K. Bile acid synthesis in humans: regulation of hepatic microsomal cholesterol 7α-hydroxylase activity. Gastroenterology. 1989;97:1498–505.
3. Ahlberg J, Angelin B, Einarsson K. Hepatic 3-hydroxy-3-methylglutaryl coenzyme A reductase activity and biliary lipid composition in man: relation to cholesterol gallstone disease and effects of cholic acid and chenodeoxycholic acid treatment. J Lipid Res. 1981;22:410–22.
4. Sahlin S, Ahlberg J, Reihnér E, Ståhlberg D, Einarsson K. Cholesterol metabolism in human gallbladder mucosa: relationship to cholesterol gallstone disease and effects of chenodeoxycholic acid and ursodeoxycholic acid treatment. Hepatology. 1992;16:320–6.
5. Nilsell K, Angelin B, Leijd B, Einarsson K. Comparative effects of ursodeoxycholic acid and chenodeoxycholic acid on bile acid kinetics and biliary lipid secretion in humans. Gastroenterology. 1983;85:1248–56.
6. Angelin B, Ewerth S, Einarsson K. Ursodeoxycholic acid treatment in cholesterol gallstone disease: effects on hepatic 3-hydroxy-3-methylglutaryl coenzyme A reductase activity, biliary lipid composition, and plasma lipid levels. J Lipid Res. 1983;24:461–8.

29
Premicellar bile salts enhance intestinal calcium absorption

A. J. SANYAL and E. W. MOORE

INTRODUCTION

Traditionally, it has been thought that the principal role of bile salts in the small intestine is to solubilize dietary lipids by incorporation into micelles[1], thereby making such lipids available to digestive enzymes and mucosal transport. Although it has long been recognized that bile is essential for normal absorption of both iron and calcium, the potential role of biliary constituents in the intestinal transport of these cations was not previously known. Specifically, the role of bile salts, the principal organic constituent of bile, was unknown.

In 1982 Moore $et\ al.$[2] demonstrated that certain bile salts had considerable Ca^{2+}-binding properties. They found that taurocholate (TC), at concentrations above the critical micellar concentration (CMC) bound Ca^{2+} with relatively low affinity ($K'f$ ~5 l/mole). However, with decreasing $[Ca^{2+}]$ below the CMC, binding affinity increased sharply, with a limiting affinity constant ($K'f$) of about 220 l/mole at very low bile salt concentrations. It was subsequently shown that such high-affinity premicellar binding required the presence of a 7- and/or 12-OH group on the cholanic ring of a given bile salt[3]. Thus, taurodehydrocholate (3-oxo,7-oxo,12-oxo cholyltaurine) with no ring OH groups, had only minimal Ca^{2+} binding properties.

During modelling studies of this high-affinity binding between Ca^{2+} and premicellar bile salts, it became apparent that the binding locus might behave as a reversible ion-exchanger where other divalent cations having hydrated atomic dimensions identical to Ca^{2+} (6 Å)[4] might be similarly bound (i.e. with high-affinity premicellar and low-affinity micellar binding). Ferrous (Fe^{2+}) iron is one such cation. Since then, we have shown this to be the case; premicellar TC bound Fe^{2+} with high affinity, while only low-affinity binding was noted at micellar TC concentrations[5]. As was predicted from the lack of binding of Ca^{2+} by TDHC, this bile salt did not show any high-affinity Fe^{2+}-binding[6].

Both inorganic calcium and iron are virtually insoluble in the alkaline milieu of the small intestinal lumen[7,8]. The limiting solubility of each cation is determined by the solubility product of the least soluble species present. For Ca^{2+} this

"

is $CaCO_3 (K_{sp} = 3.8 \times 10^{-8}\,mol/l)$[9], while that for iron is Fe_2O_3 or $Fe(OH)_3$ with similar K_{sp} values of $1.7 \times 10^{-18}\,mol/l$[10]. The substantial Fe^{2+}- and Ca^{2+}-binding properties of premicellar bile salts resulting in formation of soluble bile salt–cation complexes led us originally to hypothesize that formation of such complexes would increase the availability of these cations for uptake and transmucosal transport in small intestine[5].

In initial studies we showed that premicellar TC did produce a marked increment in Fe^{2+} uptake in isolated perfused intestinal segments in bile duct and pancreatic duct-ligated animals *in vivo*[11]. Further, using total body counting to accurately measure iron absorption, i.e. transmucosal transport rather than disappearance from intestinal lumen, we found that administration of a small dose of TC could reverse severe iron malabsorption induced by ligation of the common bile duct[12]. Also, as predicted, TDHC (having no high-affinity Fe^{2+} binding properties) had no significant effects on iron absorption. Finally, we have recently shown that administration of ursodeoxycholate (UDCA) can correct severe iron deficiency anaemia refractory to oral administration of iron supplements[13]. Thus, *bile salts clearly appear to play an important role in intestinal iron transport*. However, their role in calcium transport had not been previously characterized. In this study we examined the effects of TC and TDHC on the intestinal transport of calcium ions.

METHODS

Studies of Ca2+ uptake

The first set of studies were done to determine if TC or TDHC had any effects on intestinal calcium uptake. These were done using an isolated perfused intestinal segment model described by us previously[11]. Briefly, following sodium pentobarbital anaesthesia, adult male Sprague-Dawley rats underwent laparotomy, and the common bile duct as well as pancreatic ducts were ligated. The small intestine was divided into approximately equal proximal, mid, and distal segments, taking care to keep the vascular supply intact. Each segment was perfused simultaneously from the oral end at a constant rate (0.3 ml/min) for 40-min perfusion periods using the same perfusate solution. Effluents from each segment were collected separately in tared glass tubes. The perfusate solution contained ^{45}Ca-$CaCl_2$ (0.1–1 mmol/l) tris-hydroxymethyl aminomethane (THAM) buffer at pH 7.0, TC or TDHC (0–10 mmol/l), phenylsulphonphthalein (PSP, a non-absorbed marker), and sufficient NaCl to yield a total ionic strength (μ) of 0.15 mol/l. ^{45}Ca counts were made from both perfusates and effluent solutions, and Ca^{2+} uptake was measured as follows:

$$\text{Uptake} = \frac{\text{Amount Ca perfused} - \text{Amount Ca recovered}}{\text{Gut length} \times \text{Perfusion time} \times \text{PSP recovery}}$$

For a given animal, four randomized perfusions containing solutions of identical $[Ca^{2+}]$ were made while varying bile salt concentration from 0 to 10 mmol/l. However, for a given perfusion period, all segments were perfused with identical solutions.

Studies of Ca2+ absorption from small intestine

To determine whether changes in Ca^{2+} uptake (as measured by disappearance of
[45]Ca-CaCl$_2$ from intestinal lumen above) actually reflected changes in calcium
absorption, the proximal small intestine was selected as the region for study. This
is normally the region of maximal calcium absorption[8,14]. The proximal segment
was isolated as described above, and then divided into an orad and caudad
subsegment. In a given animal one subsegment was randomly perfused with a
control solution containing [45]Ca-CaCl$_2$, THAM (pH 7) and NaCl ($\mu = 0.15$ mol/l)
while the other was perfused with an identical solution with the exception of
added bile salt. In a group of 22 animals the orad segment was perfused with
control solution in half the animals, whereas in the other half it was perfused with
the bile salt-containing solution. At the end of a single perfusion period, during
which effluents were collected and counted as above, the intestinal segments
were washed, weighed and dissolved in a 1:2 protosol–ethanol mixture. [45]Ca
counts were obtained from perfusates, effluents, and scraped intestinal mucosa.
The amount of calcium absorbed was determined from the difference between
that lost from intestinal lumen, i.e. uptake, and that remaining in the intestinal
wall, i.e. mucosal retention.

In vitro studies of Ca2+ uptake by small intestinal brush-border vesicles

Transport of all solutes across the small intestine may theoretically occur via
paracellular or transcellular pathways. Although the studies described above
were designed to detect any changes in overall uptake or transmucosal transport,
they did not specifically address the potential pathways by which these changes
occurred. Studies of transport across isolated purified apical brush-border
vesicles from enterocytes can be used to exclude paracellular transport, and may
thus serve to directly study potential effects of bile salts on Ca^{2+} uptake by
enterocytes.

Isolated brush-border membrane vesicles (BBMV) were prepared by the
methods described by Knickelbein *et al.*[15]. Vesicle purity was determined by 20-
fold enrichment of brush-border enzyme (alkaline phosphatase) and 12-fold
de-enrichment of basolateral membrane enzyme Na^+,K^+-ATPase. Functional
integrity was confirmed by demonstration of typical overshoot of uptake of
[³H]glucose uptake in the presence of Na^+ ions.

The specific aim of these studies was to measure Ca^{2+} uptake across the brush-
border membrane both in the presence and absence of bile salts in the incubating
medium, while ensuring that vesicles remained intact during the study. To
monitor structural integrity, vesicles were loaded with [¹⁴C]inulin, and integrity
assessed by ^{14}C counts at various time intervals. Ca^{2+} uptake was simultaneously
determined from [45]Ca-CaCl$_2$ +/− bile salts. However, both [45]Ca and ^{14}C have β
emissions, and the accuracy with which each isotope can be counted in a sample
containing both isotopes depends on the ratio of the isotopes. Since the ratio of
the two isotopes at any given time point could not be predicted, and varied from
one instant to the next, the two isotopes could not be counted accurately from a
single vesicle sample.

To bypass this problem the following study design was employed. Vesicles were initially incubated in a 'preincubation medium' containing HEPES 74 mmol/l, TRIS 31 mmol/l, MES 37 mmol/l, pH 6.8, mannitol 150 mmol/l and NaCl 17 mmol/l. The vesicle suspension was then divided into two equal batches, A and B. Vesicles in batch A were loaded with [^{14}C]inulin (0.5 mmol/l) using a freeze–thaw technique[16], and those from batch B were loaded with identical concentrations of non-radiolabelled inulin. Vesicle aliquots (10 μl) from batch A were incubated with 40 μl of solutions containing non-labelled $CaCl_2$ with or without bile salts. Identical volumes of vesicle suspensions from batch B were incubated with solutions identical to those used for batch A except that the $CaCl_2$ was labelled with ^{45}Ca. Ca^{2+} uptakes were halted at various time intervals by addition of a stop solution containing (in mmol/l) HEPES/Tris/MES 74:31:34, mannitol 150, $MgCl_2$ 16, $CaCl_2$ 0.1 and NaEGTA 1. Vesicles were filtered on a Millipore (0.45 μm) membrane (Bedford, MA) and washed with a 9-fold volume of stop solution. Filters were dissolved in scintillation fluid, and ^{14}C as well as ^{45}Ca counts obtained in a Beckman beta-counter using constant-counting geometry. Proteins were measured by the method of Lowry *et al* .[17].

Data analysis

Data were analysed using a Lotus spreadsheet, and studies of significance made using appropriate Student's *t*-tests. Graphs were made with both Lotus and Harvard graphics software using an IBMPS2 personal computer.

RESULTS

Studies of TC and TDHC effects on Ca2+ uptake

The effects of TC on Ca^{2+} uptake were studied in a total of 15 animals while TDHC effects were studied in seven rats. The results of studies involving TC and TDHC are discussed separately below.

A total of 156 perfusions were made in the 15 animals where TC effects were examined. Ca^{2+} uptake in the absence of TC at perfusate [Ca^{2+}] of 0.1, 0.5 and 1 mmol/l was initially assessed. Uptake was greatest in proximal small intestine and then decreased progressively in more distal regions. This is in keeping with previous observations that the proximal small intestine is the principal site of intestinal calcium absorption.

The effects of increasing [TC] from 0 to 10 mmol/l in all regions of small intestine are shown in Fig. 1. At each [Ca^{2+}] studied, uptake was greatest in proximal small intestine as noted above. At [Ca^{2+}] 0.1 mmol/l a small insignificant increment in uptake was noted. However, in absolute terms, up to 40% increments were noted in individual animals. In sharp contrast, a marked highly significant ($p < 0.01$) increase in calcium uptake was noted at both [Ca^{2+}] of 0.5 and 1 mmol/l. Uptake increment occurred stepwise below the CMC (5 mmol/l), with only minor or no further increments noted at 10 mmol/l TC.

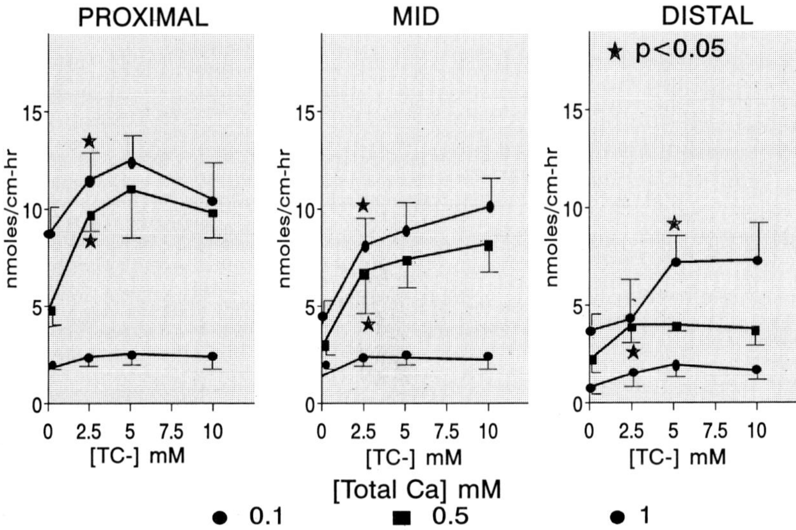

Fig. 1 Effects of increasing [TC] from 0 to 10 mmol/l in all regions of small intestine. Uptake was greatest in proximal regions and decreased progressively down the intestine. Premicellar TC produced a marked enhancement of Ca^{2+} uptake

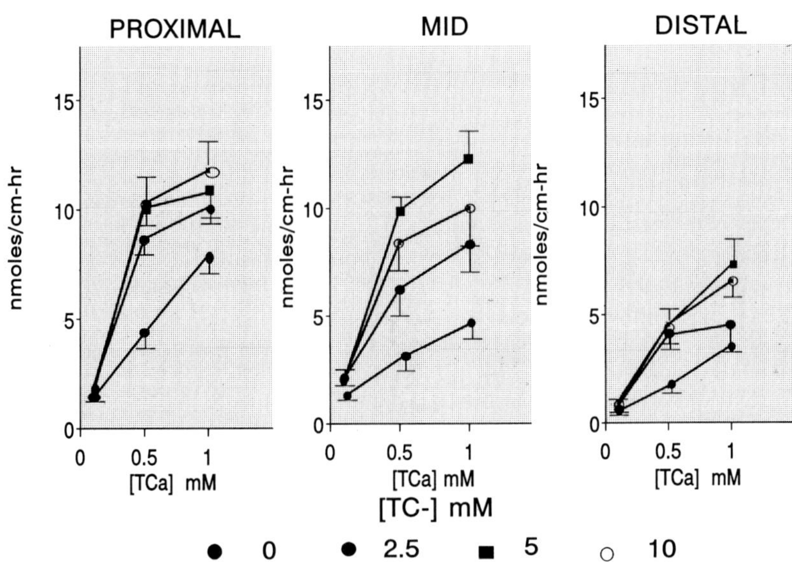

Fig. 2 Effects of TC on the kinetics of Ca^{2+} uptake. There was an upward and 'left' shift in all regions of small intestine

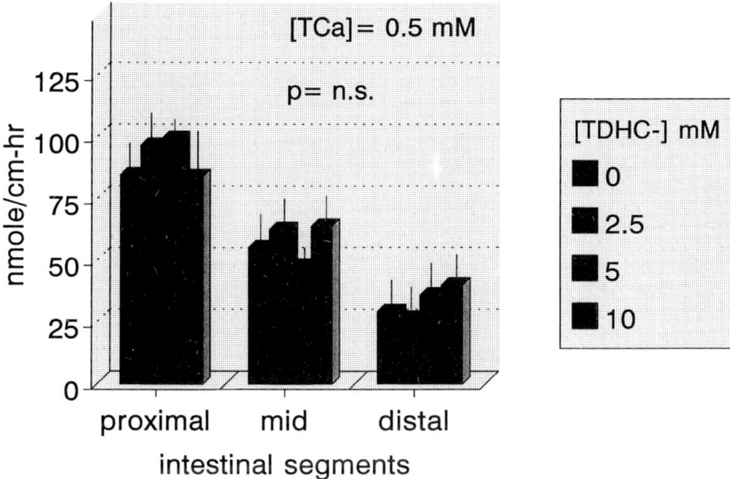

Fig. 3 Effects of TDHC on Ca^{2+} uptake from all regions of small intestine. In contrast to TC, TDHC had no significant effects

Although the results were qualitatively similar in all regions of small intestine, absolute uptake was greatest in proximal intestine.

The effects of TC on the kinetics of Ca^{2+} uptake are shown in Fig. 2. In the absence of bile salt, a plot of uptake vs perfusate $[Ca^{2+}]$ should be curvilinear, since calcium uptake normally occurs by facilitated diffusion[17]. In these studies the linear nature of the plot in the absence of TC in all regions probably reflected the low $[Ca^{2+}]$ values studied, which were physiological but below the point of inflection of the uptake vs $[Ca^{2+}]$ plot. In all regions the shape of the plot in the presence of TC became curvilinear. This was principally due to the greatest uptake-enhancement noted at 0.5 mmol/l total calcium at a given [TC]. A potential explanation of this phenomenon may be that TC moved the 'uptake curve' to the left, thereby exposing the point of inflection of the curve. Again, data from different regions of the intestine were qualitatively similar.

Figure 3 shows the effects of TDHC on intestinal calcium uptake in all regions of small intestine. Once again, uptake was greatest in proximal small intestine in the absence of bile salt. In sharp contrast to the marked uptake-increment noted with premicellar TC, no significant effects of TDHC at 2, 5 or 10 mmol/l were noted in any region of intestine.

These data clearly demonstrate that *premicellar TC, but not TDHC, markedly enhances intestinal calcium uptake in the bile duct-ligated isolated perfused small intestine* in vivo. Uptake increment was most noted at 2.5 mmol/l TC, and peak effects were usually noted at about 5–6 mmol/l TC, which corresponds closely to the CMC of TC under the study conditions[18].

Studies of TC effects on calcium absorption from small intestine

Since TDHC had no significant effects on calcium uptake, studies to determine the effects on net transmucosal transport were limited to those for TC only. In

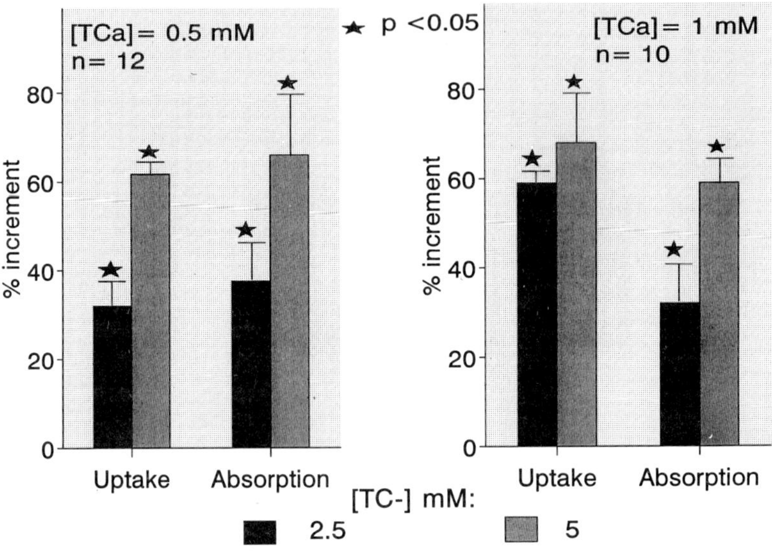

Fig. 4 Effects of TC on intestinal calcium absorption. Note that both uptake as well as true lumen-to-plasma transfer of calcium was increased by premicellar TC

these studies the effects of 2.5 and 5 mmol/l TC on calcium absorption (calculated from the difference between uptake and mucosal retention) were measured in 12 and 10 rats at $[Ca^{2+}]$ values of 0.5 and 1 mmol/l, respectively. At both calcium concentrations studied, TC induced absolute increments in both mucosal retention and lumen-to-plasma transfer of calcium (Fig. 4). In terms of percentage change, a 30–70% increment in uptake and absorption occurred ($p < 0.01$). Thus, premicellar TC not only increased calcium uptake from the lumen, but also increased the net lumen-to-plasma movement of calcium.

In vitro studies of TC effects on Ca2+ uptake across BBMV

In order to directly confirm that the observed enhancement of Ca^{2+} absorption involved transcellular pathways, the effects of TC on ^{45}Ca-$CaCl_2$ movement across BBMVs were studied. In initial studies, BBMVs were loaded with $[^{14}C]$inulin and vesicles counted for loss of inulin (indicating vesicle disruption) at varying time intervals. No significant changes were noted so long as medium osmolality remained essentially unchanged.

In controls ($[TC] = 0$ mmol/l), Ca^{2+} uptake increased curvilinearly over time, with near maximal values attained by 300 s. In initial studies, calcium uptakes from media of varying $[Ca^{2+}]$ and of increasing osmolality were measured. A plot of uptake vs the inverse of medium osmolality was linear and yielded a y-intercept near the origin (−0.2) for studies at 0.1 mmol/l $[Ca^{2+}]$, indicating that true transmembrane transport rather than non-specific adherence was being measured. In studies at 0.5 and 1 mmol/l $[Ca^{2+}]$, a positive intercept was obtained,

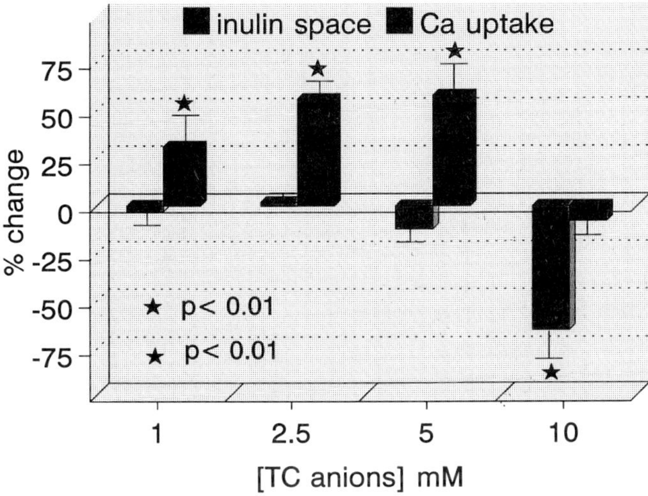

Fig. 5 Effects of TC on Ca^{2+} uptake by BBMV. At 10 mmol/l TC the degree of vesicle disruption did not allow adequate measurement of Ca^{2+} uptake. However, premicellar TC produced a significant increase in calcium uptake

indicating that considerable non-specific adsorption was also occurring. Further studies were therefore made only at 0.1 mmol/l [Ca^{2+}].

Data were obtained in triplicate in each of 12 studies of TC effects on Ca^{2+} uptake across BBMVs. There were no significant changes in [^{14}C]inulin counts at or below [TC]=2.5 mmol/l (Fig. 5). However, at 5 and 10 mmol/l TC, respective losses of 12% and 65% of inulin counts occurred, *indicating vesicle disruption by micellar bile salt*. It can be seen that calcium uptake increased in a stepwise manner up to 5 mmol/l TC, i.e. below the CMC. Uptakes could not be accurately measured at 10 mmol/l TC, due to the large fractional disruption of vesicles at this bile salt concentration.

Finally, to ascertain whether the noted increase in Ca^{2+} uptake by BBMVs reflected true transmembrane transport, as opposed to increased surface adsorption, Ca^{2+} uptakes were measured from solutions containing 0 or 2.5 mmol/l TC in media of increasing osmolality. A plot of uptake vs 1/osmolality (Fig. 6) yielded an intercept at or near the origin, indicating that TC produced a true increase in Ca^{2+} movement across small intestinal brush border.

These data indicate that premicellar TC produce a significant increase in intestinal calcium uptake and lumen-to-plasma calcium transfer, and that this involves transcellular pathways. Thus, premicellar bile salts appear to have significant effects on calcium absorption from small intestine.

DISCUSSION

The importance of bile in both intestinal iron and calcium absorption has long been recognized. As early as 1928[19], Whipple and co-workers noted that,

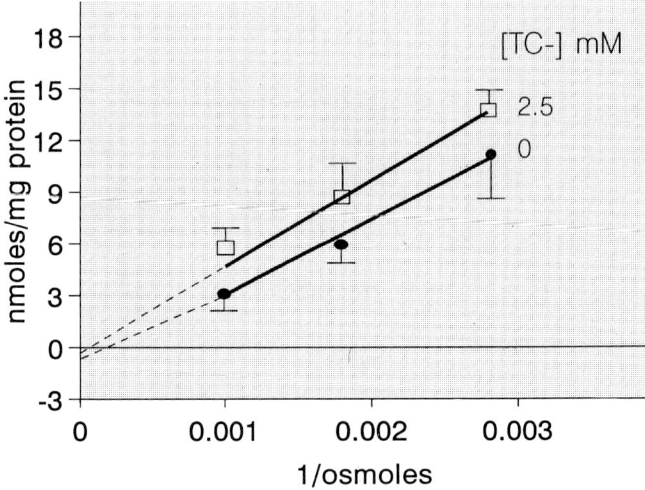

Fig. 6 Ca^{2+} uptake plotted against 1/osomoles of incubating medium. Note that the intercept essentially passes through the origin, indicating that true transmembrane transport was being measured and that TC enhance Ca^{2+} uptake across BBMV

following creation of a bile fistula, iron-deficient dogs were unable to replenish their iron stores by the simple addition of therapeutic amounts of iron in the diet. Likewise creation of a bile fistula has been shown to produce osteoporosis[20], while administration of bile with milk increased serum calcium levels transiently[21]. Intraperitoneal injections of TC also produced striking increments of incorporation of radio-labelled dietary calcium into the femur[22]. However, the specific role of bile salts on intestinal calcium absorption has not been previously quantified.

The most obvious role for bile salts in Ca^{2+} absorption relates to the ability of micellar bile salts to enhance the absorption of vitamin D, a fat-soluble vitamin. Indeed, the osteoporosis noted by Pavlov in bile-fistula dogs may have been due to vitamin D malabsorption. However, the increments in serum Ca^{2+} noted by Von Beznak were much too rapid to be mediated by vitamin D. In addition, Webling and Holdsworth noted a 2–3-fold decrease in mucosa-to-serosa calcium influx in *in vitro* gut sacs after bile duct ligation[23]. Finally, bile from vitamin D-deficient chicks was able to correct the Ca^{2+} malabsorption noted after bile duct ligation[24].

We had originally proposed that, under physiological conditions, premicellar bile salts may enhance Ca^{2+} absorption by increasing the soluble pool of calcium available for absorption. However, intestinal perfusion studies are necessarily restricted by the fact that only *soluble* calcium species could be studied, because large errors would occur if there were precipitation of calcium in the crypts. The enhancement in calcium absorption noted under conditions where all of the calcium available was in soluble form indicated that other mechanism(s) are also operative. However, it is possible that solubility considerations play an important part in the bile salt effects on calcium absorption.

One might argue that the observed uptake-enhancement of Ca^{2+} by bile salts results from injury to intestinal epithelium, with increased paracellular Ca^{2+} movement from lumen to plasma. However, several factors predicate against this possibility. First, under study conditions the electrochemical gradient favoured movement of Ca^{2+} from plasma to lumen, rather than in the opposite direction. Also, lack of carry-over effects during randomized perfusions and near-complete recovery of PSP indicate that significant non-specific permeabilization did not occur. Finally, Ca^{2+} movement across brush-border membranes was enhanced by *premicellar* bile salts, indicating that bile salts may increase Ca^{2+} uptake by enterocytes.

That bile salts may enhance calcium uptake across BBMVs is not totally unexpected. In 1979, Abramson and Shamoo showed that certain bile salts could act as calcium ionophores across black lipid membranes[25]. Further, Oelberg *et al.* have shown that premicellar bile salts may increase calcium uptake by red cell membranes[26] and model lipid membranes[27]. Our studies suggest that such effects may also occur in the intestine. The precise molecular basis for these effects, however, remains to be elucidated.

Although our studies were not designed to completely define the mechanisms by which premicellar bile salts enhance calcium absorption, the noted enhancement in BBMV studies indicates that TC has Ca^{2+} ionophoric properties in small intestine. We hypothesize that, in the lumen, bile salts bind Ca^{2+} with 2.1 stoichiometry, $Ca(BS_2)$, with Ca^{2+} resonating between the hydroxyl and carboxyl groups of the hydrophilic surfaces, leaving the hydrophobic surfaces facing outwards. Because of the interface between the hydrophobic face of the bile salt and water dipoles, this complex would be inherently unstable, but would readily partition into the lipid bilayer of the brush-border membrane. Once in the membrane, Ca^{2+} ions would be preferentially bound by calcium-binding proteins on the cellular aspect of the apical membrane, leaving a hydrophilic channel through which other calcium ions could traverse. This would represent a classical 'channel-type' ionophore. However, this remains to be experimentally verified.

In summary, it is well recognized that micellar bile salts are important for lipid absorption from small intestine. These studies show that, in addition to these effects, certain bile salts have substantial and highly significant effects on intestinal calcium and iron absorption. *To our knowledge, this is the first known potential function of* premicellar *bile salts.* Further studies are now needed to define the mechanisms of these observations, and the importance of bile salts in the normal absorption of calcium and iron from the intestine.

Acknowledgements

This work was supported by NIH grant DK 32130, and by an award from the Jeffress foundation. The authors wish to acknowledge the able technical assistance of Ms Inge Moore, Jennifer Coady, Sherri Holmes, and Sandra Walker in these studies.

References

1. Carey MC, Small DM, Bliss CM. Lipid digestion and absorption. Annu Rev Physiol. 1983; 45:651–77.
2. Moore EW, Celic L, Ostrow JD. Interactions between ionized calcium and sodium taurocholate: bile salts are important buffers for prevention of calcium-containing gallstones. Gastroenterology. 1982;83:1079–89.
3. Moore EW. The role of calcium in the pathogenesis of gallstones: Ca^{++} electrode studies of model bile salt solutions and other biologic systems. Hepatology. 1984;4:228–43S.
4. Klotz IM. Chemical thermodynamics. Englewood Cliffs, NJ: Prentice-Hall, 1950:331.
5. Sanyal AJ, Hirsch JI, Moore EW. Premicellar taurocholate avidly binds ferrous (Fe^{2+}) iron: a potential physiologic role for bile salts in iron absorption. J Lab Clin Med. 1990;116:76–86.
6. Sanyal AJ, Hirsch JI, Moore EW. High-affinity binding is essential for bile salt-induced enhancement of intestinal iron and calcium uptake. Gastroenterology. 1991;102:1997–2005.
7. Conrad ME. Iron absorption. In: Johnson L, editor. Physiology of the gastrointestinal tract. New York: Raven Press; 1993:1437–53.
8. Bronner F. Calcium absorption. In: Johnson LR, editor. Physiology of the gastrointestinal tract. New York: Raven Press; 1987:1419–35.
9. Moore EW, Verine HJ. Pathogenesis of pancreatic and biliary $CaCO_3$ lithiasis: the solubility product (K′sp) of calcite determined with the Ca^{++} electrode. J Lab Clin Med. 1985;106:611–18.
10. Forth W, Rummel W. Iron absorption. Physiol Rev. 1973;53:724–92.
11. Sanyal AJ, Hirsch JI, Moore EW. Premicellar taurocholate enhances ferrous iron uptake from all regions of rat small intestine. Gastroenterology. 1991;101:382–9.
12. Sanyal AJ, Hirsch JI, Moore EW. Evidence that bile salts are important for iron absorption. Am J Physiol. 1994;266:G318–23.
13. Sanyal AJ, Shiffman ML, Moore EW. A pilot study of ursodeoxycholate for correcting iron-deficiency refractory to oral replenishment. Hepatology. 1994 (Submitted).
14. Bronner F, Pansu D, Stein WD. An analysis of intestinal calcium transport across the intestine. Editorial review. Am J Physiol. 1986;250:G561–9.
15. Knickelbein R, Aronson PS, Atherton W, Dobbins W. Sodium and chloride transport across rabbit ileal brush border: evidence for Na^+ exchange. Am J Physiol. 1983;245:G504–10.
16. Donowitz M, Emmer E, McCullen J et al. Freeze thaw and high voltage allow macromolecule uptake into ileal brush border vesicles. Am J Physiol. 197;15:G723–35.
17. Lowry O, Rosebrough NJ, Farr AL, Randall RJ. Protein measurement with the Folin phenol reagent. J Biol Chem. 1951;193:265–75.
18. Roda A, Hofmann AF, Mysels KJ. The influence of bile salt structure on self-association in aqueous solutions. J Biol Chem. 1983;258:6362–70.
19. Hawkins WB, Robscheit-Robbins FS, Whipple GH. Hemoglobin production in anemia as influenced by the bile fistula. J Exp Med. 1938;67:89–110.
20. Pavlov IP. Experimental studies on biliary secretions. Verhandl Ges Russ Aertz. 1904;72: 314–19.
21. Von Beznak A. Der Einflußiger galle auf die Resorption des Calciums. Pflugers Arch Ges Physiol. 1931;228:604–13.
22. Lengemann FW, Dobbins JW. The role of bile in calcium absorption. J Nutr. 1958;66:45–54.
23. Webling DA, Holdsworth ES. Bile salts and calcium absorption. Biochem J. 1966;100:652–60.
24. Webling DA, Holdsworth ES. The effect of bile, bile acids, and detergents on calcium absorption in the chick. Biochem J. 1965;97:408–21.
25. Abramson JJ, Shamoo AE. Anionic detergents as divalent cation ionophores across black lipid membrane. J Membr Biol. 1979;50:241–4.
26. Oelberg DG, Dubinsky WP, Sackman JW, Wang LB, Adcock EW, Lester R. Bile salts induce calcium uptake in vitro by human erythrocytes. Hepatology. 1987;7:245–52.
27. Oelberg DG, Wang LB, Sackman JW, Adcock EW, Lester R, Dubinsky WP. Bile salt-induced calcium fluxes in artificial phospholipid vesicles. Biochim Biophys Acta. 198;937:289–99.

Section VII
Cytotoxicity and immunology of bile acids

30
Disruptive and protective interactions of bile salts, cholesterol: lecithin vesicles, and canalicular membranes

D. M. HEUMAN

INTRODUCTION

Bile salts are potent biological detergents which can disrupt lipid bilayers and solubilize structural membrane lipids and proteins. The detergency of bile salts increases with increasing relative hydrophobicity as estimated by reverse-phase high-pressure liquid chromatography (HPLC)[1,2]. The membrane-disruptive effects of bile salts may contribute to pathogenesis of liver injury in cholestatic diseases. Administration of ursodeoxycholic acid, a relatively hydrophilic bile salt, reduces liver cell injury and improves bile excretory function in many liver diseases. Studies performed in bile fistula rats[3-5] and in isolated hepatocytes[6,7] suggest that ursodeoxycholic acid is protective at the level of the hepatocyte. Ursodeoxycholate conjugates also reduce disruption of lecithin: cholesterol liposomes by more hydrophobic bile salts[8], suggesting that the hepatoprotective effect of ursodeoxycholate may have a physicochemical mechanism.

The mechanisms by which hepatocytes and biliary epithelial cells normally resist disruption by bile salts are not well understood. Although canaliculi are cholesterol-rich and relatively resistant to dissolution by bile salts, they clearly can be disrupted by bile salts at physiological biliary concentrations[9]. Recent data suggest that both lecithin–cholesterol vesicles and hydrophilic bile acids at concentrations achieved in bile may reduce the membrane-disruptive effects of more hydrophobic bile salts[10], and these findings may have relevance as regards resistance of hepatocytes to detergency of bile salts in the canalicular lumen. To address this question we have studied the protective effects of ursodeoxycholate and lecithin: cholesterol vesicles towards isolated canalicular membranes. As an index of canalicular disruption we measured solubilization of the structural canalicular ectoenzyme alkaline phosphatase.

MATERIALS AND METHODS

Sodium salts of taurine conjugated bile acids were obtained from Calbiochem-Behring, La Jolla, CA. All were >99% pure by HPLC and were employed without further purification. Egg lecithin (99% phosphatidylcholine) and highly purified cholesterol were obtained from Sigma, St Louis, MO. Radionuclides were purchased from NEN-Dupont, Boston, MA. Large unilamellar vesicles with uniform diameter of 100 nm were prepared by hydration and extrusion as described by Hope *et al.*[11], using a commercial extrusion device (Lipex Biomembranes, Vancouver, BC).

Hepatocyte plasma membranes and canalicular membrane subfractions were isolated by density gradient ultracentrifugation using the method of Meier and Boyer[12]. Disruption of canalicular membranes was quantified by measuring solubilization of alkaline phosphatase, a canalicular membrane-bound ecto-enzyme. Canalicular membranes were incubated with buffered saline containing bile salts and extruded PC:Ch vesicles at various concentrations for 15 min at 25°C, after which membranes were pelleted by rapid ultracentrifugation for 10 min at 40 000 g. The time at which supernatant was harvested was 30 min from the start of the incubations, and was carefully controlled. Alkaline phosphatase activity was determined in samples taken pre- and post-centrifugation by a colorimetric endpoint method using p-nitrophenyl phosphate as substrate, and the fraction of activity remaining in the supernatant (solubilized alkaline phosphatase) was calculated after subtraction of apparent activity remaining after acidification. The latter step was critical to control for effects of turbidity following vesicle addition.

RESULTS

The fraction of alkaline phosphatase activity eluted from canalicular membranes increased with increasing concentrations of deoxycholyl taurine (TDC), with nearly complete dissociation observed at a concentration of 6 millimolar. In contrast, ursodeoxycholyl taurine (TUDC) at concentrations as high as 24 mmol/l caused little release of alkaline phosphatase. A mixture of the two bile acids exhibited intermediate toxicity (Fig. 1).

The effect of adding TUDC to TDC is shown in Fig. 2. Concentration-dependent release of alkaline phosphatase into the supernatant caused by TDC at high concentrations was suppressed moderately by addition of tauroursodeoxycholate. In contrast, at lower TDC concentrations, below 2 mmol/l, added TUDC was not protective.

The effects of added lecithin and cholesterol ([L]=5.5 mmol/l) are shown in Fig. 3. Membrane disruption was reduced by addition of vesicles. Pure lecithin vesicles were more protective than vesicles having a Ch:L ratio of 0.5. The effect of vesicles was most striking at low bile acid concentrations.

The effect of vesicles on canalicular membrane disruption can be explained by their binding and sequestration of bile acids. Figure 4 shows the effect of large unilamellar vesicles, under the conditions employed in these studies, on the concentration of TDC as monomers and simple micelles in the aqueous phase. In

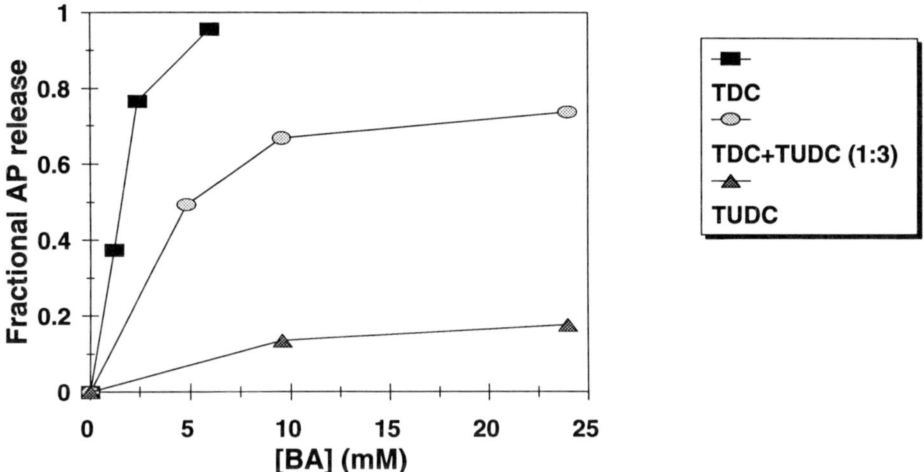

Fig. 1 Release of alkaline phosphatase from canalicular membranes: effects of different bile acids, singly and in combination. AP = alkaline phosphatase activity; TDC = deoxycholyl taurine; TUDC = ursodeoxycholyl taurine; TDC + TUDC (1:3) = combination of TDC and TUDC at mole ratio of 1 to 3. The horizontal axis indicates total bile acid concentration

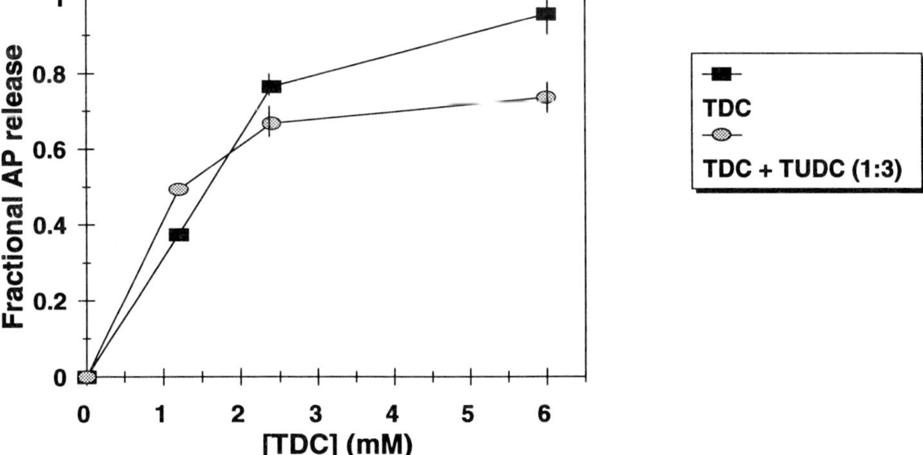

Fig. 2 Same data as Fig. 1; in this figure the horizontal axis indicates the concentration of TDC. At TDC concentrations greater than 2 mmol/l, addition of TUDC reduces AP release from canalicular membranes

these studies, [^{14}C]TDC was included in the mixture; non-lecithin associated [^{14}C]TDC, consisting of low molecular weight aggregates (monomers and simple micelles), was separated from [^{14}C]TDC in large, lecithin-associated aggregates (vesicles and mixed micelles) by rapid ultrafiltration, as described previously. Because hydrophobic bile salts adsorb strongly to membranes and large mixed micelles, the concentration of free, non-lecithin-associated bile acid in the

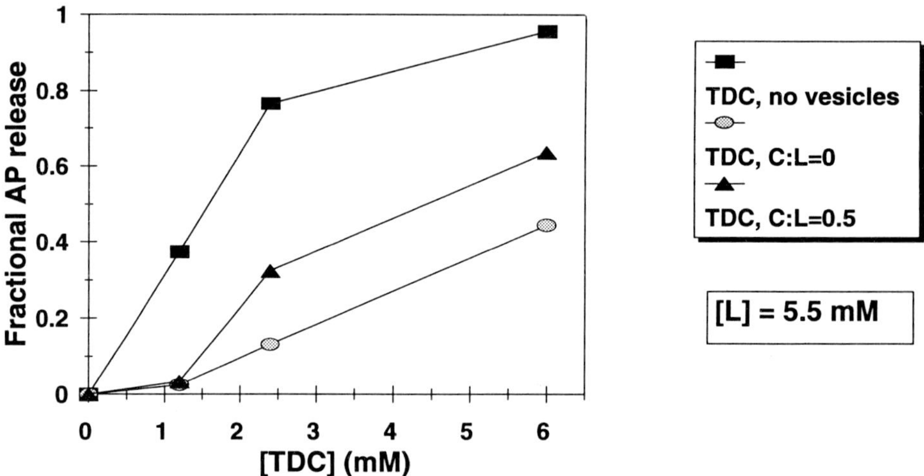

Fig. 3 Effect of added vesicles composed of lecithin (L) and cholesterol (C) on AP release from canalicular membranes following exposure to TDC. Vesicles were added to produce a final lecithin concentration of 5.5 mmol/l. The horizontal axis indicates TDC concentration. C:L=cholesterol: lecithin mole ratio in vesicles

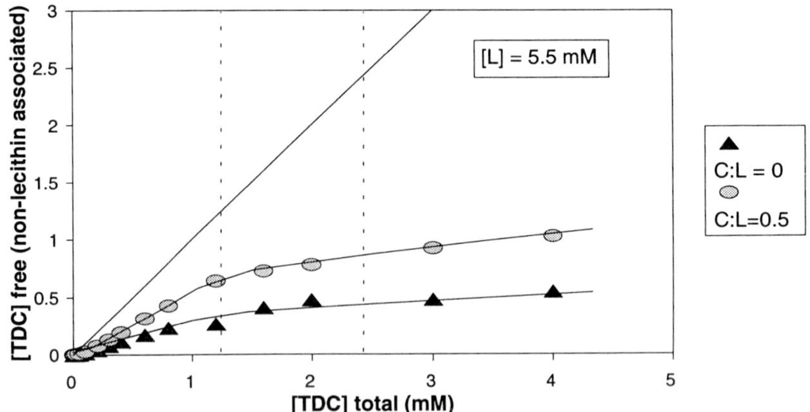

Fig. 4 Effect of vesicles on the concentration of free (non-lecithin associated) TDC. Free TDC (monomers and simple micelles) was separated from lecithin-associated TDC (vesicles and mixed micelles) by rapid ultrafiltration through 0.1 μm filters as described in ref. 18. Free TDC was reduced to a greater extent by pure lecithin vesicles than by vesicles containing cholesterol, because inclusion of cholesterol in lecithin membranes reduces affinity of bile salt adsorption

intermicellar aqueous phase decreases following addition of phospholipid. Cholesterol reduces the affinity of bile acids for lecithin membranes. The greater protection observed with addition of pure lecithin vesicles than with lecithin:cholesterol vesicles reflects the greater adsorption of bile acids with greater lowering of the intermicellar bile acid concentration.

The effect of vesicles on the protective effect of TUDC is shown in Fig. 5. In

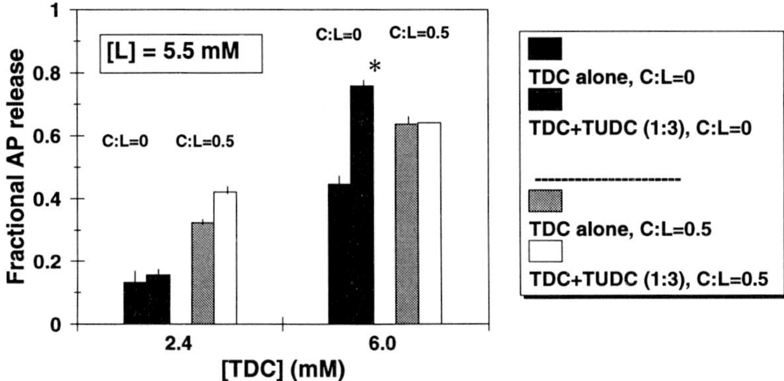

Fig. 5 Effect of TUDC on canalicular toxicity of TDC in the presence of C:L vesicles. Addition of TUDC to TDC was not protective in the presence of vesicles; at the higher concentration of TDC (6 mmol/l), in the presence of pure lecithin vesicles (C:L=0), addition of TUDC caused a significant increase in release of AP from canaliculi. *$p < 0.05$

the presence of vesicles ([L] = 5.5 mmol/l), the protective effect of TUDC was lost. Indeed, at the 6 mmol/l concentration of TDC, the addition of TUDC to TDC in the presence of pure lecithin vesicles significantly aggravated canalicular membrane disruption; this effect was not observed with cholesterol-containing vesicles.

DISCUSSION

Our data are compatible with the hypothesis that the toxicity of bile salts and the protective effect of ursodeoxycholate in cholestatic liver disease may result from physicochemical events occurring at the luminal surface of the canalicular membrane. According to a hypothesis first clearly enunciated by Coleman and associates[13], and elaborated by Hardison, Kitani, and others[5,14–16], hydrophobic bile salts at high concentrations in the canaliculus may injure the canalicular membrane via their detergent effect, possibly by disrupting tight junctions, dissolving membrane lipids, or stripping key hydrophobic proteins from the membrane outer leaflet. The physicochemical disruptive effects of bile salts towards membranes have been shown to be a function of concentration and, to a first approximation, of hydrophobicity[8]. We found previously that addition of TUDC to more hydrophobic bile salts attenuated their detergency and reduced disruption of cholesterol-rich lecithin membranes, and that the magnitudes of disruption and protection were influenced by the total concentrations of membrane lipids, as well as by the concentrations of bile salts[8].

The current studies advance our understanding of the interactions between hydrophilic and hydrophobic bile acids, vesicles, and the biliary canalicular membrane. There were two key findings. First, lecithin:cholesterol vesicles at concentrations attainable in bile markedly reduced the disruption of canaliculi by TDC. This finding complements the previous reports indicating that phospholipid can reduce cytolytic effects of bile salts towards erythrocytes[17] and hepatocytes[10]. At low bile acid concentrations in our studies the protective effect of vesicles was nearly complete, and addition of cholesterol reduced the protective effect. These findings can be explained by the fact that incorporation of hydrophobic bile acids into vesicles and mixed micelles greatly reduces the concentration of bile acid monomers and simple micelles in the aqueous phase[18] (Fig. 4). Indeed, at bile acid concentrations just above the critical micellar concentration, adsorption of bile salts to vesicles may cause the aqueous bile acid concentration to fall below the critical micellar limit. The weaker protection observed with cholesterol-containing vesicles is consistent with the observation that cholesterol reduces affinity of bile acids for membranes; thus membranes with high cholesterol content are less effective in binding TDC and lowering the non-lecithin associated [TDC]. Because TDC binds with greater affinity than TUDC, addition of lecithin also increases the overall relative hydrophilicity of non-lecithin associated bile salts, as demonstrated recently by Donovan et al.[19].

Second, we confirmed that TUDC has little intrinsic canalicular toxicity, and under some conditions may directly attenuate the toxicity of more hydrophobic bile salts such as TDC. In contrast to previous findings with model membranes composed solely of lecithin and cholesterol, the protective effect of TUDC against canalicular membrane disruption by TDC was relatively modest; it was demonstrable only at relatively high concentrations of TDC and TUDC, and was abolished by addition of vesicles. The reasons for these differences are unclear. Solubilization of alkaline phosphatase from the canalicular membrane may not invariably reflect changes in canalicular membrane lipid composition or permeability. In addition, the canalicular membrane contains a complex mixture of lipids and proteins which are distributed asymmetrically; interactions among these components may affect its susceptibility to disruption by bile salts. The modest protective effect of TUDC *in vitro* contrasts to very striking protection against bile salt hepatotoxicity *in vivo*. The *in vivo* protective effects of TUDC may result not only from direct interference with detergency of TDC and other hydrophobic bile salts, but also from dilution of more toxic bile salts via stimulation of biliary water secretion. An additional protective effect of UDC in humans may result from its ability to reduce the cholesterol:lecithin ratio of bile.

The protective effect of biliary vesicles may provide a teleological explanation for biliary lipid secretion, and particularly for the high concentration of vesicles in human bile. Most other mammalian species have much lower rates of secretion of lipid into bile; these species may normally avoid detergent injury to canalicular membranes and biliary epithelia by synthesis and secretion of a relatively hydrophilic (non-toxic) bile salt pool, or by dilution of biliary bile salts through bile salt-independent canalicular bile secretion. In humans the bile salt pool consists predominantly of relatively hydrophobic chenodeoxycholate and deoxycholate, and bile salt-independent canalicular secretion is minimal. Thus, in humans, high rates of biliary secretion of vesicles may have evolved as a major physicochemical mechanism by which bile salt toxicity is avoided.

Acknowledgements

The author gratefully acknowledges the contributions of Ms Linda Nelms and Ms Qian Lin. These studies were supported by grant PO1-DK38030 from the

National Institutes of Health and by grants from the Department of Veterans Affairs and the Ciba-Geigy Corporation.

References

1. Armstrong MJ, Carey MC. The hydrophobic–hydrophilic balance of bile salts. Inverse correlation between reverse-phase high performance liquid chromatographic mobilities and micellar cholesterol-solubilizing capacities. J Lipid Res. 1982;23:70–80.
2. Heuman DM. Quantitative estimation of the hydrophobic–hydrophilic balance of mixed bile salt solutions. J Lipid Res. 1989;30:719–30.
3. Heuman DM, Mills AS, McCall JB, Hylemon PB, Pandak WM, Vlahcevic ZR. Conjugates of ursodeoxycholate protect against cholestasis and hepatocellular necrosis caused by more hydrophobic bile salts: in vivo studies in the rat. Gastroenterology. 1991;100:203–11.
4. Kitani K, Kanai S. Tauroursodeoxycholate prevents taurocholate induced cholestasis. Life Sci. 1982;30:515–23.
5. Kitani K, Ohta M, Kanai S. Tauroursodeodycholate prevents biliary protein excretion induced by other bile salts in the rat. Am J Physiol. 1985;248:G407–17.
6. Heuman DM, Pandak WM, Hylemon PB, Vlahcevic ZR. Conjugates of ursodeoxycholate protect against toxicity of more hydrophobic bile salts: *in vitro* studies in rat hepatocytes and human erythrocytes. Hepatology. 1991;14:920–6.
7. Galle PR, Theilmann L, Raedsch R, Otto G, Stiehl A. Ursodeoxycholate reduces hepatotoxicity of bile salts in primary human hepatocytes. Hepatology. 1990;12:486–91.
8. Heuman DM, Bajaj RS. Ursodeoxycholate conjugates protect against disruption of cholesterol-rich membranes by bile salts: a possible physicochemical basis for the hepatoprotective action of ursodeoxycholate. Gastroenterology. 1994;106:1333–41.
9. Vyvoda OS, Coleman R, Holdsworth G. Effects of different bile salts upon the composition and morphology of a liver plasma membrane preparation. Deoxycholate is more membrane damaging than cholate and its conjugates. Biochim Biophys Acta. 1977;465:68–76.
10. Puglielli L, Amigo L, Arrese M et al. Protective role of biliary cholesterol and phospholipid lamellae against bile acid-induced cell damage. Gastroenterology. 1994;107:244–54.
11. Hope MJ, Bally MB, Webb G, Cullis PR. Production of large unilamellar vesicles by a rapid extrusion procedure. Characterization of size distribution, trapped volume and ability to maintain a membrane potential. Biochim Biophys Acta. 1985;812:55–65.
12. Meier PJ, Boyer JL. Preparation of basolateral (sinusoidal) and canalicular plasma membrane vesicles for the study of hepatic transport processes. Methods Enzymol. 1990;192:534–48.
13. Coleman R, Holdsworth G, Vyvoda OS. Hepatocyte surface enzymes and their appearance in bile. In: Popper H, Bianchi L, Reutter W, editors. Falk Symposium 22. Membrane alterations as basis of liver injury. Lancaster: MTP Press; 177:143–56.
14. Hardison WGM, Hatoff DE, Miyai K, Weiner RG. Nature of bile acid maximum secretory rate in rat. Am J Physiol. 1981;241:G337–43.
15. Hatoff DE, Hardison WG. Bile acid-dependent secretion of alkaline phosphatase in rat bile. Hepatology. 1982;2:433–9.
16. Kitani K, Kanai S, Ohta M, Sato Y. Differing transport maxima values for taurine-conjugated bile salts in rats and hamsters. Am J Physiol. 1986;251:G852–8.
17. Coleman R, Iqbal S, Godfrey PP, Billington D. Membranes and bile formation. Composition of several mammalian biles and their membrane-damaging properties. Biochem J. 1979;178:201–8.
18. Bajaj R, Heuman DM. Adsorption of bile salts to model membranes: effects of cholesterol and ursodeoxycholate. In: Paumgartner G, Stiehl A, Gerok W, editors. Bile acids and the hepatobiliary system. Dordrecht: Kluwer Academic Publishers; 1993:197–205.
19. Donovan JM, Jackson AA, Carey MC. Molecular species composition of inter-mixed micellar/vesicular bile salt concentrations in model bile: dependence upon hydrophilic-hydrophobic balance. J Lipid Res. 1993;34:1131–40.

31
The hydrophobic bile salt as an agent of mitochondrial toxicity

J. R. SPIVEY, R. BOTLA, S. F. BRONK and G. J. GORES

INTRODUCTION

The interaction of bile salts with cell membrane lipids has long been, and continues to be, a primary focus of research with regard to the mechanism of cell injury in cholestasis. However, the subcellular target of bile salt-induced hepatocyte injury remains unclear. An enlarging body of information supports the role of the hydrophobic bile salt as a mitochondrial toxin[1-4]. For example, enlarged, swollen mitochondria are observed in secondary biliary cirrhosis, and mitochondria isolated from rats with cholestasis have impaired respiration[2-4]. Moreover, hepatocyte necrosis during bile salt cytotoxicity is associated with ATP depletion[1]. Despite these compelling data, a unifying mechanism by which hydrophobic bile salts produce mitochondrial toxicity has not been identified.

Recent observations point to the importance of the mitochondrial membrane permeability transition (MMPT) in lethal hepatocellular injury[5-7]. The inner mitochondrial membrane is normally impermeant to solutes. However, when the mitochondrial membrane is broached via the MMPT, the inner mitochondrial membrane becomes abruptly permeable to small molecular weight compounds[7]. The MMPT results in mitochondrial swelling, loss of the mitochondrial membrane potential, and failure of oxidative phosphorylation[7]. Although the molecular mechanism by which cell necrosis results from the MMPT is unknown, the data demonstrating a relationship between the MMPT and cell necrosis are compelling and convincing[6]. Indeed, manoeuvres which prevent the MMPT also protect against necrosis of the cell[6]. Because of the recent data implicating bile salts as mitochondrial toxins, and the MMPT as a mechanism of cell necrosis, we sought to determine if toxic bile salts lead to lethal hepatocellular injury through induction of the MMPT. Additionally, we performed experiments to determine if ursodeoxycholate (UDCA) may exert its cytoprotective effect against bile salt cytotoxicity by blocking the MMPT.

We used glycochenodeoxycholate (GCDC) for our toxic, hydrophobic bile salt, based on the following rationale. First, GCDC is a primary bile salt whose serum and intrahepatic concentrations increase in cholestasis[8]. Second, GCDC is known to be toxic to human hepatocytes[9]. Finally, GCDC is the most prevalent conjugate of chenodeoxycholate in humans[10].

EXPERIMENTAL PROCEDURES

Hepatocyte isolation and culture, measurement of cell viability, and determination of ATP

Hepatocyte suspensions were isolated from adult male Sprague-Dawley rats (250–350 g) as previously described in detail[1]. Cell viability was determined in cell suspensions from the total fluorescence of propidium iodide[11]. ATP was quantitated in hepatocyte suspensions by the luciferin/luciferase assay as we have previously described in detail[12].

Measurement of mitochondrial respiration in digitonin-permeabilized cells

Hepatocytes were permeabilized with digitonin and mitochondrial respiration quantitated as we have previously described[1]. State III respiration was measured in the presence of 5 μmol/l rotenone, 5 mmol/l succinate, and 1 mmol/l adenosine diphosphate (ADP)[1]. State IV respiration was measured under identical conditions to state III except oligomycin, 1 μg/ml, was added to the buffer[1].

Mitochondrial isolation

Low calcium liver mitochondria were isolated from adult male Sprague-Dawley rats (250–350 g) and purified by sucrose–Percoll gradient centrifugation[6,13]. Briefly, the rats were anaesthetized with sodium pentobarbital, the peritoneal cavity was opened, and liver perfused *in situ* with 30–40 ml of ice-cold 0.25 mol/l sucrose containing 1 mmol/l EGTA, pH 7.4. The liver was removed and 10–12 g of the liver were minced into small pieces (less than 1 cm) using scissors. The minced liver was placed in a Teflon glass Poter-Elvehjem homogenizer (Curtin Matheson Scientific, Inc., Houston, TX) and homogenate buffer (sucrose 70 mmol/l, mannitol 220 mmol/l, EGTA 1 mmol/l and HEPES 10 mmol/l, pH 7.4 at 4°C) was added to make a 10% homogenate. The liver tissue was gently homogenized at a speed of 800 r.p.m. using six complete up-and-down strokes with a wall-mounted and speed-controlled mechanical skill drill and Teflon pestle (Electro-Craft Servo Products, Eden Prairie, MN). The homogenate was placed in 50 ml conical plastic tubes and centrifuged at 600*g* for 10 min at 4°C using a Mistral 3000i centrifuge (Curtin Matheson Scientific, Inc., Houston, TX). The postnuclear supernatant was collected and centrifuged in 50 ml polycarbonate centrifuge tubes (Beckman Instruments, Inc., Palo Alto, CA) at 700*g* for 10 min using a Beckman Centrifuge Model J2-21 M/E and JA 20 rotor (Beckman Instruments, Inc., Palo Alto, CA). Mitochondria in the pellet were further purified by sucrose–Percoll gradient centrifugation. The mitochondrial pellet was resuspended in 2 ml of homogenate buffer and 1 ml each of the resuspended pellet was carefully layered on top of 35 ml of the sucrose–Percoll gradient. The sucrose–Percoll solution was prepared by mixing 75 ml of the 0.25 mol/l sucrose containing 1 mmol/l EGTA and 25 ml of Percoll (density 1.129 g/ml); a self-generating gradient was generated by centrifuging 35 ml of the sucrose–Percoll solution at 43 000g at 4°C using a Beckman Centrifuge Model J2-21 M/E and JA 20 rotor. The clear supernatant solution was carefully aspirated with a vacuum suction, and the bottom turbid layer was resuspended in 30 ml of wash buffer at 4°C (KCl 0.1 mol/l, MOPS 5 mmol/l and EGTA 1 mmol/l at pH 7.4) and centrifuged at 7000g for 10 min at 4°C. The mitochondrial pellet was resuspended in a buffer containing sucrose, 50 mmol/l KCl, 5 mmol/l HEPES, 2 mmol/l KH_2PO_2 which had been treated with chelex-100 to remove Ca^{2+}.

Measurement of mitochondrial membrane permeability transition (MMPT) in de-energized mitochondria

MMPT was measured spectrophotometrically as described by Pastorino and co-workers[6]. This assay equates the MMPT with high-amplitude, rapid swelling of mitochondria. An increase in mitochondrial swelling results in a decrease in optical density. Isolated rat liver mitochondria were suspended (1 mg of protein/ml) in chelex-treated respiration buffer containing 0.1 mol/l NaCl and 10 mmol/l MOPS, pH 7.4 at 25°C. The optical density was monitored for a total of 10 min at 540 nm in a Beckman DU 7400 Diode Array spectrophotometer (Beckman Instruments, Inc., Palo Alto, CA) at 2°C; 1 mmol/l glutamate and malate, substrates for complex I of the respiratory chain, were added to the final volume of 3 ml to initiate respiration. Three minutes later, 5 μmol/l rotenone, an inhibitor of complex I, was added to the suspension. Two minutes following the addition of rotenone, 200 μmol/l glycochenodeoxycholic acid (GCDC) was added to the suspension. The optical density was measured for an additional 5 min after addition of GCDC. Where indicated, mitochondria were preincubated with ursodeoxycholate (100–500 μmol/l) or cyclosporin A (5 μmol/l) plus trifluoperazine (10 μmol/l) for 5 min at 25°C before initiation of the assay.

RESULTS/DISCUSSION

Fructose prevents GCDC-induced ATP depletion and loss of cell viability

GCDC, the most prevalent form of chenodeoxycholate during cholestasis, reliably resulted in cell death when added to hepatocyte suspensions. After 2 h of incubation with 250 μmol/l GCDC, the viability of cell suspensions was only 23 ± 1% (Fig. 1). In contrast, viability of cells not treated with GCDC was 89 ± 5% after 2 h of incubation. GCDC also produced rapid depletion of ATP with only 14 ± 5% of the initial ATP concentration remaining after 30 min of incubation. Because 95% of cellular ATP generation is derived from oxidative phosphorylation, these data suggest that impairment of mitochondrial function occurs during cytotoxicity by GCDC. However, the mechanistic relationship

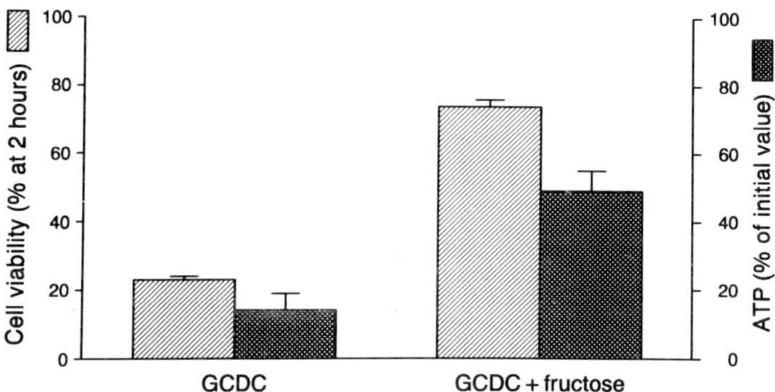

Fig. 1 Fructose prevents GCDC-induced ATP depletion and loss of cell viability. Hepatocyte suspensions were incubated in 3 ml of KRH buffer containing 1 μmol/l propidium iodide and 0.2% BSA at 37°C. Cell viability was assessed by propidium iodide fluorometry after the addition of 250 μmol/l GCDC (left axis, cross-hatched bars). Under identical conditions, ATP concentrations were quantitated using a luciferin/luciferase bioluminescence assay after the addition of 250 μmol/l GCDC and 250 μmol/l GCDC plus 20 mmol/l fructose (right axis, double cross-hatched bars). Basal concentrations of ATP were 19.8 ± nmol/10^6 cells

between the ATP depletion and hepatocyte necrosis by GCDC was unclear. To determine if ATP depletion contributes to cell necrosis by GCDC, we incubated hepatocytes with fructose during exposure to GCDC. Fructose prevents cell necrosis during mitochondrial dysfunction in anoxia by supplying ATP via glycolysis[14]. In the presence of 20 mmol/l fructose, ATP concentrations improved to 49±6% of the initial value up to 90 min after the addition of 250 μmol/l GCDC, and cell viability was maintained at 74±2% after 2 h of incubation (Fig. 1). Protection against GCDC-induced cell necrosis by glycolytic ATP generation suggests that ATP depletion contributes to loss of cell viability during incubation of hepatocytes with GCDC. Because cellular ATP can be partially maintained with glycolysis, ATP depletion during GCDC cytotoxicity appears to be due to mitochondrial dysfunction. These data raise the following question: Is GCDC a mitochondrial toxin?

GCDC results in inhibition of state III respiration in permeabilized hepatocytes

To test the hypothesis that GCDC is a direct mitochondrial toxin, we measured state III and state IV mitochondrial respiration in permeabilized hepatocytes in the presence and absence of GCDC. We chose to use permeabilized hepatocytes instead of isolated mitochondria because the permeabilized hepatocytes retain intracellular bile salt-binding proteins. The presence of intracellular bile salt-binding proteins may influence the compartmentation of the bile salts and the free bile salt concentration, rendering the experiment more applicable to cholestasis occurring *in vivo*. GCDC inhibited state III respiration in a dose-dependent manner (Table 1); however, state IV respiration was unaffected (data not shown). Although 500 μmol/l UDCA protects against the onset of cell necrosis during exposure of hepatocytes to 250 μmol/l GCDC (Fig. 2), UDCA

Table 1 Concentration dependence of glycochenodeoxycholate-mediated inhibition of state III mitochondrial respiration

Concentration of GCDC (mmol/l)	State III respiration (percentage of basal values)
0	100
250	68±3
500	54±2
750	41±1
1000	31±2

Mitochondrial respiration was measured as oxygen consumption in hepatocyte suspensions permeabilized with $10\,\mu$mol/l digitonin. Permeabilized cells were incubated with 1 mmol/l ADP, 5 mmol/l succinate, $5\,\mu$mol/l rotenone, and various concentrations of GCDC. Oxygen consumption was measured polarographically. Basal values for state III mitochondrial respiration were 181 ± 8ng $-$atm 0 min^{-1} per 10^6 cells

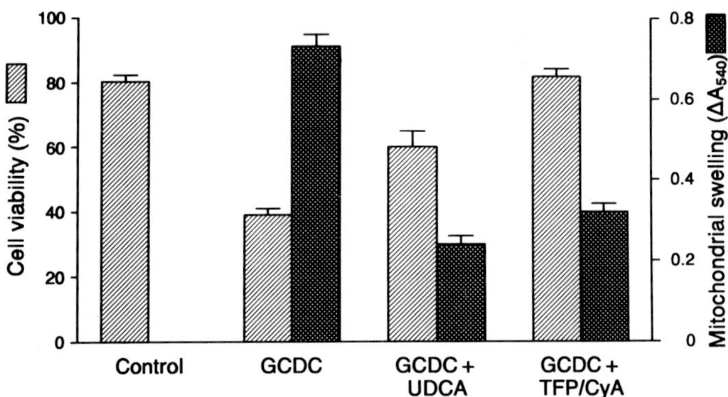

Fig. 2 Association between cytotoxicity and induction of the mitochondrial membrane permeability transition by GCDC. Hepatocyte suspensions (10^5/ml) were incubated in 3 ml of KRH buffer containing $1\,\mu$mol/l propidium iodide and 0.2% BSA at 37°C. Cell viability was assessed by propidium iodide fluorometry (left axis, cross-hatched bars). Isolated mitochondria (1 mg protein/ml) were suspended in respiration buffer at 25°C and preincubated for 5 min with $5\,\mu$mol/l cyclosporin A (CyA) plus $10\,\mu$mol/l TFP or $500\,\mu$mol/l UDC (right axis, double cross-hatched bars). Large-amplitude swelling of suspended mitochondria was measured by monitoring the optical density at 540 nm. At time zero, $200\,\mu$mol/l GCDC was added, and mitochondrial swelling was monitored for an additional 5 min

did not prevent ATP depletion or inhibition of state III mitochondrial respiration in the presence of GCDC (data not shown). These data directly demonstrate that GCDC impairs mitochondrial respiration and oxidative phosphorylation, and support the concept that toxic bile salts are direct mitochondrial toxins.

Association between cell viability and the mitochondrial membrane permeability transition

The cellular mechanisms mediating cell necrosis during loss of oxidative phosphorylation and ATP depletion remain controversial[5]. However, recent data strongly suggest the mitochondrial membrane permeability transition (MMPT) mediates cell necrosis during mitochondrial dysfunction[5–7]. The MMPT is characterized by a rapid permeability of the inner mitochondrial membrane to small molecular weight solutes, and can be measured by monitoring colloid-osmotic swelling of mitochondria spectrophotometrically[6]. Therefore, we determined whether GCDC could induce the MMPT in isolated mitochondria by monitoring mitochondria swelling in the presence and absence of GDCD. GCDC resulted in high-amplitude mitochondrial swelling at a concentration of 200 μmol/l compared to control preparations which exhibited no swelling. Thus, GDCD induced a MMPT in isolated mitochondria. The MMPT can occur by either cyclosporin A-sensitive or -insensitive mechanisms[15]. Inhibition of the MMPT by cyclosporin A is enhanced by trifluorperazine[7]. To determine the mechanism of the GCDC-induced MMPT (i.e. cyclosporin A-sensitive or insensitive mechanism), we determined the effect of cyclosporin A (5 μmol/l) and trifluoperazine (10 μmol/l) on mitochondrial swelling caused by 200 μmol/l GCDC. Cyclosporin A and trifluoperazine were extremely effective in preventing the GCDC-induced mitochondrial swelling (Fig. 2). Similarly, 500 μmol/l UDCA effectively reduced GCDC-induced mitochondrial swelling (Fig. 2). Both UDCA and cyclosporin A plus trifluoperazine also improved hepatocyte viability to 60 ± 5% and 82 ± 2%, respectively, compared to a viability of 23 ± 1% after 2 h of incubation with 250 μmol/l GCDC alone. Thus, concentrations of UDCA and cyclosporin A plus trifluoperazine which block the GCDC-induced MMPT are cytoprotective.

In composite, these data suggest that toxic bile salts cause a bioenergetic form of hepatocyte necrosis by three sequential steps. First, the toxic bile salts cause failure of oxidative phosphorylation characterized by GCDC-induced inhibition of state III respiration. Second, cellular ATP depletion results from the inhibition of oxidative phosphorylation if glycolytic substrates are unavailable to maintain cellular ATP concentrations via glycolysis (Fig. 1). However, despite ATP depletion, cell necrosis can be prevented if the MMPT does not occur (Fig. 2). Thus, the third step of hepatocyte necrosis due to toxic bile salts is the MMPT. Our data demonstrating impaired mitochondrial respiration, ATP depletion, and the MMPT by GCDC are consistent with this interpretation of the mechanisms of cell necrosis during bile salt cytotoxicity (Fig. 3). Prevention of cell necrosis with fructose demonstrates the importance of ATP depletion in contributing to bile-salt-induced hepatocyte necrosis (Figs 1 and 3). Cytoprotection with cyclosporin A plus trifluoperazine highlights the importance of the MMPT in mediating cell necrosis. Thus, multiple mechanistic steps can be identified during bile salt-induced hepatocyte necrosis, and each step can be targeted to help ameliorate hepatocyte toxicity from hydrophobic bile salts. Finally, our data suggest a new paradigm to explain cytoprotection by UDCA against cytotoxicity by hydrophobic bile salts. UDCA may protect against bile salt-induced cell necrosis by inhibiting the MMPT. Further work will be required to determine the mechanism of UDCA inhibition of the MMPT, and if these *in vitro* observations can be applied to liver injury *in vivo* during cholestasis.

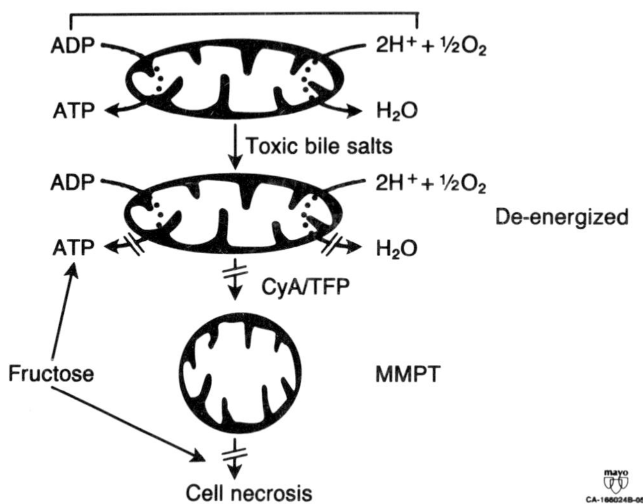

Fig. 3 Schematic representation of mitochondrial dysfunction during bile salt cytotoxicity. During physiological conditions, mitochondrial respiration is coupled to ATP synthesis. However, toxic bile salts inhibit oxidative phosphorylation, decreasing both mitochondrial respiration and mitochondrial ATP generation. The de-energized mitochondria are then prone to undergo mitochondrial membrane permeability transition (MMPT) induced by further exposure to the toxic bile salts. The onset of MMPT causes cell necrosis (cytolysis). Glycolytic substrates such as fructose can inhibit bile salt-induced necrosis by generating sufficient ATP via glycolytic pathways. In addition, agents such as cyclosporin A (Cya) plus trifluoperazine (TFP), which inhibit the onset of the MMPT, can also prevent cell necrosis despite ATP depletion

Acknowledgements

This work was supported by Grant DK 41876 from the National Institutes of Health, the Gainey Foundation, and by the Mayo Foundation.

References

1. Spivey JR, Bronk SF, Gores GJ. Glycochenodeoxycholate-induced lethal hepatocellular injury in rat hepatocytes: role of ATP depletion and cytosolic free calcium. J Clin Invest. 1993;92: 17–24.
2. Krahenbuhl S, Krahenbaul-Glauser S, Stucki J, Gehr P, Reichen J. Stereological and functional analysis of liver mitochondria from rats with secondary biliary cirrhosis: impaired mitochondrial metabolism and increased mitochondrial content per hepatocyte. Hepatology. 1992;15:1167–72.
3. Krahenbuhl S, Talos C, Fisher S, Reichen J. Toxicity of bile acids on the electron transport chain of isolated rat liver mitochondria. Hepatology. 1994;19:471–9.
4. Krahenbuhl S, Stucki J, Reichen J. Reduced activity of the electron transport chain in liver mitochondria isolated from rats with secondary biliary cirrhosis. Hepatology. 1992;15:1160–6.
5. Rosser BG, Gores GJ. Liver cell necrosis: mechanisms and clinical implications. Gastroenterology (In press).
6. Pastorino JG, Snyder JW, Serroni A, Hoek JB, Farber JL. Cyclosporin and carnitine prevent the anoxic death of cultured hepatocytes by inhibiting the mitochondrial permeability transition. J Biol Chem. 1993;268:13791–8.
7. Gunter TE, Pfeiffer DR. Mechanisms by which mitochondria transport calcium. Am J Physiol. 1990;258:C755–86.

8. Greim H, Czygan P, Schaffner F, Popper H. Determination of bile acids in needle biopsies of human liver. Biochem Med. 1973;8:280–6.
9. Miyazaki K, Nakayama F, Koga A. Effect of chenodeoxycholic and ursodeoxycholic acids on isolated adult human hepatocytes. Dig Dis Sci. 1984;12:1123–30.
10. Crosignani A, Podda M, Battezzati PM *et al*. Changes in bile acid composition in patients with primary biliary cirrhosis induced by ursodeoxycholic acid administration. Hepatology. 1991;14:1000–7.
11. Gores GJ, Nieminen A, Fleishman KE, Dawson TL, Herman B, Lemasters JJ. Extracellular acidosis delays onset of cell death in ATP-depleted hepatocytes. Am J Physiol. 1988;255: C315–22.
12. Groskreutz JL, Bronk SF, Gores GJ. Ruthenium red delays the onset of cell death during oxidative stress of rat hepatocytes. Gastroenterology. 1991;102:1030–8.
13. Sokol RJ, Devereaux M, Mierau GW, Hambridge KM, Shikes RH. Oxidative injury to hepatic mitochondrial lipids in rats with dietary copper overload. Gastroenterology. 1990;99:1061–71.
14. Anundi I, DeGroot H. Hypoxic liver cell death: critical pO_2 and dependence of viability on glycolysis. Am J Physiol. 1989;257:G58–64.
15. Broekemeier KM, Pfeiffer DR. Cyclosporin A-sensitive and insensitive mechanisms produce the permeability transition in mitochondria. Biochem Biophys Res Commun. 1989;163:561–6.

32
Effect of bile acids on expression of HLA on primary human hepatocytes

U. TÖX, J. C. ARNOLD, L. THEILMANN, G. OTTO, W. STREMMEL and A. STIEHL

Ursodeoxycholic acid (UDCA) improves liver function and survival in patients with primary biliary cirrhosis (PBC)[1] and primary sclerosing cholangitis (PSC)[2,3]. Several mechanisms are discussed as explanation for the beneficial effects of UDCA: shift of the hydrophilic–hydrophobic balance of bile acids in serum towards more hydrophilicity[4], increase of the amount of hydrophilic bile acids in the hepatocyte, direct hepatoprotective effect[5], induction of choleresis[6], and modulation of the immune system.

The concept of immunomodulation by UDCA is supported by *in vivo* and *in vitro* data. It was demonstrated that, in patients with PBC, aberrant expression of HLA I on hepatocytes is reduced under therapy with UDCA[7]. A similar effect was shown for the aberrant expression of HLA II on biliary epithelium. In addition, UDCA decreases proliferation of lymphocytes and synthesis of cytokines and immunoglobulins *in vitro*[8,9]. This suppressive effect on cytokine production is also known for other bile acids. The aim of this study was to examine the influence of chenodeoxycholic acid (CDCA) on the expression of HLA on primary human hepatocytes.

After stimulation with γ-interferon, primary human hepatocytes were incubated in various concentrations of CDCA. HLA I and HLA II were detected with a conventional immunohistochemical technique.

After stimulation with γ-interferon, HLA I and HLA II were induced on most of the cultivated primary human hepatocytes: $92\pm6.9\%$ of cells positive for HLA I, and $83\pm8.1\%$ of cells positive for HLA II (Fig. 1).

Following incubation with CDCA, HLA I and HLA II expression were significantly reduced at a concentration of $100\,\mu$mol/l and higher. The reduction of HLA II was not as marked compared to HLA I: $38\pm3.9\%$ of cells positive for HLA I, $58\pm4.0\%$ of cells positive for HLA II (CDCA $100\,\mu$mol/l) (Fig. 1).

UDCA treatment led to a more marked reduction in HLA I and HLA II expression than did CDCA.

The influence of UDCA on immunological processes is increasingly acknowledged as a further mechanism of the drug. This study demonstrates that

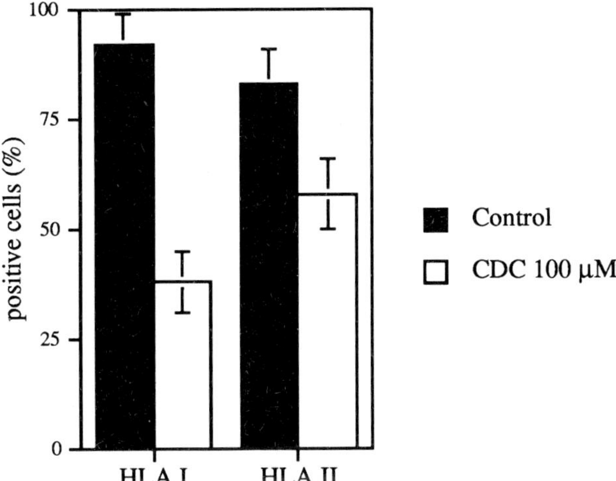

Fig. 1 Effect of chenodeoxycholic acid 100 μmol/l on the expression of HLA I and HLA II on primary human hepatocytes

CDCA also modulates immunologic processes. It was shown that CDCA has a direct suppressive effect on the induced expression of HLA I and HLA II on human primary hepatocytes.

The reduction of HLA I on hepatocytes may have important implications for the progress of chronic hepatic inflammation, as the membraneous expression of these molecules is mandatory for T-cell dependent immune reactions. In addition, the hepatocyte seems to be able to stimulate and perpetuate cellular immune reactions via HLA without the additional support of accessory cells as monocytes[10].

The mechanism reducing HLA expression on hepatocytes after incubation with CDCA is not known. This effect may be due to membraneous integration of the bile acid possibly changing the conformation of the HLA molecule. Alternatively, CDCA may decrease synthesis of HLA by intracellular signalling pathways.

References

1. Poupon RE, Balkau B, Eschwege E, Poupon R. A multicenter, controlled trial of ursodiol for the treatment of primary biliary cirrhosis. UDCAAA-PBC Study Group. N Engl J Med. 1991;324: 1548–54.
2. Stiehl A, Walker S, Stiehl L, Rudolph G, Hofmann WJ, Theilmann L. Effect of ursodeoxycholic acid on liver and bile duct disease in primary sclerosing cholangitis. A 3-year pilot study with a placebo-controlled study period. J Hepatol. 1994;20:57–64.
3. Beuers U, Spengler U, Kruis W et al. Ursodeoxycholic acid for treatment of primary sclerosing cholangitis: a placebo-controlled trial. Hepatology. 1992;16:707–14.
4. Batta AK, Salen G, Arora R et al. Effect of ursodeoxycholic acid on bile acid metabolism in primary biliary cirrhosis. Hepatology. 1989;10:414–19.
5. Galle PR, Theilmann L, Raedsch R, Otto G, Stiehl A. Ursodeoxycholate reduces hepatotoxicity of bile salts in primary human hepatocytes. Hepatology. 1990;12:486–91.

6. Renner EL, Lake JR, Cragoe EJ, Van DR, Scharschmidt BF. Ursodeoxycholic acid choleresis: relationship to biliary HCO_3^- and effects of Na^+-H^+ exchange inhibitors. Am J Physiol. 1988; 254:G232–41.
7. Calmus Y, Gane P, Rouger P, Poupon R. Hepatic expression of class I and class II major histocompatibility complex molecules in primary biliary cirrhosis: effect of ursodeoxycholic acid. Hepatology. 1990;11:12–15.
8. Yoshikawa M, Tsujii T, Matsumura K *et al*. Immunomodulatory effects of ursodeoxycholic acid on immune responses. Hepatology. 1992;16:358–64.
9. Lacaille F, Paradis K. The immunosuppressive effect of ursodeoxycholic acid: a comparative in vitro study on human peripheral blood mononuclear cells. Hepatology. 1993;18:165–72.
10. Volpes R, Desmet VJ. Can hepatocytes serve as 'activated' immunomodulating cells in the immune response? J Hepatol. 1992;16:228–40.

33
Effect of cholestasis and bile acids on interferon-induced 2′5′-oligoadenylate synthetase and natural killer activities

R. POUPON, P. PODEVIN, Y CALMUS and C. CHEREAU

Cholestasis has a profound influence on the immune system. In bile duct-ligated rats, skin and heart allograft rejection is delayed; the mixed lymphocyte reaction is suppressed; MHC class I and II molecules are overpressed in hepatocytes and cholangiocytes. These changes are least in part reproduced by chenodeoxycholic acid but not by ursodeoxycholic acid.

In the present study we evaluate the influence of cholestasis and bile acids on 2′5′-oligoadenlyate synthetase (2′5′OAS) and natural killer (NK) activities which are both involved in the antiviral properties of interferon.

2′5′OAS activity was measured using a radioenzymatic assay, consisting in measuring the amount of ^{32}P transferred from ATP to oligonucleotides. NK activity was measured using K562 target cells.

In the first series of experiments, the effect of cholestasis induced by ligation-section of the common bile duct in the rat was investigated. Cholestasis induced a time-dependent inhibition of both spleen and liver 2′5′OAS activities. Twenty-four-hour cholestasis reduced enzyme activity by 86%, 70% and 70% related to baseline, in spleen, liver, and isolated hepatocytes, respectively.

In a second series of experiments, the effects of bile acids were evaluated *in vitro* on interferon-induced 2′5′OAS activity and NK activity from fresh human mononuclear cells. Chenodeoxycholic acid and its glyco- and tauroconjugates induced a concentration-dependent inhibition on both 2′5′OAS and NK activites, while ursodeoyxholic acid and its conjugates had less inhibitory properties. In both cases, the biological activities of bile acids were closely related to their surface activity index ($r = 0.79$ and 0.68, respectively; $p = 0.002$).

In conclusion, these results show that cholestasis diminishes the biological activity of interferon. This effect is mimicked *in vitro* by chenodeoxycholic but not by ursodeoxycholic acid. Our results suggest a decrease in the antiviral defenses in cholestatic conditions.

Supported by a grant from Tokyo-Tanabe, Tokyo.

34
Dietary calcium, bile acids, and colon cancer

R. VAN DER MEER, M. J. A. P. GOVERS and J. H. KLEIBEUKER

INTRODUCTION

Colon cancer is the second most common cause of cancer deaths in Western societies. The incidence of this multifactorial disease is strongly related to age, both in high- and low-risk countries[1]. This long latency period of colon cancer probably reflects a sequence of slowly reacting cellular transformations in the protective surface layer (epithelium) of colon mucosa. Molecular-genetic studies[2] indeed indicate that colon carcinogenesis is due to a time-dependent accumulation of about six mutations in tumour suppressor and oncogenes in the colonic epithelial cell. These mutations offer a molecular explanation for the generally accepted adenoma–carcinoma sequence of colon carcinogenesis. Migrant studies and other epidemiological evidence indicate that the incidence of colon cancer is strongly associated with environmental determinants, in particular diet[3]. The intake of a typical Western diet with a high amount of animal (saturated) fat and/or red meat and a low amount of fibre and/or vegetables and fruits is especially associated with a high incidence of adenomas[4] and carcinomas[5,6]. Concerning the mechanisms it is generally hypothesized that dietary fat-dependent increases in secondary bile acids and of fatty acids in the colonic lumen are primary aetiological factors[7]. These hydrophobic and cytolytic surfactants may damage epithelial cells and thus induce a compensatory hyperproliferation of colonic crypt cells resulting in an increased risk of mutation in the oncogenes and tumour-suppressor genes, mentioned above. In addition, hyperproliferation may also promote the outgrowth of premalignant cells into tumours.

Several lines of evidence support this mechanism. A high dietary intake of fat induces colonic epithelial hyperproliferation, both in experimental animals and humans[8,9]. Colonic epithelial hyperproliferation is frequently observed in subjects with colonic adenomas (see e.g. ref. 10). Most case–control studies show no difference in total faecal bile acids. However, levels of secondary bile acids, mainly deoxycholate, are higher in serum and bile of adenoma subjects[11,12], indicating that colonic epithelial exposure to and absorption of these bile acids is

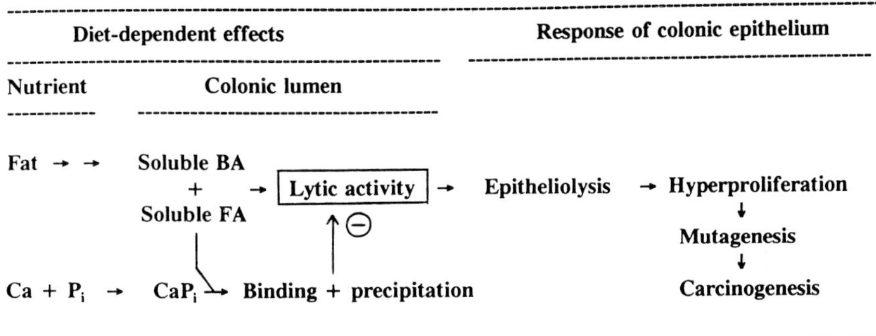

Fig. 1 Proposed mechanism of the protective effect of dietary calcium on colon cancer risk

higher in these subjects[12]. Colonic epithelial proliferation is also increased in intestinal bypass subjects[13], again suggesting that increased exposure of the colonic epithelium to bile acids and/or fatty acids is a causal factor. Newmark *et al.*[14] proposed that the effects of secondary bile acids and of fatty acids on colonic epithelium could be inhibited by soluble calcium in the colonic lumen. They hypothesized that Ca^{2+} precipitates these surfactants and thus prevents their detrimental, cytolytic effects. They further hypothesized that dietary phosphate should inhibit this favourable effect of Ca^{2+}, due to the formation of insoluble calcium phosphate. However, they did not present direct experimental evidence supporting this inhibitory effect of dietary phosphate. Because phosphate is far in excess of calcium in human diets, quantification of the proposed intestinal interactions between calcium, phosphate, bile acids and/or fatty acids is important for a proper understanding of the colonic effects of calcium. Based on our studies[15,16] of the binding of biliary micelles and bile acids to insoluble calcium phosphate, we proposed a modified hypothesis for the intestinal interactions between calcium, phosphate, bile acids and fatty acids (Fig. 1). Our working hypothesis implies that, in the intestinal lumen, dietary calcium and phosphate form an insoluble, amorphous, calcium phosphate complex (CaP_i), which precipitates and thus inactivates bile acids and fatty acids. This precipitation may decrease the surfactant-dependent cytolytic activity of the colonic contents. Consequently, epithelial hyperproliferation, as well as the expression of cellular carcinogenic mutations, may be inhibited. This chapter summarizes our research with regard to the molecular mechanisms of this modified hypothesis. First, we studied the molecular interactions between bile acids, fatty acids, calcium and phosphate *in vitro*, because these interactions are difficult, if not impossible, to study *in vivo*. Subsequently, the physiological relevance of these biochemical studies is ascertained in nutritional studies in animals. Finally the mechanisms of the colonic effects of calcium are studied in humans.

IN VITRO STUDIES

First, we determined the effects of calcium and phosphate on the solubility of different types of bile acids. Using the pH range 5.5–8.0, which is that reported

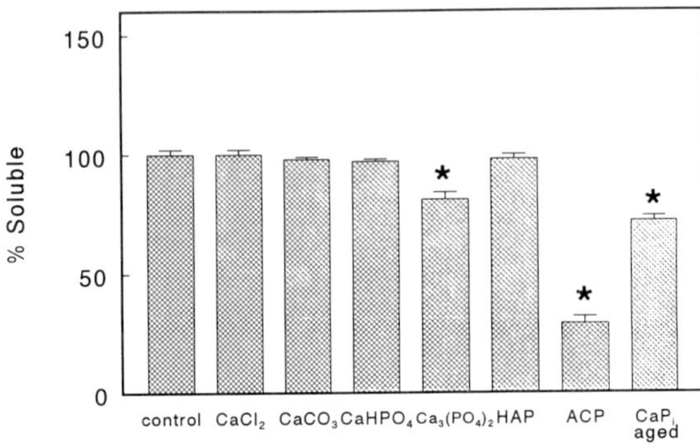

Fig. 2 Effects of calcium chloride and of various insoluble calcium salts on the solubility of GCDC. The calcium salts were preincubated (pH 7) for 10 min and subsequently incubated with 4 mmol/l GCDC for 15 min. Solubility was measured after centrifugation. HAP: hydroxyapatite; ACP: amorphous calcium phosphate; aged CaP_i: ACP preincubated for 12 h ($*p < 0.05$ vs control)

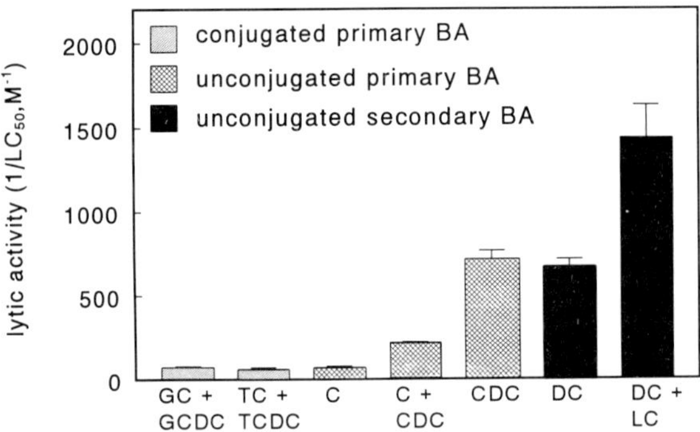

Fig. 3 Lytic activity of the physiologically relevant primary and secondary bile acids (BA). Lytic activity is defined as the reciprocal of the concentration required for 50% lysis (mean ± SD; $n = 6$)

for the human intestine[17], we found that precipitation of bile acids coincides with the formation of insoluble calcium phosphate[16]. Under these physiological conditions simple bile acids, as well as bile acids in human bile, were precipitated by calcium phosphate[16,18,19] and not by soluble Ca^{2+}. As illustrated in Fig. 2, this precipitation is an almost unique property of freshly formed, amorphous calcium phosphate (ACP) and is hardly observed with aged, more crystalline calcium phosphates and with other insoluble calcium salts. The mechanism of this binding of bile acids, mediated by hydrophobic aggregation of bile acid monomers at the ACP surface, has recently been described[19].

Subsequently, the cytolytic activity of bile acids was studied using lysis of erythrocytes as a model system. This is an adequate model, because surfactant-induced lysis of erythrocytes is analogous to that of colonic epithelial cells[20,21]. Figure 3 shows the lytic effects of different physiological mixtures of bile acids using the reciprocal of the concentration required for 50% lysis ($1/LC_{50}$) as

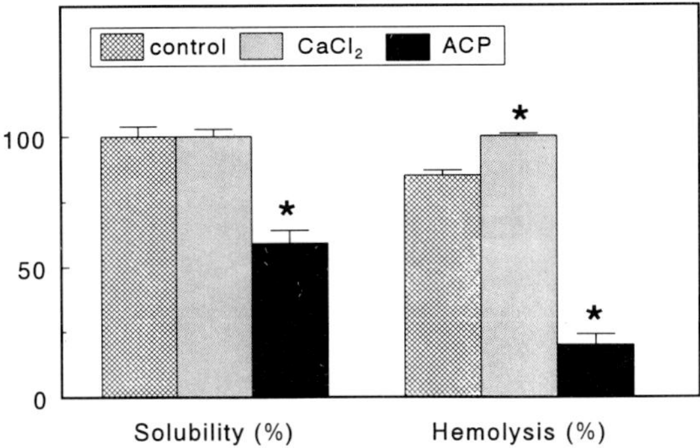

Fig. 4 Differential effects of calcium chloride and of amorphous calcium phosphate (ACP) on the solubility and cytolytic activity of deoxycholate. Total calcium concentration 10 mmol/l; total deoxycholate concentration ≈ 2 mmol/l (*$p < 0.05$ vs control)

measure for their cytolytic activity[22]. Cytolytic activity of the unconjugated, secondary bile acids was much higher than that of their conjugated, primary counterparts. These effects of bile acid structure on cytolytic activity may be of relevance for the integrity of human intestinal mucosa. For instance, bile acids in the small intestine are mainly composed of the relatively non-lytic glycine- and taurine-conjugated primary bile acids cholate (GC and TC) and chenodeoxycholate (GCDC and TCDC). These bile acids are deconjugated and dehydroxylated by colonic bacteria. Consequently, more than 90% of the colonic bile acids consists of the hydrophobic, secondary bile acids deoxycholate (DC) and lithocholate (LC), which have a high lytic activity. In similar experiments we observed also that hydrophobicity of fatty acids is an important determinant of their cytolytic activity[21]. Moreover, low submicellar concentrations of bile acids synergistically stimulate fatty acid-induced lytic activity with the same hydrophobic dependence as observed for bile acids alone.

Finally, we studied the effects of ionic calcium and of ACP on the cytolytic activity of bile acids. Amorphous calcium phosphate binds and thus precipitates bile acids. This binding inhibits the cytolytic activity, as is illustrated for the colonic bile acid deoxycholate (DC) in Fig. 4. In contrast, soluble ionic calcium does not precipitate this bile acid, but stimulates its cytolytic activity[22]. Thus, ACP binds and precipitates bile acids, and consequently decreases their cytolytic activity, consistent with the first step in our working hypothesis. This selective binding of bile acids to ACP may also be of relevance for other bile acid-related diseases[23-26].

ANIMAL STUDIES

To ascertain the physiological relevance of the effects of ACP we determined whether insoluble calcium phosphate is formed *in vivo* in the intestine of rats. Intestinal and faecal samples of rats, fed low and high calcium phosphate purified diets, were analysed[27]. We found that calcium and phosphate already precipitated

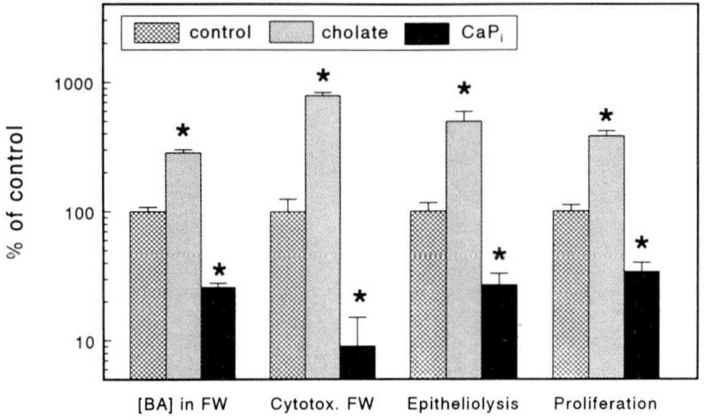

Fig. 5 Effects of dietary cholate (0.15 wt%) and dietary calcium phosphate (Ca: 0.85 wt%) on luminal parameters and response of colonic epithelium in rats (mean±SE; $n=6$; *$p<0.05$ vs control)

in the small intestine and were almost completely precipitated in colon and faeces. In addition, we observed that the solubility of intestinal calcium and phosphate is determined by the pH of its solubility product, analogous to that observed for ACP *in vitro*[28]. Similar results have been obtained in our human studies (see below). Thus, the amount of soluble Ca^{2+} is low, whereas that of ACP is high in colon of rat and humans. Comparison of the data in rat and humans also shows that the conditions in the human colon can be mimicked in rats by changing the calcium phosphate content of the diet.

Effects of dietary calcium on (pre)malignant changes in colonic epithelium have been studied predominantly in rodents. However, as far as we know, intestinal interactions between calcium, phosphate, bile acids and fatty acids were not determined in these studies. Therefore, our experiments were focused on the effects of dietary calcium on luminal parameters in relation to colonic epithelial proliferation. In these experiments we isolated faecal water to quantitate the physiologically relevant cytolytic surfactants, because only soluble surfactants are lytic (see above). As illustrated in Fig. 5, supplementation of a low-calcium, purified diet of rats with a bile acid (cholate) drastically increased the concentration of bile acids in faecal water and stimulated its cytolytic activity, measured with our haemolysis bioassay. Supplemental cholate also induced epitheliolysis, measured as the release of the epithelial cell marker alkaline phosphatase, and stimulated colonic epithelial proliferation. Increasing the amount of calcium phosphate in the diet from 20 μmol/g (which simulates a human calcium intake of about 400 mg/day) to 200 μmol/g diet drastically inhibited all luminal and epithelial parameters (Fig. 5).

In other experiments we studied the differential effects of the type of dietary fat[29], the proposed inhibitory effects of dietary phosphate[27] and the effects of different types of dietary calcium, including calcium phosphate in milk[30]. Taken together these animal experiments confirmed earlier studies that have shown that dietary calcium inhibits colonic proliferation[31,32]. They extend these studies by showing that this effect is not inhibited by phosphate, and that milk calcium has at least a similar protective effect. In addition, they show that the protective effect of calcium is mediated by a decrease in solubility of colonic surfactants, like bile acids and fatty acids, and an inhibition of epithelial cell damage and proliferation. We found that cytolytic activity of faecal water, as well as epitheliolysis, were significantly correlated with colonic epithelial proliferation ($r = 0.97$ and 0.88, respectively). Because of these high correlations, and the analogous results of our biochemical studies, we consider it most likely that this sequence of calcium-specific colonic effects reflects causal relationships, consistent with our working hypothesis.

HUMAN STUDIES

To ascertain the relevance of the results of our biochemical and animal studies for human physiology, we first studied the intestinal association of calcium, phosphate and bile acids[18]. Because in human diets phosphate is far in excess of calcium, supplemental dietary calcium (without phosphate) may stimulate complexation with phosphate and/or bile acids. This increased complexation can be measured only as an increase in faecal excretion of phosphate and bile acids, provided that the intake of phosphate is maintained constant. In healthy subjects, supplemental calcium carbonate increased the faecal excretion of both phosphate and bile acids, which indicates the intestinal formation of an insoluble complex of calcium, phosphate and bile acids. Also in humans the solubility of faecal calcium and phosphate is determined by the solubility product of ACP[33]. Using the calcium chelator EDTA, we found that resolubilization of calcium resulted in an increase of soluble phosphate and of soluble bile acids. This shows that calcium, phosphate and bile acids are present in faeces as an insoluble complex. We also studied the effects of calcium on duodenal bile acid composition. In accordance with the results of our *in vitro* studies calcium decreased the hydrophobic and cytolytic dihydroxy bile acids chenodeoxycholic and deoxycholic acid, and increased the hydrophilic, less cytolytic cholic acid. These results suggest that calcium lowers the cytolytic activity of the soluble bile acids in the intestinal lumen. In line with this we found that calcium decreased the concentration of hydrophobic surfactants in faecal water, and significantly inhibited the cytolytic activity of faecal water[33]. Similar effects of supplemental calcium on faecal bile acid excretion, duodenal bile acid composition and cytolytic activity of faecal water were obtained in patients with colonic adenomas[34].

These effects of calcium supplementation of the diet prompted us to study whether calcium in the habitual diet has similar protective effects on the luminal metabolic risk factors. In a typical Western diet about 70% of dietary calcium is derived from milk and dairy products. Therefore we studied the effects of habitual dietary calcium in a double-blind crossover experiment using specially prepared milk products[35]. During the experimental period of 2 weeks the male volunteers consumed a constant habitual diet in which all liquid dairy products were replaced by either placebo milk/yogurt or regular, high-calcium containing milk/yogurt. These products differed only in calcium content and provided 3 and 30 mmol of Ca/day for the placebo and calcium period, respectively. At the end of each period, faeces were quantitatively collected for 3 days and urine for 1 day. Minerals were measured in faeces and urine, to determine whether the total

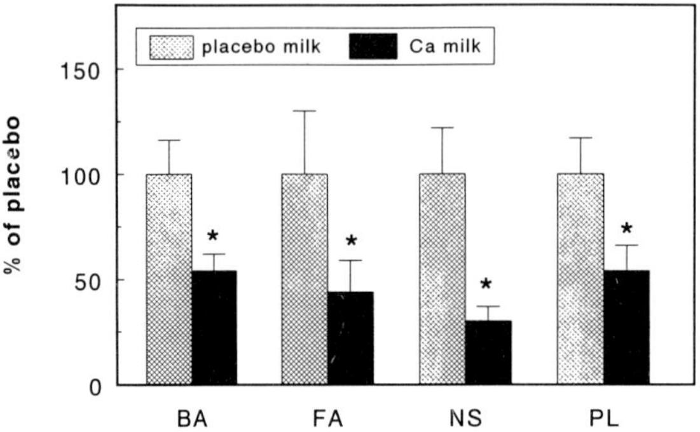

Fig. 6 Effects of calcium milk versus placebo milk in healthy subjects on bile acids (BA), fatty acids (FA), neutral sterols (NS) and phospholipids (PL) in faecal water (mean $\pm$ SE; $n = 13$; *$p < 0.05$ vs placebo)

daily output was in accordance with the designed intake of nutrients. Faecal water was prepared by centrifugation of homogenized faeces and its composition determined by standard procedures. Cytolytic activity was measured as lysis of erythrocytes by faecal water.

The registered intake of nutrients reflected a typical Western diet, and was similar for the placebo and calcium period except for calcium intake. The measured total excretion of calcium differed by 27 mmol/day, which is exactly the difference in calcium content of the supplied placebo and calcium milk products. This shows an excellent compliance with the study protocol, and indicates that effects can be attributed to this increase in dietary calcium. Milk calcium significantly increased faecal pH and the faecal excretion of phosphate, bile acids, and fatty acids, indicating intestinal calcium phosphate formation and precipitation of bile acids and fatty acids. Figure 6 shows that calcium indeed decreases the concentration of bile acids and fatty acids in faecal water, and thus precipitates these lipids. Neutral steroids and phospholipids are probably solubilized by hydrophobic bile acids and thus also precipitated by calcium. To quantitate the effects on hydrophobicity of bile acids we also determined their composition in faecal water. Figure 7 shows that faecal water bile acids mainly consist of the secondary bile acids deoxycholate and lithocholate. Calcium did not change the low concentration of hydrophilic bile acids and of chenodeoxycholate, but significantly decreased the concentration of deoxycholate and of lithocholate. Our *in-vitro* work shows that these hydrophobic secondary bile acids have very severe cytolytic effects (see Fig. 3). In line with these *in-vitro* results we found that milk calcium drastically inhibited the cytolytic activity of faecal water from $68 \pm 9\%$ to $28 \pm 12\%$.

Taken together, the results of our human studies show that dietary calcium has protective effects on the cytolytic surfactants in colonic lumen. The design of our studies is similar to that of the clinical trials studying the effect of calcium on colonic epithelial proliferation. This suggests that the mechanisms described above can be extrapolated to these trials. However, in humans, in contrast to rats, epithelial proliferation can be measured *in vitro* only by using biopsies from

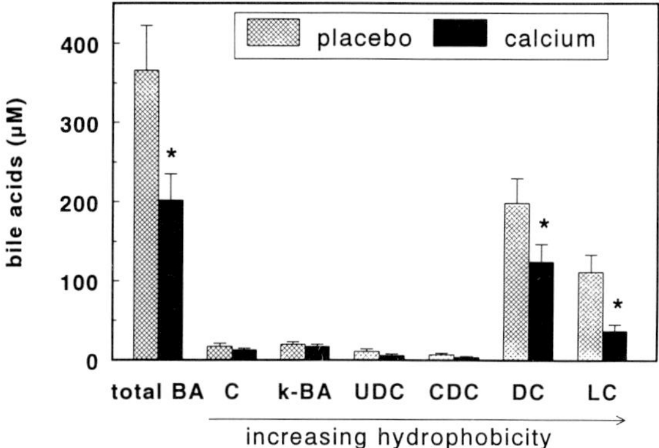

Fig. 7   Effects of calcium milk versus placebo milk in healthy subjects on the composition of faecal water bile acids (mean±SE; $n=13$ *$p<0.05$ vs placebo)

colonic mucosa. For that reason, only patients at an increased risk of colon cancer, and not healthy volunteers, have been studied. A calcium-dependent inhibition of epithelial proliferation is observed in most, but not all, clinical studies (see ref. 36 for a recent review). Whether this reflects differences in response between different patient groups or differences in the control of dietary intake is at present not known. For prevention in the general population it is also important to know whether healthy volunteers and patients differ in epithelial response to dietary calcium[37]. We therefore feel that research should also be focused on the development of *in-vivo* markers of hyperproliferation, which would considerably facilitate the study of the possible preventive effect of calcium in healthy volunteers.

SUMMARY AND CONCLUSIONS

Our *in-vitro*, animal and human studies summarized in this chapter are consistent with the model presented in Fig. 1. As shown *in vitro*, hydrophobic bile acids are preferentially precipitated by insoluble, amorphous calcium phosphate. This precipitation drastically inhibits their cytolytic activity. In rats a diet-induced increase in luminal bile acid concentration stimulates lytic activity of faecal water and epitheliolysis, resulting in an increased epithelial proliferation. The increase in luminal surfactant concentration, lytic activity of faecal water, and colonic epithelial proliferation can be counteracted by dietary calcium phosphate. In humans dietary calcium increases the formation of insoluble calcium phosphate in colonic lumen, decreases the concentration of soluble hydrophobic bile acids and fatty acids and decreases the lytic activity of faecal water. This sequence of effects offers a molecular explanation for the inhibitory effects of supplemental calcium on epithelial proliferation, observed in animals and several patient groups. Final proof, however, is not yet available, because these antiproliferative effects have not yet been studied in healthy volunteers, and are not observed in all clinical trials. Therefore, more well-designed studies in healthy volunteers and patients are needed, using a combined biochemical, nutritional and clinical approach, to elucidate the complex mechanisms of the effects of calcium on colon carcinogenesis.

Acknowledgements

The stimulating contribution of our colleagues at NIZO and the University Hospital Groningen to the studies summarized here is gratefully acknowledged. Our work has been supported by the Netherlands Organization for Scientific Research (NWO), Medical Sciences, and the Dutch Cancer Society.

References

1. Waterhouse J, Muir C, Shanmuguratman K, Powell J. Cancer incidence in five continents, Vol. 4. Lyon: IARC Scientific Publications; 1982.
2. Fearon ER, Jones PA. Progressing toward a molecular description of colorectal cancer development. FASEB J. 1992;6:2783–90.
3. Willett W. The search for the causes of breast and colon cancer. Nature. 1989;338:389–94.
4. Giovannucci E, Stampfer MJ, Colditz G, Rimm EB, Willett C. Relationship of diet to risk of colorectal adenoma in man. J Natl Cancer Inst. 1992;84:91–8.
5. Willett WC, Stampfer MJ, Colditz GA, Rosner BA, Speizer FE. Relation of meat, fat and fiber intake to the risk of colon cancer in a prospective study among women. N Engl J Med. 1990;323:1664–72.
6. Giovannucci E, Rimm EB, Stampfer MJ, Colditz GA, Ascherio A, Willett WC. Intake of fat, meat, and fiber in relation to risk of colon cancer in men. Cancer Res. 1994;54:2390–7.
7. Bruce WR. Recent hypotheses for the origin of colon cancer. Cancer Res. 1987;47:4237–42.
8. Bird RP, Medline A, Furrer R, Bruce WR. Toxicity of orally administered fat to the colonic epithelium of mice. Carcinogenesis. 1985;6:1063–6.
9. Stadler J, Stern HS, Yeung KS *et al*. Effect of high fat consumption on cell proliferation activity of colorectal mucosa and on soluble faecal bile acids. Gut. 1988;29:1326–31.
10. Lipkin M. Biomarkers of increased susceptibility to gastrointestinal cancer: new application to studies of cancer prevention in human subjects. Cancer Res. 1988;48:235–45.
11. Bayerdörffer E, Mannes GE, Richter WO *et al*. Increased serum deoxycholic acid levels in men with colorectal adenomas. Gastroenterology. 1991;104:145–51.
12. Van der Werf SDJ, Nagengast EM, Van Berg Henegouwen GP, Huijbregts AWM, Van Tongeren JHM. Colonic absorption of secondary bile acids in patients with adenomatous polyps and in matched controls. Lancet. 1982;1:759–62.
13. Steinbach G, Lupton J, Reddy BS, Kral JG, Holt PR. Effect of calcium supplementation on rectal epithelial hyperproliferation in intestinal bypass subjects. Gastroenterology. 1994;106:1162–7.
14. Newmark HL, Wargovich MJ, Bruce WR. Colon cancer and dietary fact, phosphate, and calcium: a hypothesis. J Natl Cancer Inst. 1984;72:1323–5.
15. Van der Meer R. Is the hypercholesterolemic effects of casein related to its phosphorylation state? Atherosclerosis. 1983;49:339–41.
16. Van der Meer R, De Vries HT. Differential binding of glycine- and taurine-conjugated bile acids to insoluble calcium phosphate. Biochem J. 1985;229:265–8.
17. Fordtran JS, Locklear TW. Ionic constituents and osmolality of gastric and small-intestinal fluids after eating. Am J Dig Dis. 1966;11:503–21.
18. Van der Meer R, Welberg JWM, Kuipers F *et al*. Effects of supplemental dietary calcium on the intestinal association of calcium, phosphate, and bile acids. Gastroenterology. 1990;99:1653–9.
19. Govers MJAP, Termont DSML, Van Aken GA, Van der Meer R. Characterization of the adsorption of conjugated and unconjugated bile acids to insoluble, amorphous calcium phosphate. J Lipid Res. 1994;35:741–8.
20. Velardi ALM, Groen AK, Oude Elferink RPJ, Van der Meer R, Palasciano G, Tytgat GNJ. Cell-type dependent effect of phospholipid and cholesterol on bile salt cytotoxicity. Gastroenterology. 1991;101:457–64.

21. Lapré JA, Termont DSML, Groen AK, Van der Meer R. Lytic effects of mixed micelles of fatty acids and bile acids. Am J Physiol. 1992;263:G333–7.
22. Van der Meer R, Termont DSML, De Vries HT. Differential effects of calcium ions and calcium phosphate on cytotoxicity of bile acids. Am J Physiol. 1991;260:G142–7.
23. Van der Meer R, Vonk RJ, Kuipers F. Cholestasis and the interactions of sulfated glyco- and taurolithocholate with calcium. Am J Physiol. 1988;254:G644–9.
24. Kuipers F, Hardonk MJ, Vonk RJ, Van der Meer R. Bile secretion of sulfated glycolithocholic acid is required for its cholestatic action in rats. Am J Physiol. 1992;262:G267–73.
25. Castleden WM, Detchon P, Misso NLA. Biliary bile acids in cholelithiasis and colon cancer. Gut. 1989;30:860–5.
26. Qui S-M, Wen G, Hirakawa N, Soloway RD, Hong N-K, Crowther RS. Glycochenodeoxycholic acid inhibits calcium phosphate precipitation in vitro by preventing the transformation of amorphous calcium phosphate to calcium hydroxyapatite. J Clin Invest. 1991;88:1265–71.
27. Govers MJAP, Van der Meer R. Effects of dietary calcium and phosphate on the intestinal interactions between calcium, phosphate, fatty acids, and bile acids. Gut. 1993;34:365–70.
28. Lapré JA, De Vries HT, Van der Meer R. Dietary calcium phosphate inhibits intestinal cytotoxicity. Am J Physiol. 1991;261:G907–12.
29. Lapré JA, De Vries HT, Koeman JH, Van der Meer R. The anti-proliferative effect of dietary calcium on colonic epithelium is mediated by luminal surfactants and dependent on the type of dietary fat. Cancer Res. 1993;53:784–9.
30. Govers MJAP, Termont DSML, Van der Meer R. The mechanism of the antiproliferative effect of milk mineral and other calcium supplements on colonic epithelium. Caner Res. 1994;54:95–100.
31. Caderni G, Stuart EW, Bruce WR. Dietary factors affecting the proliferation of epithelial cells in the mouse colon. Nutr Cancer. 1988;11:147–53.
32. Wargovich MJ, Lynch PM, Levin B. Modulating effects of calcium in animal models of colon carcinogenesis and short-term studies in subjects at increased risk for colon cancer. Am J Clin Nutr. 1991;54:202–5S.
33. Lapré JA, De Vries HT, Termont DSML, Kleibeuker JH, De Vries EGE, Van der Meer R. Mechanism of the protective effects of supplementary dietary calcium on cytolytic activity of fecal water. Cancer Res. 1993;53:248–53.
34. Welberg JWM, Kleibeuker JH, Van der Meer R et al. Effects of oral calcium supplementation on intestinal bile acids and cytolytic activity of fecal water in patients with adenomatous polyps of the colon. Eur J Clin Invest. 1993;23:63–8.
35. Govers M, Lapré J, Kleibeuker J, Vonk R, Van der Meer R. Calcium in milk products precipitates intestinal surfactants and inhibits luminal cytolytic activity in healthy subjects. Gastroenterology. 1994;106:A388.
36. Kleibeuker JH, Cats A, Van der Meer R, Lapré JA, De Vries EGE. Calcium supplementation as prophylaxis against colon cancer? Dig Dis. 1994;12:85–97.
37. Paraskava C. Colorectal cancer and dietary intervention. Lancet. 1992;339:869–70.

Section VIII
Bile acids and biliary stone disease

35
Effect of phospholipid fatty acid composition on cholesterol nucleation and crystal growth

S. TAZUMA, H. OCHI, K. HORIKAWA, H. MIURA, T. OHYA,
G. KAJIYAMA and K. ITOH

INTRODUCTION

Lecithin-cholesterol vesicle is present in human bile and supersaturated model bile solutions, and plays an important role in the pathogenesis of cholesterol gallstone formation[1-3]. Cholesterol nucleation is believed to occur from non-micellar fractions, especially vesicle, and such a vesicular cholesterol metastability is seemingly regulated by the storage of cholesterol within a bilayer; the ratio of cholesterol to phospholipids in vesicle[4,5]. In contrast, recent investigations indicate that cholesterol packing density within a bilayer is modulated by the balance between hydrophobicity and hydrophilicity of lecithin[6,7], and such a balance is possibly associated with the degree of fatty acyl chain unsaturation. Therefore, the aim of the present study was to determine the effect of the degree of acyl chain unsaturation in biliary lecithin on vesicular cholesterol packing density as reflected by cholesterol crystal nucleation.

METHODS

Preparation of supersaturated model bile solutions

Supersaturated model bile (MB) solutions (total lipid concentration, 9 g/dl; cholesterol 7.7 mol%, bile salt/lecithin ratio, 3.7; theoretical cholesterol saturation index, 1.2) were prepared according to a previously described method[8], using sodium taurocholate, cholesterol, and egg-yolk lecithin (EYL-MB), soybean lecithin (SBL-MB), and synthetic lecithins; dipalmitoyl lecithin (DPL-MB), sn-1: palmitoyl, sn-2: linoleoyl lecithin (PLL-MB), and dilinoleoyl lecithin (DLL-MB). Hepes/NaCl (10 mmol/l/150 mmol/l) buffer containing 4 mmol/l EDTA and 0.02% NaN_3 (pH 7.5) was used for resolubilization of lyophilized and stored MB samples.

Conventional nucleation time study

Nucleation time was determined essentially as previously described[9]. Samples were observed every 12 h under a differential interference contrast microscope (Labophoto-2, Nikon, Tokyo, Japan) for 600 h to detect the formation of cholesterol crystals.

Cholesterol crystal growth assay

The growth of cholesterol crystals nucleated in sample solutions was quantitatively assayed using a modification of the recently developed method[10]. A 40-ml aliquot of each MB solution was sampled and diluted with a standard buffer containing 30 mmol/l sodium taurodeoxycholate. After 20 min the absorbance was measured at a wavelength of 900 nm using a spectrophotometer (UV-160, Shimadzu, Kyoto, Japan) over a period of 600 h.

Dimensions of vesicles

The dimensions of vesicles present in MB solutions were determined using a laser diffraction particle size analyser (SALD-2000, Shimadzu, Kyoto, Japan) as previously described[11]. This apparatus analyses the diffraction and scattering patterns of laser light to measure the particle size ranging from 0.03 mm to 280 mm.

Lipid analysis

Concentrations of cholesterol, bile salts, and phospholipids were determined enzymatically. The lecithin hydrophobic–hydrophilic balance was determined by the retention factors calculated from retention times in reversed-phase–high-performance liquid chromatography (HPLC, Shimadzu LC-6A system, Shimadzu Instruments, Tokyo) as previously described[12]. Lecithins were separated into molecular species in a Shimadzu Ultrasphere ODC column (5 mm particle size, 4.5×250 mm). The mobile phase was 20 mmol/l choline chloride in methanol–water–acetonitrile 90.5:7:2.5, at a flow rate of 2.0 ml/min. The hydrophobic index of each lecithin was indexed by the relative retention factors which were determined by retention times.

RESULTS

Nucleation time study and cholesterol crystal growth assay

The ranking order of nucleation time of the MB solution composed of various lecithin species was DPL-MB (>500 h)>EYL-MB (70 h)>PLL-MB (10 h) >SBL-MB (5 h)>DLL-MB (2 h).

Cholesterol crystal growth assay

Cholesterol crystal growth curves of MB solutions were non-linearly sigmoidal. DPL-MB showed no nucleation, and therefore, no growth was observed for 500h. The growth rate of each MB solution was; EYL-MB, 0.005 O.D.(optical density)/h; PLL-MB, 0.046 O.D./h; SBL-MB, 0.061 O.D./h; DLL-MB, 0.161 O.D./h.

The relative hydrophobicity of various lecithin species by HPLC

The order of hydrophobicity (hydrophobic index calculated by HPLC, HI) of the lecithin species was DPL (2.5)>EYL (1.4)>PLL (1.)>SB (0.9)>DLL (0.8).

The dimension of vesicles in various MB solutions

The order of median diameter of vesicles determined by a laser diffraction particle analyser was DPL-MB > EYL-MB > PLL-MB > SBL-MB > DLL-MB.

SUMMARY AND CONCLUSION

In the present study the possible relationship between the net balance of hydrophobicity and hydrophilicity of lecithin and bile metastability as reflected by nucleation time and time for growth of cholesterol crystals was evaluated. The model bile solution consisting of hydrophilic lecithin showed a rapid nucleation time and growth of cholesterol crystals, whereas the solution consisting of the hydrophobic lecithin showed a slow nucleation time and growth of cholesterol crystals. Further, the dimension of vesicles was correlated with the degree of lecithin hydrophobicity. Thus, a hydrophobic lecithin with a high degree of fatty acyl chain saturation binds tightly to cholesterol to form stable cholesterol–lecithin aggregates with a high cholesterol-packing density, whereas a hydrophilic lecithin with a high degree of fatty acyl chain unsaturation binds less tightly to cholesterol with a lower cholesterol-packing density. These results indicate that the balance between hydrophobicity and hydrophilicity of lecithin species influences the structure and properties of vesicles, accordingly regulating bile metastability as reflected by cholesterol nucleation. In conclusion, lecithin species play a role in the process of cholesterol crystal nucleation and growth.

Acknowledgements

This study was supported, in part, by the ministry of Education of the Japanese Government, awarded to Dr Tazuma (No. 06670557).

References

1. Somjen GJ, Gillat T. A non-micellar mode of cholesterol transport in human bile. FEBS Lett. 1983;156:265–8.

2. Halpern Z, Dudley MA, Kibe A, Lynn MP, Breuer AC, Holzbach RT. Rapid vesicle formation and aggregation in abnormal human bile. Gastroenterology. 1986;90:875–85.
3. Lee SP, Park HZ, Madani H, Kaler EW. Partial characterization of a nonmicellar system of cholesterol solubilization in bile. Am J Physiol. 1987;252:G374–84.
4. Halpern Z, Dudley MA, Lynn MP, Nader JM, Breuer AC, Holzbach RT. Vesicle aggregation in model systems of supersaturated bile: relation to crystal nucleation and lipid composition of the vesicular phase. J Lipid Res. 1986;27:295–306.
5. Harvey PRC, Somjen G, Lichtenberg MS, Petrunka C, Gilat T, Strasberg SM. Nucleation of cholesterol from vesicles isolated from bile of patients with and without cholesterol gallstones. Biochim Biophys Acta. 1987;921:198–204.
6. Cohen DE, Carey MC. Acyl chain unsaturation modulates distribution of lecithin molecular species between mixed micelles and vesicles in model bile. Implications for particle structure and metastable cholesterol solubilities. J Lipid Res. 1991;32:1291–302.
7. Tao S, Tazuma S, Kajiyama G. Fatty acid composition of lecithin is a key factor in bile metastability in supersaturated model bile systems. Biochim Biophys Acta. 1993;1167:142–6.
8. Tazuma S, Holzbach RT. Transport of conjugated bilirubin and other organic anions in bile: relation to biliary lipid structures. Proc Natl Acad Sci USA. 1987;84:2052–6.
9. Holan KR, Holzbach RT, Hermann RE, Coopermann AM, Claffey WJ. Nucleation time: a key factor in the pathogenesis of cholesterol gallstone disease. Gastroenterology. 1979;77:611–17.
10. Busch N, Tokumo H, Holzbach RT. A sensitive method for determination of cholesterol crystal growth using model solutions of supersaturated bile. J Lipid Res. 1990;31:1903–9.
11. Tazuma S, Ochi H, Teramen K *et al*. Degree of fatty acyl chain unsaturation in biliary lecithin dictates cholesterol nucleation and crystal growth. Biochim Biophys Acta. 1994 (In press).
12. Patton GM, Fasulo JM, Robins SJ. Separation of phospholipids and individual molecular species of phospholipids by high-performance liquid chromatography. J Lipid Res. 1982;23:190–6.

36
Octreotide prolongs intestinal transit and increases biliary deoxycholic acid and cholesterol saturation – key steps in gallbladder stone formation

S. H. HUSSAINI, S. P. PEREIRA, C. KENNEDY, P. JENKINS,
G. M. MURPHY, J. A. H. WASS and R. H. DOWLING

BACKGROUND

Octreotide (OT), a long-acting analogue of somatostatin, suppresses growth hormone release and is an effective treatment for acromegaly. However, long-term OT therapy induces gallbladder stones (GBS) in 13–60% of patients after 3–51 months treatment[1,2]. We have shown recently that most of these stones are cholesterol-rich[3].

In non-acromegalic patients, 'conventional' cholesterol gallstones develop when at least three abnormalities coexist – the so-called triple defect[4]: (a) supersaturation of gallbladder bile with cholesterol, (b) rapid nucleation of cholesterol microcrystals and (c) retention of these crystals within the gallbladder, as a result of crystal trapping by excess mucus glycoprotein secretion from the gallbladder mucosa and/or stasis due to gallbladder motor dysfunction.

We[5], and others[6,7], have shown that OT treatment impairs gallbladder emptying – due mainly to inhibition of meal-stimulated cholecystokinin release from the intestine[6,7]. Until recently the resultant stasis of bile within the gallbladder was considered to be the principal, and possibly the sole, mechanism for the OT-induced gallstones[2].

However, we reported recently[8] that, in addition to gallbladder stasis, OT-treated acromegalic patients have multiple abnormalities in their bile lipid and bile acid composition, and in the physical chemistry of fresh gallbladder bile. Thus, gallbladder bile from acromegalic patients with OT-associated GBS: (a) was supersaturated in cholesterol and had (b) a higher percentage of the total biliary cholesterol in the vesicular fraction; (c) a high cholesterol:phospholipid molar ratio in the vesicles (suggesting vesicular instability and vulnerability to aggregation, fusion and precipitation of cholesterol microcrystals); and (d) pathologically rapid crystal nucleation times. These abnormalities were comparable to those seen in a disease control group with 'conventional' gallstone disease (unrelated to acromegaly and OT treatment) and were significantly different from the results in stone-free acromegalic control patients untreated with OT. Furthermore, we found that the amount of deoxycholic acid (DCA) in bile, expressed as a percentage of total biliary bile acids, was significantly greater in the acromegalic patients with OT-associated stones and in the non-acromegalic patients with conventional cholesterol-rich GBS, than in the stone-free acromegalic patients who had not been treated with OT[8].

These findings were presented, in preliminary form, at the 1992 International Bile Acid Meeting[9,10]. At that time we suggested that the high percentage of biliary deoxycholate might play a major role in the pathogenesis of OT-induced GBS.

The present study extends this previous work by describing the results of paired studies of bile acid composition and biliary cholesterol saturation in gallbladder bile from acromegalic patients examined before and during OT treatment.

Having found that, independent of gallstone formation, OT treatment resulted in a two-fold increase in the percentage of deoxycholate in gallbladder bile, we went on to explore possible mechanisms for the induced changes in biliary bile acid composition. Since the proportion of biliary DCA is affected by intestinal transit[11], and OT prolongs mouth-to-caecum transit time (MCTT) in non-acromegalic patients[12,13], we also examined the effect of OT on small (MCTT) and large bowel transit times (LBTT), in both acromegalic patients and controls.

PATIENTS AND METHODS

Bile composition and physical chemistry

Patients

In the paired studies, five acromegalic patients (mean age 43, range 29–64 years), three of whom were women, were examined before and during 3–24 months OT therapy (300–400 μg/day). One of the five developed gallstones during treatment.

Bile sampling

Of the 10 samples, nine were fresh gallbladder bile obtained by ultrasound-guided percutaneous transhepatic fine-needle puncture[14,15]. The tenth sample was obtained by duodenal drainage after stimulating gallbladder contraction with intravenous cholecystokinin.

Bile analyses

Biliary cholesterol[16], total phospholipids[17] and total bile acids[18] were measured using standard enzymatic assays. The cholesterol saturation indices (CSI) were then calculated using a polynomial equation[19].

Micelles were separated from vesicles by sucrose density gradient ultracentrifugation[20]. The vesicular fraction was arbitrarily defined as that with a density of < 1.06 g/ml sucrose[21]. In this fraction, the following parameters were measured: (a) the vesicular cholesterol expressed as a percentage of the total biliary cholesterol, (b) the molar ratio of cholesterol:phospholipid (CH:PL) – an index of vesicular stability/instability[22] and (c) the cholesterol microcrystal nucleation time[23]. The concentrations of the individual bile acid conjugates were also determined, using reverse-phase high-performance liquid chromatography[24], and expressed as a percentage of total bile acids.

Mouth-to-caecum transit time (MCTT)

Patients

Six non-acromegalic control subjects (mean age 31 ±SEM 2.0; range 25–36 years) were studied, three of whom were men. Their mean body mass index was 22.4±1.4 (range 18.2–27.8). A further 10 acromegalic patients (mean age 51±4.4; range 27–67 years) were studied, six of whom were men. Their mean body mass index was 29.0±1.63 (range 22.1–38.0). All patients were stone-free, as judged by ultrasound of the gallbladder and biliary tree, and none of the acromegalic patients had previously been treated with OT.

Protocol

A randomized, double-blind, placebo-controlled, crossover design was used to study the non-acromegalic control subjects and the acromegalic patients.

A subcutaneous injection of either placebo (saline) or 50 μg OT was given 30 min before the subjects drank 250 ml of a fat-rich liquid test meal ('Ensure') containing 20 ml of lactulose, after which small-bowel transit time was measured by the breath hydrogen technique[25,26]. The study was repeated 1–3 weeks later when the alternative subcutaneous injection – saline or OT as appropriate – was given. One of the control subjects, and one of the acromegalic patients, did not attend for the second part of the study.

Large bowel transit time (LBTT)

Patients

For the studies of large bowel transit there have, as yet, been no paired studies. Instead, we examined three groups of patients: (a) 11 controls, of whom nine were men (mean age 38±3.5, range 23–57 years); (b) nine acromegalic patients untreated with OT (five men, mean age 57±3.3, range 41–67 years); and (c) four acromegalic patients (two men, mean age 48±3.7, range 40–58 years) who had been treated with OT in a dose of 300–600 μg/day for 3 months or more (mean 12±8 months).

Protocol

Large bowel transit time was assessed by the radiopaque marker shape technique of Metcalf et al.[27]. On three successive mornings, the volunteers ingested 20

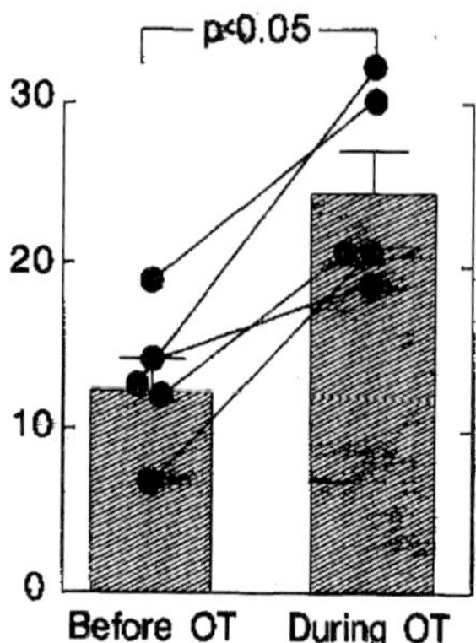

Fig. 1 Paired data for the proportion of DCA conjugates (percentage of total biliary bile acids) in bile before and during OT treatment (300–400 μg/day for a mean of 8 months). The shaded bars show the mean values ± SEM and the solid circles represent individual data points

marker shapes (maximum size 6×6 mm), contained in a single gelatine capsule, with breakfast. A plain abdominal radiograph was taken on day four. The number of markers present on the abdominal X-ray, multiplied by a factor of 1.2, was taken as the LBTT in hours[27].

Ethical considerations

The use of ultrasound-guided gallbladder puncture, and the studies of small and large bowel transit, were approved by the Research Ethics Committee of St Bartholomew's Hospital and by the Ethics Committee of Guy's Hospital. All patients gave their written informed consent.

Statistical analysis

The statistical significance of differences in results between the patient groups, and in the paired studies, was tested with the Mann–Whitney non-parametric method using 'Minitab' software version 2.0 (Minitab Inc., State College, Pennsylvania, USA). Values of $p < 0.05$ were considered to be statistically significant.

RESULTS

Bile composition and physical chemistry

In the paired studies, the results for the percentage of DCA conjugates in bile are shown in Fig. 1. Octreotide treatment resulted in an 87% increase in the mean proportion of biliary DCA which rose from 13.3 ± 2.1% before, to 24.9 ± 2.7% during, treatment ($p < 0.03$). There was a corresponding reduction in the mean

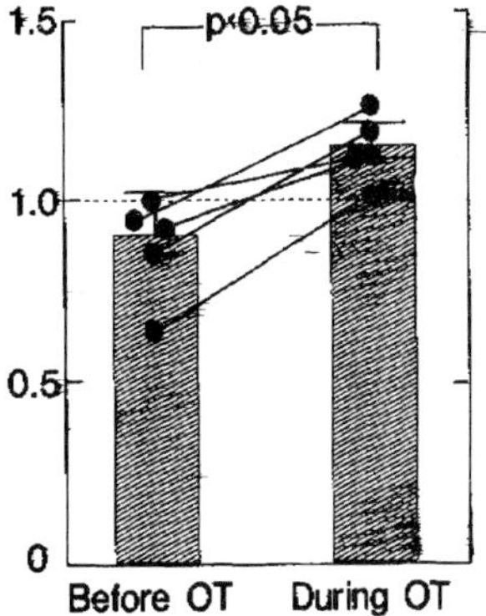

Fig. 2 Paired data for the cholesterol saturation indices in bile before and during OT treatment (300–400µg/day for 8 months; see legend to Fig. 1)

proportion of cholic acid (CA), which fell from 49.6±3.4% before, to 41.5±3.8% during, treatment (n.s.). However, the mean percentages of chenodeoxycholic acid (35.6+1.2% before, and 32.6±2.5% during, OT), ursodeoxycholic acid (1.1±0.4% and 0.2±0.1%), and lithocholic acid (0.4 ±0.2% and 0.9±0.8%, respectively) did not change significantly.

The effect of OT treatment on the cholesterol saturation indices is shown in Fig. 2. In the paired studies, the CSI values rose in all five individuals with a mean increase of 26% ($p < 0.02$). Moreover, the percentage of total biliary cholesterol found in the vesicular fraction also rose, from 36.1±6.2% to 50.4±6.2%, as did the molar ratio of CH:PL in the vesicles (from 0.53±0.07 to 0.72±0.08), although these differences were not statistically significant.

In the acromegalic patient who developed gallstones while on OT treatment, the nucleation time changed from 21 days before treatment to 1 day during therapy. In the remaining three patients whose gallbladder bile was sampled (none of whom developed stones on treatment), the nucleation time remained unchanged in two patients but decreased in one, from 21 to 12 days. As a result, the 34% reduction in the mean value during OT treatment was statistically significant ($p < 0.05$).

Intestinal transit

Mouth-to-caecum transit time (MCTT)

The results for the MCTT in the control subjects and the acromegalic patients given either saline or OT before the lactulose-containing meal, are given in Table 1. In the control subjects, the mean MCTT after the saline injection was just over 1¾h but after a single injection of 50µg OT the MCTT increased in every case – the mean value being 113% greater than that seen after saline (p<0.01).

In the untreated acromegalic patients (saline placebo), the mean MCTT of

Table 1 Mouth-to-caecum transit time, measured by the breath-hydrogen technique, in control subjects and acromegalic patients given either saline or 50 µg OT, 30 min before a lactulose-containing, fat-rich liquid test meal

	Mouth-to-caecum transit time (min)		
Subjects	Saline	Octreotide	p-value
Non-acromegalic controls	108 ± 22.9 ($n = 5$)	230 ± 20.4 ($n = 6$)	< 0.01
Acromegalic patients	165 ± 14.7 ($n = 10$)	285 ± 11.7 ($n = 9$)	< 0.002

Table 2 Large bowel transit time, measured with radiopaque marker shapes, in control subjects, acromegalic patients untreated with OT and acromegalics treated with OT for more than 3 months

Subjects	Large bowel transit time (h)
Non-acromegalic controls	21 ± 3.2 ($n = 11$)*
Acromegalic patients untreated with OT	39 ± 7.5 ($n = 9$)
Acromegalics treated long-term with OT	49 ± 9.8 ($n = 4$)*

*p value for difference between groups < 0.03

2¾h was 53% greater than that seen in the saline-injected controls (n.s.). However, after OT, the MCTT again increased in every case, and the 73% increase in the mean value was significantly greater ($p < 0.002$) than that seen in the same patients given saline. In fact, in seven of the nine acromegalic patients given OT, there had been no rise in the breath hydrogen excretion at 300 min when the observations were abandoned.

Large bowel transit time (LBTT)

The results for LBTT in the three groups of patients studied are given in Table 2. In the non-acromegalic control subjects the mean LBTT was just under 24 h. Just as small bowel transit (MCTT) was greater in acromegalic patients than in controls, so the mean LBTT was also 46% greater in the non-OT-treated acromegalic patients, than in controls. However, given the large scatter of results in the acromegalic patients (2–66 h), this difference was not statistically significant. Furthermore, in the four acromegalic patients on long-term OT, the mean LBTT of just over 48 h was significantly greater ($p < 0.05$) than that in control subjects, but not than that in non-OT-treated acromegalic patients.

DISCUSSION

The present results extend our previous studies of bile composition and physical chemistry in acromegalic patients developing GBS as a complication of long-term OT treatment. The paired, before-and-during OT treatment studies clearly show that the increases in the percentage DCA conjugates in bile, and in biliary cholesterol saturation, seen in patients with OT-induced GBS, are due to the OT treatment itself, and not to changes in bile composition as a consequence of developing gallstones. Furthermore, the fact that OT treatment prolongs both small and large bowel transit in acromegalic patients is compatible with our hypothesis that the increase in the percentage DCA in bile seen during chronic OT therapy, is due to increased bacterial 7α-dehydroxylation of cholic acid (CA) to form DCA in the intestine.

The present findings are important not only in the small group of acromegalic patients who have the misfortune to develop iatrogenic gallstones as a complication of their chronic OT treatment, but also in 'conventional' gallstone disease. They extend the results of a study by Heaton *et al.*[28], and suggest that, by countering the prolonged intestinal transit and/or by stimulating gallbladder contraction, it may be possible to prevent both primary (conventional and OT-induced) and secondary (recurrent) gallstone formation.

Mechanism for the OT-induced increase in percentage biliary DCA

There is a number of possible mechanisms by which OT may induce an increase in the percentage biliary DCA, and thus in lithogenic changes in bile composition and physical chemistry. First, as noted above, OT could prolong intestinal transit. Second, it could increase the absolute number of micro-organisms in the intestine. Third, it could increase the ratio of anaerobic:aerobic bacteria in the bowel which, in turn, could increase the total amount of bacterial 7α-dehydroxylase activity in the intestinal lumen. Fourth, it could induce bacterial 7α-dehydroxylase enzyme-specific activity, while leaving the number and type of intestinal micro-organisms unchanged. Fifth, the impaired gallbladder emptying induced by OT could result in the sequestration of much of the bile acid pool within the gallbladder, with more rapid than normal enterohepatic cycling of the remaining pool. A similar increase in enterohepatic cycling has been described after cholecystectomy – where there is also a greater than normal percentage of DCA in the hepatic bile[29].

Despite the many possible mechanisms for the increase in the percentage of DCA conjugates in bile during OT treatment, as previously discussed, the results of the present study provide strong indirect evidence that a major mechanism is prolongation of intestinal transit. Previous observations have shown that both native somatostatin[30–33], and its analogue OT[12,13,34,35], prolong the MCTT in control subjects. We have now shown that a single injection of OT prolongs the MCTT in acromegalic patients. However, the conversion of CA to DCA occurs predominantly in the caecum and ascending colon – rather than in the small bowel[36–38]. Therefore, we need to consolidate and extend our present results by showing, in paired studies of a larger number of patients, that OT slows colonic, as well as small bowel, transit. To date our results for LBTT in acromegalic patients treated long-term with OT are not significantly greater than those in acromegalic patients untreated with OT, although this lack of statistical significance may be a type II error.

Effect of OT on gastrointestinal motility

The effect of OT on intestinal motility is different when patients are fasted, from that seen after food. Thus, during fasting, OT stimulates interdigestive small bowel motility by increasing the frequency of migrating motor complexes[39] while, after a meal, it inhibits intestinal transit[40].

There are at least two explanations for OT's inhibitory effect on postprandial motility. First, it may act directly on intestinal somatostatin receptors since, in dogs, an intra-arterial infusion of somatostatin induces phase III migrating motor complexes[41]. Second, it may act indirectly by inhibiting the meal-stimulated release of intestinal peptides which influence gastrointestinal motor function – such as pancreatic polypeptide, cholecystokinin, motilin, neurotensin and peptide YY[12,34].

Role of biliary deoxycholate in gallstone pathogenesis

There is good epidemiological and physicochemical evidence to implicate biliary DCA in the pathogenesis of gallstones. Thus, in a review by Marcus and Heaton[42], in 19 of 20 studies the proportion of biliary DCA was greater in gallstone patients than in controls. The mechanisms whereby increased proportions of biliary DCA favour gallstone formation are complex. Carulli *et al.*[43] showed that when hepatic bile was enriched with DCA (by intraduodenal infusion of DCA in post-cholecystectomy T-tube patients), biliary cholesterol secretion increased. Moreover, we[44] and others[45,46] found that there are significant linear correlations between the percentage DCA and: (a) the moles% cholesterol, (b) the CSI and (c) the amount of arachidonic acid-rich phospholipids, in bile. In turn, increased proportions of arachidonic acid-rich phospholipids may lead to excess mucus glycoprotein synthesis and secretion by, and hypomotility of, the gallbladder[47]. We have recently shown that OT significantly increases the proportion of arachidonic acid-rich phospholipids in bile[48]. Furthermore, in patients with rapid nucleation of cholesterol microcrystals (<5 days), the mean percentage DCA in bile was approximately twice as great ($p<0.05$) as that in individuals with normal nucleation times (>10 days)[44]. Whether this difference is due directly to the increased percentage DCA in bile, or indirectly to induced increases in biliary cholesterol saturation, and in the proportion of arachidonic acid-rich phospholipids in bile, is unknown. However, Stolk and colleagues have recently shown that model biles containing hydrophobic bile acids, such as DCA, have more rapid nucleation of cholesterol microcrystals than those containing hydrophilic bile acids, such as CA[49].

Intestinal transit and biliary deoxycholic acid

Supporting evidence that changes in the percentage DCA in bile may be a consequence of altered intestinal transit, comes from studies by Marcus and Heaton[11]. These authors showed that prolongation of intestinal transit resulted in increases in both the percentage DCA in bile and in biliary cholesterol saturation.

Furthermore, from a study of 23 women with gallstones, Berr *et al.*[50] found that in a subgroup of eight who had 'loss of the gallbladder reservoir' (due to a blocked cystic duct in five and a shrunken gallbladder in three), there were significant increases in the conversion of CA to DCA, and in the pool size of DCA. These authors speculated that, in this subgroup of patients, the bile acid changes may have been due to *rapid* (rather than slow) small bowel transit. However, no formal measurements of small or large bowel transit were reported by these authors.

Experimental design

In the present study, as in previous reports on the effects of OT on intestinal motility[12,13], MCTT was measured by the lactulose-breath hydrogen technique. This is based on the concept that when the head of a test meal, containing lactulose, reaches the bacteria-rich part of the intestine, hydrogen is liberated, absorbed and excreted in the breath. It also assumes that high counts of bacteria, capable of degrading lactulose to hydrogen and other metabolites, are not found until the caecum. Although this assumption can be criticized, we[26] and others[51,52] have validated the method by showing, in the same individuals, that MCTT measured by the lactulose-breath hydrogen technique gives comparable results to those obtained by radionuclide scanning.

In theory, the timing of the rise in breath hydrogen excretion after a lactulose-containing meal could be influenced by redistribution of bacteria within the gut. Thus, if OT induced stasis in the small bowel, it could result in secondary bacterial overgrowth and displacement of the bacteria-rich part of the intestine from the caecum, to a more proximal site. If this were to happen, the rise in breath hydrogen excretion would occur before the test meal reached the large bowel, in which case the prolongation in MCTT seen in the present study would actually *underestimate* the magnitude of OT's effect on intestinal transit.

Although the results of the paired studies suggest that the percentage DCA conjugates in bile doubles as a result of OT treatment, the mean percentage DCA value found during therapy was still within the normal range quoted by others. Therefore, to *prove* that OT increases the conversion of CA to DCA, we would need to use isotope dilution techniques to measure the conversion rate of $[^{14}C]$- or $[^{13}C]$cholic acid to deoxycholic acid, and the pool size and synthesis rates of both bile acids. Such studies are now in progress.

Further studies to consolidate the link between OT, intestinal transit, DCA and gallstone formation

There are several possible experimental approaches which could be adopted to provide indirect support for our hypothesis. First, in short-term studies at least, we could combine OT with broad-spectrum antibiotic treatment with the aim of inhibiting the bacterial 7α-dehydroxylation of CA. This approach has been used in the past when studying the effects of CA administration on bile composition[53]. Normally, during CA therapy, there is a marked increase in DCA formation and absorption. Therefore, to study the primary effect of CA on bile composition (rather than the secondary effect of is bacterial metabolite, DCA), CA and antibiotics have been administered together[53,54]. While such an approach might be adopted in the short term, the adaptation of this technique to long-term prophylaxis of OT-induced stones is unlikely to be acceptable.

Second, we could consider treatment with prokinetic agents which might overcome the inhibitory effects of OT on intestinal transit. Candidate regimes include the use of: (a) non-antibiotic analogues of erythromycin which are motilin agonists[55,56], (b) bran-enriched high fibre diets[57], (c) long-term lactulose treatment[11], (d) purgative drugs such as senna and its derivatives[11], and (e) the 5-HT3 antagonist/5-HT4 agonist, cisapride. If we opt for a trial of one of these agents, we first need to show that such treatment will, indeed, overcome the inhibitory effects of OT on intestinal transit. We then need to demonstrate that, by doing so, we can prevent the OT-induced increase in the percentage DCA conjugates in bile, and the corresponding changes in bile composition and physical chemistry. Finally, we need to prove, in long-term prospective trials, that the use of these prokinetic agents will prevent iatrogenic gallstone formation as a result of chronic treatment – either with OT itself or with one of the new long-acting derivatives of OT currently being developed. Again, such studies are now in progress.

Acknowledgements

We thank Mehran Maghsoudloo PhD, for his help in performing the HPLC determinations of bile acid composition, the study patients for their time, and the Special Trustees of Guy's Hospital and Sandoz Pharma Ltd for their financial support.

References

1. Ho KY, Weissberger AJ, Marbach P, Lazarus L. Therapeutic efficacy of the somatostatin analog SMS 201-995 (octreotide) in acromegaly. Ann Intern Med. 1990;112:173–81.
2. Dowling RH, Hussaini SH, Murphy GM, Besser GM, Wass JAH. Gallstones during octreotide therapy. Metabolism. 1992;41(S2):22–33.
3. Hussaini SH, Pereira SP, Murphy GM et al.. Composition of octreotide-associated gallbladder stones: response to oral ursodeoxycholic acid. Gut. 1995;36:126–32.
4. Dowling RH,Gleeson D, Ruppin DC, Murphy GM. Gallstone recurrence and post-dissolution management. In: Paumgartner G, Stiehl A, Gerok W, editors. Enterohepatic circulation of bile acids and sterol metabolism. Lancaster: MTP Press; 1984:361–70.
5. Hussaini SH, Pereira SP, Kennedy C et al. Effect of octreotide on gallbladder emptying, small bowel and colonic motility. J Endocrinol. 1994;140(S):60 (abstr.).
6. Stolk MFJ, van Erpecum KJ, Koppeschaar HPF et al. Postprandial gallbladder motility and hormone release during intermittent and continuous subcutaneous octreotide treatment in acromegaly. Gut. 1993;34:808–13.
7. van Liessum PA, Hopman WP, Pieters GF et al. Post prandial gallbladder motility during long term treatment with the long-acting somatostatin analogue SMS 201-955 in acromegaly. J Clin Endocrinol Metab. 1989;69:557–62.
8. Hussaini SH, Murphy GM, Kennedy C, Besser GM, Wass JAH, Dowling RH. The role of bile composition and physical chemistry in the pathogenesis of octreotide-associated gallbladder stones. Gastroenterology. 1994 ;107:1503–13.
9. Hussaini SH, Maghsoudloo M, Murphy GM, Kennedy C, Wass JAH, Dowling RH. Biliary deoxycholic acid (DCA): further evidence that DCA plays a central role in the pathogenesis of

cholesterol (CH) gallbladder stones (GBs). XII International Bile Acid Meeting (Basel, Switzerland). Bile acids and the hepatobiliary system: from basic science to clinical practice. Falk Symposium No. 68, 1992, Abstract 84.

10. Hussaini SH, Maghsoudloo M, Murphy GM, Kennedy C, Wass JAH, Dowling RH. Octreotide (OT) increases the proportion of deoxycholic acid (DCA) in gallbladder (GB) bile – the prime mover in the pathogenesis of OT-induced gallbladder stones (GBS)? XII International Bile Acid Meeting (Basel, Switzerland). Bile acids and the hepatobiliary system: from basic science to clinical practice. Falk Symposium No. 68, 1992, Abstract 85.

11. Marcus SN, Heaton KW. Intestinal transit, deoxycholic acid and the cholesterol saturation of bile: three inter-related factors. Gut. 1986;27:550–8.

12. Fuessl HS, Carolan G, Williams G, Bloom SR. Effect of a long-acting somatostatin analogue (SMS 201-995) on postprandial gastric emptying of 99mTc-tin colloid and mouth-to-caecum transit time in man. Digestion. 1987;36:101–7.

13. O'Donnell LJD, Watson AJM, Cameron D, Farthing MJG. Effect of octreotide on mouth-to-caecum transit time in healthy subjects and in the irritable bowel syndrome. Aliment Pharmacol Ther. 1990;4:177–82.

14. Swobodnik W, Hagert N, Janowitz P, Wenk H. Diagnostic fine needle puncture of the gallbladder with US guidance. Radiology. 1991;178:755–8.

15 Hussaini SH, Kennedy C, Pereira SP, Wass JAH, Dowling RH. Ultrasound-guided percutaneous fine needle puncture of the gallbladder for studies of bile composition. Br J Radiol. 1995;68:271–6.

16. Roschlau P, Bernt E, Gruber W. Enzymatic determination of total cholesterol in serum. Z Clin Biochem. 1974;12:403–7.

17. Qureshi MY, Murphy GM, Dowling RH. The enzymatic determination of total phospholipids in bile and bile-rich duodenal aspirates. Clin Chim Acta. 1980;105:407–10.

18. Talalay P. Enzymatic analysis of steroid hormones. Meth Biochem Anal. 1960;8:119–43.

19. Thomas PJ, Hofmann AF. A simple calculation of the lithogenic index of bile: expressing biliary lipid composition on rectangular co-ordinates. Gastroenterology. 1972;65:698–700.

20. Sahlin S, Thyberg P, Ahlberg J, Angelin B, Einarsson K. Distribution of cholesterol between vesicles and micelles in human gallbladder bile: influence of treatment with chenodeoxycholic acid and ursodeoxycholic acid. Hepatology. 1991;13:104–10.

21. Ulloa N, Garrido J, Nervi F. Ultracentrifugal isolation of vesicular carriers of biliary cholesterol in native human and rat bile. Hepatology. 1987;7:235–44.

22. Halpern Z, Dudley MA, Lynn MP, Nader JM, Breuer AC, Holzbach RT. Vesicle aggregation in model systems of supersaturated bile: relation to crystal nucleation and lipid composition of the vesicular phase. J Lipid Res. 1986;27:295–306.

23. Holan KR, Holzbach RT, Hermann RE, Cooperman AM, Claffey NJ. Nucleation time: a key factor in the pathogenesis of cholesterol gallstone disease. Gastroenterology. 1979;77:611–17.

24. Wildegrube HJ, Fussel U, Lauer H, Stockhausen H. Measurement of conjugated bile acids by ion-pair high performance liquid chromatography. J Chromatogr. 1983;282:603–8.

25. Bond JH, Levitt MD. Investigation of small bowel transit time in man utilizing pulmonary hydrogen measurements. J Lab Clin Med. 1974;85:546–56.

26. Howard PJ, Lazarus C, Maisey MN, Dowling RH. Interpretation of postprandial breath hydrogen excretion in relation to small bowel transit and ileocecal flow patterns of a radiolabeled solid meal in man. J Gastrointest Motil. 1990;2:194–201.

27. Metcalf AM, Phillips SF, Zinsmeister AR, MacCarty RL, Beart RW, Wolff BG. Simplified assessment of segmental colonic transit. Gastroenterology. 1987;92:40–7.

28. Heaton KW, Emmett PM, Symes CL, Braddon FEM. An explanation for gallstones in normal-weight women: slow intestinal transit. Lancet. 1993;341:8–10.

29. Roda E, Aldini R, Mazzela G et al. Enterohepatic circulation of bile acids after cholecystectomy. Gut. 1978;19:640–9.

30. Efendic S, Mattsson O. Effect of somatostatin on intestinal motility. Acta Radiol. 1978;19:348–52.

31. Johansson C, Efendic S, Wisen O, Uvnas-Wallensten K, Luft R. Effects of short time somatostatin infusion on gastric and intestinal propulsion in humans. Scand J Gastroenterol. 1978;13:481–3.

32. Konturek SJ. Somatostatin and gastrointestinal secretion and motility. Adv Exp Med Biol. 1978;106:227–34.

33. Johansson C, Efendic S, Wisen O, Uvnas-Wallensten K. Effects of somatostatin on gastrointestinal propagation and absorption of oral glucose in man. Digestion. 1981;22:126–37.
34. Lembcke B, Creutzfeldt S, Schlesser R, Ebert R, Shaw C, Koop I. Effect of the somatostatin analogue (SMS 201-995) on gastrointestinal, pancreatic and biliary function and hormone release in normal man. Digestion. 1987;36:108–24.
35. Møller N, Petrany G, Cassidy D, Sheldon WJ, Johnston DG, Laker MF. Effects of the somatostatin analogue SMS 201-995 (sandostatin) on mouth-to-caecum transit time and absorption of fat and carbohydrates in normal man. Clin Sci. 1988;75:345–50.
36. MacDonald IA, Bokkenheuser VD, Winter J, McLernon AM, Mosbach EH. Degradation of steroids in the human gut. J Lipid Res. 1983;24:675–700.
37. Morris JS, Low-Beer TS, Heaton KW. Bile salt metabolism in the colon. Scand J Gastroenterol. 1973;8:425–31.
38. Yahiro K, Setoguchi T, Katsuki T. Effect of caecum and appendix on 7 alpha-dehydroxylation and 7 beta-epimerization of chenodeoxycholic acid in the rabbit. J Lipid Res. 1980;21:215–22.
39. Soudah HC, Hasler WL, Owyang C. Effect of octreotide on intestinal motility and bacterial overgrowth in scleroderma. N Engl J Med. 1991;325:1461–7.
40. Richards WO, Geer R, O'Dorisio TM et al. Octreotide acetate induces fasting small bowel motility in patients with the dumping syndrome. J Surg Res. 1990;49:483–7.
41. Hostein J, Janssens J, Vantrappen G, Peeters TL, Vandeweerd M, Leman G. Somatostatin induces ectopic activity fronts of the migrating motor complex via a local intestinal mechanism. Gastroenterology. 1984;87:1004–8.
42. Marcus SN, Heaton KW. Deoxycholic acid and the pathogenesis of gallstones. Gut. 1988;29:522–3.
43. Carulli N, Loria P, Bertolotti M. Effects of acute changes in bile acid pool composition on biliary lipid secretion. J Clin Invest. 1985;74:616–24.
44. Hussaini SH, Maghsoudloo M, Murphy GM, Kennedy C, Wass JAH, Dowling RH. The roles of biliary deoxycholic acid (DCA) and vesicular cholesterol (CH) in the pathogenesis of CH gallbladder stones (GBS). Gut. 1992;33:S57 (abstr.).
45. Hofmann AF, Grundy SM, Lachin JM et al. Pre-treatment lipid composition in white patients with gallstones in the National Cooperative Gallstone Study. Gastroenterology. 1982;83:738–52.
46. van Berge Henegouwen GP, van der Werf SDG, Ruben AT. Fatty acid composition of phospholipids in bile in man: promoting effect of deoxycholate on arachidonate. Clin Chim Acta. 1987;165:27–37.
47. Carey MC, Cahalane MJ. Whither biliary sludge? Gastroenterology. 1988;95:508–23.
48. Pereira SP, Hussaini SH, Cassell TB, Murphy GM, Wass JAH, Dowling RH. Octreotide increases the proportions of arachidonic acid-rich phospholipids in gallbladder bile. Gut. 1993;34(S3):S32 (abstr.).
49. Stolk MFJ, van de Heijning BJM, van Erpecum KJ, van den Broek AMWC, Renooij W, van Berge Henegouwen GP. The effect of bile salt hydrophobicity on nucleation of several types of cholesterol crystals from model bile vesicles. J Hepatol. 1994 ;20:802–10.
50. Berr F, Pratschke E, Fisher S, Paumgartner G. Disorders of bile acid metabolism in cholesterol gallstone disease. J Clin Invest. 1992;90:859–68.
51. Read NW, Miles CA, Fisher D et al. Transit of a meal through the stomach, small intestine, and colon in normal subjects and its role in the pathogenesis of diarrhoea. Gastroenterology. 1980;79:1276–82.
52. Caride VJ, Prokop EK, Troncale FJ, Buddoura W, Winchenbach K, McCallum RW. Scintigraphic determination of small intestinal transit time; comparison with the hydrogen breath technique. Gastroenterology. 1984;86:714–20.
53. Samuel P, Holtzman CM, Meilman E, Sekowski I. Effect of neomycin and other antibiotics on serum cholesterol levels and on 7 alpha-dehydroxylation of bile acids by the fecal bacterial flora in man. Circ Res. 1973;33:393–402.
54. Ponz de Leon M, Carulli N. The influence of bile acid pool composition on the regulation of cholesterol transport. In: Paumgartner G, Stiehl A, Gerok W, editors. Falk Symposium No. 29: Bile acids and lipids. Lancaster: MTP Press; 1980:133–40.
55. Kawamura O, Sekiguchi T, Itoh Z, Omura S. Effect of erythromycin derivative EM523L on human interdigestive gastrointestinal tract. Dig Dis Sci. 1993;38:1026–31.
56. Peeters TL. Erythromycin and other macrolides as prokinetic agents. Gastroenterology. 1993;105:1886–99.
57. Pomare EW, Heaton KW, Low-Beer TS, Espiner HJ. The effect of wheat bran upon bile salt metabolism and upon lipid composition of bile in gallstone patients. Am J Dig Dis. 1976;21:521–6.

Section IX
Bile acids in therapy

37
Inborn errors of bile acid biosynthesis: clinical and therapeutic aspects

W. F. BALISTRERI

INTRODUCTION

An important development over recent years has been the delineation of a new category of metabolic liver disease – inborn errors of bile acid biosynthesis. Recognition of these disorders not only provides insight into normal hepatobiliary physiology but also offers the clinician a treatable form of liver injury. The dramatic clinical response to bile acid replacement therapy in the disorders recognized to date should serve as a stimulus to carry out precise and widespread screening of patients with cholestatic diseases, as well as further investigation into their pathophysiology. In this chapter we will discuss the clinical presentation of patients with defects in bile acid biosynthesis and summarize their response to therapy. Details regarding screening methodology and the biochemical aspects are presented elsewhere in this volume.

BILE ACID BIOSYNTHESIS

The primary bile acids, cholic and chenodeoxycholic acid, are synthesized in the liver from cholesterol through a sequential enzymatic cascade involving multiple different enzymatic reactions (Table 1)[1]. The bile acid biosynthetic pathway involves two major structural alterations to cholesterol: (1) modification of the cyclopentanoperhydrophenanthrene *ring* structure or nucleus (Fig. 1) and (2) oxidation and shortening of the eight carbon atom *side-chain* of the sterol (Fig. 2). Detailed descriptions of the biochemistry and regulation of bile acid biosynthesis have recently been published[1,2]. Improper functioning of any of these enzymatic reactions could give rise to clinically manifest hepatobiliary dysfunction.

Defective bile acid biosynthesis may occur in the presence of a primary enzyme deficiency or may arise secondary to specific organelle dysfunction (Table 2)[3,4].

Table 1 Enzymes involved in bile acid biosynthesis

Enzyme	Reaction mediated	Subcellular localization	Comments
1 Cholesterol 7α-hydroxylase	C-7 hydroxylation	ER	Cytochrome P450, liver specific
2 3β-hydroxy-Δ^5-C$_{27}$-steroid oxidoreductase	Oxidation 3β-OH$\rightarrow$3-oxo and $\Delta^5\rightarrow\Delta^4$	ER	Multiple isozymes, bile acid enzyme cDNA not yet cloned
3 Sterol 12α-hydroxylase	C-12 hydroxylation (cholic acid)	ER	Cytochrome P450
4 Δ^4-3-Oxosteroid 5β–reductase	Reduction of $\Delta^4\rightarrow5\beta$(H)	Cytoplasm	Present in many tissues
5 3α-Hydroxysteroid dehydrogenase	Reduction of 3-oxo$\rightarrow$3α-OH	Cytoplasm	Aldehyde/aldose reductase family
6 Sterol 27-hydroxylase	Side-chain hydroxylation	Mitochondria	Cytochrome P 450, present in many tissues
7 Alcohol dehydrogenase	Side-chain oxidaation$\rightarrow$C-26 COOH	Cytoplasm	Multiple isozymes
8 Aldehyde dehydrogenase	Side-chain oxidation$\rightarrow$C-26 COOH	Cytoplasm	Multiple isozymes, bile acid enzyme not yet identified
9 Bile acid coenzyme A ligase	Side-chain oxidation$\rightarrow$C-26 COOH	ER	Distinct from fatty acid CoA ligase
10 Bile acid oxidase	Side-chain oxidation$\rightarrow$C-26 COOH	Peroxisome	Liver specific, distinct from fatty acid oxidase
11 Bile acid hydratase/dehydrogenase	Side-chain oxidation$\rightarrow$C-26 COOH	Peroxisome	Bifunctional enzyme, relation to fatty acid peroxisomal β-oxidation enzyme known
12 Bile acid thiolase	Side-chain oxidation$\rightarrow$C-26 COOH	Peroxisome	May be the same as fatty acid peroxisomal β-oxidation enzyme

Numbers in column 1 refer to Figs 1 and 2. ER=endoplasmic reticulum; steps 7–12 (side-chain oxidation) form a multiple step procedure involving formation of CoA derivative, hydroxylation at C-24, and β-oxidation
Modified from ref. 1

PRIMARY DEFECTS

Bile acids have a central role in generating bile flow and in serving as apparent trophic factors on the developing hepatobiliary system[3,5,6]. It is therefore intuitive that defective bile acid biosynthesis or transport could be an initiating or perpetuating factor in neonatal cholestatic disorders[4,6–8]. We have attempted to define a subset of children with cholestatic disorders in whom defective bile acid biosynthesis was present. Our hypothesis was that primary inborn errors in bile acid biosynthesis, resulting from an inherent enzyme deficiency, will lead to the underproduction of the normal trophic and choleretic primary bile acids as well as overproduction of potential hepatotoxic primitive bile acid metabolites[3,4].

An analogy should be drawn to the congenital adrenal hyperplasia (CAH) syndromes, which can be caused by a disorder at *any* point in the complex series of enzymatic conversions involved in steroid hormone synthesis from cholesterol. The resultant clinical manifestations of CAH are due either to absence of a critical steroid or accumulation of compounds which exert adverse effects.

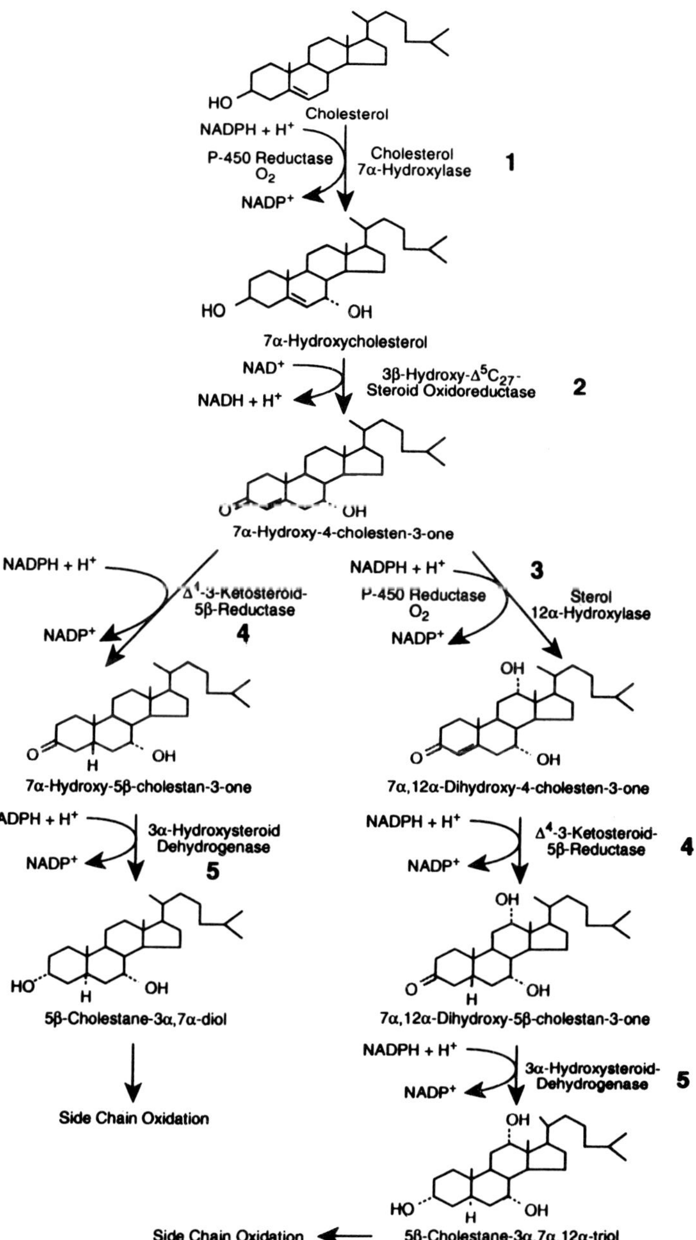

Fig. 1 Modifications to the sterol *ring* structures (nucleus) in bile acid biosynthesis. Reactions are numbered in bold type. Enzymes and cofactors that catalyse a particular reaction are indicated next to the arrows. *Note:* Reaction 4 is catalysed by a Δ⁴-3-*oxo*steroid 5β-reductase. Reproduced from ref. 1

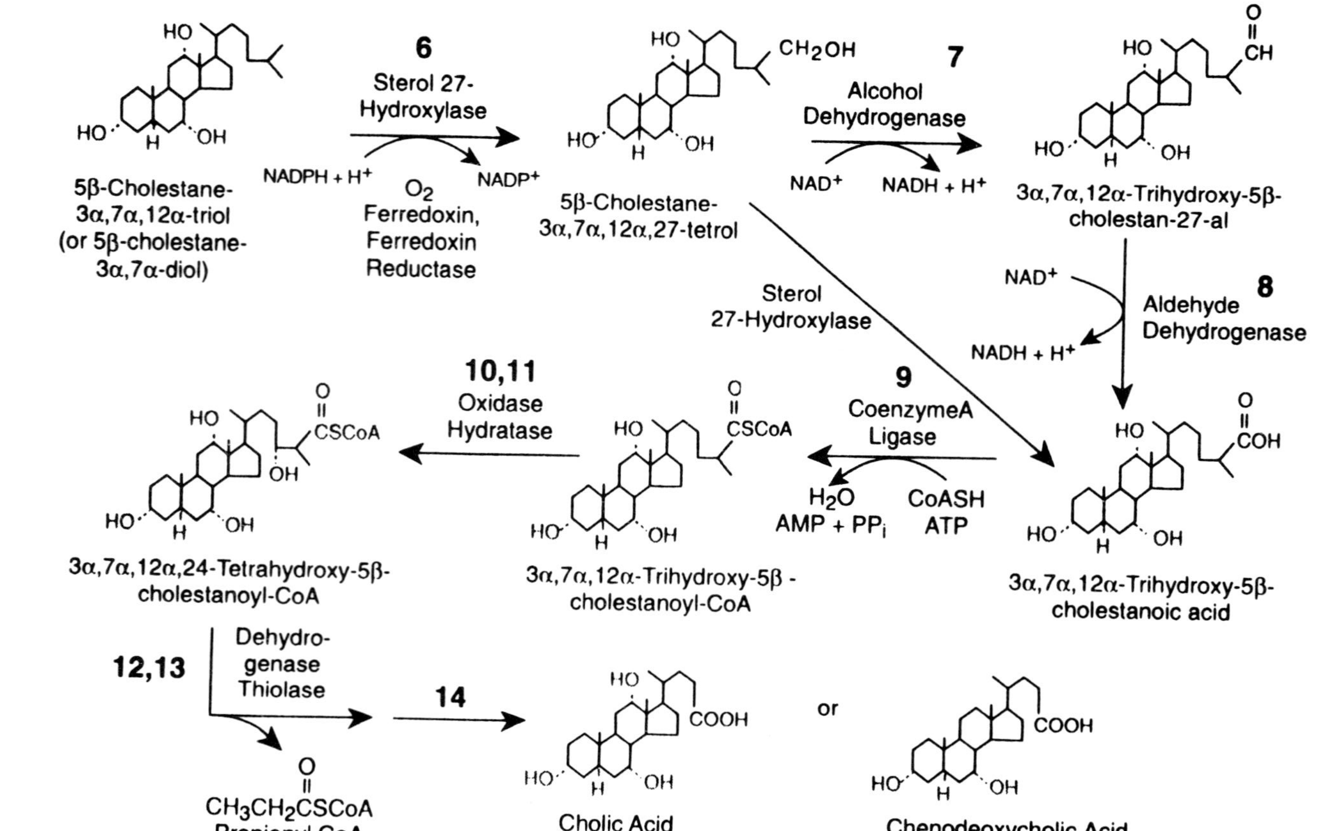

Fig. 2 Modifications to the sterol *side-chain* in bile acid biosynthesis. Reactions are numbered in bold type. Enzymes and cofactors that participate in a particular reaction are indicated next to the arrows. Reproduced from ref. 1

Table 2 Inborn errors of bile acid biosynthesis and transport

A. Defective biosynthesis
  1. Primary defects (enzymopathies)
    (a) Defective degradation of cholesterol side-chain
      (1) Cerebrotendinous xanthomatosis[54,55]
    (b) Defective transformation of steroid nucleus:
      (1) 3β-hydroxy-ΔC_{27} steroid dehydrogenase/isomerase deficiency[12]
      (2) Δ^4-3-oxosteroid 5β-reductase deficiency[13]

  2. Secondary defects (due to organelle damage)
    (i) Specific peroxisomal disorders[34–38]
      (1) Disorders of peroxisome biogenesis with *general* loss of peroxisomal function
        (a)   Zellweger's (cerebrohepatorenal) syndrome
        (b)   Neonatal adrenoleukodystrophy
        (c)   Infantile Refsum's disease[56]
        (d)   Hyperpipecolic acidaemia
        (e)   Leber's congenital amaurosis[57]
      (2) Disorders with loss of *limited* number of peroxisomal functions (structure intact)
        (a)   Rhizomelic chondrodysplasia punctata
        (b)   Zellweger-like syndrome[40]
      (3) Disorders with loss of a *single* peroxisomal function (structure intact)
        (a)   Adrenoleukodystrophy (X-linked)
        (b)   Thiolase deficiency (pseudo-Zellweger's syndrome)[58]
        (c)   Bifunctional protein deficiency[59]
        (d)   Acyl-CoA oxidase deficiency (pseudo-neonatal adrenoleukodystrophy)[33]
        (e)   Hyperoxaluria type I
        (f)   Acatalasaemia
    (ii) Generalized hepatic synthetic dysfunction:
      (1)   Tyrosinaemia
      (2)   Neonatal iron storage disease
      (3)   Fulminant hepatic failure (multiple aetiologies)

B. Defective transport
  1. Byler's syndrome[30,31]
  2. Alagille syndrome[3]

Modified from ref. 3

Development of replacement therapy for each of the CAH syndromes followed an understanding of the adrenal steroidogenic pathways and the enzymes that mediate steroid hormone synthesis[9]. The heterogeneity of clinical manifestations in both bile acid biosynthetic and adrenal steroid biosynthetic disorders may be related to how much functional enzyme is produced. Therefore, every patient requires individual evaluation and periodic monitoring and tailoring of replacement therapy.

Each of the reactions listed in Table 1 is a potential site of a primary inborn error in bile acid biosynthesis. Specific defects have been defined following the application of methodological advances such as fast atom bombardment ionization–mass spectrometry (FAB-MS) and gas chromatography–mass spectrometry (GC-MS) in the screening for inborn errors of bile acid biosynthesis and in the delineation of specific disorders[10,11]. Patients affected by these disorders have previously been considered to have idiopathic disease, such as 'idiopathic' neonatal hepatitis or intrahepatic cholestasis. Recognition has allowed the sub-segmentation of those broader categories[10,12,13]. At present two distinct disorders related to defective transformation of the steroid nucleus have been described: (1) Δ^4-3-oxosteroid 5β-reductase deficiency and (2) 3β-hydroxy-C_{27}-steroid dehydrogenase/isomerase deficiency. Sporadic case reports of somewhat disparate phenotypes of these disorders have been published. It is possible that these defects account for up to 5% of patients with idiopathic intrahepatic cholestatic disorders; however, the true incidence is not known. The limitation to greater recognition is the lack of widespread availability of sensitive and specific screening methodology such as FAB-MS[10,11,14,15].

Δ^4-3-Oxosteroid 5β-reductase deficiency

History

Deficiency of 5β-reductase was first described in monochorionic male twins with marked cholestasis noted in the first few days of life; a similarly affected sibling had died at 4 months of age[4,13,16]. These patients presented with elevated serum aminotransferase levels, conjugated hyperbilirubinaemia, and severe coagulopathy. The liver biopsy revealed a pattern typical of 'idiopathic' neonatal hepatitis, namely lobular disarray, pseudoacinar transformation of hepatocytes, hepatocellular and canalicular bile stasis and extramedullary haematopoiesis; however, assessment of hepatic ultrastructure by electron microscopy demonstrated unique canalicular abnormalities (Fig. 3)[16]. Screening of the urine samples by FAB-MS indicated the presence of elevated amounts of taurine conjugates of oxo bile acids (hydroxy-oxo-cholenoic and dihydroxy-oxo-cholenoic acids). Their structure was confirmed by GC-MS to be 3-oxo-7α-hydroxy-4-cholenoic acid and 3-oxo-7α,12α-dihydroxy-4-cholenoic acid; Δ^4-oxo-bile acids represented the major urinary bile acids[13]. In these patients, bile obtained from the gallbladder contained only trace amounts of bile acids ($<2\,\mu$mol/l). The bile acid synthetic rate, estimated from the daily urinary excretion, indicated a marked reduction in the rate of synthesis of the primary bile acids (<3 mg/day).

Enzymology

These data suggested that these patients were affected by a defect in hepatic bile acid biosynthesis in which the conversion of the 3-oxo intermediates to the corresponding 3α-hydroxy-5β (H) structures was inoperative. This reaction, step 4 in the bile acid biosynthetic pathway (see Fig. 1) is catalysed by cytosolic Δ^4-3-oxosteroid 5β-reductase. This enzyme has been purified to homogeneity by Onishi *et al.*[17,18]; the molecular weight is 38 kDa. Using antibodies and oligonucleotides as probes, a cDNA which contained an $\sim$980 bp long open reading frame encoding 326 amino acid residues was isolated[17,18]. The rat and human cDNAs encoding the enzyme have been sequenced and expressed in cell lines[19]. This enzyme exists only in the liver; it is not expressed in fibroblasts[17,18]. Immunoblot analysis of the cytosolic fraction of liver samples from patients with 5β-reductase deficiency using monoclonal antibody directed against rat liver Δ^4-3-oxosteroid 5β-reductase[17,18] demonstrated the absence of 38 kDa protein in the liver of affected patients[1].

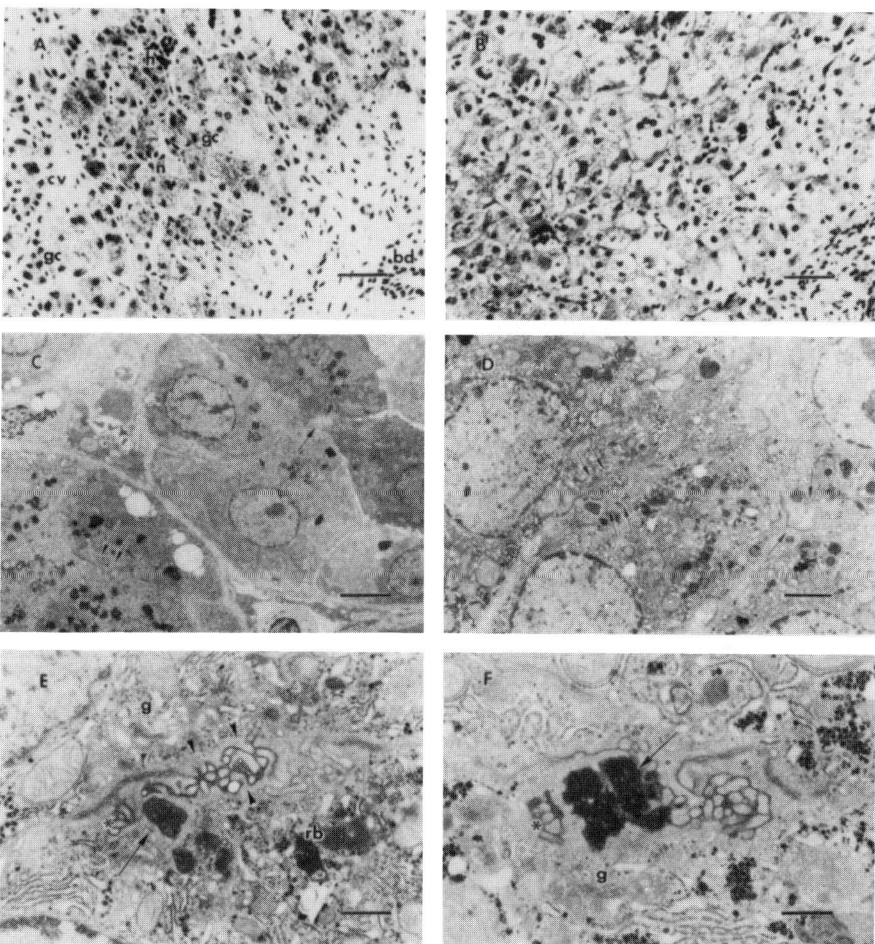

Fig. 3 Liver morphology in patients with Δ⁴-3-oxosteroid 5β-reductase deficiency. **A**: Light micrograph, obtained from a patient (one of the twins) at 4 weeks of age before treatment with bile acids, shows intensive cytoplasmic cholestasis with nodules of giant-cell transformation (gc), extramedullary haematopoiesis (h) and hepatocellular necrosis (n). Bile ductules (bd) in general were unremarkable. Only rare, tiny, canalicular bile plugs (arrow) were apparent. CV, central vein. Bar, 50 μm. **B**: Light micrograph of biopsy obtained from another patient (younger sibling of the twins) at 5 days of age shows panlobar giant-cell transformation, along with the other features noted in **A**. Bar, 50 μm. **C**: Low-magnification electron micrograph obtained at 4 weeks of age from patient shown in **A**, illustrates the tendency of hepatocytes to form clusters. In one cluster (arrow), the normal canaliculus is empty and undistended, and there are few pericanalicular residual bodies. The abnormal canaliculus (double arrows) in the other cluster of hepatocytes is surrounded by abundant electron-dense residual body pigment. Bar, 6 μm. **D**: Higher magnification (7 weeks of age) shows a similar alternating pattern of normal and abnormal canaliculi with a normal canaliculus (or canaliculi [single arrows]) adjacent to an abnormal canaliculus (double arrows). Bar, 2.8 μm. **E**: Abnormal bile canaliculus collapsed, with granular electron-dense contents outlining a portion of the profile (arrowheads) and adjacent accumulation of a similar substance (arrow) in a diverticulum or isolated vesicle. The frequency of such profiles, sometimes clearly connected as diverticula, and convoluted membrane contours (*) (which may represent collapsed diverticula) suggest increased complexity of canalicular shape. g, Golgi apparatus; rb, residual body. Bar, 1.0 μm. **F**: Another partly collapsed canaliculus contains an electron-dense plug (arrow) with adjacent convoluted membrane contours (*). Similar profiles sometimes appear empty. g, Golgi apparatus. Bar, 0.8 μm. Reproduced from ref. 16

Clinical features

Patients with 5β-reductase deficiency described to date have presented with severe neonatal cholestasis, as described above, accompanied by a coagulopathy. This phenotype resembles other forms of severe neonatal metabolic liver disease including tyrosinaemia and neonatal iron storage disease; there are, however, distinguishing features (Table 3). The histology is that of 'giant cell' neonatal hepatitis, as described above. Despite exhibiting a pattern of cholestatic injury seen in other forms of cholestasis, patients with 5β-reductase deficiency could be distinguished from patients with other forms of neonatal hepatitis and biliary atresia by the presence of uniform mosaic of altered and unaltered canaliculi, the relative lack of large bile plugs and the generalized complex membrane contours and canalicular diverticula[16].

Diagnosis

The diagnosis is suggested by FAB-MS screening of urine, which will detect an increased total bile acid excretion, with a predominance of conjugates whose molecular weight is consistent with unsaturated oxo-hydroxy cholenoic acid and oxo-dihydroxy cholenoic acids[13]. The identity of these compounds can be confirmed by GC-MS. While Δ^4-3-oxo bile acids may be present in urine samples from patients with other forms of liver disease[15], in patients with 5β-reductase deficiency there is an increased ratio of Δ^4-3-oxo bile acids relative to primary bile acids and significant amounts of allo (5α-H) bile acids are detectable[1].

Pathophysiology

The mechanism of liver injury is unclear; hepatocellular and bile ductular injury may be directly attributable to the accumulation of hepatotoxic Δ^4-3-oxo bile acids or due to inadequate synthesis of the primary bile acids needed to generate bile acid-dependent bile flow.

Treatment

Oral cholic acid therapy was instituted to specifically *replace* the absent primary bile acids; this was combined with ursodeoxycholic acid to *displace* the hepatotoxic compounds and thereby aid in reversal of hepatic injury. We hypothesized that: (1) cholic acid would down-regulate endogenous bile acid synthesis via feedback inhibition of cholesterol 7α-hydroxylase and thereby prevent the further accumulation of potentially hepatotoxic Δ^4-3-oxo bile acids, and (2) ursodeoxycholic acid would offer cytoprotective and choleretic effects. When this drug combination was given orally to the first patients (twins) diagnosed to have 5β-reductase deficiency, we noted suppression of Δ^4-3-oxo bile acid synthesis and normalization of liver function tests (Table 4)[7,10,16]. The same rationale has been utilized in subsequently diagnosed children, including the newborn sibling of the index cases.

In these patients, hepatocellular cholestasis and giant cell transformation resolved in parallel with clinical and biochemical recovery during oral bile acid

Table 3 Differential features of neonatal cholestatic disorders

	5β-Reductase deficiency	3B-HSD deficiency	Tyrosinaemia (acute form)	Neonatal storage disease	ECHO virus	Shock
Neonatal liver failure	+	?	+	+	+	+
Neonatal cholestasis	+	+	+	+	+	+
Synthetic dysfunction	+	?	++	+	+	±
Coagulopathy	+	?	+	+	+	±
γ-GGTP	↑	N	↑	↑	↑	↑
Serum bile acid	N	N	↑	↑	↑	↓
Succinylacetone	Mild ↑	?	++++	+	+	?
MRI (extrahepatic siderosis)	–	–	–	++++	–	–
Serum ferritin	↑	?	↑	↑↑↑	↑	↑

MRI = magnetic resonance imaging; + = present, N = normal; – = absent; ↑ = elevated (to varying degrees as signified by abundance of symbols); ? = not studied

Table 4 Representative clinical data – effect of bile acid therapy in one patient with 5β-reductase deficiency

	Total/direct bilirubin (mg/dl)	AST (IU/l)	Serum bile acids		Urine bile acids	
Age			Percentage oxo	Total (μmol/l)	Percentage oxo	Total (μmol/l)
1 week	6/7	103	—	—	—	—
4 weeks	20/14	106	17	52	92	46
7 weeks	23/18	167	0.2	191	8	40
12 weeks	19/17	139	0.2	298	4	136
8–9 months	8/6	74	—	—	—	—
13 months	10/7	74	—	—	8	134
15 months	1/0	69	—	—	—	—
>24 months	<1/0	55	—	—	—	—

AST = aspartate aminotransferase
Modified from ref. 16

administration[16]. In the first two patients studied (twins), stable portal fibrosis of a mild degree was present in the most recent biopsy; they remain healthy at 7 years of age. The follow-up biopsy in their younger brother (at 8 months of age) was *normal* (Fig. 4); he remains healthy at 4 years of age. Hepatic ultrastructural alterations initially noted in all three (abnormalities of bile canaliculi including small bile plugs, diverticula and lattice-like elaborations of hepatocellular membranes adjacent to bile canaliculi) resolved completely on subsequent biopsies[16]. Figure 5 shows a photograph of the three brothers, all of whom are doing well on replacement therapy.

Conclusion

These patients represent a subset of familial 'idiopathic' neonatal hepatitis[3,6]; the proportion of such cases explained by 5β-reductase deficiency and the variability

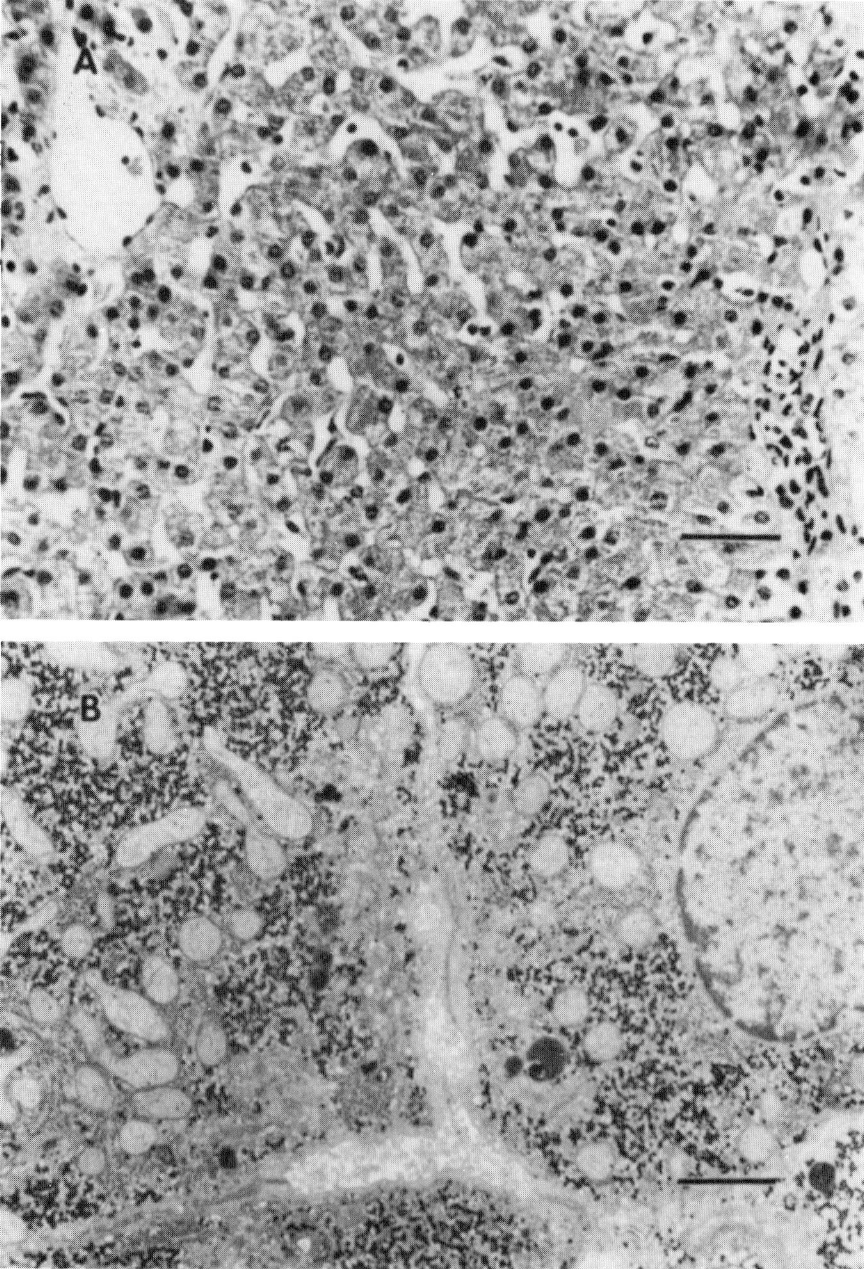

Fig. 4 Follow-up biopsy: **A**: Histological appearance of the liver of a patient with 5β-reductase deficiency receiving bile acid therapy is essentially normal at 8 months of age. Bar, 50 μm. **B**: Bile canaliculi and ultrastructural features are also normal. Bar, 2.2 μm. Modified from ref. 16

of presentation of the defect remain to be defined[16]. Eight additional cases have been identified by screening of urine samples; six, detected late in their disease, have died. Two others, who are receiving bile acid therapy are alive – for a total of seven deaths, untreated, and five survivors on therapy[16]. Figure 6 shows a picture of Thomas, a brother of the three boys shown in Fig. 5. The diagnosis was not made, and he died at 4 months. The picture was taken a few weeks before his death. This favourable outcome indicates that treatment is *lifesaving* and that early treatment prevents the development of liver failure.

3β-Hydroxy-C_{27}-steroid dehydrogenase/isomerase (3β-HSD) deficiency

History

Clayton *et al.* described a 3-month-old Saudi Arabian boy with neonatal cholestasis who excreted monosulphates of $3\beta,7\alpha$-dihydroxy and $3\beta,7\alpha,12\alpha$-trihydroxy-5-cholenoic acid and their glycine conjugates in urine[12]. Cholic and chenodeoxycholic acid were undetectable. These findings suggested that the cholestasis was related to an inborn error affecting 3β-hydroxy-C_{27}-steroid dehydrogenase/isomerase (oxidoreductase), an enzyme which catalyses the second step in bile acid biosynthesis (see Fig. 1). This child, the product of a consanguineous marriage, was one of three siblings with 'giant cell hepatitis'; the siblings died as a result of end-stage liver disease. Since description of this family several additional cases have been reported[20-26].

Enzymology

The reaction: 7α-hydroxycholesterol $\rightarrow$ 7α-hydroxy-4-cholesten-3-one is catalysed by microsomal 3β-hydroxy-C_{27}-steroid dehydrogenase/isomerase, a C_{27} sterol-specific isoenzyme[1]. In the absence of enzyme activity accumulated 7α-hydroxycholesterol is metabolized to C_{24} bile acids which retain the 3β-hydroxy Δ-5 structure. This isoenzyme has not yet been purified to homogeneity; however, the enzyme is expressed in fibroblasts[27]. Cultured skin fibroblasts obtained from the patient described by Clayton *et al.* were utilized to document *complete absence* of 3β-hydroxy-Δ^5-C_{27}-steroid dehydrogenase/isomerase activity in this phenotype[27]. In addition fibroblasts obtained from his parents exhibited reduced activity, suggesting a heterozygous genotype. This observation established that the primary nature of the biochemical defect was an inborn error involving a specific enzyme required for bile acid biosynthesis.

Clinical features

Reported patients have presented at various ages with jaundice, hepatomegaly, and elevated aminotransferase levels. They may have malabsorption of fat and fat-soluble vitamins and poor growth[23]; pruritus is surprisingly uncommon[26]. There appears to be bimodal presentation either as neonatal hepatitis or chronic hepatitis in older children. The γ-glutamyltranspeptidase (γ-GGTP) and serum bile acid levels are normal despite elevated conjugated bilirubin levels, which is

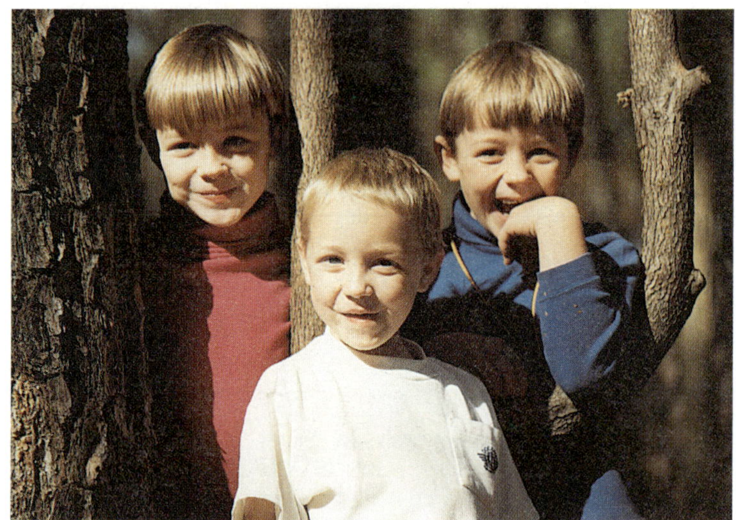

Fig. 5 (left to right) Seth, Will and Josh

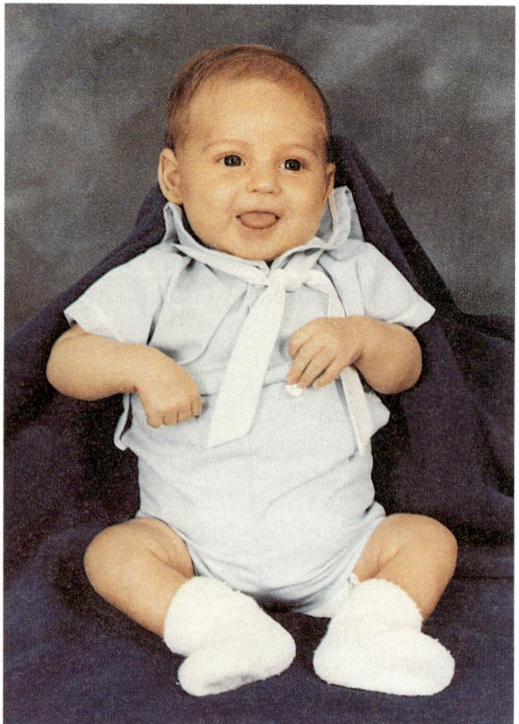

Fig. 6 Thomas

in contrast to most forms of neonatal cholestasis (Table 3). The serum cholesterol levels may also be low[26]. Liver biopsy specimens are heterogeneous – ranging from giant cell hepatitis to micronodular cirrhosis[23]. In many documented cases a similar clinical picture is present in siblings. There is an association with consanguinity. The disorder may be transmitted in an autosomal recessive fashion.

Diagnosis

The diagnosis of 3β-hydroxy-C_{27}-steroid dehydrogenase/isomerase deficiency is initiated by screening of urine by FAB-MS which will reveal a quantitative increase in total bile acid excretion; however, qualitatively there will be an absence of normal glycine and taurine conjugates of the primary bile acids. Sulphate and glycosulphate conjugates of (unsaturated) di- and tri-hydroxy cholenoic acids accumulate in the place of the primary bile acids[12,20–26]; these compounds are bile acids formed from precursors in which normal conversion of the 3β-hydroxy-Δ^5 structure to the 3α-hydroxy-5β(H) structure has not occurred. The absence of primary bile acids presumably explains the failure to generate bile acid-dependent bile flow and the absence of a critical micellar concentration of bile acids in the proximal intestinal lumen.

The biochemical diagnosis can be confirmed by GC-MS analysis of urine which will reveal $3\beta,7\alpha$-dihydroxy-5-cholenoic acid and $3\beta,7\alpha,12\alpha$-trihydroxy-5-cholenoic acid, and of serum, which will demonstrate the accumulation of 7α-hydroxycholesterol. Since the enzyme activity is expressed in cultured skin fibroblasts, 7α-hydroxycholesterol can be utilized as a substrate to probe for the presence of the enzyme[27]. In homozygotes there will be no detectable enzyme.

Pathophysiology

The liver injury may be related to the absent choleretic effect of the primary bile acids or the cholestatic effect of the atypical bile acids; $3\beta,7\alpha$-dihydroxy-5-cholenoic acid is normally metabolized rapidly to chenodeoxycholic acid by 3β-hydroxy-C_{27}-steroid dehydrogenase/isomerase; this will not occur in patients with deficiency of this enzyme.

Treatment

The therapeutic rationale is that primary bile acids, given orally, will enter the enterohepatic circulation and down-regulate the activity of 7α-hydroxylase (the rate-limiting enzyme) thereby reducing the production of 'hepatotoxic' 3β-hydroxy-Δ^5 bile acids. In addition primary bile acids will drive bile flow and facilitate fat absorption. In the initial reports chenodeoxycholic acid was utilized in an empiric dose (125–150 mg/day), based on the monitoring of levels of endogenous bile acids; the dose was titrated versus disappearance of the abnormal 3β-hydroxy-Δ^5 bile acids.

The effects of bile acid therapy in a child with hepatic 3β-hydroxy-C_{27}-steroid dehydrogenase/isomerase deficiency were described by Ichimiya *et al.*[23,24]. Initial empirical therapy, begun at approximately 4 years of age, consisted of chenodeoxycholic acid (125 mg twice daily; 18 mg/kg); the dose was reduced to

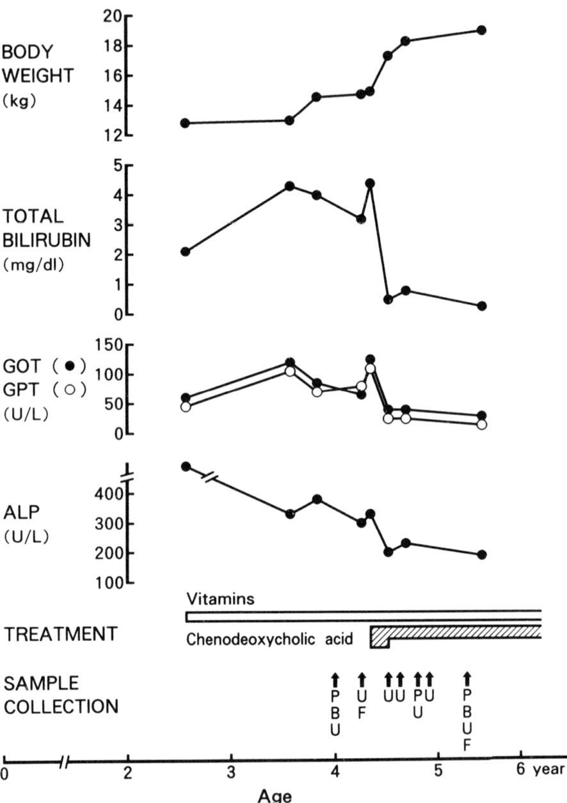

Fig. 7 Clinical, laboratory data, and times of sampling of urine (U), plasma (P), bile (B), and faeces (F) before and during treatment of patients with 3β-hydroxy-Δ^5-C_{27}-steroid dehydrogenase/isomerase deficiency with chenodeoxycholic acid. Modified from ref. 24

125 mg daily after 2 months. At baseline the biliary bile acids predominantly consisted of glycocholic acid (25%) and of sulphated and glycine-conjugated di- and trihydroxycholenoic acids (55%), along with two C_{27} bile acids and sulphated bile alcohols all having $3\beta,7\alpha$-dihydroxy-Δ^5 or $3\beta,7\alpha,12\alpha$-trihydroxy-Δ^5 ring structures. Treatment with chenodeoxycholic acid resulted in marked clinical improvement (abatement of pruritus and improved weight gain) along with normalization of liver function tests (Fig. 7). The plasma bile acid concentration decreased and urinary excretion decreased. Chenodeoxycholic and ursodeoxycholic acids became predominant in all samples (Fig. 8)[23,24].

An additional child with this disorder was described by Horslen *et al.*[25]. This child, also born to a consanguineous marriage, was noted to have neonatal cholestasis. At 4 months of age the patient remained jaundiced, but otherwise appeared well. Treatment with chenodeoxycholic acid (125 mg daily; 12 mg/kg per day) was begun at 11.5 months of age. The plasma bile acid profiles before and after 4 months of bile acid therapy are shown in Table 5. Aminotransferase levels declined over this 4-week period and normalized by 6 weeks. A repeat

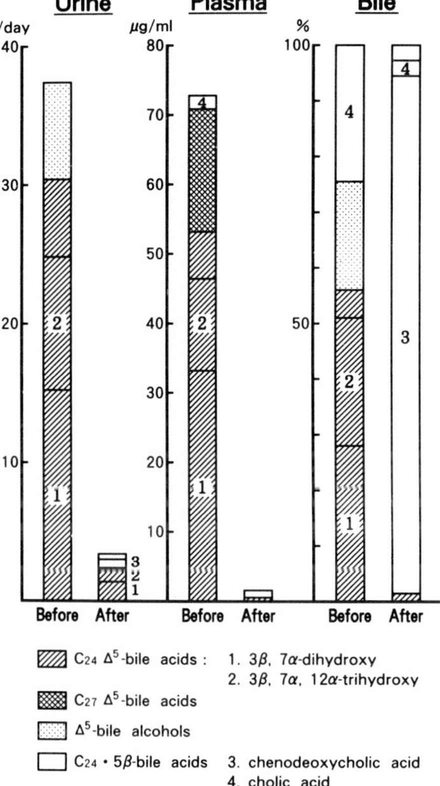

Fig. 8 Concentrations and composition of bile acids and bile alcohols determined by GLC analyses of urine, plasma and bile collected before and during (after) treatment of patients with 3β-hydroxy-Δ^5-C_{27}-steroid dehydrogenase/isomerase deficiency with chenodeoxycholic acid. Modified from ref. 24

liver biopsy after 4 months of therapy demonstrated a reduction in the inflammatory infiltrate and resolution of individual hepatocyte necrosis[25].

Jacquemin *et al.* successfully treated five patients with 3β-hydroxy-C_{27}-steroid dehydrogenase/isomerase deficiency with ursodeoxycholic acids *alone* ($600\,\text{mg/m}^2$ per day, by mouth)[26]. However, they suggested that *replacement* therapy, using primary bile acids, should be co-administered in order to suppress endogenous bile acid synthesis and prevent synthesis of atypical 3β-hydroxy-Δ^5 bile acids[26].

DEFECTIVE BILE ACID BIOSYNTHESIS IN OTHER CHOLESTATIC DISEASES

Byler's disease (progressive familial intrahepatic cholestasis)

Byler's disease is a relatively discrete disorder characterized by unrelenting progressive intrahepatic cholestasis; clinical findings include pruritus, fat

Table 5 Plasma bile acid profile of a patient with 3β-hydroxy-Δ^5-C_{27}-steroid dehydrogenase/isomerase deficiency before and after (4 months) chenodeoxycholic acid therapy

	Plasma concentration ($\mu mol/l$)		
Bile acid	Pre-treatment	Post-treatment	Normal
Chenodeoxycholic acid	0.08	8.4	0.22–12.4
Cholic acid	0.21	0.01	0.05–4.6
Ursodeoxycholic acid	n.d.	0.85	n.d.–2.9
$3\beta,7\alpha$-Dihydroxy-5-cholenoic acid	1.5	0.07	n.d.
$3\beta,7\alpha,12\alpha$-Trihydroxy-5-cholenoic acid	0.06	n.d.	n.d.
$3\beta,7\alpha$-Dihydroxy-5-cholestenoic acid	3.2	0.23	n.d.–0.05

n.d. = not detectable
Modified from ref. 25

Table 6 Bile acid concentration and composition in patients with Byler's disease compared to patients with other forms of cholestasis

	Byler's disease	Other cholestatic diseases
Serum	($n=7$)	($n=5$)
Total (mmol/l)*	0.3	0.2 n.s.
CDC (%)	44	32
C (%)	37	62
Bile	($n=7$)	($n=8$)
Total (mmol/l)	1.1	88.9 $p<0.001$
CDC (%)	9	28
C (%)	56	71

*Healthy controls = 0.008 mmol/l; CDC = chenodeoxycholic acid; C = cholic acid
Modified from ref. 31

malabsorption, and low γ-GGTP levels[28,29]. There are clear biochemical features which differentiate patients with Byler's disease from patients with 3β-hydroxy-C_{27}-steroid dehydrogenase/isomerase deficiency[26]; however, the clinical similarities between these two groups of patients led to a search for specific defects in bile acid biosynthesis in patients with Byler's disease. To date no specific inborn error in biosynthesis has been described; however, there does appear to be a difference in *compartmentalization* of individual bile acids between serum, urine, and bile (Table 6)[30,31]. The biliary bile acid concentrations are low, with a predominance of cholic acid. However, chenodeoxycholic acid predominates in serum and in urine, suggesting a defect in canalicular excretion.

Neonatal iron storage disease

A recent interesting observation was made by Shneider *et al.* of 5β-reductase deficiency in the presence of neonatal liver failure and haemochromatosis[32]. Two infants with liver failure were found to have increased iron in the salivary glands, suggesting neonatal iron storage disease (NISD). NISD or perinatal haemochromatosis is a rare clinicopathological entity characterized by recurrence in siblings, severe and generally fatal liver disease of intrauterine onset, and extrahepatic siderosis that spares reticuloendothelial elements (haemochromatotic siderosis)[33]. Intrauterine growth retardation, premature birth, and severe hypoglycaemia, probably secondary to liver dysfunction, are frequent. Antemortem diagnosis is based on the demonstration of iron deposits at extrahepatic sites by biopsy, or via magnetic resonance imaging of the liver, heart, pancreas, and spleen. At autopsy, many organs (pituitary, thyroid, pancreas, heart) contain increased amounts of stainable iron; however, unlike haemolytic or transfusional siderosis, reticuloendothelial elements are spared. Hepatocellular giant cell transformation is common.

It remains unclear whether NISD is a heritable disorder of iron handling or the result of fetal liver disease of various unknown aetiologies. To date the diagnosis of NISD is one of exclusion. By definition, primary hepatic structural abnormalities, identifiable intrauterine infections, exposure to toxic agents, and metabolic disorders are not present.

The serum ferritin levels in the patients reported by Shneider *et al.* were markedly elevated (> 1000 μg/l)[32]. Screening of the urine with FAB-MS revealed a paucity of primary bile acids and predominance of 7α-hydroxy-3-oxo-4-cholenoic and 7α,12α-dihydroxy-3-oxo-4-cholenoic acids, suggesting Δ^4-3-oxosteroid 5β-reductase deficiency. Bile acid therapy was started at day 38 in one patient; however, the patient died on day 47. Treatment was started in the second patient at approximately day 50; the patient underwent a liver transplantation. In the explanted liver there was extensive iron deposition. Western blot of the liver from both patients, using monoclonal antibody versus 5β-reductase, revealed truncated protein in the first patient and the absence of protein in the second[32].

What is the relationship of 5β-reductase to NISD? It is possible that a primary defect in bile acid biosynthesis leads to diffuse haemosiderosis with liver injury, and the absence of primary bile acids leads to impaired iron excretion. Alternatively, there may be genetic linkage of the two defects, or iron overload may inhibit 5β-reductase activity[32]. Further study is required.

SECONDARY DEFECTS

Peroxisomes are essential for cellular metabolism, including bile acid β-oxidation. Defective bile acid biosynthesis has been described as a *secondary* feature of various peroxisomal disorders (Table 2)[34–40]. The bile acid intermediates detected in serum, bile, and urine of patients with peroxisomal disorders, polyhydroxylated cholestanoic acid derivatives, reflect deficiency of the final steps in the bile acid biosynthetic pathway (see Fig. 2; reactions 10–13)[1].

Zellweger's syndrome

Clinical features

Zellweger (cerebrohepatorenal) syndrome is manifest clinically by profound psychomotor retardation, hypotonia, characteristic facies, cortical cysts of the kidneys and intrahepatic cholestasis[41,42]. Hepatic histological features in early life include variable degrees of cholestasis, lobular disarray, and focal liver cell necrosis, often with paucity of intrahepatic ducts[41–43]. Mitochondrial abnormalities are also present[44,45]. Hepatomegaly is noted along with jaundice in the first 2–3 weeks of life. This disease is rapidly fatal; affected patients usually die by 6 months of age. At autopsy diffuse micronodular cirrhosis is noted. In Zellweger's syndrome there is virtual absence of hepatic peroxisomes. Biochemical features reflecting absent peroxisomal function are excessive urinary excretion of $3\alpha,7\alpha,12\alpha$-trihydroxy 5β-cholestanoic acid (THCA) and $3\alpha,7\alpha$-dihydroxy 5β-cholestanoic acid (DHCA), all precursors of primary bile acids which have not undergone side-chain oxidation[46]. Increased concentration of C_{27} bile acid intermediates is present in serum and bile[47–50].

Pathophysiology

The biochemical defect caused by absence of peroxisomal function involves inadequate synthesis of the primary bile acids and failure of side-chain oxidation of DHCA and THCA; these compounds accumulate. It is likely that THCA and other bile acid precursors contribute to the hepatic pathology. It has been noted that infusion of THCA into experimental models will cause haemolysis and hepatic injury; the ultrastructural features of the latter are similar to those seen in patients with Zellweger's syndrome[51].

Treatment

Attempts to reverse the hepatic pathology in Zellweger's syndrome with bile acid therapy have been reported[52]. When cholic and chenodeoxycholic acid (100 mg each per day) were given orally, a significant improvement in biochemical indices of liver function occurred and there was histological improvement (decreased inflammation and bile duct proliferation and disappearance of canalicular plugs). It is doubtful that bile acid therapy will affect the long-term outcome in view of the severe, irreversible neurological disease.

'Zellweger-like' syndrome with detectable hepatic peroxisomes

There exists a subgroup of disorders in which clinical and biochemical features similar to those seen in Zellweger's syndrome are noted; however, hepatic peroxisomes are detectable by electron microscopy[38,40]. Abnormalities in bile acid biosynthesis are present, similar to those seen in patients with Zellweger syndrome.

Other peroxisomal disorders

Another subset of disorders is characterized by defective peroxisomal *biogenesis*. Similar to patients with Zellweger's syndrome there is aberrant peroxisomal chain shortening function. These disorders are characterized by either general loss of peroxisomal function or specific loss of certain peroxisomal functions (Table 2). The role of bile acid therapy in these disorders has not been defined.

SUMMARY

With sophisticated technology we are now able to delineate defective bile acid biosynthesis, metabolism, and transport in a wide variety of disease states. Recognition of specific aberrations, such as the two documented inborn errors in bile acid biosynthesis manifesting as neonatal cholestasis, offers new opportunities for therapeutic interventions[53]. Future studies should determine the incidence of bile acid biosynthetic defects in patients with enigmatic and unexplained liver diseases[3,4].

Acknowledgement

Original studies funded, in part, by a grant (FDR-000357) from the Food and Drug Administration, Department of Health and Human Services. We thank the parents of the patients for permission to reproduce the photographs.

References

1. Russell DW, Setchell KDR. Bile acid biosynthesis. Biochemistry. 1992;31:4737–49.
2. Vlahcevic ZR, Heuman DM, Hylemon PB. Regulation of bile acid synthesis. Hepatology. 1991;13:590–600.
3. Balistreri WF, Schubert WK. Liver disease in infancy and childhood. In: Schiff L, Schiff ER, editors. Diseases of the liver, 7th edn. Philadelphia: PA: J.B. Lippincott; 1994:1099–203.
4. Balistreri WF. Fetal and bile acid synthesis and metabolism: clinical implications. J Inher Metab Dis. 1991;14:459–77.
5. Nathanson MH, Boyer JL. Mechanisms and regulation of bile secretion. Hepatology. 1991;14:551–66.
6. Balistreri WF. Neonatal cholestasis: Lessons from the past issues from the future. In: Balistreri WF, editor. Seminars in liver disease. New York: Thieme; 1987 (Foreword).
7. Balistreri WF, Hofmann AF, A-Kader HH, Setchell KDR. Successful bile acid therapy in 3 siblings with neonatal hepatitis due to an inborn error of bile acid biosynthesis. Pediatr Res. 1991;29:99A.
8. Balistreri WF, Setchell KDR. Clinical implications of bile acid metabolism. In: Silverberg M, Daum F, editors. Textbook of pediatric gastroenterology. Chicago: Year Book Medical; 1987:72–89.
9. Miller WL. Congenital adrenal hyperplasias. Endocrinol Metab Clin N Am. 1991;20:721–49.
10. Setchell KDR, Street JM. Inborn errors of bile acid synthesis. Semin Liver Dis. 1987;7:85–9.
11. Setchell KDR, O'Connell NC. Inborn errors of bile acid metabolism. In: Suchy FJ, editor. Liver disease in children. Boston, MA: Mosby; 1994:835–51.
12. Clayton PT, Leonard JV, Lawson AM *et al.* Familial giant cell hepatitis associated with synthesis of $3\beta,7\alpha$-dihydroxy and $3\beta,7\alpha,12\alpha$-trihydroxy-5-cholenoic acids. J Clin Invest. 1987;79:1031–8.

13. Setchell KDR, Suchy FJ, Welsh MB, Zimmer-Nechemias L, Heubi J, Balistreri WF. Δ^4-3-oxosteroid 5β-reductase deficiency described in identical twins with neonatal hepatitis: a new inborn error in bile acid synthesis. J Clin Invest. 1988;82:2148–57.

14. Evans JE, Ghosh A, Evans BA, Natowicz MB. Screening techniques for the detection of inborn errors of bile acid metabolism by direct injection and micro-high performance liquid chromatography continuous flow/fast atom bombardment mass spectrometry. Biol Mass Spectrometry. 1993;22:331–7.

15. Libert R, Hermans D, Draye JP, Van Hoof F, Sokal E, de Hoffmann E. Bile acids and conjugates identified in metabolic disorders by fast atom bombardment and tandem mass spectrometry. Clin Chem. 1991;37:2102–10.

16. Daugherty CC, Setchell KDR, Heubi JE, Balistreri WF. Resolution of hepatic biopsy alterations in 3 siblings with bile acid treatment of an inborn error of bile acid metabolism (Δ^4-3-oxosteroid 5β-reductase deficiency). Hepatology. 1993;18:1096–101.

17. Onishi Y, Noshiro M, Shimosato T, Okuda K. Δ^4-3-oxosteroid 5β-reductase. Structure and function. Biol Chem Hoppe-Seyler. 1991;372:1039–49.

18. Onishi Y, Noshiro M, Shimosato T, Okuda K. Molecular cloning and sequence analysis of cDNA encoding Δ^4-3-ketosteroid 5β-reductase of rat liver. FEBS. 1991;283:215–18.

19. Kondo KH, Kai MH, Setoguchi YS et al. Cloning and expression of cDNA of human Δ^4-3-oxosteroid 5β-reductase and substrate specificity of the expressed enzyme. Eur J Biochem. 1994;219:357–63.

20. Clayton PT. Inborn errors of bile acid metabolism. J Inher Metab Dis. 1991;14:478–96.

21. Witzleben CL, Piccoli DA, Setchell KDR. Case 3: A new category of causes of intrahepatic cholestasis. Pediatr Pathol. 1992;12:269–74.

22. Setchell KDR, Balistreri WF, Piccoli DA, Clerici C. Oral bile acid therapy in the treatment of inborn erors in bile acid synthesis associated with liver disease. In: Paumgartner G, Stiehl A, Gerok W, editors. Bile acids as therapeutic agents. From basic science to clinical practice. Boston, MA: Kluwer; 1990:367–73.

23. Ichimiya H, Nazer H, Gunasekaran T, Clayton P, Sjovall J. Treatment of chronic liver disease caused by 3β-hydroxy-Δ^5-C_{27}-steroid hydrogenase deficiency with chenodeoxycholic acid. Arch Dis Child. 1990;65:1121–4.

24. Ichimiya H, Egestad B, Nazer H, Baginski ES, Clayton PT, Sjovall J. Bile acids and bile alcohols in a child with hepatic 3β-hydroxy-Δ^5-C_{27}-steroid dehydrogenase deficiency: effects of chenodeoxycholic acid treatment. J Lipid Res. 1991;32:829–41.

25. Horslen SP, Lawson AM, Malone M, Clayton PT. 3β-Hydroxy-Δ^5-C_{27} steroid dehydrogenase deficiency; effect of chenodeoxycholic acid therapy on liver histology. J Inher Metab Dis. 1992;15:38–46.

26. Jacquemin E, Setchell KDR, O'Connell NC et al. A new cause of progressive intrahepatic cholestasis: 3β-hydroxy-C_{27}-steroid dehydrogenase/isomerase deficiency. J Pediatr. 1994;125:379–84.

27. Buchmann MS, Kvittingen EA, Nazer H et al. Lack of 3β-hydroxy-Δ^5-C_{27}-steroid dehydrogenase/isomerase in fibroblasts from a child with urinary excretion of 3β-hydroxy-Δ^5-bile acids: a new inborn error of metabolism. J Clin Invest. 1990;86:2034–7.

28. Alonso EM, Snover DC, Montag A, Freese DK, Whitington PF. Histologic pathology of the liver in progressive familial intrahepatic cholestasis. J Pediatr Gastroenterol Nutr. 1994;18:128–33.

29. Whitington PF, Freese DK, Alonso EM, Schwarzenberg SJ, Sharp JL. Clinical and biochemical findings in progressive familial intrahepatic cholestasis. J Pediatr Gastroenterol Nutr. 1994;18:134–41.

30. Tazawa Y, Yamada M, Nakagawa M, Konno T, Tada K. Bile acid profiles in siblings with progressive intrahepatic cholestasis: absence of biliary chenodeoxycholate. J Pediatr Gastroenterol Nutr. 1985;4:32–7.

31. Jacquemin E, Dumont M, Bernard O, Erlinger S, Hadchouel M. Evidence for defective primary bile acid secretion in children with progressive familial intrahepatic cholestasis (Byler disease). Eur J Pediatr. 1994;153:424–4.

32. Shneider BL, Setchell KDR, Whitington PF, Nielson KA, Suchy FA. Δ^4-3-Oxosteroid 5β-reductase deficiency causing neonatal liver failure and hemochromatosis. J Pediatr. 1994;124:234–8.

33. Knisely AS. Neonatal hemochromatosis. Adv Pediatr. 1992;39:383–403.

34. van den Bosch H, Schutgens RHB, Wanders RJA, Tager JM. Biochemistry of peroxisomes. Annu Rev Biochem. 1992;61:157–97.

35. Christensen E, Van Eldere J, Brandt NJ, Schutgens RHB, Wanders RJA, Eyssen HJ. A new peroxisomal disorder: di and trihydroxycholestanaemia due to a presumed trihydroxycholestanoyl-CoA oxidase deficiency. J Inher Metab Dis. 1990;13:363-6.
36. Clayton PT, Patel E, Lawson AM, Carruthers RA, Collins J. Bile acid profiles in peroxisomal 3-oxoacyl-coenzyme A thiolase deficiency. J Clin Invest. 1990;85:1267-73.
37. Moser HW. Peroxisomal diseases. Adv Pediatr. 1989;36:1-38.
38. Schutgens RBH, Schrakamp G, Wanders RJA, Heymans HSA, Tager JM, van den Bosch H. Prenatal and perinatal diagnosis of peroxisomal disorders. J Inher Metab Dis. 1989;12:118-34.
39. Singh I, Johnson GH, Brown FR. Peroxisomal disorders. Am J Dis Child. 1988;142:1297-301.
40. Suzuki Y, Shiozawa N, Ori T et al. Zellweger-like syndrome with detectable hepatic peroxisomes: a variant form of peroxisomal disorder. J Pediatr. 1988;113:841-5.
41. Passarge E, McAdams AJ. Cerebro-hepato-renal syndrome. J Pediatr. 1967;71:691.
42. Smith DW et al. A syndrome of multiple developmental defects including polycystic kidneys and intrahepatic biliary dysgenesis in 2 siblings. J Pediatr. 1965;67:617.
43. Gilchrist KW, Gilbert EF, Goldfarb S, Goll U, Spranger JW, Opitz JM. Studies of malformation syndromes of man: XIB. The cerebro-hepato-renal syndrome of Zellweger: comparative pathology. Eur J Pediatr. 1976;121:99-118.
44. Goldfisher S, Moore CL, Johnson AB et al. Peroxisomal and mitochondrial defects in the cerebro-hepato-renal syndrome. Science. 1973;182:62-4.
45. Mooi WJ, Dingemans KP, van den Bergh Weerman MA. Ultrastructure of the liver in cerebrohepatorenal syndrome of Zellweger. Ultrastruct Pathol. 1983;5:135.
46. Hanson RF, Isenberg JN, Williams GC et al. The metabolism of 3 alpha, 7 alpha, 12 alpha, trihydroxy-5 beta-cholestan-26 oic acid in two siblings with cholestasis due to intrahepatic bile duct anomalies. J Clin Invest. 1975;56:577.
47. Bjorkhem I, Blomstrands S, Haga P et al. Urinary excretion of dicarboxylic acids from patients with the Zellweger syndrome: importance of peroxisomes in beta-oxidation of dicarboxylic acids. Biochim Biophys Acta. 1984;795:15.
48. Datta NS, Wilson GN, Hajra AK. Deficiency of enzymes catalyzing the biosynthesis of glycerol-ether lipids in Zellweger syndrome. N Engl J Med. 1984;311:1080.
49. Eyssen H, Eggermont F, Van Eldere J, Jaeken J, Parmentier G, Janssen G. Bile acid abnormalities and the diagnosis of cerebro-hepato-renal syndrome (Zellweger syndrome). Acta Paediatr Scand. 1985;74:539-44.
50. Heymans HSA, Schutgens RBH, Tan R, van den Bosch H, Borst P. Severe plasmalogen deficiency in tissues of infants without peroxisomes (Zellweger syndrome). Nature. 1983;306:69.
51. Hanson RF, Williams GC, Hachey D, Sharp HL. Hepatic lesions and hemolysis following administration of 3 alpha, 7 alpha, 12 alpha-trihydroxy-5 beta-cholestan-26 oyl taurine in rats. J Lab Clin Med. 1977;90:536.
52. Setchell KDR, Bragetti P, Zimmer-Nechemias Z et al. Oral bile acid treatment and the patient with Zellweger syndrome. Hepatology. 1992;15:198-207.
53. Suchy FJ. Bile acids for babies? Diagnosis and treatment of a new category of metabolic liver disease (Editorial). Hepatology. 1993;18:1274-7.
54. Peynet J, Laurent A, de Liege P et al. Cerebrotendinous xanthomatosis: treatments with simvastatin, lovastatin, and chenodeoxycholic acid in 3 siblings. Neurology. 1991;41:434-6.
55. Setoguchi T, Salen G, Tint GS, Mosbach EH. A biochemical abnormality in cerebrotendinous xanthomatosis. Impairment of bile acid biosynthesis associated with complete degradation of cholesterol side-chain. J Clin Invest. 1974;53:1393-401.
56. Budden SS, Kennaway NG, Phil D, Buist NRM, Poulos A, Weleber RG. Dysmorphic syndrome with phytanic acid oxidase deficiency, abnormal very long chain fatty acids, and pipecolic acidemia: studies in four children. J Pediatr. 1986;108:33-9.
57. Elk J, Kase BF, Reith A, Bjorkhem I, Pedersen JI. Peroxisomal dysfunction in a boy with neurologic symptoms and amaurosis (Leber disease): clinical and biochemical findings similar to those observed in Zellweger syndrome. J Pediatr. 1986;108:19-24.
58. Goldfisher S, Collins J, Rappin I et al. Pseudo-Zellweger syndrome: deficiencies in several peroxisomal oxidative activities. J Pediatr. 1986;108:25-32.
59. Watkins PA, Chen WW, Harris CJ et al. Peroxisomal bi-functional enzyme deficiency. J Clin Invest. 1989;83:771-7.

38
Effect of UDCA on bile acid and cholesterol metabolism

E. RODA, A. CIPOLLA, N. VILLANOVA, P. PARINI, C. POLIMENI, C. CERRÉ and G. MAZZELLA

Over 30 years have gone by since it was recognized that cholesterol gallstone patients have supersaturated bile due to an excessive concentration of cholesterol with respect to its natural detergents, bile acids and phospholipids. For over 20 years bile acid therapy, first with chenodeoxycholic acid (CDCA) and then with ursodeoxycholic acid (UDCA), has been used to correct this metabolic defect and thus to desaturate bile[1,2]. Over the years many studies have shed light on this problem in terms of cholesterol gallstone dissolution therapy. Unfortunately, the exact mechanisms that bring about cholesterol supersaturation and the effects of CDCA and UDCA administration are still not fully understood.

The present paper will look into the effects of chronic administration of UDCA on bile acid and cholesterol metabolism using several different human models which differ with regards to basal conditions. The models that will be discussed are those that have been studied by our group over the last few years.

Cholesterol gallstone patients;
Non-familial hypercholesterolaemia before and during treatment with UDCA and/or simvastatin, an inhibitor of cholesterol synthesis;
I–III stage primary biliary cirrhosis (PBC) before and after UDCA therapy;
Obese patients before and after rapid weight loss with simvastatin or UDCA therapy.

In patients with cholesterol gallstones we demonstrated[3], differently from other authors, that the principal metabolic alteration in this group of patients is the presence of an increased biliary secretion of cholesterol that leads to supersaturation of bile. Moreover, we, like others, demonstrated that the chronic administration of CDCA and UDCA induces a reduction in the cholesterol secretion rate without influencing the secretion of bile acids and phospholipids[4-6]. The enrichment in bile of the administered bile acids (90% CDCA; 30–40% UDCA) leads to a consequent reduction in the molar percentage of endogenous bile acids and in particular of deoxycholic acid (DCA). UDCA, but not CDCA, is also able to induce an increase in the fractional turnover rate (FTR) of primary bile acids.

The studies in hyperlipidaemic (IIb) subjects[7] demonstrated that UDCA is able to reduce the hepatic secretion rate of cholesterol and cholesterol saturation index (CSI) significantly even in this condition where there are important changes in body cholesterol metabolism. Simvastatin administration also induced the same effects, indicating that cholesterol secretion is closely related to cholesterol synthesis. The combination of the two drugs induced a greater decrease than that obtained by the single administration, suggesting a synergistic effect by two different routes. An increase in FTR was observed only after UDCA administration, in accordance with others[4,5,8] who observed that UDCA induces bile acid malabsorption. Furthermore, another mechanism by which UDCA reduces cholesterol secretion may be through intestinal cholesterol malabsorption[9,10].

In patients with cholestatic liver diseases such as PBC the bile acid pool is distributed abnormally between the enterohepatic and systemic circulations. This inefficiency of the enterohepatic circulation (EHC) is due to the metabolic alterations present in PBC that regard uptake, transport and secretion of bile acids. We studied patients with I–III stage PBC before and after UDCA therapy in order to determine the pathophysiological biliary alterations and the effects of endogenous bile acid administration in this disease[11,12]. This study showed a slight but significant reduction in biliary lipid secretion rate in these patients. The administration of UDCA even in this condition was able to lower the cholesterol secretion rate. Furthermore, UDCA replaced endogenous, potentially more toxic (DCA), bile acids in the EHC by increasing primary bile acid FTR without a concomitant increase in their synthesis rates.

The most recent human model that we have studied is that of obese patients before and after rapid weight loss with simvastatin or UDCA therapy. The diet (1042 Cal) was lipid-enriched to maintain adequate gallbladder motility. During rapid weight loss there are profound changes in the metabolism of cholesterol with release of cholesterol from deposits and inhibition of its synthesis. The results of the study showed that during diet alone CSI increased mainly due to a decrease in bile acid secretion. Cholesterol secretion was also reduced but not to the same extent and thus the net balance moved towards supersaturation of bile. Simvastatin administration reduced cholesterol secretion but reduced bile acid secretion due to diet persisted and thus CSI was not significantly modified with respect to basal conditions. Only UDCA during weight loss lowered CSI due to a reduction in cholesterol output and a maintained bile acid secretion. Cholic acid pool size was significantly reduced and turnover increased after all 3 treatment periods. Diet and diet plus simvastatin induced a reduction in cholic acid synthesis, while ursodeoxycholic acid plus diet did not have any effect with respect to baseline thus suggesting that it is able to sustain bile acid secretion and synthesis even in these conditions.

From these studies it is clear that the presence of a hydrophilic bile acid such as UDCA in the EHC is able to induce constant even if monotonous effects on biliary cholesterol and bile acid metabolism. These effects can be summarized as such:

UDCA desaturates bile by suppression of cholesterol output;
UDCA increases FTR of primary bile acids;

UDCA displaces DCA in the EHC;
UDCA does not suppress bile acid synthesis.

In conclusion these studies suggest that by manipulating cholesterol synthesis (e.g. by simvastatin therapy) changes in biliary secretion of cholesterol may be induced. Furthermore, sustained bile acid flow and synthesis as observed during UDCA administration may in part account for the decrease it induces in cholesterol output.

References

1. Barbara L, Roda E, Roda A, Sama C, Festi D, Mazzella G, Aldini R. The medical treatment of cholesterol gallstones: Experience with chenodeoxycholic acid. Digestion. 1976;14:209–19.
2. Roda E, Bazzoli F, Morselli Labate AM, Mazzella G, Roda A, Sama C, Festi D, Aldini R, Taroni F, Barbara L. Ursodeoxycholic acid vs chenodeoxycholic acid as cholesterol gallstone dissolving agent. A comparative randomized study. Hepatology. 1982;2:804–10.
3. Roda E, Bazzoli F, Mazzella G, Villanova N, Simoni P, Festi D, Frabboni R, Ronchi M, Barbara L. Effect of age and sex on bile acid metabolism and biliary lipid secretion in normal subjects and gallstone patients. In: Paumgartner G, Stiehl A, Gerok W, editors. Bile acids and liver. Lancaster: MTP Press; 1986:225–7.
4. Roda E, Roda A, Sama C, Festi D, Mazzella G, Aldini R, Barbara L. Effect of ursodeoxycholic acid administration on biliary lipid composition and bile acid kinetics in cholesterol gallstone patients. Dig Dis Sci. 1979;24:123–8.
5. Nilsell K, Angelin B, Leijd B, Einarsson K. Comparative effects of ursodeoxycholic acid and chenodeoxycholic acid on bile acid kinetics and biliary lipid secretion in humans. Gastroenterology. 1983;85:1248–56.
6. Stiehl A, Raedach R, Czygan P. Effects of biliary bile acid composition on biliary cholesterol saturation in gallstone patients treated with chenodeoxycholic acid and/or ursodeoxycholic acid. Gastroenterology. 1970;79:1192–6.
7. Mazzella G, Parini P, Festi D, Bazzoli F, Aldini R, Roda A, Tonelli D, Cipolla A, Salzetta A, Roda E. Effect of simvastatin, ursodeoxycholic acid and simvastatin plus ursodeoxycholic acid on biliary lipid secretion and cholic acid kinetics in non-familial hypercholesterolemia. Hepatology. 1992;15:1072–8.
8. Stiehl A, Raedsch R, Rudolph G. Acute effects of ursodeoxycholic and chenodeoxycholic acid on the small intestinal absorption of bile acids. Gastroenterology. 1990;98:424–8.
9. Leiss O, von Bergmann K, Streicher U, Strotkoetter H. Effect of three different dihydroxy bile acids on intestinal cholesterol absorption in normal volunteers. Gastroenterology. 1980;78:214–19.
10. Hardison WGM, Grundy SM. Effect of ursodeoxycholate and its taurine conjugate on bile acid synthesis and cholesterol absorption. Gastroenterology. 1984;87:130–5.
11. Roda E, Mazzella G, Bazzoli F, Villanova N, Minutello A, Simoni P, Ronchi M, Poggi C, Festi D, Aldini R, Roda A. Effect of ursodeoxycholic acid administration on biliary lipid secretion in primary biliary cirrhosis. Dig Dis Sci. 1989;34(12)suppl:52s–58s.
12. Mazzella G, Parini P, Bazzoli F, Villanova N, Festi D, Aldini R, Roda A, Cipolla A, Polimeni C, Tonelli D, Roda E. Ursodeoxycholic acid administration on bile acid metabolism in patients with primary biliary cirrhosis. Dig Dis Sci. 1993;38:896–902.

39
Ursodeoxycholic acid prevents gallstone formation in patients undergoing rapid weight reduction

M. L. SHIFFMAN, H. J. SUGERMAN, G. D. KAPLAN and
F. F. VICKERS

INTRODUCTION

The development of cholesterol gallstones is associated with several well-defined risk factors[1-4]. One of the most important of these factors appears to be rapid weight reduction. Approximately 10–25% of persons will develop gallstones while participating in a very low calorie diet programme[5-9]; and 35% of patients with morbid obesity will develop gallstones following bariatric surgery[10-13]. Preliminary studies have demonstrated that ursodeoxycholic acid (UDCA) could reduce the incidence of gallstone formation in persons participating in a very low calorie diet programme[7] and following bariatric bypass surgery[13]. These preliminary reports inspired the present multicentre, randomized, double-blind, placebo-controlled trials to determine the optimum dose by which UDCA could prevent gallstone formation in patients undergoing rapid weight reduction. These studies were conducted at 31 affiliated Health Management Resources (HMR) weight loss centres and 10 centres specializing in the surgical treatment of morbid obesity.

METHODS

Patient population

To enter the diet trial patients had to have a body mass index (BMI) $\geq 38\,\mathrm{kg/m^2}$, essentially normal serum chemistries, be of age 18–70 years and be willing to participate in the HMR diet programme for 16 weeks. Patients in the surgical arm of the trial had to have a BMI $\geq 40\,\mathrm{kg/m^2}$ and be accepted as a candidate to undergo gastric bypass surgery. Exclusion criteria for both the diet and surgical arms included: prior cholecystectomy, the presence of gallstones or gallbladder sludge by ultrasonography, an eating disorder or other psychological problem which would interfere with participation in the study, and the use of oral bile salt preparations, non-steroidal anti-inflammatory drugs (NSAIDs), or antihyperlipidaemic agents. Informed consent to participate in this trial was obtained from all participants prior to study entry.

Dietary study design

All patients accepted into the diet study were randomly assigned to one of four groups to receive either placebo, 300, 600 or 1200 mg/day of UDCA administered twice daily. Medication started on the first day on which each patient began the HMR diet plan and was continued throughout the entire 16-week programme. The HMR diet provided 520 kcal/day of a liquid protein diet containing 50 g of protein, 79 g of carbohydrate and 1–3 g of fat (depending upon the particular HMR preparation). All participants in this plan consumed this diet, supplemented with vitamins and minerals, for 16 weeks. Gallbladder ultrasonography was repeated after 8 and 16 weeks of dieting and/or when the patient separated from the trial. If a patient was found to have developed gallstones participation in the trial was complete. Gallbladder sludge was not considered a primary endpoint. Patients who developed sludge were continued in the trial.

Surgical study design

All patients accepted as candidates for the surgical trial underwent Roux-en-Y proximal gastric bypass as described previously[14]. At the time of surgery, intra-operative ultrasonography was performed, and if gallstones or gallbladder sludge was present the patient was advanced to a puréed diet. This typically occurred by the fourth day. If study medication could not be started by postoperative day 10 the patient was dropped from the trial. As in the diet trial, patients were randomized to receive either placebo or UDCA at doses of 300, 600 or 1200 mg/day. Transabdominal ultrasonography was performed 2, 4 and 6 months following gastric bypass. If a patient was found to have developed gallstones participation in the trial was complete. As in the diet trial, gallbladder sludge was not considered an endpoint.

Statistical analysis

All randomized patients who had a normal baseline gallbladder ultrasonogram and at least one post-baseline ultrasound were included in the final 'intent-to-treat' analysis. Data from each patient group were expressed as the mean $\pm$ standard deviation (SD). Body mass index (BMI) was expressed as kg/m^2. The χ^2 test was utilized to determine if the rates of gallstone and gallbladder sludge formation in the various treatment groups were significantly different.

Table 1 Characteristics of patients

	Diet	*Surgery*
Number of patients enrolled	1004	312
Number (percentage) of patients eligible for analysis	788 (78%)	233 (75%)
Age (years)	40.1±9.1	36.7±8.7
Sex (percentage female)	66%	79%
Race (percentage white)	88%	70%
Initial body weight (kg)	128.2±23.3	139.3±28.1
Initial body mass index (kg/m^2)	44.2±6.0	49.5±8.6
Maximum weight loss (kg)	24.9±9.8	39.4±10.5

Values are given as mean±SD

RESULTS

Patient population

A total of 1004 patients were enrolled in the HMR diet trial and 312 in the surgical study. Of these, 404 patients dropped out of the diet trial without obtaining any follow up ultrasound examination. No follow-up ultrasound data were available from 79 patients who entered the surgical trial. All the remaining 788 patients in the diet study, and 233 patients in the surgical study, had at least one follow-up ultrasound and were included in the final 'intent-to-treat' analysis. Compliance with study medication was 93% and 83% in the diet and surgical studies respectively. No difference in compliance was evident between placebo and UDCA-treated patients in either the diet or surgical studies.

The age, sex and race of the 1021 patients included in the 'intent-to-treat' analysis of this trial are presented in Table 1. No differences existed with regard to sex, race or age between any of the diet or surgical treatment groups. Mean initial body weight, prior to starting the diet, was 128.2±23.3 kg (range 87.7–217.7 kg). Mean initial BMI was 44.2±6.0 g/m^2 (range 35–83 kg/m^2). No significant differences in absolute body weight or BMI existed between the four treatment groups prior to the start of dieting. For patients in the surgical study, mean initial body weight and BMI were 139.3±28.1 and 49.5±8.6 respectively (Table 1). Mean maximum weight loss figures for patients in the diet and surgical trials were 24.9±9.8 and 39.4±10.5 kg respectively. No significant differences in mean weight reduction existed between placebo and UDCA-treated patients in either arm of the trial.

Gallstone formation

The percentage of patients who developed gallstones during this trial is illustrated in Fig. 1. Overall, 285 of patients who received placebo in the diet programme and 32% of placebo-treated patients in the surgical study developed gallstones. In contrast, gallstones developed in only 8%, 3% and 2% of patients treated with 300, 600 and 1200 mg/day of UDCA in the diet trial, and 13%, 2% and 6% of UDCA-treated patients in the surgical study respectively. The rate of

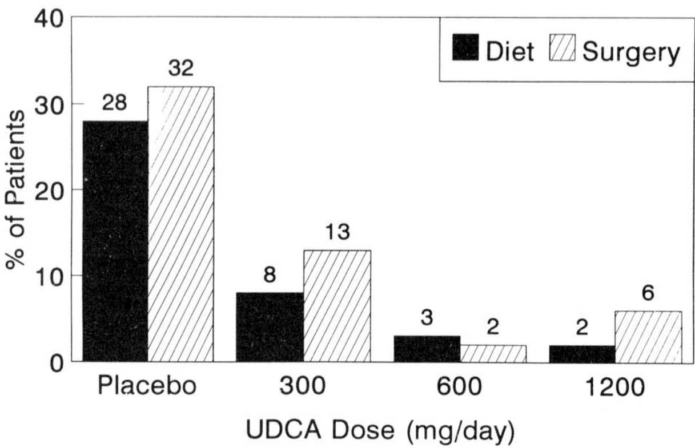

Fig. 1 Percentage of patients who developed gallstones during dietary and surgically induced weight reduction. Patients treated with 600 and 1200 mg/day of UDCA had a significantly reduced incidence for gallstone formation compared to placebo

gallstone formation in all patient groups treated with UDCA was significantly less than that observed for placebo-treated patients. In addition, the rate of gallstone formation was significantly less in patients treated with 600 mg/day of UDCA when compared to 300 mg/day.

Gallstone formation and weight reduction

The relationship between rate of weight reduction and gallstone formation for placebo-treated females is illustrated in Fig. 2. In both the diet and surgical patients the rate of gallstone formation increased stepwise with increasing rate of weight loss. In contrast, no relationship was evident between rate of weight loss and gallstone formation in placebo-treated males. On average 22% of men in the diet programme and 31% of males in the surgical trial developed gallstones. Since so few of the UDCA-treated patients developed gallstones, no relationship between degree of weight reduction and gallstone formation was apparent during UDCA treatment.

DISCUSSION

The present study has demonstrated that 28% of persons who participate in a very low calorie weight reduction programme, and 325 of morbidly obese patients undergoing proximal gastric bypass surgery, will develop gallstones. Prophylactic UDCA at a dose of 600 mg/day significantly reduced the incidence of gallstone formation in these patients to under 5%. These results confirm previous observations in smaller studies conducted in patients undergoing rapid weight loss through very low calorie diet programmes[7] and following bariatric surgery[13].

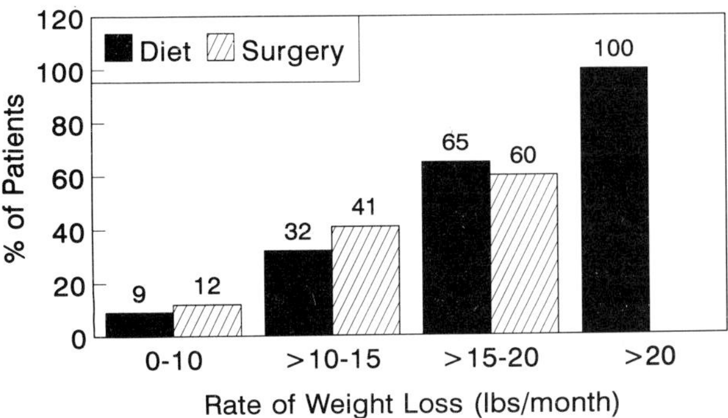

Fig. 2 Relationship between rate of weight loss and gallstone formation in placebo-treated females during dietary and surgically induced weight reduction

Several factors are thought to be important in the pathogenesis of cholesterol gallstones in these patients. Weight reduction enhances cholesterol secretion into bile and increases bile lithogenicity[15]. In addition, the very low calorie weight loss programme provided only 0.3 g of fat a day, and therefore offered little stimulus for gallbladder contraction[16]. Gallbladder motility is also significantly reduced following gastric surgery[17]. Finally, gallbladder mucin, a glycoprotein which enhances cholesterol nucleation from supersaturated bile, increases during dieting[7,18] and following bariatric surgery[19,20].

UDCA may prevent gallstone formation during weight reduction by several factors. UDCA reduces cholesterol secretion into bile and thereby reduces cholesterol saturation[21,22]. Recent data from our laboratory also suggest that UDCA reduces the concentration of gallbladder mucin in gallbladder bile, thereby eliminating a potential cholesterol nucleation factor. In contrast, UDCA does not appear to affect gallbladder motility[23].

Approximately 12% of the adult Western population have gallstones[1]. The majority of such persons have well-defined risk factors for developing gallstones including obesity, and a history of weight reduction[1-4]. Prophylaxis against gallstone formation during these high-risk activities may significantly reduce the worldwide incidence of gallstone disease. Yet to be determined is the long-term effectiveness of short-term prophylaxis during such high-risk periods, and the possible cost–benefits of such treatment.

Acknowledgements

This study was supported by Ciba-Geigy Pharmaceutical Co, and NIH first award DK43264 (M.L.S.) from the National Institutes of Digestive and Kidney Diseases. The following individuals were responsible for the conduct of these trials at the various HMR-affiliated weight loss centres and surgical treatment centres listed: J. W. Anderson, Lexington, KY; M. P. Basista, Bloomfield, NJ; L. J. Bennion, Sunnyvale, CA; G. A. Charnock, Valencia, CA; R. P. Chiles, Austin, TX; J. B. Collins, Spokane, WA; R. L. Cullen, Norfolk, VA;

D. P. Derleth, Wenatchee, WA; J. L. Early, Peoria, IL; S. C. Fox, Hackensack, NJ; M. Gottlieb, Chestnut Hills, MA; A. M. Gundry, Long Beach, CA; E. Gutowitz, La Mesa, CA; G. J. Hotchko, Jr, Yakima, WA; I. Jackson, Providence, RI; R E. Kleinmann, Charlotte, NC; D. Kremer, Portland, OR; J. D. Mancini, Winter Park, FL; T. A. McAfee, Seattle, WA; R. B. Miller, Palm Springs, CA; D. J. Morin, Bristol, TN; T. J. Meyers, Houston, TX; L. B. Nilsen, Phoenix, AZ; E. B. Noland, Salem, VA; J. Saxton, San Francisco, CA; V. Skul, Chicago, IL; A. Sussman, Renton, WA; M. Thompson, Redondo Beach, CA; G. R. Weine, Morristown, NJ; J. H. Wheeler, Atlanta, GA; J. W. Wright, Lynchburg, VA; B. D. Schirmer, Charlottesville, VA; R. E. Brolin, Brunswick, NJ; A. M. MacGregor, Gainesville, FL; M. A. L. Fobi, Los Angeles, CA; L. F. Martin, Hershey, PA; J. H. Linner, Mineapolis, MN; J. C. Oram-Smith, Colorado Springs, CO; K. G. MacDonald, Greenville, NC; D. Popoola, Los Angeles, CA.

References

1. Diehl AK. Epidemiology and natural history of gallstone disease. Gastroenterol Clin N Am. 1991;20:1–19.
2. Bennion LJ, Grundy SM. Risk factors for the development of cholelithiasis in man. N Engl J Med. 1978;299:1212–27.
3. The Rome group for epidemiology and prevention of cholelithiasis (GREPCO). The epidemiology of gallstone disease in Rome, Italy. Part II, Factors associated with the disease. Hepatology. 1988;8:907–13.
4. Jorgensen T. Gallstones in a Danish population. Relation to weight, physical activity, smoking, coffee consumption and diabetes mellitus. Gut. 1989;30:528–34.
5. Thijs C, Knipschild P, Leffers P. Is gallstone disease caused by obesity or by dieting? Am J Epidemiol. 1992;135:274–80.
6. Everhart JE. Contributions of obesity and weight loss to gallstone disease. Ann Intern Med. 1993;119:1029–35.
7. Broomfield PH, Chopra R, Sheinbaum RC et al. Effects of ursodeoxycholic acid and aspirin on the formation of lithogenic bile and gallstones during loss of weight. N Engl J Med. 1988;319:1567–72.
8. Liddle RA, Goldstein RB, Saxton J. Gallstone formation during weight-reduction dieting. Arch Intern Med. 1989;149:1750–3.
9. Yang H, Peterson GM, Roth MP, Schoenfield LJ, Marks JW. Risk factors for gallstone formation during rapid loss of weight. Dig Dis Sci. 1992;37:912–18.
10. Wattchow DA, Hall JC, Whiting MJ, Bradley B, Iannos J, Watts JM. Prevalence and treatment of gallstones after gastric bypass surgery for morbid obesity. Br Med J. 1983;286:763.
11. Amaral JF, Thompson WR. Gallbladder disease in the morbidly obese. Am J Surg. 1985;149:551–7.
12. Shiffman ML, Sugerman HJ, Kellum JM, Brewer WH, Moore EW. Gallstone formation after rapid weight loss: a prospective study in patients undergoing gastric bypass surgery for treatment of morbid obesity. Am J Gastroenterol. 1991;86:1000–5.
13. Worbobetz LJ, Inglis FG, Shaffer EA. The effect of ursodeoxycholic acid therapy on gallstone formation in the morbidly obese during rapid weight loss. Am J Gastroenterol. 1993;88:1705–10.
14. Sugerman HJ. Gastric bypass. Surg Rounds. 1993;16:169–80.
15. Bennion LJ, Grundy SM. Effects of obesity and caloric intake on biliary lipid metabolism in man. J Clin Invest. 1975;56:996–1011.
16. Stone BG, Ansel HJ, Peterson FJ, Gebhard RL. Gallbladder emptying stimuli in obese and normal-weight subjects. Hepatology. 1992;15:795–8.
17. Inoue K, Fuchigami A, Higashide S et al. Gallbladder sludge and stone formation in relation to contractile function after gastrectomy. Ann Surg. 1992;215:19–26.

18. Marks JW, Bonorris GG, Albers G, Schoenfield LJ. The sequence of biliary events preceding the formation of gallstones in humans. Gastroenterology. 1992;103:566–70.
19. Shiffman ML, Shamburek RD, Schwartz CC, Sugerman HJ, Kellum JM, Moore EW. Gallbladder mucin, arachidonic acid and bile lipids in patients who develop gallstones during weight reduction. Gastroenterology. 1993;105:1200–8.
20. Shiffman ML, Sugerman HJ, Kellum JM, Moore EW. Changes in the composition of gallbladder bile following weight reduction and gallstone formation. Gastroenterology. 1992;103:214–21.
21. Maton PN, Murphy GM, Dowling RH. Ursodeoxycholic acid treatment of gallstones: Dose-response study and possible mechanism of action. Lancet. 1977;2:1297–301.
22. Salen G, Colalillo A, Verga D *et al.* The effects of high and low doses of ursodeoxycholic acid on gallstone dissolution in humans. Gastroenterology. 1980;78:1412–18.
23. Forgacs IC, Maisey MN, Murphy GM, Dowling RH. Influence of gallstones and ursodeoxycholic acid therapy on gallbladder emptying. Gastroenterology. 1984;87:299–307.

40
Ursodeoxycholic acid for the therapy of chronic cholestatic liver disease: European experience

M. PODDA, A. CROSIGNANI, P. M. BATTEZZATI, P. INVERNIZZI,
C. COLOMBO, K. D. R. SETCHELL and M. ZUIN

INTRODUCTION

In Europe, ursodeoxycholic acid (UDCA) has been extensively investigated in chronic liver disease since the initial reports of Leuschner[1,2] and Poupon's pilot study[3]. The rationale underlying the usage of UDCA for liver disease has been reviewed elsewhere[4]. Recent experimental data supporting the favourable effects of UDCA on the liver are also reported in other chapters in the present volume.

Several European studies have also included necroinflammatory liver diseases, such as chronic active and alcoholic hepatitis, on the assumption that some degree of cholestasis is part of their clinical, biochemical and histological features with some relevance for their outcome[5].

However, as expected, the most interesting results were obtained in those diseases in which cholestasis is largely predominant, because they originate from a lesion of the bile ducts: primary biliary cirrhosis (PBC), primary sclerosing cholangitis (PSC) and cystic fibrosis-associated liver disease (CF).

Other cholestatic syndromes which are associated with particular conditions such as total parenteral nutrition[6] or cholestasis of pregnancy[7] have been studied in only a few patients, with encouraging results. Another interesting clinical condition, for its similarities with PBC, is liver involvement in graft-versus-host disease, which has also been investigated with success[8] and is the subject of another chapter in this volume. Finally, treatment of rejection after liver transplantation has been approached by one group of investigators with promising results[9,10] that need to be confirmed in controlled studies.

The purpose of this chapter is to briefly review the European experience with UDCA in PBC, PSC and CF, and to report some data from our group which are aimed at improving the efficacy of UDCA in PBC.

Table 1 European experience on UDCA for chronic cholestatic liver diseases (0: not assessed; +: improvement)

	PBC	CF	PSC
Patients (no.)	475	189	57
End-points			
liver function tests	+	+	+
histology	+	0	+
survival	+	0	0

EUROPEAN EXPERIENCE WITH UDCA IN CHRONIC CHOLESTATIC LIVER DISEASE

In Table 1 a summary is reported of the European experience on UDCA treatment for the three cholestatic conditions for which larger clinical data are available. In this table the number of patients studied included patients enrolled in both controlled and uncontrolled studies.

Primary biliary cirrhosis

Data from four randomized controlled trials have so far been published, in which 291 patients were evaluated[11–14]. Data consistently indicate improvement of liver function tests and minimal side-effects. In one study a significant increase of prealbumin serum levels, that is a parameter related to hepatic synthesis, has also been shown during UDCA administration[13].

Significant improvement of immunological markers has been reported: a decrease of serum IgM concentrations has been consistently observed, and in one study a reduction of AMA antibodies titres has also been found.

Conversely conflicting results on symptoms have been described, and a placebo effect on pruritus could not be ruled out[13].

Histological features significantly improved in only one study[12]. However, when individual components of liver histology were evaluated separately, only features related to cholestasis and inflammation improved, while no significant decrease in liver fibrosis was observed during UDCA administration[12].

Poupon and colleagues have shown that UDCA treatment is also able to slow deterioration of the Mayo risk score, a previously validated prognostic index[15], compared to placebo[12].

Only one study is available on the long-term observation of the effects of UDCA treatment to PBC patients in comparison to placebo[16]. One hundred and forty-five patients were evaluated, and comparison was made between patients administered UDCA (13–15 mg/kg body weight) for 4 years and patients treated with placebo for 2 years followed by UDCA for 2 years. The group of patients administered UDCA for 4 years showed a lower risk of death, need for orthotopic liver transplantation or major complications (Fig. 1). High bilirubin levels, low albumin levels and splenomegaly were associated with poor response to UDCA therapy.

Cystic fibrosis-associated liver disease

Clinical experience on UDCA treatment for CF-associated liver disease started several years later compared with PBC. Therefore, fewer data coming from controlled trials and focusing on histology and on clinically relevant end-points are so far available. All studies, uncontrolled and controlled, reported a significant improvement of serum liver enzyme concentrations. One hundred and five patients have been evaluated in three randomized controlled trials[17–19] of which only one has been published as a peer paper[18]. In none of these studies has histological evaluation been performed, since the typical hepatic lesion of CF-associated liver disease (focal biliary cirrhosis) may lead to large sampling errors and consequently, liver histology may be useless in assessing the efficacy of any medical treatment for liver disease in CF patients.

However, CF-associated liver disease seems to be one of the more promising indications for UDCA therapy in chronic liver diseases. A lower deterioration of a clinically relevant parameter, that is the Schwachman score, has been reported in patients administered UDCA, compared to placebo[19]. In addition, a significant improvement of hepatic excretory function has been clearly shown by an uncontrolled study[20], and improvement of nutritional status has been also reported in a group of adult CF patients during UDCA administration[21].

Taurine supplementation has been suggested to counteract taurine depletion induced by UDCA administration[22].

Primary sclerosing cholangitis

Primary sclerosing cholangitis is a less common disease compared to PBC. Only 44 patients have been enrolled in the two published European randomized clinical trials[23,24]. A consistent improvement in serum enzymes related to cholestasis and cytolysis has been reported, while a significant improvement of liver histology compared to placebo occurring during UDCA administration has been observed in only one study[23]. However, the small number of patients evaluated in this last study indicates that the effect of UDCA on liver histology in PSC needs further evaluation.

PROBLEMS WITH UDCA IN THE TREATMENT OF PBC

As reported in the previous sections of this chapter, data on UDCA treatment for chronic cholestatic liver disease coming from large patient populations are available only for PBC. In addition UDCA was suggested to improve survival only by a study performed on PBC patients[15]. Therefore discussion in this chapter will be limited to this disease.

The main problem for UDCA therapy in PBC is the timing of starting treatment. UDCA was clearly shown to be ineffective in patients with more severe disease, for whom the only effective therapeutic approach is liver transplantation, and we have previously shown that serum bilirubin concentrations higher than 2 mg/dl, and presence of liver cirrhosis, are associated with a lower response to UDCA administration[25]. On the other hand, it is questionable whether asymptomatic PBC patients who are expected to have long survival[26] may benefit from UDCA administration, and cost-effectiveness evaluation is needed.

In addition, using data so far available, UDCA was shown to be able to slow but not halt the progression of PBC. Therefore strategies aimed at improving the efficacy of UDCA therapy for PBC are warranted.

UDCA FOR PBC: HOW TO IMPROVE EFFICACY

Optimal dose and schedule

To improve the efficacy of UDCA treatment for PBC different approaches may be considered. The easiest method is to search for the optimal dose and schedule. A dose-ranging study, performed by our group, has shown that daily doses as low as 4 mg/kg body weight consistently improve serum liver enzyme levels and further improvements, as well as higher enrichment of the bile with UDCA (32 –37%) are achieved with doses up to 12 mg/kg a day[27]. During treatment, UDCA increases in bile mainly at the expense of cholic acid (CA), while hydrophobic bile acids do not decrease during treatment[28], and some unusual bile acids (i.e. homocholic and homochenodeoxycholic acids) decrease substantially[28]. On the basis of the changes induced on serum liver enzymes and on biliary bile acid composition by UDCA administration, we have suggested[27] that the optimal daily dose of the drug may range between 8 and 12 mg/kg. Therefore, all UDCA doses used in the randomized controlled trials so far published[11–14] are adequate to achieve optimal biochemical response.

Conversely, no data are available on different schedules of oral UDCA administration; UDCA has been generally administered in two divided daily doses. Data from experimental studies performed in patients with extrahepatic biliary obstruction and bile drainage indicate that a single dose of 600 mg of UDCA is absorbed for only 60%[29]. Strategies aimed at improving the rate of UDCA absorption may also improve its clinical efficacy. Since active ileal bile acid transport is easily saturated by a small amount of bile acids, the same amount of UDCA might be more efficiently absorbed when administered in multiple divided doses. Studies aimed at comparing different treatment schedules are therefore warranted, since multiple divided doses may be more efficiently absorbed, compared to the schedule currently used.

Tauroursodeoxycholic acid

Tauroursodeoxycholic acid (TUDCA) is more hydrophilic than unconjugated UDCA, and studies in animal models indicate that TUDCA has a greater cytoprotective effect than UDCA[30–32]. It may therefore be potentially more effective than UDCA therapy for PBC. We designed a randomized dose–response study aimed at assessing the safety and effects on liver biochemistries and on serum and biliary bile acid composition of different doses of TUDCA in 24

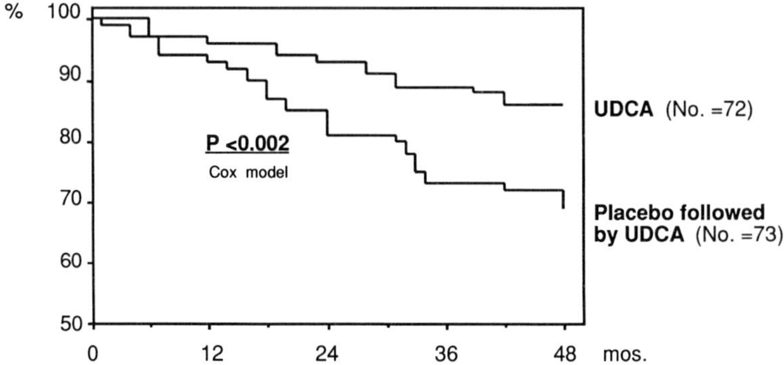

Fig. 1 Probability of response to long-term treatment with UDCA in 145 patients with PBC (modified from ref. 16)

patients with PBC. A significant improvement of serum liver enzyme levels, similar to that achieved with comparable doses of UDCA, was obtained after 6 months of TUDCA administration[33]. However, bile acid analysis performed by GC-MS suggests a potential advantage compared to unconjugated UDCA with regard to the changes induced in bile acid composition. We have previously shown that during UDCA administration lithocholic acid, measured by GC-MS, significantly increased in serum (from 1.8 to 5.0 μmol/l) and in bile (from 0.7% to 2.8%). Conversely, with TUDCA no significant increase was seen using the same methodology. This observation is of interest, since the accumulation of lithocholic acid was suggested to offset the beneficial effects of UDCA during long-term treatment[34]. However, further studies are warranted to establish the clinical relevance of such findings.

Combination therapy

Several studies have been published, or are in progress, on combination therapy for the treatment of PBC[25,35–38]. Immunosuppressive agents and a drug with antifibrotic properties, such as colchicine, were suggested to potentially exert a synergistic effect when added to UDCA.

Improvement of serum liver enzyme levels in eight patients responding insufficiently to UDCA monotherapy has been reported[36], after addition of methotrexate at the daily dose of 2.5 mg.

Conflicting data, coming from studies in which few PBC patients have been enrolled, are available on the potential synergistic effect of UDCA and colchicine[25,37,38]. In January 1990 we started a double-blind randomized controlled trial aimed at comparing UDCA alone to the combination therapy, UDCA plus colchicine. Ninety symptomatic PBC patients on UDCA for periods of 3–24 months were enrolled in six centres between January and December 1990. They were stratified according to duration of UDCA administration and were randomly and double-blindly assigned to receive colchicine (1 mg daily) or placebo. Treatment failures have been defined as follows: death or liver transplantation, development of major complication of cirrhosis (i.e. variceal bleeding, hepatic encephalopathy, intractable ascites); doubling of serum bilirubin values to levels higher than 4 mg/dl; severe impairment of symptoms and development of major side-effects. The results of a blinded interim analysis showing no significant difference between the two groups have been previously reported[25]. However, in the final analysis performed after 3 years of treatment, we have shown that treatment failures occurred more frequently in patients administered UDCA alone, as compared to patients administered UDCA plus colchicine ($p=0.056$; log-rank test). Therefore a 3-year course of colchicine associated with UDCA in patients with symptomatic PBC seems to have a moderate beneficial effect on the progression of the disease compared to UDCA monotherapy.

CONCLUSIONS

Though several questions concerning the use of UDCA in PBC need to be answered, the results obtained so far in Europe are very encouraging. It is possible that combination of UDCA with other agents might further increase its efficacy, and extend the number of patients who may benefit from this treatment.

For PSC, and especially CF-associated liver disease, the available clinical experience is satisfactory: further studies on clinically relevant end-points in large patient populations are now in progress.

REFERENCES

1. Leuschner U, Leuschner M, Sieratzki J, Kurtz W, Hubner K. Gallstone dissolution with ursodeoxycholic acid in patients with chronic active hepatitis and two years follow-up. A pilot study. Dig Dis Sci. 1985;3:642–9.
2. David R, Kurtz W, Strohm WD, Leuschner U. Die Wirkung von Ursodeoxycholsaure bei chronischen Leberkrankheiten. Eine Pilotstudie (Abstract). Z Gastroenterol. 1985;23:420.
3. Poupon R, Chretien Y, Poupon RE, Ballet F, Calmus Y, Darnis F. Is ursodeoxycholic acid an effective treatment for primary biliary cirrhosis? Lancet. 1987;1:834–6.
4. Rubin RA, Kowalsky TE, Khandelwal M, Malet IF. Ursodiol for hepatobiliary disorders. Ann Intern Med. 1994;121:207–18.
5. Bellentani S, Podda M, Tiribelli C *et al.* Ursodiol for the long-term treatment of chronic hepatitis: a double blind multicenter clinical trial. J Hepatol. 1993;19:459–64.
6. Beau P, Labat-Labourdette J, Ingrand P, Beauchant M. Is ursodeoxycholic acid an effective therapy for total parenteral nutrition-related liver disease? J Hepatol. 1994;20:240–4.
7. Mazzella G, Rizzo N, Salzetta A, Iampieri R, Bovicelli L, Roda E. Management of intrahepatic cholestasis in pregnancy. Lancet. 1991;338:1594–5.
8. Fried RH, Murakami CS, Fisher LD, Willson RA, Sullivan M, McDonald GB. Ursodeoxycholic acid treatment of refractory graft-versus-host disease of the liver. Ann Intern Med. 1992; 116: 624–9.
9. Persson H, Friman S, Scherstén T, Svanvik J, Karlberg I. Ursodeoxycholic acid for prevention of acute rejection in liver transplant recipients. Lancet. 1990;336:52–3.
10. Friman S, Persson H, Scherstén T, Svanvik J, Karlberg I. Adjuvant treatment with ursodeoxycholic acid reduces acute rejection after liver transplantation. Transplant Proc. 1992;24:389–90.
11. Leuschner U, Fischer H, Kurtz W *et al.* Ursodeoxycholic acid in primary biliary cirrhosis: results of a controlled double-blind trial. Gastroenterology. 1989;97:1268–74.
12. Poupon RE, Balkau B, Eschwege E, Poupon R and the UDCA-PBC Study Group. A multicenter,

controlled trial of ursodiol for the treatment of primary biliary cirrhosis. N Engl J Med. 1991; 324:1548–54.

13. Battezzati PM, Podda M, Bianchi FB *et al.* Ursodeoxycholic acid for symptomatic primary biliary cirrhosis. Preliminary analysis of a double-blind multicentre trial. J Hepatol. 1993;17: 332–8.

14. Turner IA, Myszor M, Mitchison HC, Bennett MK, Burt AD, James OFW. A two year controlled trial examining the effectiveness of ursodeoxycholic acid in primary biliary cirrhosis. J Gastroenterol Hepatol. 1994;9:162–8.

15. Dickson ER, Grambsch PM, Fleming TR *et al.* Prognosis in primary biliary cirrhosis: model for decision making. Hepatology. 1989;10:1.

16. Poupon RR, Poupon R, Balkau B and the UDCA-PBC Study Group. Ursodiol for long-term treatment of primary biliary cirrhosis. N Engl J Med. 1994;330:1342–7.

17. Bittner P, Posselt HG, Sailer T *et al.* The effect of treatment with ursodeoxycholic acid in cystic fibrosis and hepatopathy: results of a placebo-controlled study. In: Paumgartner G, Stiehl A, Gerok W, editors. Bile acids as therapeutic agents – from basic science to clinical practice. Dordrecht: Kluwer; 1991:345–8 (Proceedings of the 58th Falk Symposium).

18. O'Brien S, Fitzgerald MX, Hegarty JE. A controlled trial of ursodeoxycholic acid treatment in cystic fibrosis-related liver disease. Eur J Gastroenterol Hepatol. 1992;4:857–63.

19. Colombo C, Podda M, Battezati PM *et al.* Ursodeoxycholic acid for cystic fibrosis-associated liver disease: final report of a multicenter trial. Hepatology. 1993;18:142A (abstract).

20. Colombo C, Castellani MR, Balistreri WF, Seregni E, Assaisso ML, Giunta A. Scintigraphic documentation of an improvement in hepatobiliary excretory function after treatment with ursodeoxycholic acid in patients with cystic fibrosis and associated liver disease. Hepatology. 1992;15:677–84.

21. Cotting J, Lentze M, Reichen J. Effects of ursodeoxycholic acid treatment on nutrition and liver function in patients with cystic fibrosis and longstanding cholestasis. Gut. 1990;31:918–21.

22. Colombo C, Setchell KDR, Podda M *et al.* Effects of ursodeoxycholic acid therapy for liver disease associated with cystic fibrosis. J Pediatr. 1990;117:482–9.

23. Beuers U, Spengler U, Kruis W *et al.* Ursodeoxycholic acid for treatment of primary sclerosing cholangitis: a placebo-controlled trial. Hepatology. 1992;16:707–14.

24. Stiehl A, Walker S, Stiehl L, Rudolph G, Hofmann J, Theilmann L. Effect of ursodeoxycholic acid on liver and bile duct disease in primary sclerosing cholangitis. A 3-year pilot study with a placebo-controlled study period. J Hepatol. 1994;20:57–64.

25. Podda M, Almasio P, Battezzati PM *et al.* Long-term effect of the administration of ursodeoxycholic acid alone or with colchicine in patients with primary biliary cirrhosis: a double-blind multicentre study. In: Paumgartner G, Stiehl A, Gerok W, editors. Bile acids and the hepatobiliary system. Dordrecht: Kluwer; 1993:310–15.

26. Beswick DR, Kaltskin G, Boyer JL. Asymptomatic primary biliary cirrhosis: long-term follow-up and natural history. Gastroenterology. 1985;89:267.

27. Podda M, Ghezzi C, Battezzati PM *et al.* Effect of different doses of ursodeoxycholic acid in chronic liver disease. Dig Dis Sci. 1989;34:59s–65s.

28. Crosignani A, Podda M, Battezzati PM *et al.* Changes in bile acid composition in patients with primary biliary cirrhosis induced by ursodeoxycholic acid administration. Hepatology. 1991;14:1000–7.

29. Walker S, Rudolph G, Raedsch R, Stiehl A. Intestinal absorption of ursodeoxycholic acid in patients with extrahepatic biliary obstruction and bile drainage. Gastroenterology. 1992;102: 810–15.

30. Armstrong MJ, Carey MC. The hydrophobic/hydrophilic balance of bile salts. Inverse correlation between reverse-phase high performance liquid chromatographic mobilities and micellar cholesterol-solubilizing capacities. J Lipid Res. 1982;23:70–80.

31. Attili AF, Angelico M, Cantafora A, Alvaro D, Capocaccia L. Bile acid-induced liver toxicity: relation to the hydrophobic–hydrophilic balance of bile acids. Med Hypotheses. 1986;19: 57–69.

32. Heuman DM. Quantitative estimation of the hydrophobic-hydrophilic balance of mixed bile salt solutions. J Lipid Res. 1989;30:719–30.

33. Crosignani A, Battezzati PM, Camisasca M *et al.* Tauroursodeoxycholic acid for the treatment of primary biliary cirrhosis: a dose–response study. Hepatology. 1993;18:176A (abstract).

34. Javitt NB. Ursodeoxycholic acid therapy: the baby and the bathwater. Hosp Pract. 15 March 1992:12–16.

35. Kaplan MM. The therapeutic effects of ursodiol and methotrexate are additive and well tolerated in primary biliary cirrhosis. Hepatology. 1992;16:92A.
36. Buscher HP, Zietzchmann Y, Gerok W. Positive responses to methotrexate and ursodeoxycholic acid in patients with primary biliary cirrhosis responding insufficiently to ursodeoxycholic acid alone. J Hepatol. 1993;18:9-14.
37. Shibata J, Fujiyama S, Honda Y, Sato T. Combination therapy with ursodeoxycholic acid and colchicine for primary biliary cirrhosis. J Gastroenterol Hepatol. 1992;7:277-82.
38. Raedsch R, Stiehl A, Walker S *et al*. Controlled study on the effects of a combined ursodeoxycholic acid plus colchicine treatment in primary biliary cirrhosis. In: Paumgartner G, Stiehl A, Gerok W, editors. Bile acids and the hepatobiliary system. Dordrecht: Kluwer; 1993:303-9.

41
Bile acid metabolism and biliary secretion in PSC: effect of ursodeoxycholic acid treatment

A. STIEHL, P. SAUER AND G. RUDOLPH

INTRODUCTION

Treatment of patients with primary sclerosing cholangitis (PSC) with ursodeoxycholic acid (UDCA) leads to improvement of liver enzymes and in part also of serum bilirubin[1-6]. In two studies an improvement of liver histology was also observed, due mainly to a decrease of inflammation in portal triads[5,6]. Recently an effect on survival without liver transplantation has also been reported[7]. The mechanism of action is still unclear. Six principal effects seem possible: (1) change in balance between hydrophilic and hydrophobic bile acids in favour of less toxic hydrophilic bile acids, (2) direct hepatoprotective effect, (3) decrease of hepatocellular concentrations of hepatotoxic bile acids, (4) immunomodulatory effect, (5) choleretic effect with an increased secretion of potentially toxic substances, (6) increased biliary secretion of phospholipids which prevent toxicity of bile acids.

In the present study we examined the possibility that UDCA might influence bile acid metabolism, and as a consequence biliary secretion of bile acids and lipids.

POOL SIZE, SYNTHESIS AND TURNOVER OF BILE ACIDS IN PSC

In PSC the plasma concentrations of bile acids are elevated but the pool sizes of cholic acid and chenodeoxycholic acid are very small (Figs 1 and 2)[8]. Obviously there is an increased spillover of bile acids from the enterohepatic circulation into the peripheral blood and a decrease of bile acids in the enterohepatic circulation. The hepatic synthesis rates of cholic acid and chenodeoxycholic acid on average were somewhat reduced in comparison to healthy controls but the difference was not statistically significant[8]. The synthesis rates of cholic acid were smaller than those of chenodeoxycholic acid. It can be expected that in

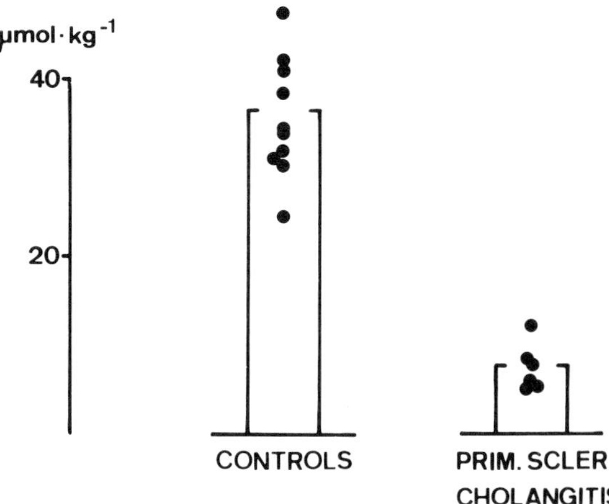

Fig. 1 Pool sizes of cholic acid in healthy controls and in patients with primary sclerosing cholangitis (from Hepatology. 1993;17:1028–32[8])

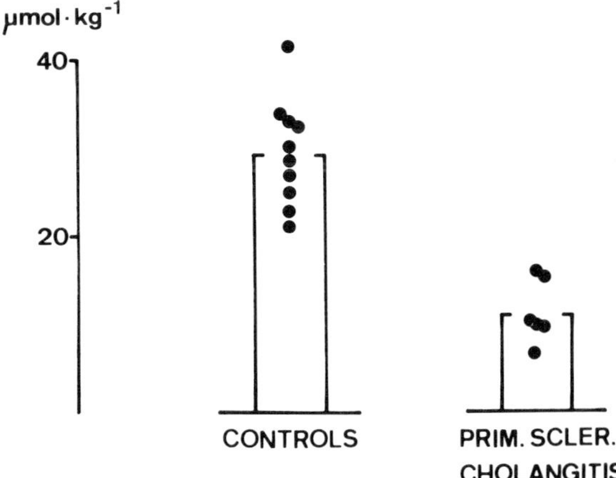

Fig. 2 Pool sizes of chenodeoxycholic acid in healthy controls and in patients with primary sclerosing cholangitis (from Hepatology. 1993;17:1028–32[8])

patients with more severe cholestasis the synthesis rates will be more markedly reduced, but in such patients it is not possible to study bile acid kinetics on the basis of a one pool system and therefore such data are not available.

The fractional turnover rates of cholic acid and chenodeoxycholic acid were somewhat increased, but the difference in comparison to healthy controls was not significant[8]. Since most patients with PSC have ulcerative colitis, with the consequence of increased bile acid losses via the intestine, the tendency towards an increased fractional turnover rate is as expected.

EFFECT OF UDCA ON POOL SIZES SYNTHESIS AND TURNOVER RATES

Following UDCA treatment for 3 months the serum concentrations of endogenous bile acids decreased, but the pool sizes of cholic and chenodeoxycholic acid were unchanged[8]. This indicates that pool sizes of both primary bile acids are shifted from the peripheral circulation into the enterohepatic circulation. Since the spillover of bile acids into the peripheral circulation is due to cholestasis, the observed reduction of this spillover seems to indicate improved enterohepatic circulation as a consequence of decreased cholestasis.

Hepatic synthesis rates of cholic acid increased in all patients after UDCA, whereas the synthesis of chenodeoxycholic acid was unchanged. The decreased intestinal absorption of cholic acid after UDCA may be responsible for its increased hepatic synthesis[9]. For chenodeoxycholic acid the evaluation of its hepatic synthesis is more difficult due to the possible transformation of UDCA to chenodeoxycholic acid. However, the overall formation of chenodeoxycholic acid did not increase, and as a consequence it seems unlikely that substantial amounts of UDCA were transformed to chenodeoxycholic acid.

After UDCA the fractional turnover of both cholic and chenodeoxycholic acid increased. The most likely explanation for this is the fact that UDCA inhibits the absorption of bile acids in the ileum[9].

EFFECT OF UDCA ON BILIARY SECRETION OF BILE ACIDS AND LIPIDS

Following UDCA treatment of patients with PSC, biliary secretion of total bile acids and phospholipids was increased, and secretion of cholesterol on average was unchanged[10]. In patients with cholestasis secretion of endogenous bile acids and of cholesterol was also increased after UDCA[10], indicating an improved biliary secretory capacity after UDCA. The increased biliary secretion of cholesterol is probably responsible for the decrease of plasma cholesterol in cholestatic patients. The increased biliary secretion of phospholipids may be related to the beneficial effect of UDCA, since phospholipids may prevent bile acid-induced liver damage in mice[11].

CONCLUSION

The changes in bile acid metabolism and biliary secretion after UDCA may reflect the cause or the consequence of an improvement of cholestatic liver disease in PSC. UDCA treatment seems to induce an improvement of the excretory capacity of the liver in patients with PSC.

References

1. Stiehl A, Radsch R, Kommerell B. The effect of ursodeoxycholic acid in primary sclerosing cholangitis: a comparison to primary biliary cirrhosis. Gastroenterology. 1988;94:A595 (abstract).

2. Hyashi H, Hihuchi T, Ichimiya H, Hishida N, Sakamoto N. Asymptomatic primary sclerosing cholangitis: brief report. Gastroenterology. 1990;99:533–5.
3. Chazouilleres O, Poupon R, Capron J-P *et al.* Ursodeoxycholic acid for primary sclerosing cholangitis. J Hepatol. 1990;11:120–3.
4. O'Brien CB, Senior JR, Arora-Merchandani R, Batta A, Salen G. Ursodeoxycholic acid for the treatment of primary sclerosing cholangitis: a 30 month pilot study. Hepatology. 1991;14:838–47.
5. Beuers U, Spengler U, Kruis W *et al.* Ursodeoxycholic acid for treatment of primary sclerosing cholangitis: a placebo controlled trial. Hepatology. 1992;16:707–14.
6. Stiehl A, Walker S, Stiehl L *et al.* Effect of ursodeoxycholic acid on liver and bile duct disease in primary sclerosing cholangitis. A 3 year pilot study with a placebo controlled study period. J Hepatol. 1994;20:57–64.
7. Stiehl A. Ursodeoxycholic acid therapy in treatment of primary sclerosing cholangitis. Scand J Gastroenterol. 1994;29(Suppl. 204):59–61.
8. Rudolph G, Endele R, Senn M, Stiehl A. Effect of ursodeoxycholic acid on the kinetics of cholic acid and chenodeoxycholic acid in patients with primary sclerosing cholangitis. Hepatology. 1993;17:1028–32.
9. Stiehl A, Raedsch R, Rudolph G. Acute effects of ursodeoxycholic and chenodeoxycholic acid on the small intestinal absorption of bile acids. Gastroenterology. 1990;98:424–8.
10. Stiehl A, Sauer R, Rudolph G. Effect of ursodeoxycholic acid on biliary secretion of bile acids and lipids in PSC. Gastroenterology. 1994;106:A989 (abstract).
11. Smit JJM, Schinkel OH, Oude Elferink RPJ *et al.* Homozygous disruption of the murine mdr 2-P-glycoprotein gene lends to a complete absence of phospholipid from bile and to liver disease. Cell. 1993;75:451–62.

42
Ursodiol and interferon-α for the treatment of chronic hepatitis C

C. B. O'BRIEN, B. S. HENZEL, W. B. LONG, L. WOLFE, A. YODER and R. A. RUBIN

INTRODUCTION

Interferon-α2b is approved as treatment for chronic hepatitis C (HCV) infection in the United States. Normalization of serum transaminases has been seen in approximately 50% of patients treated for 6 months. However, biochemical relapse occurs in the majority of patients following withdrawal of therapy[1,2]. Detection of HCV RNA in serum by reverse transcriptase polymerase chain reaction (RT-PCR) has been shown to correlate with normalization of serum transaminases on treatment, and has also been shown to precede biochemical relapse once therapy is withdrawn[3,4]. Researchers continue to devise new therapies to improve the low response rates. Higher interferon doses[5], more prolonged treatment duration[6], different species of interferon[7,8], and adjuvant therapeutic phlebotomy to remove excess iron[9] have all been tried, with various degrees of success.

In an Italian trial, Angelico first reported the use of ursodiol as adjunct therapy with interferon-α for the treatment of patients with chronic hepatitis C. These investigators found that a combination of the two agents produced a better response rate (41%) than in those patients who received interferon-α alone (17%)[10]. There was some difficulty in the interpretation of these data since the authors defined response as serum transaminases less than 1.5 times the upper limits of normal. There was also no correlation with the changes in serum transaminases and serum HCV RNA.

We wanted to determine whether the combination of ursodiol and interferon-α would increase the probability to achieve normal liver function tests (LFT) both on and off therapy. Since there were questions as to whether this effect was simply an artifact due to a non-specific lowering of serum aminotransferases, we also planned to compare the changes in the LFT with loss of HCV RNA in the patient's serum.

METHODS

Subjects

A total of 85 patients between the ages of 21 and 70 (58 males and 27 females) with liver disease of >1 year duration were followed at the Liver Center of the Hospital of the University of Pennsylvania between 1989 and 1993. All patients had a positive HCV antibody by the ELISA II or RIBA II assay. Liver biopsy was graded according to standard criteria and was consistent with a diagnosis of chronic hepatitis C in all cases. Patients were excluded from the study if they had more than one type of liver disease; a history of active alcohol or drug abuse; history of malignancy; significant renal, cardiac or pulmonary disease limiting life expectancy; or had normal LFT. All patients had the following tests drawn to exclude other known causes of chronic liver disease: hepatitis B surface antigen, hepatitis B core antibody, hepatitis B surface antibody, caeruloplasmin and serum copper if <age 30, serum iron, total iron-binding capacity, serum ferritin, α_1-antitrypsin level, antinuclear antibody, antimitochondrial antibody, and antismooth muscle antibody.

Planned duration of therapy was 9 months. Patients who were withdrawn from treatment were followed for at least a 6-month period. Patients were stratified into treatment groups based on patient selection of physician. Within the interferon-α group, patients >70kg received 5MIU s.c. three times a week, patients <70kg received 3MIU s.c. three times a week. Patients in the combination therapy group received interferon-α (dosed as above) and ursodiol 300mg by mouth twice a day. Patients were seen approximately every 2 months while on treatment and during the follow-up period. Routine blood analysis was obtained monthly while on therapy, and every other month during the follow-up period. Blood tests included serum total and direct bilirubin, alkaline phosphatase, γ-glutamyl transferase, alanine and aspartate aminotransferases, total protein, albumin and complete blood counts with platelet counts. Therapy was stopped if the patient's alanine aminotransferase (ALT) and aspartate aminotransferase (AST) did not fall within the normal range in 3 months.

Therapy was also withdrawn if ALT and AST remained abnormal for >2 months in a row. Complete response was defined as normalization of HCV RNA and liver transaminases at the end of the follow-up period.

RT-PCR

Serum was collected in serum separator (BD SST) tubes. Within 2h of blood draw the blood tubes were centrifuged at 1500*g* for 20min. Serum was collected immediately and stored at −70°C. Frozen serum was shipped in batches on dry ice to Roche Molecular Systems, Somerville, NJ, for analysis. The HCV RNAbassay was a prototype PCR-based assay using a single primer pair (biotinylated downstream primer) from the 5'-untranslated region of HCV. Uracil-*N*-glycosylase was incorporated to prevent amplicon contamination. The HCV target RNA was reverse transcribed and amplified in a single-tube reaction using the enzyme rTth DNA polymerase in the presence of Mn^{2+}. After amplification the products were alkaline-denatured and hybridized to a HCV-specific probe.

Table 1 Demographics and baseline histologies

	Age*	Sex	Duration*	CAH	Fibrosis	Cirrhosis
Interferon and ursodiol	44±10	33M/15F	10±8	87%	62%	30%
Interferon-α	50±12	25M/12F	12±9	88%	76%	54%
p=	0.01†	n.s.‡	n.s.‡	n.s.‡	n.s.‡	0.03‡

*Means±SD in years
†t-test for independent samples
‡Chi-squared test for differences

Detection was carried out in a 96-microwell format using avidin–horseradish peroxidase. The results of the assay were expressed in A_{450} units as detected on a standard microwell plate reader.

Statistical analysis

Comparisons between groups were done by independent or paired Student's t-test, and chi-squared tests, as appropriate, with a Statistica™ program version 4.1 (Statsoft Corporation).

RESULTS

We studied a total of 85 patients with chronic hepatitis C. Forty-eight consecutive patients (33 males and 15 females) were treated with interferon-α alone, and 37 consecutive patients (25 males and 12 females) were treated with both interferon-α and ursodiol. The two groups were comparable at baseline in terms of mean duration of disease and sex distribution. There was a tendency for the monotherapy group to have older patients, which was statistically significant ($p=0.01$). Histology at baseline was also comparable in the distribution of chronic active hepatitis and fibrosis between the two groups. However, there was a statistically meaningful increase in cirrhosis in the monotherapy group in comparison to the combination therapy group ($p=0.03$). For details of baseline comparison between groups, see Table 1.

Serum liver function tests

The group receiving combination therapy developed more rapid normalization of their serum transaminases than patients receiving monotherapy, which was statistically significant at the end of treatment ($p=0.001$). Combination therapy patients also maintained their LFT in the normal range for longer duration, and relapsed less when compared with the monotherapy group. At the end of follow-up, 33% of patients receiving combination therapy and 8% of patients receiving interferon-α alone had normal LFT ($p=0.0002$). Table 2 shows the number and percentage of patients achieving normal serum transaminases, with p values both at the end of the treatment and at the end of follow-up.

Table 2 Comparison of LFT and HCV RNA at the end of treatment and the end of follow-up

	NI LFT end-Rx	(–)PCR end-Rx	NI LFT off Rx	(–)PCR off Rx
Interferon and ursodiol	21/48 (44%)	15/27 (56%)	14/43 (33%)	13/36 (36%)
Interferon-α	4/37 (11%)		3/37 (8%)	
$p^* =$	0.001		0.002	

*Chi-squared differences between treatment groups

Serum HCV RNA

Patients in the interferon-α alone group had completed treatment prior to our ability to obtain HCV RNA. The patients in the combination group lost detectable HCV RNA in almost the same percentage as they developed normal serum transaminases. At the end of the treatment period, 15 out of the 27 patients (56%) had no detectable HCV RNA. The remaining 12 patients in the combination group (all with abnormal LFT) were lost to follow-up.

Interferon dose received

The monotherapy group received a mean interferon-α dose of 3.4 MIU three times a week, and a mean cumulative dose of 239 MIU. In comparison, the patients treated with both interferon-α and ursodiol received higher interferon doses with a mean interferon-α dose of 4.4 MIU three times a week and a mean cumulative dose of 428 MIU. This difference in dose was explained by the patients in the combination therapy group normalizing their transaminases more quickly, and maintaining normal LFT more frequently and for a longer duration of time.

Side-effects and adverse experiences

Ursodiol was well tolerated. The combination therapy group had a similar number of adverse events as the monotherapy group of interferon-α.

DISCUSSION

These results demonstrate the patients receiving combination therapy normalized serum transaminases and showed a lack of detectable HCV RNA more frequently than those patients on monotherapy with interferon-α.

The mechanism of clearance of the hepatitis C virus is still unclear. Shirai, from the National Cancer Institute, has demonstrated that CD8(+) cytotoxic lymphocytes recognize a non-structural protein with homology to RNA polymerase expressed in association with a HLA class I antigen[11]. Because of its stimulation of the immune system, interferon-α therapy has been used in many trials for treatment of chronic hepatitis C; the overall success rate is only 15–20%. A search has ensued for various means to boost the response rate.

Ursodiol has recently been studied as a potential therapy for primary sclerosing cholangitis[12], primary biliary cirrhosis[13,14], primary graft dysfunction after orthotopic liver transplant[15], biliary atresia[16] and cystic-fibrosis-associated liver disease[17]. Chronic obstruction to bile flow results in the accumulation of the hydrophobic bile acids: chenodeoxycholic, and to a lesser extent, deoxycholic, and lithocholic. These bile acids are toxic in high levels to the liver[18–20]. Chenodeoxycholic acid has been shown to cause liver injury in animals[21]. The pattern is different from the mainly cholestatic effect of lithocholic acid[22]. In humans, high concentrations of both chenodeoxycholic acid[23] and deoxycholic acid[24] can cause elevations of the serum transaminases. Stiehl *et al.*[25] and Heuman[26] have demonstrated that ursodiol protects isolated human hepatocyte membranes against cytolysis by toxic bile acids. Podda *et al.* proposed that the mechanism of ursodiol's action may be to increase the overall hydrophilicity of the bile acid pool[27].

Ursodiol's mechanism of action may also include modification of the human immune system. Ursodiol suppresses human leukocyte antigen (HLA) class I and class II expression in patients with primary biliary cirrhosis, as well as reducing cytokine and immunoglobulin production by peripheral mononuclear cells *in vitro*[24]. Stiehl and colleagues have recently demonstrated that ursodiol reduces intracellular adhesion molecule (ICAM-1) expression on normal human hepatocytes *in vitro*. Their data also suggested that ursodiol suppresses T-cell mediated cytotoxicity[28]. Poupon's group in Paris found that the administration of ursodiol has less inhibition on the 2-5'-oligoadenylate synthetase pathway and natural killer (NK) cell activity than equivalent levels of chenodeoxycholic acid found in patients with cholestasis[29].

Because of this success in multiple types of liver disease, and its effect on the human immune system, several investigators have tried ursodiol as monotherapy for the treatment of chronic hepatitis C. Bellentani reported in a double-blind placebo-controlled trial ($n=60$), that, after 1 year, ursodiol lowered serum ALT and AST but had no effect on histology of follow-up liver biopsies[30]. Lu from the Republic of China reported that ursodiol at the dose of 600 mg daily had no response on serum ALT, HCV RNA and the cytokine levels of TNF-α and IL-6[31].

Other groups have reported their results using combination therapy of interferon-α and ursodiol for HCV. Mazzella found that the addition of ursodiol would induce normal LFT in an additional 31% patients with whom treatment by interferon-α alone was ineffective. Unfortunately, the authors did not provide information regarding relapse rate and HCV RNA[32]. Boucher *et al.* discovered that combination therapy did not improve final cure rates as measured by loss of HCV RNA or percentage of patients with normal LFT at 1 year after the withdrawal of therapy. Their results concluded that the addition of ursodiol did significantly prolong the normalization of serum ALT levels[33]. In comparison, a Japanese group studied 70 patients treated with interferon-α 2a, 6 MIU three times a week for 6 months. They found that, 6 months after discontinuation of therapy, the loss of HCV RNA was higher in the combination therapy group (37%) than the monotherapy group (20%). There was no significant difference between these two groups as measured by the changes in percentage of patients with normal LFT (34% vs. 37%)[34]. Angelico has recently published in an abstract the results of combination therapy in 40 patients. These authors found that there was no significant difference in the loss of detectable HCV RNA between the two groups both at the end of the treatment period and at the end of the follow-up period. They did note a greater improvement in histology in the group of patients receiving combination therapy[35].

The success rate in our interferon-α monotherapy group was less than that reported in the literature for interferon-α therapy of chronic hepatitis C. We feel that the very high percentage of our patients with fibrosis (76%) and cirrhosis (54%) caused a poorer outcome in this cohort compared with results reported by other investigators. Interferon-α may cause mild hepatotoxicity with elevation of ALT and AST (4–15%)[36]. We speculate that the addition of ursodiol to interferon-α therapy of HCV prevents the interferon from causing abnormal transaminases; therefore, the patients continue to receive interferon-α since their transaminases remain in the normal range.

In summary, we have shown that the combination of ursodiol and interferon-α is more successful in the treatment of patients with chronic hepatitis C than standard therapy of interferon-α alone. Patients receiving both ursodiol and interferon-α normalized serum transaminases, and HCV RNA was undetected more frequently than in those patients on monotherapy. Adjunct ursodiol may be used if direct measurements of HCV RNA levels are not available and standard aminotransferases are used to follow therapy.

References

1. Davis GL, Balart LA, Schiff ER *et al*. Treatment of chronic hepatitis C with recombinant interferon alfa: a multicenter randomized, controlled trial. N Engl J Med. 1989;321:1501–6.
2. Di Bisceglie AM, Martin P, Kassianides C *et al*. Recombinant interferon alpha therapy for chronic hepatitis C: a randomized, double-blind, placebo-controlled trial. N Engl J Med. 1989;321:1506–10.
3. Farci P, Alter HJ, Wong D *et al*. A long term study of hepatitis C virus replication in non-A, non-B hepatitis. N Engl J Med. 1991;325:98–104.
4. Shindo M, Di Bisceglie AM, Cheung L *et al*. Decrease in serum hepatitis C viral RNA during alpha-interferon therapy for chronic hepatitis. Ann Intern Med. 1991;115:700–4.
5. Watson AR, Bartlome P. High-dose interferon alfa-2A for the treatment of chronic hepatitis C. [Review] Ann Pharmacother. 1994;28:341–2.
6. Gomez-Rubio M, Porres JC, Castillo I, Quiroga JA, Moreno A, Carreno V. Prolonged treatment (18 months) of chronic hepatitis C with recombinant alpha-interferon in comparison with a control group. J Hepatol. 1990;11(Suppl. 1):S63–7.
7. Saez-Royuela F, Porres JC, Moreno A *et al*. High doses of recombinant alpha-interferon or gamma-interferon for chronic hepatitis C: a randomized, controlled trial. Hepatology. 1991;13:327–31.
8. Nakano Y, Kiyosawa K, Sodeyama T, Tanaka E. Comparative study of clinical, histological, and immunological responses to interferon therapy in type non-A, non-B, and type B chronic hepatitis. Am J Gastroenterol. 1990;85:24–9.
9. Hayashi H, Takikawa T, Nishimura N, Yano M, Isomura T, Sakamoto N. Improvement of serum aminotransferase levels after phlebotomy in patients with chronic active hepatitis C and excess hepatic iron. Am J Gastroenterol. 1994;89:970–3.
10. Angelico M, Gandin C, Gofferdo F, Pescarmona E, Del Vecchio C, Capocaccia L. A combination of interferon-alfa and ursodeoxycholic acid is more effective than interferon-alfa alone in anti-HCV positive chronic hepatitis: a randomized, histology-controlled, clinical trial. Gastroenterology. 1992;102:A775.
11. Shirai M, Akatsuka T, Pendleton CD *et al*. Induction of cytotoxic T cells to a cross-reactive

epitope in the hepatitis C virus nonstructural RNA polymerase-like protein. J Virol. 1992;66:4098–106.

12. O'Brien CB, Senior JR, Arora R, Batta AK, Goin JE, Salen G. Ursodeoxycholic acid for the treatment of primary sclerosing cholangitis: a 30-month pilot study. Hepatology. 1991;14: 838–47.

13. Leuschner U, Fischer H, Kurtz W et al. Ursodeoxycholic acid in primary biliary cirrhosis: results of a controlled double-blind trial. Gastroenterology. 1989;97:1268–74.

14. Poupon RE, Balkau B, Eschwège E, Poupon R, and the UDCA-PBC study group. A multicenter, controlled trial of ursodiol for treatment of primary biliary cirrhosis. N Engl J Med. 1991;324:1548–54.

15. Friman S, Persson H, Schersten T, Svanvik J, Karlberg I. Adjuvant treatment with ursodeoxycholic acid reduces acute rejection after liver transplantation. Transplant Proc. 1992;24:389–90.

16. Balistreri WF, Heubi JE, Whitington P, Perrault J, Bancroft J, Setchell KDR. Ursodeoxycholic acid (UDCA) therapy in pediatric hepatobiliary disease. Hepatology. 1989;10:602(abstract 136).

17. Colombo C, Crosignani A, Assaisso M et al. Ursodeoxycholic acid therapy in cystic fibrosis-associated liver disease: a dose–response study. Hepatology. 1992;16:924–30.

18. Heuman DM, Mills AS, McCall J, Hylemon PB, Pandak WM, Vlahcevic ZR. Conjugates of ursodeoxycholate protect against cholestasis and hepatocellular necrosis caused by more hydrophobic bile salts: *in vivo* studies in the rat. Gastroenterology. 1991;120:203–11.

19. Heuman DM, Pandak WM, Hylemon PB, Vlahcevic ZR. Conjugates of ursodeoxycholate protect against cytotoxicity of more hydrophobic bile salts: *in vitro* studies in rat hepatocytes and human erythrocytes. Hepatology. 1991;14:920–6.

20. Marcus SN, Schteingart CD, Marquez ML et al. Active absorption of conjugated bile acids in vivo: kinetic parameters and molecular specificity of the ileal transport system in the rat. Gastroenterology. 1991;100:212–21.

21. Schölmerich J, Becher MS, Schmidt K et al. Influence of hydroxylation and conjugation of bile salts on their membrane-damaging properties – studies on isolated hepatocytes and lipid membrane vesicles. Hepatology. 1984;4:661–6.

22. Miyai K, Price VM, Fisher MM. Bile acid metabolism in mammals: ultrastructural studies on the intrahepatic cholestasis induced by lithocholic and chenodeoxycholic acids in the rat. Lab Invest. 1971;24:292–302.

23. Mok HYI, Bell GD, Dowling RH. Effect of different doses of chenodeoxycholic acid on bile-lipid composition and on frequency of side-effects in patients with gallstones. Lancet. 1974;2:253–7.

24. LaRusso NF, Szczepanik PA, Hofmann AF, Coffin SB. Effect of deoxycholic acid ingestion on bile acid metabolism and biliary secretion in normal subjects. Gastroenterology. 1977;72: 132–40.

25. Galle PR, Theilmann L, Kohl B, Raedsch R, Otto G, Stiehl A. Ursodeoxycholate reduces hepatotoxicity of bile salts in primary human hepatocytes. Hepatology. 1990;12:486–91.

26. Heuman DM. Hepatoprotective properties of ursodeoxycholic acid. Gastroenterology. 1993;104:1865–70.

27. Podda M, Ghezzi C, Battezzati PM et al. Ursodeoxycholic acid for chronic liver disease. J Clin Gastroenterol. 1988;10(Suppl. 2):S25–31.

28. Tox U, Arnold JC, Otto G, Theilmann L, Kommerell B, Stiehl A. Differences in the effect of ursodeoxycholic acid and chenodeoxycholic acid on the expression of HLA-molecules on human primary hepatocytes. In: Hofmann AF, Paumgartner G, Stiehl A, editors. Bile acids in gastroenterology: basic and clinical aspects. Thirteenth International Bile Acid Meeting; 30 Sept –2 Oct 1994, San Diego.

29. Poupon R, Podevin P, Calmus Y, Chereau C. Effects of cholestasis and bile acids on interferon-induced 2′5-oligoadenylated synthetase and natural killer activities. In: Hofmann AF, Paumgartner G, Stiehl A, editors. Bile acids in gastroenterology: basic and clinical aspects. Thirteenth International Bile Acid Meeting; 30 Sept–2 Oct 1994, San Diego.

30. Bellentani S, Podda M, Tiribelli C et al. Ursodiol in the long-term treatment of chronic hepatitis: a double-blind multicenter clinical trial. J Hepatol. 1993;19:459–64.

31. Lu CL, Chan CY, Hwang SJ, Lu RH, Lee SD, Lo KJ. The efficacy of ursodeoxycholic acid in the treatment of patients with chronic hepatitis C. Hepatology. 1994;20:372A.

32. Marzella G, Cipolla A, Novelli V et al. Can UDCA increase response to interferon in chronic hepatitis C? Gastroenterology. 1994;106:A941.

33. Boucher E, André P, Jouanolle H *et al*. Treatment of chronic viral C hepatitis by interferon plus ursodeoxycholic acid: results from a controlled randomized trial in 80 patients. Hepatology. 1994;20:291A.
34. Imai Y, Tamura S, Inada M *et al*.. Efficacy of combination therapy of interferon with ursodeoxycholic acid (UDCA) in chronic hepatitis C: sustained clearance of viremia after interferon discontinuation. Hepatology. 1994;20:363A.
35. Anqelico M, Gandin C, Pescarmona E *et al*. Interferon-alfa with or without ursodeoxycholic acid (UDCA) in the treatment of chronic hepatitis C: final report of a randomized, controlled, clinical trial. Gastroenterology. 1993;104:A871.
36. Product Information: Interferon alfa-2b recombinant for injection. Schering-Plough Corporation. 1994.

43
Ursodeoxycholic acid for the treatment of refractory chronic graft-versus-host-disease of the liver

R. FRIED, A. GRATWOHL and G. STALDER

INTRODUCTION

Chronic graft-versus-host-disease of the liver (GVHD) occurs 80–400 days after allogeneic bone marrow transplantation (BMT) and affects 20–40% of long-term survivors[1]. It is associated with a 'dry gland syndrome', GVHD of the skin and gastrointestinal tract[1,2]. Liver disease caused by chronic GVHD is primarily cholestatic with elevations in serum alkaline phosphatase levels and jaundice[2,3]. GVHD is similar to primary biliary cirrhosis; both diseases are characterized by degenerative changes in the small bile ducts, involve immune-mediated mechanisms, and progress to cirrhosis[4]. Although jaundice and elevation of liver enzymes may persist for years, portal hypertension and liver failure have been observed rarely[4–7]. The shortest documented period for the progression of chronic GVHD of the liver to cirrhosis with liver failure has been 2 years[7]. A combination of cyclosporin A, steroids and azathioprine has been the treatment of choice, and is effective in 50–80% of patients with chronic GVHD[8,9]. Hepatic GVHD does respond less to treatment, and in many patients becomes the dominant feature of GVHD.

Chronic GVHD is a purely immunological disease which shares many clinical, biochemical and histological features of PBC[4]. GVHD, however, is an iatrogenic disease, and may be regarded as a unique *in vivo* model for the study of chronic cholestatic liver disease such as PBC. It is seen in a homogeneous patient population and its course can be observed prospectively[10]. Unlike PBC, patients at risk (namely patients after an allogeneic BMT) can be followed before the disease develops and the exact moment of its beginning is easily recognized.

Several studies have demonstrated the efficacy of UDCA for the treatment of primary biliary cirrhosis (PBC)[11–13]. It appears to increase bile flow and to reduce the hepatic toxicity of endogenous hydrophobic bile salts by replacing them. Recently, the possibility of additional effects of UDCA as an immunological modulator has become an important topic of ongoing research[14–16].

We have demonstrated in an earlier study that treatment with UDCA decreases elevated biochemical markers of cholestasis in patients with chronic GVHD refractory to classic immunosuppressive therapy[17] within a few weeks. Following withdrawal of the drug, liver enzymes again rose to pre-treatment levels. The present study was undertaken to examine the efficacy and safety of long-term UDCA treatment of chronic GVHD of the liver not responding satisfactorily to immunosuppressive treatment alone.

METHODS

Patient selection

We studied seven patients (mean age 34.4 years; range 9–51) who after allogeneic bone marrow transplantation (BMT) had been diagnosed with chronic GVHD of the liver and had persistent elevation of liver enzymes despite immunosuppressive therapy with cyclosporin A and steroids. The mean interval after BMT was 188 days (range 47–320). The principal diagnosis was acute myelocytic leukaemia in three patients, and acute lymphocytic leukaemia, chronic myelocytic leukaemia, multiple myeloma and severe aplastic anaemia in one patient each, respectively. The diagnosis of chronic GVHD was based on published criteria[2]. Liver involvement was defined as serum alkaline phosphatase and bilirubin levels more than twice the upper normal limit of 108 U/l and 26 μmol/l, respectively. Liver biopsy samples showing histological changes of chronic GVHD were available for six patients. All patients were clinically stable without signs of decompensated liver disease. Ultrasound imaging of liver, gallbladder and biliary tree was normal.

Study design

Baseline data included a physical examination, red blood count, white blood count, thrombocytes, prothrombin time, alanine aminotransferase (ALAT) level, aspartate aminotransferase (ASAT) level, alkaline phosphatase level, gamma-glutamyltransferase (GGT) level, total serum bilirubin, creatinine, and blood urea nitrogen. Laboratory examinations were repeated at monthly intervals; clinical follow-up was every 3 months.

Ursodeoxycholic acid (Ursofalk®, supplied by Phardi AG, Ettingen, Switzerland) was given orally in divided doses of 10–15 mg/kg per day. Immunosuppressive drugs were continued, and dosage was adapted according to clinical response.

RESULTS

Median length of treatment was 18.6 months (range 6–36). No side-effects were observed. Two patients had pruritus which improved during treatment. Biochemical markers of cholestasis decreased significantly in all patients (Fig. 1a–d). The main treatment effect was observed after 1–3 months, and this was

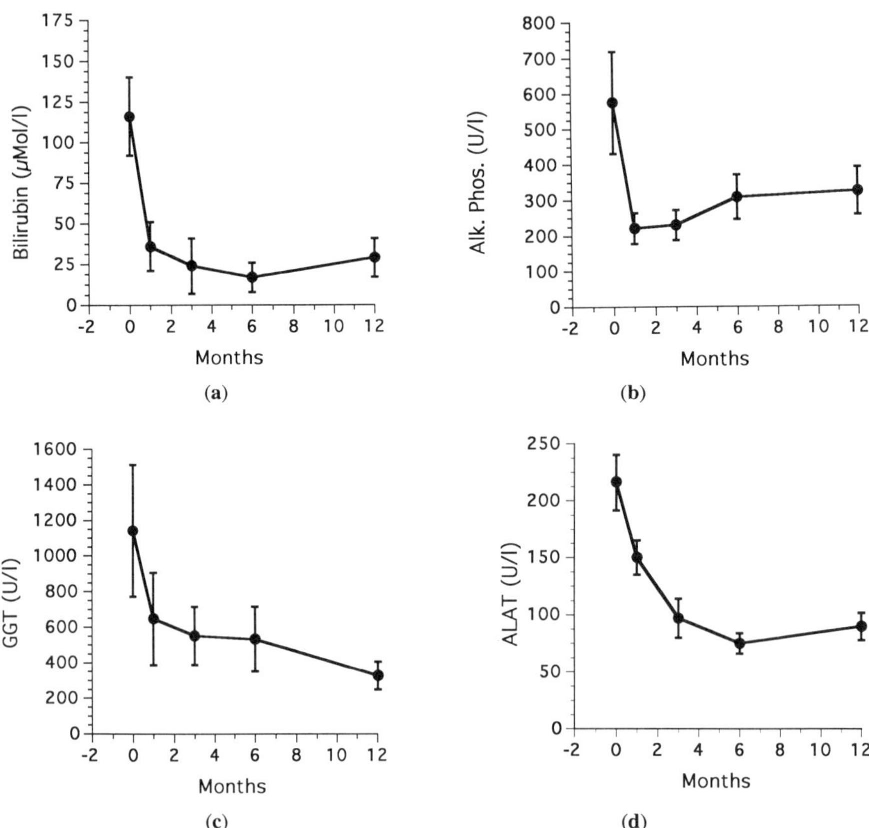

Fig. 1 Changes in bilirubin (**a**), alkaline phosphatase (Alk. Phos., **b**), gamma-glutamyltransferase (GGT, **c**), and alanine aminotransferase (ALAT, **d**) for seven patients with chronic graft-versus-host disease during UDCA therapy. Results represent mean ± SEM

Table 1 Biochemical markers of cholestasis before and at the end of ursodeoxycholic acid therapy

Variable	Values before UDCA therapy	Values at the end of UDCA therapy
Bilirubin (μmol/l)	116 ± 37	9 ± 3
Alkaline phosphatase (U/l)	575 ± 144	227 ± 33
GGT (U/l)	1142 ± 370	169 ± 60
ASAT (U/l)	121 ± 24	33 ± 4
ALAT (U/l)	216 ± 38	50 ± 8

UDCA = ursodeoxycholic acid, GGT = gamma-glutamyltransferase, ASAT = aspartate aminotransferase, ALAT = alanine aminotransferase

sustained during long-term therapy. Changes in laboratory values from baseline to the end of treatment are shown in Table 1. A significant improvement was noted for all values. Bilirubin decreased by 92%, alkaline phosphatase by 60%, GGT by 85%, ASAT by 73%, and ALAT by 77%. Mean values for bilirubin,

ALAT and ASAT reached normal levels, while alkaline phosphatase and GGT did not decrease below values equal to twice the upper normal limit.

DISCUSSION

Chronic GVHD causes significantly morbidity in survivors of allogeneic bone marrow transplantation[1]. The cholestatic liver disease of extensive chronic GVHD is less responsive to therapy than other manifestations of the disorder. Although jaundice and elevation of liver enzymes may persist for years, portal hypertension and liver failure have been observed only rarely[5-7]. The number of patients with chronic liver disease progressing to biliary cirrhosis in whom the original haematological malignancy is in complete remission, however, is expected to increase because of prolonged survival after allogeneic BMT. This study enrolled patients who had chronic GVHD of the liver unresponsive to treatment with cyclosporin A and steroids. While doses of immunosuppressive agents remained constant initially, UDCA therapy resulted in significant improvement of biochemical markers of cholestasis within the first 3 months. The treatment effect was sustained during long-term therapy. The drug was well tolerated and had a positive effect on pruritus in two patients. Because the study was conducted in an open-label fashion without a placebo control, we cannot be certain that the treatment effects observed were due to UDCA therapy alone. The striking effect of UDCA therapy on biochemical markers of cholestasis within the first month already in patients initially unresponsive to immunosuppressive therapy does, however, point to an important additive effect of UDCA.

Several long-term, double-blind controlled trials of UDCA for treatment of patients with primary biliary cirrhosis showed improvement in biochemical markers of cholestasis and histological findings in UDCA-treated patients[11-13]. The beneficial effects are more evident in patients with early stages of primary biliary cirrhosis. Long-term UDCA therapy slowed the progression of primary biliary cirrhosis and reduced the need for liver transplantation in one study[11].

The mechanisms by which UDCA exerts its effect in cholestatic liver disease are not completely understood[18]. Although the initial bile ductular damage in GVHD as well as in PBC may be immune-mediated, the progression of liver cell damage may be caused by retention of hydrophobic and more hepatotoxic bile acids upstream from the site of injury. Induction of choleresis may protect hepatocytes from cholestatic injury[19]. This may prevent the retention of more hepatotoxic bile acids such as chenodeoxycholic acid and lithocholic acid. When given orally to humans, UDCA replaces the native, more hydrophobic bile acids and becomes the predominant bile acid. One explanation for this effect is that UDCA inhibits the ileal resorption of potentially toxic bile acids[20]. UDCA binds to membranes and may stabilize them against disruption by more toxic bile salts[15].

Several investigators have postulated additional immunomodulatory effects of UDCA. Calmus et al.[14] have found a reduction of class I HLA antigen expression on hepatocytes from patients with PBC. Reduction in hepatocyte HLA class I expression could block immune-mediated hepatocellular necrosis by suppressing the cytotoxic T-cell target. In an in vitro study, Lacaille and Paradis found that

UDCA inhibited human mononuclear cell proliferation stimulated by mitogens[16]. In one part of the experiments, where cyclosporin A showed only partial suppression of a mitogenic response, UDCA had an additive inhibitory effect. The mechanism of this effect remains unknown.

In summary, UDCA appears to be safe and effective in the long-term treatment of chronic GVHD of the liver. An additive effect is observed in patients whose disease responds unsatisfactorily to immunosuppressive therapy. It is not known whether this form of therapy alters the natural history of chronic GVHD of the liver, or slows its progression to biliary cirrhosis. UDCA therapy may lessen the impact of cholestasis in a disease with a primarily immunological pathogenesis. In addition, immunomodulatory effects of UDCA may play a role. Finally, our results also lend support to the concept that UDCA treatment early in the course of cholestatic liver disease is most effective.

Acknowledgement

This work was supported by a grant-in-aid from Phardi AG, Ettingen, Switzerland.

References

1. Sullivan KM, Agura E, Appelbaum F *et al*. Chronic graft-versus-host disease and other late complications of bone marrow transplantation. Semin Hematol. 1991;28:249–58.
2. Shulman HM, Sullivan KM, Weiden PL *et al*. Chronic graft-versus-host syndrome in man: a long-term clinicopathologic study of 29 Seattle patients. Am J Med. 1980;69:204–17.
3. Shulman HM, Sharma P, Amos D, Fenster LF, McDonald GB. A coded histologic study of hepatic graft-versus-host-disease after human bone marrow transplantation. Hepatology. 1988;8: 463–70.
4. Epstein O, Thomas HC, Sherlock S. Primary biliary cirrhosis is a dry gland syndrome with features of chronic graft-versus-host disease. Lancet. 1980;1:166–8.
5. Yau JC, Zander AR, Srigley JR *et al*. Chronic graft-versus-host-disease complicated by micronodular cirrhosis and esophageal varices. Transplantation. 1986;41:129–30.
6. Knapp AB, Crawford JM, Rappeport JM, Gollan JL. Cirrhosis as a consequence of graft-versus-host disease. Gastroenterology. 1987;92:513–19.
7. Stechschulte DJ, Fishback JL, Emami A *et al*. Secondary biliary cirrhosis as a consequence of graft-versus-host disease. Gastroenterology. 1990;98:223–5.
8. Sullivan KM, Witherspoon RP, Storb R *et al*. Alternating day cyclosporine. Blood. 1988;72: 555–61.
9. Sullivan KM, Witherspoon RP, Storb R *et al*. Prednisone and azathioprine compared with prednisone and placebo for treatment of chronic graft-versus-host disease. Blood. 1988;72:546–54.
10. Shulman HM. Graft-versus-host-induced cirrhosis: possible mechanisms. Hepatology. 1987;7: 1385–6.
11. Poupon RE, Poupon R, Balkau B *et al*. Ursodiol for the long-term treatment of primary biliary cirrhosis. N Engl J Med. 1994;330:1342–7.
12. Lindor KD, Dickson ER, Baldus WP *et al*. Ursodeoxycholic acid treatment of primary biliary cirrhosis. Gastroenterology. 1994;106:1284–90.
13. Leuschner U, Güldütuna S, Imhof M, Hübner K, Benjaminov A, Leuschner K. Effects of ursodeoxycholic acid after 4 to 12 years of therapy in early and late stages of primary biliary cirrhosis. J Hepatol. 1994;21:624–33.
14. Calmus Y, Gane P, Rouger P, Poupon R. Hepatic expression of Class I and Class II major histocompatibility complex molecules in primary biliary cirrhosis: effect of ursodeoxycholic acid. Hepatology. 1990;11:12–15.

15. Heuman DM. Hepatoprotective properties of ursodeoxycholic acid. Gastroenterology. 1993;104:1865–70.
16. Lacaille F, Paradis K. The immunosuppressive effect of ursodeoxycholic acid: a comparative *in vitro* study on human peripheral blood mononuclear cells. Hepatology. 1993;18:165–72.
17. Fried RH, Murakami CS, Fisher LD, Willson RA, Sullivan KM, McDonald GB. Ursodeoxycholic acid treatment of refractory chronic graft-versus-host disease of the liver. Ann Intern Med. 1992;116:624–9.
18. Hofmann AF. Bile acid hepatotoxicity and the rationale for UDCA therapy in chronic cholestatic liver disease: some hypotheses. In Paumgartner G, Stiehl A, Barbara L, Roda E, editors. Strategies for the treatment of hepatobiliary diseases. Dordrecht: Kluwer; 1990:13–33.
19. Erlinger S. Hypercholeretic bile acids: a clue to mechanism? Hepatology. 1990;11:888–90.
20. Marteau P, Chazouilleres O, Myara A, Jian R, Rambaud JC, Poupon R. Effect of chronic administration of ursodeoxycholic acid on ileal absorption of endogenous bile acids in man. Hepatology. 190;12:1206–8.

Index

therapy   27
   action mechanism in PSC   372
   in cholestasis   364–9
   in cystic fibrosis-associated liver disease
      366, 369
   in GVHD   384–3, 384–8
   in 3β-HSD deficiency   347
   in PBC   365, 366–9, 384
   in PSC   366, 369, 372, 374
   in 5β-reductase deficiency   340–1, 342
   toxic bile acid ileal resorption inhibition
      387
   see also 6-FUDCA; 6-MUDCA
ursodeoxycholylsarcosine, intestinal
      cholesterol absorption inhibition, study
      methods/materials   262–4
ursodiol
   immune system modification   380
   interferon-α combination therapy
      in chronic hepatitis C   376–81
      efficacy   381
   side-effects/adverse reactions   379
   therapeutic applications   380

valproic acid, biliary lipid secretion inhibition
      236
vasoactive intestinal polypeptide (VIP)   176
vesicles
   fusion   176
      and hepatocyte bile acid transport   162
      see also exocytosis

retrieval   176
structure, phase map   48, 51–3, 54
transcytotic pathway, micotubule-dependent
   177
vesiculization, biliary lipids   233
vincristine   247
vitamin D absorption, micellar bile salt effects
   278
Vlahcevic, Z R
   Adolf Windaus prizewinner 1994   81–4
   early US career   85–6
vulpecholic acid   16

weight reduction, rapid
   dietary study design   358
   gallstone formation, prevention by UDCA
      357–61
   statistical analysis of study   358
   surgical study design   358
Windaus, Adolf, prize, 1994   81–4
Wolff-Kishner reduction, Huang-Minlon
   modification   12

x-ray, small angle scattering   42
xanthomatosis, cerebrotendinous   104, 129

Zellweger-like syndrome, with detectable
   hepatic peroxisomes   350
Zellweger's syndrome   350
zinc borohydride   12, 13

Falk Symposium Series

43. Reutter W, Popper H, Arias IM, Heinrich PC, Keppler D, Landmann L, eds.: *Modulation of Liver Cell Expression*. Falk Symposium No. 43. 1987   ISBN: 0-85200-677-2*

44. Boyer JL, Bianchi L, eds.: *Liver Cirrhosis*. Falk Symposium No. 44. 1987
ISBN: 0-85200-993-3*

45. Paumgartner G, Stiehl A, Gerok W, eds.: *Bile Acids and the Liver*. Falk Symposium No. 45. 1987   ISBN: 0-85200-675-6*

46. Goebell H, Peskar BM, Malchow H, eds.: *Inflammatory Bowel Diseases – Basic Research & Clinical Implications*. Falk Symposium No. 46. 1988   ISBN: 0-7462-0067-6*

47. Bianchi L, Holt P, James OFW, Butler RN, eds.: *Aging in Liver and Gastrointestinal Tract*. Falk Symposium No. 47. 1988   ISBN: 0-7462-0066-8*

48. Heilmann C, ed.: *Calcium-Dependent Processes in the Liver*. Falk Symposium No. 48. 1988   ISBN: 0-7462-0075-7*

50. Singer MV, Goebell H, eds.: *Nerves and the Gastrointestinal Tract*. Falk Symposium No. 50. 1989   ISBN: 0-7462-0114-1

51. Bannasch P, Keppler D, Weber G, eds.: *Liver Cell Carcinoma*. Falk Symposium No. 51. 1989   ISBN: 0-7462-0111-7

52. Paumgartner G, Stiehl A, Gerok W, eds.: *Trends in Bile Acid Research*. Falk Symposium No. 52. 1989   ISBN: 0-7462-0112-5

53. Paumgartner G, Stiehl A, Barbara L, Roda E, eds.: *Strategies for the Treatment of Hepatobiliary Diseases*. Falk Symposium No. 53. 1990   ISBN: 0-7923-8903-4

54. Bianchi L, Gerok W, Maier K-P, Deinhardt F, eds.: *Infectious Diseases of the Liver*. Falk Symposium No. 54. 1990   ISBN: 0-7923-8902-6

55. Falk Symposium No. 55 not published

55B. Hadziselimovic F, Herzog B, Bürgin-Wolff A, eds.: *Inflammatory Bowel Disease and Coeliac Disease in Children*. International Falk Symposium. 1990 ISBN 0-7462-0125-7

56. Williams CN, eds.: *Trends in Inflammatory Bowel Disease Therapy*. Falk Symposium No. 56. 1990   ISBN: 0-7923-8952-2

57. Bock KW, Gerok W, Matern S, Schmid R, eds.: *Hepatic Metabolism and Disposition of Endo- and Xenobiotics*. Falk Symposium No. 57. 1991   ISBN: 0-7923-8953-0

58. Paumgartner G, Stiehl A, Gerok W, eds.: *Bile Acids as Therapeutic Agents: From Basic Science to Clinical Practice*. Falk Symposium No. 58. 1991   ISBN: 0-7923-8954-9

59. Halter F, Garner A, Tytgat GNJ, eds.: *Mechanisms of Peptic Ulcer Healing*. Falk Symposium No. 59. 1991   ISBN: 0-7923-8955-7

60. Goebell H, Ewe K, Malchow H, Koelbel Ch, eds.: *Inflammatory Bowel Diseases – Progress in Basic Research and Clinical Implications*. Falk Symposium No. 60. 1991
ISBN: 0-7923-8956-5

61. Falk Symposium No. 61 not published

62. Dowling RH, Folsch UR, Löser Ch, eds.: *Polyamines in the Gastrointestinal Tract*. Falk Symposium No. 62. 1992   ISBN: 0-7923-8976-X

63. Lentze MJ, Reichen J, eds.: *Paediatric Cholestasis: Novel Approaches to Treatment*. Falk Symposium No. 63. 1992   ISBN: 0-7923-8977-8

64. Demling L, Frühmorgen P, eds.: *Non-Neoplastic Diseases of the Anorectum*. Falk Symposium No. 64. 1992   ISBN: 0-7923-8979-4

64B. Gressner AM, Ramadori G, eds.: *Molecular and Cell Biology of Liver Fibrogenesis*. International Falk Symposium. 1992   ISBN: 0-7923-8980-8

*These titles were published under the MTP Press imprint.

Falk Symposium Series

65. Hadziselimovic F, Herzog B, eds.: *Inflammatory Bowel Diseases and Morbus Hirschprung*. Falk Symposium No. 65. 1992   ISBN: 0-7923-8995-6

66. Martin F, McLeod RS, Sutherland LR, Williams CN, eds.: *Trends in Inflammatory Bowel Disease Therapy*. Falk Symposium No. 66. 1993   ISBN: 0-7923-8827-5

67. Schölmerich J, Kruis W, Goebell H, Hohenberger W, Gross V, eds.: *Inflammatory Bowel Diseases – Pathophysiology as Basis of Treatment*. Falk Symposium No. 67. 1993   ISBN: 0-7923-8996-4

68. Paumgartner G, Stiehl A, Gerok W, eds.: *Bile Acids and The Hepatobiliary System: From Basic Science to Clinical Practice*. Falk Symposium No. 68. 1993   ISBN: 0-7923-8829-1

69. Schmid R, Bianchi L, Gerok W, Maier K-P, eds.: *Extrahepatic Manifestations in Liver Diseases*. Falk Symposium No. 69. 1993   ISBN: 0-7923-8821-6

70. Meyer zum Büschenfelde K-H, Hoofnagle J, Manns M, eds.: *Immunology and Liver*. Falk Symposium No. 70. 1993   ISBN: 0-7923-8830-5

71. Surrenti C, Casini A, Milani S, Pinzani M , eds.: *Fat-Storing Cells and Liver Fibrosis*. Falk Symposium No. 71. 1994   ISBN: 0-7923-8842-9

72. Rachmilewitz D, ed.: *Inflammatory Bowel Diseases – 1994*. Falk Symposium No. 72. 1994   ISBN: 0-7923-8845-3

73. Binder HJ, Cummings J, Soergel KH, eds.: *Short Chain Fatty Acids*. Falk Symposium No. 73. 1994   ISBN: 0-7923-8849-6

74. Keppler D, Jungermann K, eds.: *Transport in the Liver*. Falk Symposium No. 74. 1994   ISBN: 0-7923-8858-5

74B. Stange EF, ed.: *Chronic Inflammatory Bowel Disease*. Falk Symposium. 1995   ISBN: 0-7923-8876-3

75. van Berge Henegouwen GP, van Hoek B, De Groote J, Matern S, Stockbrügger RW, eds.: *Cholestatic Liver Diseases: New Strategies for Prevention and Treatment of Hepatobiliary and Cholestatic Liver Diseases*. Falk Symposium 75. 1994.   ISBN: 0-7923-8867-4

76. Monteiro E, Tavarela Veloso F, eds.: *Inflammatory Bowel Diseases: New Insights into Mechanisms of Inflammation and Challenges in Diagnosis and Treatment*. Falk Symposium 76. 1995.   ISBN 0-7923-8884-4

77. Singer MV, Ziegler R, Rohr G, eds.: *Gastrointestinal Tract and Endocrine System*. Falk Symposium 77. 1995.   ISBN 0-7923-8877-1

78. Decker K, Gerok W, Andus T, Gross V, eds.: *Cytokines and the Liver*. Falk Symposium 78. 1995.   ISBN 0-7923-8878-X

79. Holstege A, Schölmerich J, Hahn EG, eds.: *Portal Hypertension*. Falk Symposium 79. 1995.   ISBN 0-7923-8879-8

80. Hofmann AF, Paumgartner G, Stiehl A, eds.: *Bile Acids in Gastroenterology: Basic and Clinical Aspects*. Falk Symposium 80.   ISBN 0-7923-8880-1